USMLE Step 2 CK Plus

USMLE Step 2 CK Plus

ABDILLAHI M. OMAR, MD, MBA candidate
Department of Radiology
Detroit Medical Center
Wayne State University
Detroit, Michigan, United States

ELSEVIER

Elsevier
1600 John F. Kennedy Blvd.
Ste 1800
Philadelphia, PA 19103-2899

USMLE Step 2 CK Plus

ISBN: 9780323829861

Notice

Practitioners and researchers must always rely on their own experience and knowledge in evaluating and using any information, methods, compounds or experiments described herein. Because of rapid advances in the medical sciences, in particular, independent verification of diagnoses and drug dosages should be made. To the fullest extent of the law, no responsibility is assumed by Elsevier, authors, editors or contributors for any injury and/or damage to persons or property as a matter of products liability, negligence or otherwise, or from any use or operation of any methods, products, instructions, or ideas contained in the material herein.

International Standard Book Number: 9780323829861

Content Strategist: James Merritt
Content Development Manager: Somodatta Roy Choudhury
Publishing Services Manager: Shereen Jameel
Project Manager: Shereen Jameel
Design Direction: Bridget Hoette

Printed in India

Last digit is the print number: 9 8 7 6 5 4 3 2 1

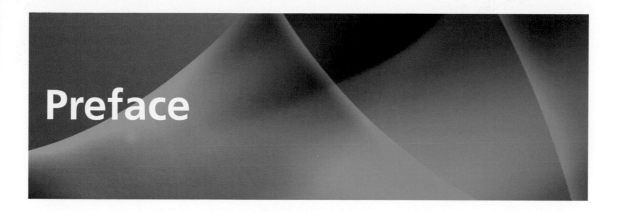

Preface

The purpose of this book is to provide those studying for the USMLE Step 2 a comprehensive review source that can be used to study for the individual NBME shelf examinations as well as the USMLE Step II exam.

Hope you enjoy and best of luck.

The reason I decided to write this book was because during my studying it was made more difficult having to use multiple resources for each of the different shelf examinations, each with its own approach to presenting the material and a different focus. Unlike the USMLE Step I, where there is a consensus, comprehensive review source (First Aid), such a resource does not exist for the USMLE. This book attempts to fill that void so that students have the one-stop frame of reference resource, similar to the USMLE Step 1.

Having personally done well in the USMLE Step 2 (278, >99th percentile), I felt I was well qualified to write such a book. The book is organized into the main shelf examination topics (internal medicine, obstetrics/gynecology, pediatrics, psychiatry, and surgery) allowing for focused studying for each of these examinations as they approach.

Throughout the book you will notice several topics will repeat in more than one subsection due to the integrated nature of medicine today. Therefore, a topic that is repeated in multiple sections is likely important to be familiar with as it can be tested from multiple perspectives.

One of the best preparations to do well on the USMLE Step 2 is to have a strong basic science foundation. Although the basic science topics are primarily tested in the USMLE Step 1, they are frequently brought up throughout this book to provide greater integration of knowledge from a basic science to a clinical science perspective. This facilitates greater understanding, less rote memorization, and, therefore, long-term retention of the material. In addition, for each of the disease processes that are discussed, the information is presented in a way that is tested in the actual examination. For example, the common questions that are often related to the most likely diagnosis, risk factors, pathophysiology, diagnostic testing, management, and complications." Each of these possible questions is directly addressed for every topic allowing for easy recall during the USMLE Step 2 exam.

I have also made extensive use of tables to allow for easier differentiation of disease processes that are similar or are commonly tested together. Furthermore, you will notice several images are added after the text for several disease processes to provide a visual representation of the topic, to allow for increased memory via reading and visual learners. Seeing information in different formats allows for increased likelihood of retention.

Sincerely,
Abdillahi Mohamed Omar

Contents

CHAPTER 1 Preventative Medicine

Smoking
- Pathophysiology: chronic inflammation → metaplasia → dysplasia → cancer
- Associations
  - Vascular
    - Coronary artery disease, cerebrovascular accident (CVA), peripheral artery disease
    - Aortic aneurysm
    - Buerger disease
  - HEENT
    - Tongue, larynx, adenoid, and vocal cord cancer
    - Leukoplakia
  - Pulmonary
    - Chronic obstructive pulmonary disease
    - Squamous and small cell carcinoma of the lung
    - Asthma
    - Bronchiectasis
  - Gastrointestinal
    - Esophageal, stomach, and pancreatic cancer
    - Peptic ulcer disease
  - Genitourinary
    - Kidney, ureteral, and bladder cancer
    - Cervical, penis, and vaginal cancer
  - Musculoskeletal
    - Osteoporosis
    - Arthritis
- Management
  - Nonpharmacologic
    - Behavioral modification (avoid associated activities)
    - Motivational interviewing
  - Pharmacologic
    - Nicotine replacement (lozenges, gums, patches)
    - Bupropion
      - Norepinephrine-dopamine reuptake inhibitor
      - Avoid in anorexia nervosa and seizure disorder
  - Varenicline
    - Partial nicotine acetylcholine receptor agonist
    - Associated with vivid dreams

Body mass index (BMI) may be overestimated in athletic individuals (increased muscle mass) and underestimated in the elderly (increased adipose tissue).

Obesity
- Definition: body mass index (BMI) >95th percentile for age and sex
- Risk factors
  - Western diet
  - Sedentary lifestyle
  - Family history
  - Endocrine abnormalities (hypothyroidism, hypercortisolism)

TABLE 1-1   Screening Guidelines

Osteoporosis	All women >65 yr old with dual-energy x-ray absorptiometry (DEXA) scan
Hypertension	Start at age 18 with every annual office visit
Dyslipidemia	Men start at age 35, women start at age 45; screen every 5 yr
Breast cancer	Start at age 50 every 2 yr with mammograms. Varies depending on different subspecialty governing societies.
Cervical cancer	Start at age 21 every 3 yr with Pap smear Age 30–65 every 5 yr with Pap smear and HPV DNA testing

More details about specific screening guidelines are discussed in the corresponding sections.

- • Genetic syndromes (Prader-Willi, Beckwith-Wiedemann)
- • Medications (glucocorticoids)
- – Associations
  - • Coronary artery disease, CVA
  - • Type II diabetes
  - • Dyslipidemia
  - • Hypertension
  - • Obstructive sleep apnea, obesity hypoventilation syndrome
  - • Osteoarthritis
  - • Nonalcoholic steatohepatitis
- – Management
  - • Lifestyle modifications
    - ▪ Exercise: aerobic (30 minutes/day, 5×/week) and weight-based training
    - ▪ Healthy diet: low calorie, low fat, low carbohydrate
  - • Pharmacologic
    - ▪ Orlistat
      - ○ Pancreatic lipase inhibitor
      - ○ Promotes malabsorption resulting in fatty diarrhea, abdominal cramps, flatus
      - ○ Requires nutritional supplementation
    - ▪ Topiramate-phentermine
    - ▪ Lorcaserin (serotonin agonist)
    - ▪ Liraglutide (GLP-1 receptor agonist)
  - • Surgical
    - ▪ Laparoscopic banding: decreases stomach size
    - ▪ Gastric bypass: increased risk of dumping syndrome, vitamin deficiencies

Monitor for B12 deficiency in patients with gastric bypass as intrinsic factor is made by parietal cells located in the stomach.

Cancer and general health screenings (Table 1-1) are a major component of preventative medicine as they allow for early detection of disease, increasing the probability of curative and minimally invasive treatment. This decreases overall morbidity, mortality, and health care costs.

CHAPTER 2 Neurology

I. Neuroanatomy
A. Key Principles
1. The signs and symptoms produced from brain lesions occur due to loss of normal function of the affected brain region (Table 2-1).
2. Lesions commonly occur due to trauma, infection, infarction, or hemorrhage.

II. Stroke
A. Definition: loss of blood supply to the brain in a vascular distribution resulting in focal neurologic deficits (Figs. 2-1, 2-2, 2-3)
B. Risk factors
1. Hypertension
2. Diabetes mellitus
3. Dyslipidemia
4. Smoking
5. Less common risk factors
   a. Inherited hypercoagulability
   b. Amyloid angiopathy: deposition of amyloid protein weakens blood vessel walls
   c. Vascular dissection (trauma)
   d. Global hypotension (infarcts in watershed areas)
   e. Anticoagulant therapy
   f. Connective tissue disorders (Marfan, Ehlers-Danlos)
C. Pathophysiology
1. Thrombotic
   a. Carotid artery atherosclerotic disease
   b. Most common cause overall
   c. May be preceded by prodrome of transient visual (amaurosis fugax) or neurologic (transient ischemic attack) deficits that self-resolve
2. Cardioembolic
   a. Atrial fibrillation, endocarditis, paradoxical deep vein thrombosis
   b. Sudden onset of symptoms
3. Hemorrhagic
   a. Hypertension
   b. Subarachnoid hemorrhage
   c. Cerebral amyloid angiopathy
D. Signs and symptoms: depends on the area of infarction with symptoms occurring contralateral to the side of infarction
1. Middle cerebral artery (MCA)
   a. Weakness of face, arms, and legs
   b. Homonymous hemianopsia
   c. Eyes look toward the side of lesion if frontal eye fields are involved since frontal eye fields normally stimulate the eyes to look away from the side of stimulation
   d. Aphasia if dominant hemisphere is affected
2. Anterior cerebral artery (ACA)
   a. Weakness of lower limb > upper limbs
   b. Urinary incontinence (micturition center affected)
   c. Personality change (frontal lobe involvement)
3. Posterior cerebral artery (PCA)
   a. Visual deficits with macular sparing (due to collaterals from MCA)
   b. Weber and Benedikt (penetrating branches of the PCA)

3

TABLE 2-1   Disorders and Associated Symptomatology Caused by Lesions in Key Brain Structures

LOCATION OF LESION	SIGNS AND SYMPTOMS	
Frontal lobe	Broca aphasia (inferior frontal lobe): • Comprehension intact • Loss of repetition • Loss of fluency	• Personality changes • Loss of executive functioning • Social disinhibition • Lack of impulse control
Temporal lobe	Wernicke aphasia (superior temporal lobe): • Loss of comprehension • Loss of repetition • Fluency intact ("word salad")	• Auditory hallucinations mimicking schizophrenia • Common foci for epileptic seizures • Superior quadrantanopia
Parietal lobe	Gerstmann syndrome (dominant parietal lobe): • Agraphia • Acalculia • Finger agnosia • Left-right disorientation	• Nondominant parietal lobe (hemispatial neglect)—agnosia of left side of the body • Inferior quadrantanopia
Occipital lobe	• Visual field deficits	
Amygdala	Kluver-Bucy syndrome: • Hyperphagia • Hyperorality • Hypersexuality	
Hippocampus	• Alzheimer dementia	
Mamillary bodies	• Wernicke-Korsacoff: secondary to vitamin B1 deficiency • Wernicke: triad of ataxia, ophthalmoplegia, confusion • Korsacoff: Wernicke plus confabulation and memory deficits	
Cerebellum	• Fall to the side of the lesion • Dysdiadochokinesia • Fail finger-to-nose and heel-to-shin test • Intention tremor	
Arcuate fasciculus	• Conduction aphasia (disconnect between Wernicke and Broca area) • Intact comprehension • Loss of repetition • Intact fluency	
Subthalamic nucleus	• Hemiballismus: wild flailing of the contralateral limb	

- Ipsilateral cranial nerve (CN) III palsy
- Contralateral ataxia

4. Vertebrobasilar
   a. Loss of consciousness
   b. Ataxia
5. Wallenberg syndrome (posterior inferior cerebellar artery)
   a. Ipsilateral face sensory loss
   b. Ataxia
   c. Dysarthria, dysphagia
   d. Vertigo
   e. Horner syndrome (involvement of descending sympathetic fibers)
E. Diagnostics
   1. Noncontrast computed tomography (CT) brain: detects the presence of blood to determine whether thrombolytics should be administered
   2. Magnetic resonance imaging (MRI) brain
      a. Performed after noncontrast CT since it takes longer to perform and therefore unsuitable in the acute setting where it must be determined if blood is present or absent in the brain
      b. Sensitive for subtle ischemic changes
   3. Evaluating etiology of stroke
      a. Carotid duplex ultrasound: stenosis and flow through carotid artery
      b. Echocardiogram: valvular abnormalities, thrombus
      c. Electrocardiogram: arrhythmias (particularly atrial fibrillation)
      d. Prothrombin time, partial thromboplastin time: coagulopathies
      e. +/− CT angiography/MR angiography: evaluate for areas of stenosis

Cortical vascular territories

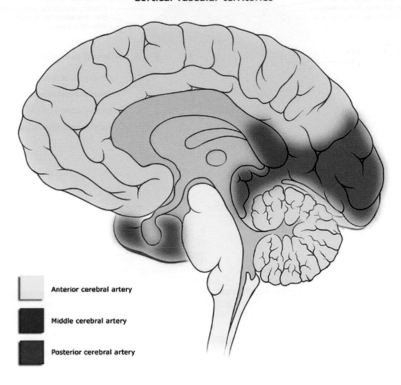

Figure 2-1: Vascular territories of the major intracranial blood vessels on midline view. (Image courtesy Frank Gaillard; CC BY-SA [https://creativecommons.org/licenses/by-sa/3.0])

Cortical vascular territories

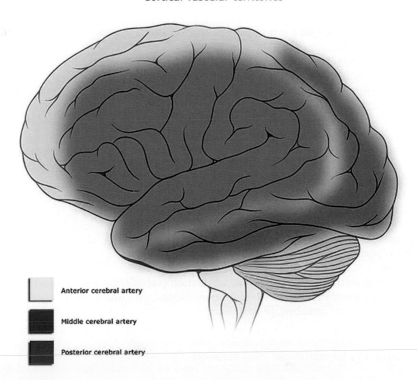

Figure 2-2: Vascular territories of the major intracranial blood vessels on lateral view. (Image courtesy Frank Gaillard; CC BY-SA [https://creativecommons.org/licenses/by-sa/3.0])

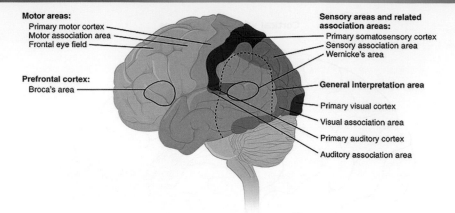

Figure 2-3: Cortical anatomy and associated functions. (Image courtesy OpenStax College; CC BY-SA [https://creativecommons.org/licenses/by-sa/3.0])

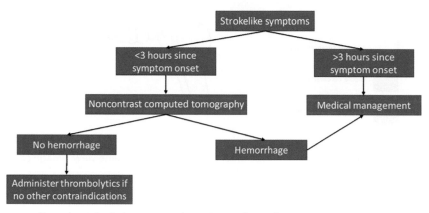

Figure 2-4: Summary flow chart depicting approach to the stroke patient.

    F. Management: depends on the time of presentation after symptom onset and absence or presence of hemorrhage (Fig. 2-4)
      1. <3 hours: thrombolytics
      2. >3 hours: aspirin
        a. Administer within the first 24–48 hours
        b. Add dipyridamole if patient is already on aspirin
        c. Clopidogrel if patient is allergic to aspirin
        d. Ticlopidine if patient is allergic to both aspirin and clopidogrel
      3. Thrombolytics should not be given regardless of timing if blood is present on noncontrast CT
    G. Complications
      1. Cerebral edema
      2. Seizures
      3. Conversion to hemorrhagic stroke
    H. Prevention
      1. Optimize medical management of risk factors
      2. Aspirin
      3. Heparin to warfarin bridge for atrial fibrillation (valvular or nonvalvular)
        a. Direct thrombin inhibitors (argatroban, dabigatran, bivalirudin)
        b. Xa inhibitors (apixaban, rivaroxaban)

Direct thrombin inhibitors and Xa inhibtors only for nonvalvular atrial fibriation.

      4. Carotid endarterectomy if symptomatic and >70% carotid artery stenosis

Contraindications to thrombolytics:
- **Presence of blood on noncontrast CT:** the only absolute contraindication, all others are relative contraindications
- Bleeding disorders or on anticoagulation
- Recent hemorrhage
- Recent surgery or trauma
- Uncontrolled hypertension (>185/110)

I. Contraindications to thrombolytics:
1. Definition: occlusion of the small lacunar arteries (small branches off MCA) penetrating the brain parenchyma resulting in motor and sensory symptoms without cortical dysfunction
2. Cause: hypertension (most common cause)
3. Pathophysiology: lipohyalinosis and microatheroma
4. Types of lacunar stroke syndromes
   a. Motor
      - Most common type overall
      - Pure motor hemiparesis
      - Internal capsule stroke
   b. Sensory
      - Pure sensory deficits
      - Thalamic stroke: may be complicated by thalamic pain syndrome (hemisensory loss or pain weeks to months after stroke)
   c. Ataxic
      - Weakness with predominant ataxic gait and deviation to affected side
      - Pons stroke
   d. Dysarthria clumsy hand syndrome: facial involvement (dysarthria, dysphagia), clumsy hand

III. **Spinal Cord Lesions**

A thorough neurologic exam can help localize the location of a particular spinal cord lesion as the different spinal cord tracts (Figs. 2-5 and 2-6) each provide unique sensory and motor functions (Tables 2-2 and 2-3).

A. Vitamin B12 deficiency
   1. Risk factors
      a. Long-term pure vegan without adequate B12 supplementation
      b. Pernicious anemia (antibodies against intrinsic factor)
      c. Postgastric bypass, terminal ileum disease (resection, Crohn's disease)
      d. Drugs
         - Nitrous oxide
         - Metformin
         - Alcohol
   2. Infections: Diphyllobothrium latum
   3. Signs and symptoms: secondary to loss of dorsal column-medial lemiscus (DCML), spinocerebellar, and corticospinal tract
   4. Diagnostics
      a. Low serum vitamin B12
      b. Elevated methylmalonic acid
   5. Management: parenteral vitamin B12 replacement
B. Syringomyelia
   1. Definition: cyst within the spinal cord
   2. Risk factors
      a. Cervical spine trauma (motor vehicle accident with whiplash)
      b. Arnold Chiari malformation
   3. Signs and symptoms: secondary to loss of spinothalamic tract in the upper extremities
   4. Diagnostics: MRI
   5. Management: surgery
C. Tabes dorsalis
   1. Pathophysiology: neurosyphilis infection
   2. Signs and symptoms: secondary to loss of DCML
   3. Associations
      a. Argyll-Robertson pupils (accommodate but do not react to light)

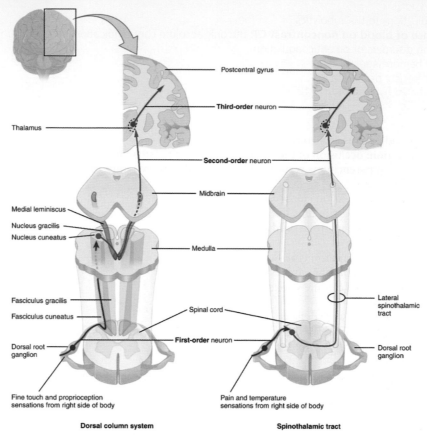

Figure 2-5: Ascending pathways of the spinal cord. (Image courtesy of OpenStax College; CC BY-SA [https://creativecommons.org/licenses/by-sa/3.0])

     b. Charcot joint: destruction of joint due to lack of awareness in space; also common in diabetics

  4. Diagnostics

     a. Cerebrospinal fluid (CSF) Veneral Disease Research Laboratory rapid plasma reagin

     b. Fluorescent treponemal antibody absorption

  5. Management: penicillin (desensitization if penicillin allergic)

D. Anterior spinal artery (ASA) occlusion

  1. Risk factors

     a. Hypotension: thoracic ASA is a watershed area (lower thoracic spinal cord is supplied by artery of Adamkiewicz)

     b. Aortic dissection, aneurysm

     c. Thoracic surgery

  2. Signs and symptoms: lesion involving the entire spinal cord, sparing the DCML

     a. Loss of corticospinal tract with both upper and lower motor neuron signs

     b. Loss of spinothalamic tract

  3. Diagnostics: MRI

  4. Management

     a. Treat underlying cause

     b. Supportive management

E. Posterior spinal artery (PSA) occlusion

  1. Risk factors: similar to ASA occlusion; however, less at risk than ASA due to receiving blood supply from two PSA compared to one ASA

  2. Signs and symptoms: secondary to loss of DCML

  3. Diagnostics: MRI

  4. Management

     a. Treat underlying cause

     b. Supportive management

Conus medullaris and cauda equina syndrome involve lesions at the distal spinal cord or nerve roots resulting in contrasting signs and symptoms (Table 2-4).

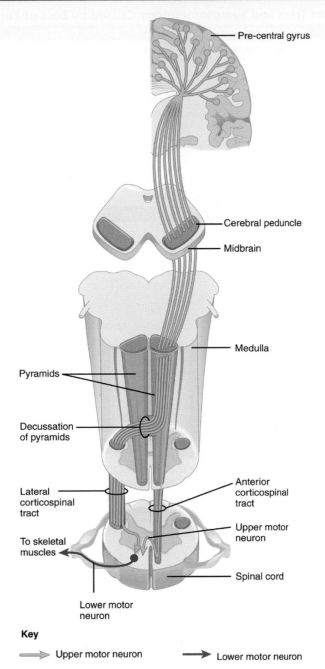

Figure 2-6: Descending corticospinal tract anatomy. (Image courtesy OpenStax College; CC BY-SA [https://creative-commons.org/licenses/by-sa/3.0])

TABLE 2-2 Review of Spinal Cord Tract Course and Their Functions

SPINAL CORD TRACTS	COURSE	FUNCTION
Dorsal column medial lemniscus	Enter dorsal column → ascend ipsilaterally to synapse at cuneate/gracile nucleus → decussate at medulla → ascend at medial lemniscus → VPL thalamus → sensory cortex	Two-point discrimination Vibration Fine touch Proprioception
Spinothalamic	Enter dorsal column → immediately decussate via anterior white commissure → ascend via spinothalamic tract → VPL thalamus → sensory cortex	Pain and temperature Crude touch
Corticospinal	Motor cortex → decussate at medullary pyramids → synapse at anterior horn → leaves spinal cord to stimulate muscle contraction	Voluntary motor movements

Magnetic resonance imaging is the diagnostic test of choice for evaluation of spinal cord lesions.
VPL, Ventral posterolateral nucleus.

TABLE 2-3   Spinal Cord Tract and Symptomatology Caused by Loss of Function

SPINAL CORD TRACT	SIGNS AND SYMPTOMS ASSOCIATED WITH LOSS OF FUNCTION
Dorsal column medial lemniscus	• Loss of fine touch, proprioception, vibration, two-point discrimination
Spinocerebellar	• Ataxia, fall to the side of the lesion
Corticospinal	• Upper motor neuron signs (hyperreflexia, positive Babinski, pronator drift) • Lower motor neuron signs at the level of lesion (flaccid paralysis, fasciculations, decreased deep tendon reflexes)
Spinothalamic	• Loss of pain and temperature, crude touch

TABLE 2-4   Conus Medullaris Versus Cauda Equina

CONUS MEDULLARIS	CAUDA EQUINA
Lesion at the termination of the spinal cord (L1–L2)	Lesion of lumbosacral nerve roots below the level of the spinal cord
Back pain	Radicular pain
Perianal anesthesia	Saddle anesthesia
Early bowel and bladder symptoms	Late bladder and bowel symptoms
Symmetric weakness	Asymmetric weakness
UMN and LMN signs	LMN signs only

LMN, Lower motor neuron; *UMN,* upper motor neuron.

IV. **Seizures**
   A. Types of seizure
      1. Simple: seizure without loss of consciousness
      2. Complex: seizure with loss of consciousness
      3. Partial: seizure arising from discrete foci in the brain
      4. Generalized: seizure arising from the entire brain
   B. Definition: abnormal firing of neurons resulting in abnormal movements and change in consciousness with associated postictal state
   C. Etiologies
      1. Metabolic
         a. Hypo/hypernatremia
         b. Hypo/hyperglycemia
         c. Hypo/hypercalcemia
         d. Hypomagnesemia
         e. Uremia
         f. Hyperammonemia
         g. Hypoxia
         h. Thyroid storm
      2. Infectious
         a. Meningitis
         b. Encephalitis
         c. Brain abscess
      3. Drugs
         a. Discontinuation of anticonvulsant
         b. Cocaine
         c. Alcohol/benzodiazepine withdrawal
         d. Theophylline
         e. Imipenem
         f. Lithium
      4. Vascular: vasculitis, stroke
      5. Eclampsia
   D. Signs and symptoms
      1. Aura: abnormal sensation preceding seizure onset (abnormal smell/taste, Jacksonian march, déjà vu, visual disturbances, paresthesias)
      2. Loss of conscious

3. Tongue biting
4. Bladder and bowel dysfunction
5. Tonic-clonic contractions
6. Postictal phase: period of confusion after seizure has resolved
E. Diagnostics
1. Workup underlying cause
a. Head CT
b. Complete blood count, comprehensive metabolic panel
c. Urine toxicology
d. Anticonvulsant drug levels: determine if patient is compliant and the levels are within therapeutic window

Todd paralysis—focal neurologic deficits that self-resolve after a seizure.

2. Electroencephalogram (EEG) if no cause is identified
F. Management: treat underlying cause; no need to start anticonvulsant therapy if cause of seizure is identified and reversible
1. Long-term antiepileptics are only used for first-time status epilepticus or patient has recurrent seizures without discernible etiology and therefore diagnosed with epilepsy.
2. Most anticonvulsants are teratogenic (category D or X) due to their antifolate effects resulting in neural tube defects, and therefore should be used with caution in pregnant women.
3. Anticonvulsants work by blocking Na channels, increasing gamma-aminobutyric acid (GABA) levels, or blocking T-type Ca channels.
4. Choice of therapy is based on side effect profile and patient comorbidities since they all have similar efficacy (Table 2-5).
G. Complications
1. Status epilepticus
2. Cerebral anoxia
3. Intellectual disability

TABLE 2-5 Anticonvulsant Pharmacology

DRUG	SIDE EFFECTS	OTHER FEATURES
Carbamazepine	• Agranulocytosis • SIADH • CYP-450 inducer	• Used in treatment of trigeminal neuralgia
Ethosuximide	• Stevens-Johnson syndrome (less common than lamotrigine)	• First line for absence seizures
Lamotrigine	• Stevens-Johnson syndrome	• Used in depressive episodes of bipolar disorder
Levetiracetam	• May unmask underlying anxiety	• Fewest adverse effects of all anticonvulsants
Phenobarbital	• Respiratory depression	• Used in neonates • Last line of treatment in status epilepticus
Phenytoin	• Gingival hyperplasia • Hirsutism • SLE-like syndrome • Megaloblastic anemia • Fetal hydantoin syndrome (cleft lip/palate, nail hypoplasia) • Hypotension and/or AV block when given intravenously	• Used in status epilepticus if patient is unresponsive to benzodiazepine
Topiramate	• Nephrolithiasis • Weight loss	• Migraine prophylaxis
Valproic acid	• Hepatoxicity • Thrombocytopenia • Weight gain	• Alternative to ethosuximide for absence seizures • Used in maintenance treatment of bipolar disorder • First line for myoclonic seizures

AV, Atrioventricular; *SIADH,* syndrome of inappropriate antidiuretic hormone; *SLE,* systemic lupus erythematosus. (Image courtesy of Stage2sleep.svg: User:Neocadre.ljustam at en.wikipediaderivative work: Neocadre.)

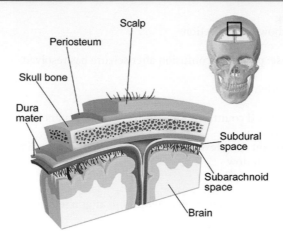

Layers covering the Brain

Figure 2-7: Layers covering the brain. (Image courtesy of Blausen Medical BruceBlaus; CC BY-SA [https://creative-commons.org/licenses/by-sa/4.0])

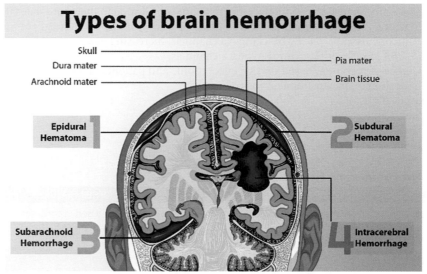

Figure 2-8: Types of brain hemorrhage. (Image courtesy of https://www.myupchar.com/en)

V. **Hemorrhage**

   Intracranial hemorrhage can involve many different spaces of the brain such as subdural, epidural, subarachnoid, or intraparenchymal (Figs. 2-7 and 2-8). Each of these produces a unique set of imaging findings and potential complications (Table 2-6).

VI. **Headache**

   A. Primary headaches
      1. Tension
         a. Signs and symptoms
            • Bandlike tightness around the head
            • Frontooccipital distribution
            • Neck soreness
            • Worsened by stress, lack of sleep, anxiety
            • Worsens throughout the day
         b. Management
            • Nonsteroidal antiinflammatory drugs (NSAIDs), acetaminophen (pregnancy)
            • Avoid stressors
      2. Migraine
         a. Risk factors
            • Females

TABLE 2-6   Differentiating Types of Brain Hemorrhage

	EPIDURAL HEMATOMA	SUBDURAL HEMATOMA	SUBARACHNOID HEMORRHAGE (SAH)
Pathophysiology	• Temporal bone trauma resulting in rupture of the middle meningeal artery	• Rupture of bridging veins	• Rupture of cerebral aneurysm
Clinical presentation	• Trauma resulting in loss of consciousness followed by lucid interval, and then rapid clinical deterioration (nausea, vomiting, coma)	• Chronic worsening headache and confusion over days to weeks • May or may not recall minor trauma • Focal neurologic deficits due to mass effect • Elderly, chronic alcoholic	• Sentinel headache that occurs days to weeks prior to SAH • Sudden onset severe headache • Meningismus symptoms • Loss of consciousness
Diagnosis	• Noncontrast computed tomography (CT): lens-shaped hyperdensity that does not cross suture lines	• Noncontrast CT: crescent-shaped density that crosses suture lines	• Noncontrast CT: hyperdensity filling the subarachnoid space
Management	• Surgical evacuation and decompression	• Surgical evacuation and decompression	• Coiling or embolization • Nimodipine to prevent vasospasm
Complications	• Transtentorial herniation • Ipsilateral pupillary dilation (due to compression of extrinsic portion of CN III) • "Down and out pupil" (loss of CN III extraocular muscle function) • Ipsilateral hemiparesis (compression of contralateral crus)	• Herniation	• Vasospasm • Seizures • Hydrocephalus
Imaging	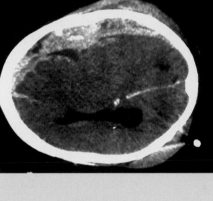	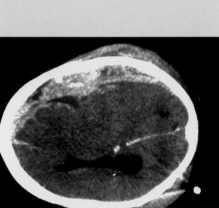	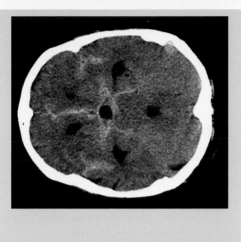

- Family history
- Worsened by certain foods (chocolate, wine, cheese), changes in weather, sleep, menses (catamenial migraines)
  b. Signs and symptoms
  - Photophobia, phonophobia
  - Aura: visual/sensory disturbances prior to migraine onset
  - Nausea, vomiting
  - Lasts 4–72 hours
  c. Subtypes
  - Basilar
  - Complicated
  - Status
  d. Management
  - Acute
    - Triptans (sumatriptan, rizatriptan)
    - NSAIDs
    - Dopamine antagonist antiemetics (chlorpromazine, metoclopramide, prochlorperazine)
  - Prophylaxis (if >4/month or lasts >12 hours): consider pharmacotherapy based on patient comorbidities
    - Propranolol, timolol, metoprolol
    - Venlafaxine, amitriptyline
    - Topiramate, valproate
  - Prevention: avoid exacerbating factors
3. Cluster
  a. Risk factors
  - Males
  - Smokers
  b. Signs and symptoms
  - Severe unilateral retroorbital pain
  - Lacrimation
  - Conjunctival injection
  - Partial Horner syndrome (ptosis, miosis)
  - Attacks occur at the same time every day for weeks followed by a period of remission
  c. Management
  - Acute
    - 100% oxygen
    - Subcutaneous triptans
  - Prophylaxis
    - Verapamil
    - Alternatives: prednisone, lithium, topiramate
  - Prevention: smoking cessation
B. Secondary headaches
  1. Often have worrisome and refractory symptoms
    a. Worsening headaches
    b. Worse in the morning and improves throughout the day
    c. Wakes patient up from sleep
    d. Sudden onset
    e. Altered mental status
    f. Seizures
  2. Causes
    a. Pseudotumor cerebri (benign intracranial hypertension)
    b. Meningitis
    c. Glaucoma
    d. Giant cell arteritis
    e. Hemorrhage
    f. Stroke
    g. Hypertension
    h. Tumor
    i. Trauma
  3. Diagnostics/management: based on history and physical exam

C. Pseudotumor cerebri (benign intracranial hypertension)
   1. Risk factors
      a. Obesity
      b. Medications (vitamin A, tetracyclines, oral contraceptive pills)
      c. Young female
   2. Sign and symptoms
      a. Visual disturbances
      b. Papilledema
      c. Enlarging blind spot
      d. Nausea, vomiting
   3. Diagnostics
      a. Exclude intracranial pathology with MRI or CT
      b. Lumbar puncture: negative except for increased opening pressure
   4. Management
      a. Weight loss
      b. Acetazolamide, furosemide
      c. Refractory
         • Ventriculoperitoneal shunt
         • Optic nerve fenestration (allows CSF to drain via optic nerve sheath)
   5. Complications: blindness

Summary of other causes of secondary headaches:
• Meningitis: fever, headache, neck stiffness
• Glaucoma: eye pain, conjunctival injection, halos
• Giant cell arteritis: jaw claudication, tender/palpable temporal artery, blindness, polymyalgia rheumatica in 50%
• Hemorrhage: see previous section on hemorrhage (epidural, subdural, subarachnoid)
• Stroke: focal neurologic deficits, aphasia, altered mental status
• Hypertension: >180/100, dizziness, visual disturbances
• Tumor: mass effect, symptoms depend on location of mass +/- focal neurologic deficits
• Concussion: amnesia, history of trauma

VII. **Multiple Sclerosis (MS)**
   A. MS facts
      1. Risk factors
         a. Female, white
         b. North of the equator, lack of sunlight
         c. Viral infection (Epstein-Barr virus [EBV])
      2. Pathophysiology: T-cell–mediated type IV hypersensitivity reaction against myelin basic protein resulting in demyelinating disorder affecting white matter of the central nervous system (CNS)
      3. Signs and symptoms
         a. Symptoms worsen during stressful events such as infection, trauma, heat (Uhthoff phenomenon)
         b. Symptoms improve during pregnancy
         c. Waxing and waning motor and sensory deficits that self-resolve over days to weeks (Fig. 2-9)
         d. Optic neuritis (afferent pupillary defect)
         e. Cerebellar ataxia
         f. Bladder/bowel incontinence
         g. Internuclear ophthalmoplegia (medial longitudinal fasciculus lesion)—lesion of crossing fibers connecting ipsilateral CN VI nuclei to contralateral CN III nuclei (Figs. 2-10 and 2-11)
         h. Scanning speech
         i. Spasticity
         j. Less common findings
            • Cognitive dysfunction
            • Lhermitte sign (shocklike sensation radiating down the spine upon flexion of head)
            • Trigeminal neuralgia
      4. Diagnostics
         a. MRI
            • Old and new (time and space) demyelinating white matter lesions
            • Dawson fingers: periventricular lesions
         b. Lumbar puncture: oligoclonal bands (due to production of antibodies from plasma cells)

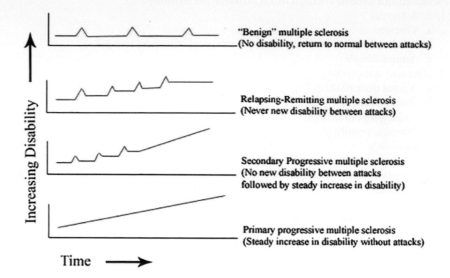

Figure 2-9: Subtypes of multiple sclerosis and their progression over time. (Image courtesy of Garrondo at en.wikipedia.)

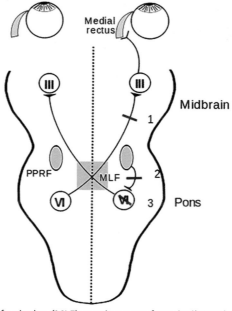

Figure 2-10: Medial longitudinal fasciculus *(MLF)* crossing over from ipsilateral cranial nerve (CN) VI to contralateral CN III. Loss of the MLF results in impaired adduction past midline of the ipsilateral eye. *PPRF,* Paramedian pontine reticular formation. (Image courtesy of Suraj Rajan; CC BY-SA [https://creativecommons.org/licenses/by-sa/3.0])

5. Management: goal of therapy is to slow progression of disease and treat symptoms as they arise
   a. Acute: high-dose steroids
   b. Maintenance
      • Interferon-beta
        ▪ Side effects
          - Flulike symptoms
          - Worsening depression
          - Leukopenia, thrombocytopenia
      • Glatiramer acetate
      • Natalizumab
        ▪ Integrin inhibitor
        ▪ May result in reactivation of John Cunningham (JC) virus → progressive multifocal leukoencephalopathy (PML)

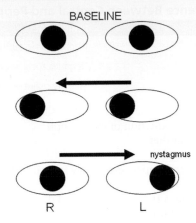

Figure 2-11: Patient with right internuclear ophthalmoplegia demonstrating impaired adduction of the right-sided past midline on contralateral gaze. (Image courtesy of Samir; CC BY-SA 3.0 [http://creativecommons.org/licenses/by-sa/3.0/])

- Fingolimod
  - Sphingosine analogue: prevents lymphocytes from proliferating outside the lymph nodes
  - Side effects
    - Cardiotoxicity
    - Macular edema (worse in diabetics)
- Teriflunomide
  - Mitoxantrone: may result in cardiotoxicity, secondary acute myelogenous leukemia
- Dimethyl fumarate
- Azathioprine
- Smoking cessation
- Symptomatic
  - Spasticity: baclofen (GABA agonist)
  - Urinary incontinence
    - Urge: oxybutynin, tolterodine
    - Retention: bethanechol
  - Walking difficulties: dalfampridine (K-channel blocker)
  - Fatigue: amantadine, modafinil
  - Trigeminal neuralgia: carbamazepine

B. Neuromyelitis optica (NMO)
  1. Similar presentation to MS
  2. Causes bilateral optic neuropathy (MS causes unilateral) and lesions in cervical spinal cord
  3. Spares brain, unlike MS
  4. Diagnostics: NMO–IgG

VIII. **Vertigo**
  A. Vertigo principles
    1. Presents as sensation of the room spinning, dizziness, tilting, or swaying
    2. Can present similarly to presyncope (lightheadedness, palpitations, weakness)
    3. Divided into central vs peripheral causes (Table 2-7)
    4. Associated with nystagmus depending on central vs peripheral vertigo
    5. Differentiated based on duration, position, frequency of episodes, and associated symptoms

If isolated tinnitus, consider aspirin overdose, multiple sclerosis, or foreign body.

IX. **Peripheral Vertigo**
  A. Meniere disease
    1. Pathophysiology: overproduction of endolymph → increased perilymphatic pressure → stimulation of vestibular apparatus and abnormal vestibular function
    2. Signs and symptoms
      a. Triad of tinnitus, vertigo, unilateral sensory hearing loss
      b. Waxing and waning symptoms depending on endolymph pressure

TABLE 2-7 Summary of Difference Between Central and Peripheral Vertigo

CENTRAL	PERIPHERAL
Vertical nystagmus	Horizontal nystagmus
Neurologic deficits	Negative focal neurologic deficits
Significant instability when walking	Stability maintained when walking

       3. Management: decrease production of endolymph
         a. Diuretics plus low-salt diet
     B. Labyrinthitis
       1. Pathophysiology: postviral upper respiratory tract infection
       2. Signs and symptoms
         a. Sudden onset of acute vertigo lasting several days and can last for hours (vs Meniere vertigo attacks that last for minutes)
         b. Nausea, vomiting
         c. Hearing loss, tinnitus
       3. Diagnostics: head thrust test
         a. When head is turned to affected side, the patient is unable to maintain visual fixation
       4. Management: supportive
         a. Steroid taper for acute treatment: shown to improve short-term outcomes
         b. Meclizine
         c. Antiemetics (promethazine, metoclopramide), anticholinergic (scopolamine, diphenhydramine)
         d. Surgery: for refractory case; however, results in deafness as it obliterates the vestibular apparatus

If similar presentation as labyrinthitis but hearing is preserved, then the diagnosis is vestibular neuritis.

     C. Benign position peripheral vertigo
       1. Pathophysiology: loose calcium crystals in the semicircular canals that strike sensitive nerve endings resulting in discrepant signaling from the semicircular canal and producing symptoms of nystagmus and vertigo
       2. Signs and symptoms
         a. Vertigo worsened by changes with position and head movements
         b. Episodic symptoms that last seconds occurring over several days
         c. No tinnitus or hearing loss
       3. Diagnostics: Dix-Hallpike test
         a. With the patient sitting up, abruptly lay the patient down and rotate the head 45 degrees to one side and watch for nystagmus
         b. Putting patient's head in different position will activate the semicircular canals
         c. Should elicit nystagmus with fast phase toward the affected ear
       4. Management: Epley maneuver
         a. Repositions the otoliths in the semicircular canal
     D. Perilymphatic fistula
       1. Pathophysiology: trauma (barotrauma, blunt) resulting in rupture of bony capsule in the inner ear and leakage of perilymph into middle ear
       2. Signs and symptoms: vertigo associated with increased pressure maneuvers (Valsalva, straining, coughing, sneezing, scuba diving)
       3. Diagnostics: clinical
       4. Management: supportive (meclizine +/− diazepam)
     E. Vestibular schwannoma
       1. Tumor of CN VIII resulting in unilateral hearing loss (if bilateral, consider neurofibromatosis type 2)
     F. Cogan syndrome
       1. Autoimmune disease associated with interstitial keratitis and vestibuloauditory symptoms
X. Central vertigo
     A. Key principles (Fig 2-12)
       1. Occurs due to primary CNS pathology, most commonly cerebellar
       2. Present with ataxia, diplopia, dysarthria, dysphagia, or vertical nystagmus
       3. Requires CNS imaging, MRI better than CT for visualizing posterior fossa

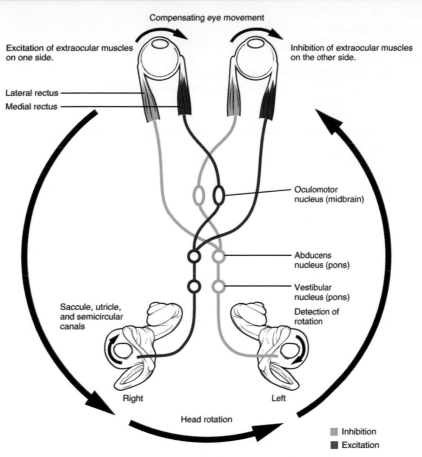

Figure 2-12: Vestibular ocular reflex in a patient turning the head to the left. Vestibular system and cranial nerves work together to keep the eyes centered on a visual stimulus. During head movements, the eyes move in the opposite direction allowing the patient to maintain focus and center the visualized object. (Image courtesy of Samir; CC BY-SA 3.0 [https://creativecommons.org/licenses/by-sa/3.0])

B. CNS causes of vertigo
   1. Tumors: medulloblastomas, meningioma
   2. Arnold-Chiari: cerebellar tonsil herniation below the foramen magnum; vertigo induced by neck extension
   3. Vascular
      a. Wallenberg
         • Occlusion of posterior inferior cerebellar artery → infarction of the lateral medulla
         • Loss of pain and temperature, bulbar muscle weakness, vertigo, nystagmus, and Horner syndrome
      b. Vertebrobasilar insufficiency: atherosclerosis of the posterior circulation
      c. Subclavian steal syndrome
         • Stenosis of the subclavian artery
         • Flow reversal in ipsilateral vertebral artery during ipsilateral upper extremity exertion → vertebrobasilar ischemia
   4. Hemorrhage
   5. Multiple sclerosis
      a. Relapsing remitting symptoms
      b. Symptoms due to lesions involving the vestibular nuclei
   6. Vestibular migraine: migraine and vertigo symptoms that resolve when migraine resolves
   7. Aminoglycoside toxicity
      a. Damages cochlear and hair cells resulting in hearing loss and vertigo
      b. Oscillopsia: sensation of objects moving when looking in any direction
      c. Abnormal head thrust test: while looking at a fixed target, rapid head movement away from the target will result in patient inability to maintain gaze on the target object; when eyes move away and return to object, the patient will develop a horizontal saccade

XI. Tremors

  A. Huntington disease

    1. Risk factors: family history (autosomal dominant inheritance)

    2. Pathophysiology

      a. CAG trinucleotide repeats on chromosome 4

      b. Decreased GABA and acetylcholine, increased dopamine

    3. Signs and symptoms

      a. Chorea, athetosis

      b. Personality changes: social disinhibition, anxiety, depression, psychosis, suicidality, dementia

      c. Gait instability, dyskinesia

    4. Diagnostics

      a. Brain MRI/CT: atrophy of caudate nucleus (results in enlarged lateral ventricles)

      b. Genetic testing (CAG trinucleotide repeats)

    5. Management: symptomatic

      a. Psychosis: haloperidol, quetiapine

      b. Chorea, athetosis: long-acting benzodiazepines (diazepam, clonazepam)

      c. Dyskinesia: tetrabenazine

      d. Depression, anxiety: selective serotonin reuptake inhibitors (SSRIs)

Anticipation: expansion in the number of trinucleotides repeat in subsequent generations resulting in earlier disease presentation.

  B. Parkinson's disease

    1. Causes

      a. Idiopathic

      b. Trauma (boxing)

      c. Drugs: result in parkinsonian symptoms

        • Typical antipsychotics (haloperidol, fluphenazine)

        • Metoclopramide

        • Alpha-methyldopa

        • MPTP (converted to toxic metabolites by the enzyme monoamine oxidase B, which destroys cells in the basal ganglia)

        • Carbon monoxide, cyanide, manganese poisoning

    2. Pathophysiology: degeneration of dopaminergic neurons in the substantia nigra

    3. Signs and symptoms: related to basal ganglia dysfunction

      a. Pill-rolling resting tremor (often the first manifestation of disease)

      b. Cogwheel rigidity, postural instability

      c. Bradykinesia, shuffling gait (slowing of movements)

      d. Dysarthria, dysphagia

      e. Micrographia (small handwriting)

      f. Masked facies (expressionless face)

      g. Dementia in advanced disease

    4. Diagnostics

      a. Clinical: signs and symptoms plus response to treatment

      b. Definitive diagnosis made on autopsy

    5. Management: goal is to increase dopamine and decrease acetylcholine, which will slow disease progression and relieve symptoms

      a. Levodopa carbidopa

        • First-line treatment for Parkinson's disease

        • Levodopa: precursor to dopamine, which can cross the blood brain barrier (BBB) and be converted to dopamine

        • Carbidopa: peripheral DOPA decarboxylase inhibitor that prevents metabolism of levodopa into dopamine, which cannot cross the BBB. This allows the maximum amount of levodopa to cross the BBB and maximize its effects in the CNS

        • Side effects

          ▪ Dyskinesias, hallucinations, nausea, and vomiting

          ▪ "On-off" phenomenon: characterized by episodes of dyskinesia and akinesia due to fluctuation in response to treatment after long-term use; this occurs due to disease progression and narrowing therapeutic window

b. Bromocriptine, pramipexole, apomorphine, rotigotine
- Dopamine receptor agonists
- Apomorphine: subcutaneous injection, used as rescue therapy for sudden akinetic episode
- Rotigotine: transdermal patch

c. Amantadine
- Increases the release and prevents uptake of dopamine
- Previously used to treat influenza; however, no longer used due to increased resistance
- Side effects: ataxia, livedo reticularis

d. Selegiline
- Monoamine oxidase B inhibitor preventing metabolism of dopamine

e. Tolcapone, entacapone
- Catechol-O-methyltransferase inhibitors
- Used to prolong the effects of carbidopa by blocking the metabolism of dopamine

f. Benztropine, trihexyphenidyl
- Anticholinergic
- Useful in patients who primarily have tremors and mild disease (can still manage the activities of daily living)
- Side effects
  - Avoid in elderly, preexisting glaucoma, benign prostate hyperplasia
  - Dry mouth, constipation

g. Surgery
- Last resort when patient is refractory to medication
- Deep brain stimulation in the subthalamic nucleus or globus pallidus

C. Parkinson-plus syndromes: present similarly to Parkinson's disease; however, does not respond to traditional treatment
  1. Supernuclear palsy
    a. Parkinson plus vertical gaze palsy (due to degeneration in the midbrain where vertical gaze centers are located)
    b. Axial dystonia
  2. Multisystem atrophy (Shy-Drager syndrome): Parkinson plus autonomic dysfunction (orthostatic hypotension)
  3. Lewy body dementia
    a. Parkinson plus visual hallucinations
    b. Rapid eye movement (REM)–related sleep disorder
    c. Hypersensitivity to neuroleptics
  4. Olivopontocerebellar degeneration: Parkinson plus ataxia
  5. Corticobasilar degeneration: alien hand syndrome (sensation that the limb is foreign to patient as the ability to control its movements is lost)

D. Essential tremor
  1. Risk factors: family history (autosomal dominant inheritance)
  2. Signs and symptoms
    a. Tremor that occurs at rest and with intention
    b. Primarily affects the hands
    c. Worsened by stimulants such as caffeine, relieved by depressants such as alcohol
    d. Distinguished from other causes of tremor due to lack of associated symptoms
  3. Diagnostics: clinical
  4. Management: only treat if it is affecting the patient's ability to function
    a. Propranolol: first line
    b. Primidone, alprazolam, clozapine
    c. Deep brain stimulation

The type of tremor (Table 2-8), along with factors that improve or worsen the tremor, can help localize the location of the lesion.

XII. **Dementia/Delirium**

Delirium and dementia are two clinical presentations that may appear very similar when viewed during a single patient encounter; however, based on the acuity of presentation and thorough evaluation of potential triggers these can be easily differentiated (Table 2-9).

A. Specific causes of dementia
  1. Reversible causes
    a. Hypothyroidism
      - Causes

TABLE 2-8   Types of Tremors

TYPE OF TREMOR	SYMPTOMATOLOGY	ASSOCIATED CONDITIONS
Physiologic	Normal, low amplitude tremor not readily visualized	Anxiety, adrenergic agents, caffeine
Intention	Tremor worsened with movement, absent at rest	Cerebellar lesion
Resting	Tremor that improves with movement, present at rest	Parkinson's disease

TABLE 2-9   Delirium Versus Dementia

	DEMENTIA	DELIRIUM
Onset	• Insidious	• Acute
Progression	• Slowly progressive symptoms over months to years	• Rapidly worsening symptoms with waxing and waning course
Triggers	• Family history • Elderly	• Drugs (benzodiazepines, narcotics, anticholinergics, steroids, antipsychotics) • Infection (urinary tract infections) • Metabolic (electrolytes, glucose) • Medical (stroke, seizures, carbon dioxide narcosis) • Prolonged hospital stay with intensive care unit admission (circadian rhythm disruption)
Symptoms	• Memory deficits • Confabulation • Poor insight into nature of cognitive changes	• Agitation • Combativeness • Hallucinations
Management	• Often irreversible	• Removal and treatment of causative factor • Reorientation • Reassurance • If necessary: antipsychotics +/- restraints

- Autoimmune thyroiditis (Hashimoto thyroiditis)
        - Iatrogenic (postthyroidectomy)
        - Drugs (lithium, amiodarone)
    - Key features
        - Weight gain, lethargy, depression
        - Hypercholesterolemia, bradycardia, hypothermia
        - Menorrhagia, constipation
        - Decreased reflexes, muscle aches
        - Hair loss, myxedema
    - Management: thyroid replacement with thyroxine
  b. B12 deficiency
    - Causes
        - Vegan
        - Pernicious anemia
        - Terminal ileal disease (Crohn's disease)
        - Postsurgical (gastric bypass, gastrectomy)
    - Key features
        - Memory deficits
        - Neurologic deficits (corticospinal tract, spinothalamic tract, spinocerebellar)
    - Management: parenteral B12 replacement, treatment of underlying cause
  c. Syphilis
    - Cause: treponema pallidum infection
    - Key features: only tertiary syphilis presents with neurologic symptoms
        - Dementia
        - Meningitis
        - Tabes dorsalis (loss of vibratory and position sensation)
        - Argyll Robertson pupils (pupils accommodate but do not react to light)
    - Management: penicillin
  d. Lyme disease
    - Cause: Ixodes tick (located in the northeastern United States)
    - Key features: only stage II and III Lyme disease typically involves the CNS

- Meningitis, encephalitis
- Cranial nerve deficits
- Altered mental status
- Management: IV ceftriaxone; doxycycline for early disease

e. Normal pressure hydrocephalus
  - Cause: interference with absorption of CSF at the level of the arachnoid granulations → enlargement of the ventricles and stretching of the corona radiata fibers
  - Key features
    - Dementia
    - Gait disturbance
    - Urinary incontinence
  - Management: ventriculoperitoneal shunt; improvement in symptoms after lumbar puncture and release of CSF

f. Pseudodementia
  - Cause: depression
  - Key features: commonly seen in elderly patients who present with memory deficits and nonspecific symptoms inconsistent with other causes of dementia
    - Lethargy
    - Sleep disturbance
    - Slowed mentation, forgetfulness
    - Decreased energy
    - Weight changes
  - Management: SSRIs

g. Wernicke-Korsacoff
  - Cause: thiamine (B1) deficiency due to chronic alcohol use and malnutrition
  - Key features
    - Triad of ataxia, confusion, ophthalmoplegia
    - Can progress to Korsakoff syndrome with addition of amnesia, personality changes, and confabulation
  - Management: vitamin B1 (thiamine) followed by glucose
    - Administering glucose before thiamine can induce encephalopathy due to depletion of thiamine

2. Irreversible causes of dementia
  a. Alzheimer disease
    - Pathophysiology: chronic cortical atrophy, deposition of amyloid plaques and neurofibrillary tangles resulting in neuronal dysfunction and memory loss
    - Risk factors
      - Trisomy 21 (due to three copies of amyloid precursor protein)
      - *apoE4* gene
      - Advanced age
    - Signs and symptoms: often recognized by family members
      - Early disease
        - Cognitive impairment
        - Memory and visual-spatial deficits
        - Loss of executive function
      - Advanced disease
        - Personality changes
        - Loss of social graces
        - Hallucinations
    - Diagnostics: clinical
      - Rule out reversible causes of dementia
      - Neuroimaging: preferential atrophy of the temporal and parietal lobes (Figs. 2-13 and 2-14)
      - Mini-Mental Status Examination (MMSE)
      - Definitive diagnosis on autopsy
    - Management: targeted to slow disease progression
      - Acetylcholinesterase inhibitors (donepezil, rivastigmine, galantamine)
        - Prevent breakdown of acetylcholine at the neuromuscular junction increasing levels of acetylcholine in the CNS
        - Side effects: hypotension, bradycardia
      - N-methyl-D-aspartate (NMDA) antagonist (memantine): decreases neuronal excitotoxicity

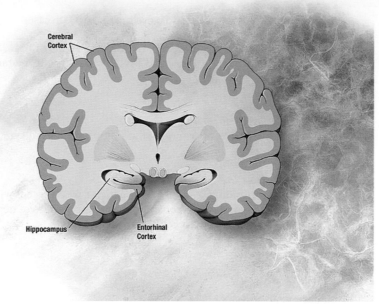

Figure 2-13: Normal brain anatomy and cortex. (Image courtesy of Samir; CC BY-SA 3.0 [https://creativecommons.org/licenses/by-sa/3.0])

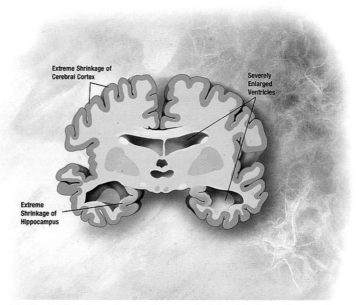

Figure 2-14: Compared with Fig. 2.13, this patient is diagnosed with Alzheimer disease. (Image courtesy ADEAR: Alzheimer Disease Education and Referral Center, a service of the National Institute on Aging; CC BY-SA [https://creativecommons.org/licenses/by-sa/3.0])

  b. Vascular dementia
   • Pathophysiology: multiple, chronic, cortical subclinical infarcts due to vascular disease (hypertension, diabetes, dyslipidemia, smoking)
   • Signs and symptoms: chronic stepwise decline in cognitive function
     ▪ Focal neurologic deficits consistent with strokes in various parts of the brain
     ▪ Dysarthria, dysphasia
     ▪ Hyperreflexia
     ▪ Gait disturbances
   • Diagnostics
     ▪ Clinical
     ▪ MRI brain
   • Management: control underlying vascular disease

    c. Frontotemporal dementia
- Dementia primarily involving the frontal and temporal lobes
- Emotional and personality changes, loss of social inhibitions, memory loss later in disease

    d. Lewy body dementia
- Dementia associated with Parkinson's disease
- Dementia occurs before or around the same time as parkinsonian symptoms
- Associated with visual hallucinations, REM sleep disorder, constructional apraxia
- Unresponsive to parkinsonian medications
- Hypersensitivity to neuroleptics

    e. Creutzfeldt-Jakob disease
- Rapidly progressive dementia due to transmission of prions
- EEG: sharp, triphasic synchronous discharges
- Myoclonic jerks, ataxia
- CSF positive for 14-3-3 protein

XIII. Neuromuscular Disorders

A. The neuromuscular junction is a complex structure involving the use of different ion channels, axons, and cells (Fig. 2-15). Pathology at any of these sites can produce unique symptomatology.

Myasthenia gravis

1. Epidemiology
   a. Age 20–30 s in women
   b. Age 60–80 s in men
   c. History of other autoimmune diseases
2. Pathophysiology: autoantibodies against nicotinic acetylcholine receptors at the neuromuscular junction resulting in complement activation and receptor destruction (Fig. 2-16)
3. Signs and symptoms
   a. Fluctuating muscle weakness that worsens with use
   b. Diplopia with normal pupillary response
      - Often the earliest complaint due to constant use of these muscles and relatively increased density of acetylcholine receptors
   c. Difficulty chewing, slurred speech, dysarthria, dysphagia
   d. Nasal sounding speech
   e. Trident tongue (one central and two lateral longitudinal furrows of the tongue)
   f. No sensory deficits
4. Diagnostics: clinical plus serology
   a. Serology
      - Acetylcholine receptor antibodies
      - Antimuscle-specific kinase antibodies for patients who are acetylcholine receptor antibody negative

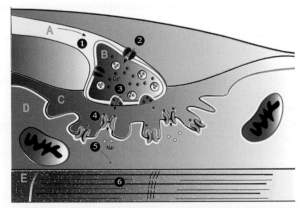

Figure 2-15: Normal neuromuscular junction physiology. *A,* Motor neuron axon; *B,* axon terminal; *C,* synaptic cleft; *D,* muscle cell; *E,* part of a myofibril. *1,* The action potential reaches the axon terminal; *2,* voltage-dependent calcium gates open, allowing calcium to enter the axon terminal; *3,* neurotransmitter vesicles fuse with the presynaptic membrane and acetylcholine (ACh) is released into the synaptic cleft via exocytosis; *4,* ACh binds to postsynaptic receptors on the sarcolemma; *5,* this binding causes ion channels to open and allows sodium ions to flow across the membrane into the muscle cell; *6,* the flow of sodium ions across the membrane into the muscle cell generates an action potential, which travels to the myofibril and results in muscle contraction. (Image and caption courtesy of Elliejellybelly13; CC BY-SA [https://creativecommons.org/licenses/by-sa/4.0].)

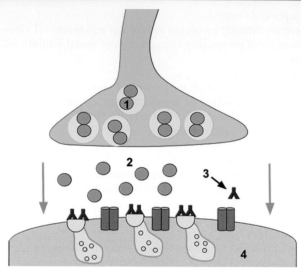

Figure 2-16: Pathophysiology of myasthenia gravis: Acetylcholine (Ach) *(1)* is released into the synapse *(2)* but cannot bind to ACh receptors on the muscle fiber due to antibodies *(3)* on the receptors blocking entry of Ach. Triggering of the muscle fiber *(4)* is inhibited, resulting in muscle weakness and ACh deficiencies. (Image and caption courtesy of Libbyspek.)

5. Other supporting diagnoses
   a. Ice pack test: placement of ice pack over the patient's eyelids for several minutes often results in an improvement in ptosis and diplopia due to the cold temperature inhibiting breakdown of acetylcholine at the neuromuscular junction
   b. Edrophonium test: short-acting acetylcholinesterase inhibitor resulting in rapid improvement in muscle weakness
   c. Electromyography (EMG): decreased response to repetitive stimulation
   d. CT chest: thymoma present in 15% of cases
      • Appears as an anterior mediastinal mass
6. Management
   a. Acetylcholinesterase inhibitors (first line)
      • Inhibits acetylcholinesterase at the neuromuscular junction prolonging the effects of acetylcholine and outcompeting the autoantibodies
      • Examples: neostigmine, pyridostigmine
      • Side effects: due to excess acetylcholine
         ▪ Salivation, lacrimation
         ▪ Emesis
         ▪ Bronchoconstriction
         ▪ Urinary incontinence, diarrhea
   b. Thymectomy: may provide complete relief of symptoms due to autoantibodies originating from the thymus
   c. Immunosuppressive agents: for patients nonresponsive to acetylcholinesterase inhibitors and thymectomy; they take several weeks to reach their efficacy
      • Corticosteroids
      • Steroid-sparing agents (azathioprine, cyclosporine, tacrolimus, cyclophosphamide, mycophenolate)
7. Complications: myasthenic crisis
   a. MS exacerbation presenting with severe muscle weakness with involvement of diaphragmatic muscles resulting in respiratory compromise
   b. May be triggered by underlying infection or stress (surgery, medication, pregnancy)
   c. Treat with plasmapheresis or IV immunoglobulin (IVIG)

If pupils are involved, then consider other causes such as botulinum toxicity. In botulinum toxicity, patient will have dilated pupils, and repetitive nerve stimulation on electromyography will show incremental increase in muscle response.

Aminoglycosides in patients with myasthenia gravis should be avoided due to their side effect of preventing the release of acetylcholine from the presynaptic cleft.

B. Lambert-Eaton syndrome
1. Pathophysiology: paraneoplastic syndrome characterized by autoantibodies against presynaptic voltage-gated calcium channels and preventing release of acetylcholine into the neuromuscular junction
2. Signs and symptoms
   a. Muscle weakness that improves with use—repetitive use will build up gradient of calcium outside the presynaptic voltage-gated channel that eventually outcompetes the autoantibody
   b. Proximal muscle weakness
   c. Decreased deep tendon reflexes (DTRs)
   d. Normal pupils
3. Diagnostics
   a. Serology: voltage-gated calcium channel antibodies
   b. EMG
   c. Chest CT looking for lung cancer if this is the first presenting symptom
4. Associations
   a. Small cell lung cancer
   b. Lymphoproliferative disorders (Hodgkin lymphoma)
5. Management: treatment of underlying malignancy

Other paraneoplastic symptoms associated with small cell lung cancer include syndrome of inappropriate antidiuretic hormone and Cushing syndrome (due to ectopic production adrenocorticotropic hormone).

C. Amyotrophic lateral sclerosis
1. Pathophysiology
   a. Neurodegenerative disorder of unknown etiology affecting upper and lower motor neurons
   b. Superoxide dismutase mutation in familial cases
2. Signs and symptoms
   a. Upper motor neuron signs
      • Increased DTRs
      • Spasticity
      • Pronator drift
      • Clasp knife reflex
   b. Lower motor neuron signs
      • Fasciculations
      • Atrophy
      • Hypotonia
      • Decreased DTRs
   c. Asymmetric limb weakness, nasal speech, cramping, stiffness
   d. Corticobulbar involvement: difficulty chewing, swallowing (decreased gag reflex), coughing (decreased cough reflex)
   e. Sensation intact
3. Diagnostics: clinical and electrical evidence
   a. EMG
      • Diffuse axonal injury
      • Loss of neural innervation involving multiple muscle groups
   b. Postmortem stain of the spine: confirmatory test
4. Management: symptomatic
   a. Riluzole: glutamate modulator (NMDA inhibitor) shown to decrease progression of the disease
      • Increases survival for up to six months longer by preventing glutamate-induced excitotoxicity and neuronal destruction
      • Side effects: dizziness, weakness, granulocytopenia
   b. Antispastics agents (baclofen, tizanidine, cyclobenzaprine)
   c. Respiratory support

5. Complications
   a. Aspiration pneumonia: secondary to decreased cough and gag reflex
   b. Respiratory failure due to involvement of diaphragmatic muscles—most common cause of death

---

Myelin helps with saltatory conduction to allow jumping from one node of Ranvier to the next.

D. Pseudobulbar affect syndrome
   1. Inappropriate/involuntary laughing, crying, and/or yawning
E. Guillain-Barré syndrome (GBS)
   1. Pathophysiology: autoimmune disorder targeting myelin sheath of peripheral nerves secondary to molecular mimicry after an upper respiratory or gastrointestinal (GI) infection (Campylobacter)
   2. Other associations
      a. Cytomegalovirus, human immunodeficiency virus (HIV), EBV, herpes simplex virus (HSV)
      b. Mycoplasma
      c. Postvaccination
      d. Systemic lupus erythematosus
      e. Lymphoma
   3. Signs and symptoms
      a. Ascending muscle weakness
      b. Decreased DTRs
      c. Difficulty breathing secondary to involvement of diaphragm
      d. Autonomic dysfunction
         • Hypotension/hypertension
         • Tachyarrhythmias
         • Diaphoresis
      e. May have sensory involvement: pain and dysesthesias due to loss of large unmyelinated fibers carrying proprioception
   4. Diagnostics: clinical and electrical evidence
      a. EMG
         • Demyelination and decreased conduction speed
         • Small or absent F response
      b. Lumbar puncture: albuminocytologic dissociation (elevated protein with normal cell count)
   5. Management: symptomatic plus monitoring for complications
      a. IVIG or plasmapheresis: both shown to shorten time to independent walking by 50%
      b. Overall good prognosis as myelin regenerates (80% recover completely)
   6. Complications: respiratory failure
      a. Important to periodically check the patient's forced vital capacity and peak inspiratory pressure to determine involvement of respiratory muscles and if necessary, escalate level of care
F. Miller Fisher variant
   1. No ascending muscle weakness
   2. Bulbar and facial involvement: difficulty speaking and swallowing, ophthalmoplegia, ataxia
   3. Anti-GQ1B antibody
G. Chronic inflammatory demyelinating polyneuropathy
   1. Presents as GBS that does not resolve after 8 weeks
   2. Chronic, insidious, and slowly progressive
   3. Sensorimotor involvement
   4. Management: glucocorticoids; may also use IVIG or plasmapheresis similar to GBS

F Response: When a stimulus is given it should travel anterograde (to the muscle) and retrograde (to the cell body then back to the muscle). This loop is called the F response and is diminished in demyelinating disease.

TABLE 2-10   Neuropathies and Their Associated Deficits

NERVE	FUNCTION	DEFICITS	ASSOCIATIONS
Axillary	• Motor: deltoid, teres minor • Sensory: deltoid	• Weakness of abduction from 15 to 90 degrees (supraspinatus abducts from 0–15 degrees)	• Improper use of crutches • Fracture of surgical neck of humerus • Anterior shoulder dislocation
Musculocutaneous	• Motor: biceps, brachialis, coracobrachialis • Sensory: lateral forearm	• Weakness of flexion and supination at the elbow • Loss of biceps reflex	• Rarely injured due to presence of biceps muscle
Radial	• Motor: posterior compartment of the arm and forearm • Sensory: posterior arm, forearm, dorsum of the hand and lateral 3.5 fingers excluding nail beds	• Weakness of elbow and wrist extension (wrist drop) • Loss of triceps reflex	• Saturday night palsy • Fracture of shaft of humerus • Prolonged use of tourniquets
Median	• Motor: anterior compartment forearm (except flexor carpi ulnaris and medial aspect of flexor digitorum profundus, which are supplied by ulnar nerve), some intrinsic muscles of the hand • Sensory: lateral portion of the palmar hand, lateral 3.5 fingers, including nail beds	• Weakness of wrist flexion, abduction • Loss of sensation over thenar eminence • Hand of benediction: inability to flex index or middle finger due to unopposed extension	• Supracondylar fracture of the humerus • Carpal tunnel syndrome • Self-inflicted wrist laceration
Ulnar	• Motor: majority of intrinsic muscles of the hand • Sensory: medial 1.5 fingers on the dorsal and palmar surfaces of the hand including nail beds	• Loss of sensation over hypothenar eminence and wasting of intrinsic muscles of hand • Claw hand: inability to extend ring or pinky finger due to unopposed flexion	• Supracondylar fracture of humerus • Fracture of medial condyle • Compression at Guyon canal
Lateral cutaneous nerve of the thigh	• Motor: N/A • Sensory: lateral thigh	• Loss of sensation over lateral thigh	• Sitting with legs crossed, tight pants
Peroneal (also known as fibular nerve)	• Motor: lateral compartment (superficial fibular nerve) and anterior compartment of the leg (deep fibular nerve) • Sensory: lateral leg and dorsum of the foot	• Loss of dorsiflexion (foot drop), eversion, extension of digits	• Fracture of fibula • Tight cast of the lower limb

XIV. Neuropathies

Injury to the various peripheral nerves (Table 2-10), brachial plexus (Figs. 2-17 and 2-18), and lumbar plexus (Figs. 2-19 and 2-20) results in reproducible sensory and motor deficits based on the dermatomes and muscles they enervate.

A. Other peripheral neuropathies
  1. Lead poisoning
    a. Signs and symptoms
      • Initially asymptomatic
      • GI: abdominal pain, constipation
      • Neurologic
        ▪ Irritability, insomnia
        ▪ Headache
        ▪ Behavioural changes
        ▪ Motor and sensory deficits
      • Hematologic: microcytic anemia, pallor
      • Renal: hypertension, nephropathy
    b. Diagnostics
      • Elevated blood lead levels and serum zinc protoporphyrin
      • Peripheral smear: basophilic stippling, microcytic anemia
      • X-ray: lead lines in long bones

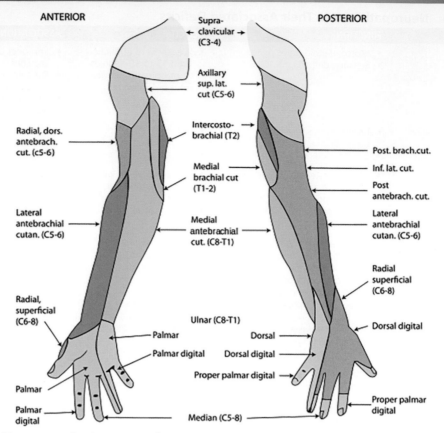

Figure 2-17: Upper extremity dermatomes. (Image courtesy Henry Vandyke Carter)

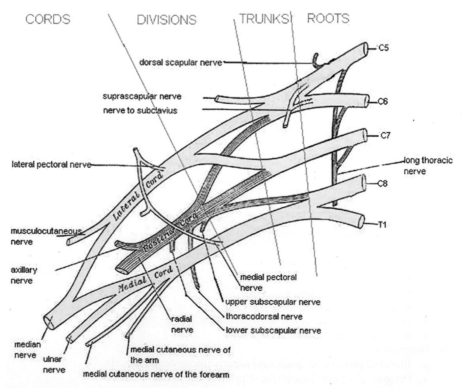

Figure 2-18: Branches of the brachial plexus. (Image courtesy of de:Benutzer:Uwe Gille.)

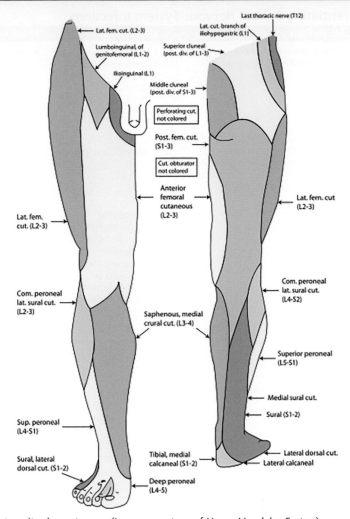

Figure 2-19: Lower extremity dermatomes. (Image courtesy of Henry Vandyke Carter.)

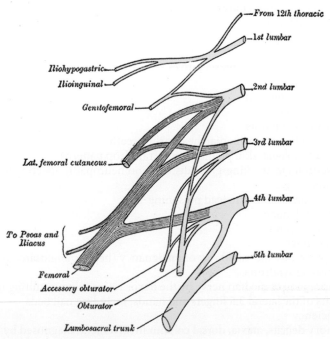

Figure 2-20: Branches of the lumbar trunk. (Image courtesy of Gray.)

TABLE 2-11 Differentiating Central Nervous System Infections

	MENINGITIS	ENCEPHALITIS	BRAIN ABSCESS
Signs and symptoms	• Headache, fever, neck stiffness • Positive Kernig and Brudzinski signs	• Similar to meningitis with addition of confusion, focal neurologic deficits, and personality changes	• Fever, progressively worsening headache • Presence of risk factors (recent neurosurgery, otitis media, sinusitis, endocarditis)
Microbiology	• Differs according to age of patient and risk factors; however, most common cause in adults is *Streptococcus pneumonia*	• Herpes simplex virus	• Polymicrobial with gram negatives and anaerobes
Diagnostics	• Lumbar puncture	• Computed tomography scan first due to symptoms • Lumbar puncture followed by viral polymerase chain reaction of cerebrospinal fluid	• Stereotactic brain biopsy and aspiration • If patient is HIV positive, then treat empirically for Toxoplasma, and if brain abscess resolves then retrospective diagnosis can be made
Management	• Ceftriaxone, vancomycin, and steroids empirically until lumbar puncture results come back. Discontinue steroids if *S. pneumonia* is not the cause • Add ampicillin for suspected listeria in elderly (>50 yr old), neonates, pregnant, and immunocompromised	• Acyclovir	• Metronidazole and third-generation cephalosporin • For HIV positive: pyrimethamine and sulfadiazine. If abscess does not get smaller after reimaging in 5–7 days, then it must be biopsied to exclude CNS lymphoma

Computed tomography scan before lumbar puncture should be done in the following scenarios: confusion, focal neurologic deficits, seizures, papilledema.
CNS, Central nervous system; *HIV*, human immunodeficiency virus.

     c. Management: chelation
- Succimer: best choice for children
- Dimercaprol: best choice for encephalopathy
- Ethylenediaminetetraacetic acid
- Penicillamine

  2. Arsenic poisoning
    a. Risk factors
- Exposure to wood preservatives
- Pesticides
- Coal combustion
- Well water

    b. Signs and symptoms
- GI: abdominal pain, diarrhea, garlic breath
- Dermatologic: skin pigmentation (raindrop pattern)
- Neurologic: stocking-glove distribution neuropathy affecting legs more than hands

    c. Management: similar to lead poisoning
- Penicillamine
- Dimercaprol
- Succimer

    d. Complications: increased risk of malignancy (hepatic angiosarcoma)

  3. Carpal tunnel syndrome
    a. Compression of median nerve by the flexor retinaculum resulting in motor and sensory deficits of the lateral 3.5 fingers and hands, including nail beds

  4. B12 deficiency
    a. Memory deficits, ataxia, dorsal column involvement; diagnosed by low B12 and elevated methylmalonic acid levels; treat with parenteral B12

5. Drug induced
  a. Chemotherapeutics
    • Vincristine
    • Cisplatin
    • Paclitaxel
  b. HIV drugs
    • Stavudine
    • Didanosine
  c. Antibiotics
    • Linezolid
    • Isoniazid
  d. Amiodarone
  e. Phenytoin
  f. Chronic alcoholism
6. Infection
  a. HSV/varicella zoster virus reactivation (shingles)
7. Systemic diseases
  a. Cryoglobulinemia
  b. Amyloidosis
  c. Diabetes mellitus
  d. Vasculitis (polyarteritis nodosa)
  e. Waldenström macroglobulinemia
  f. Wilson disease

XV. Infections

The three main CNS infections include meningitis (inflammation of the leptomeninges), encephalitis (inflammation of the brain parenchyma), and brain abscess (pus collection within the brain parenchyma) (Table 2-11). These are differentiated based on their signs and symptoms due to the different brain spaces they involve. Additionally, the microbiologic organism often differs and can be determined using a CSF analysis (Table 2-12).

Additional notes regarding central nervous system infections:
• Steroids are shown to decrease mortality in *Streptococcus pneumoniae* meningitis as they decrease inflammation, brain edema, and subsequent herniation caused by the robust immune response.
• Complications of meningitis include hydrocephalus, CN VIII palsy, and herniation.
• Less common causes of viral encephalitis include arbovirus, varicella zoster virus, West Nile, measles, coxsackie, and mumps.

Causes of meningitis based on age and risk factors:
• 0–3 months old: group B strep, *Escherichia coli*, listeria
• 3 months–18 years old: *Neisseria meningitidis, Streptococcus pneumonia, Haemophilus influenzae*
• 18–50 years old: *S. pneumonia, N. meningitidis, H influenza*
• >50 years old: *S. pneumonia, N. meningitidis, H. influenza*, listeria
• Recent immigrant: tuberculosis
• Human immunodeficiency virus: Cryptococcus

TABLE 2-12 Lumbar Puncture Cerebrospinal Fluid Analysis

	CELLS	GLUCOSE	PROTEIN	OPENING PRESSURE
Bacterial	Polymorphonuclear cells	Decreased	Increased	Increased
Viral	Lymphocytes	Normal	Normal	Normal
Tuberculosis	Lymphocytes	Decreased	Increased	Increased

Other common CNS infections have unique clinical presentations, risk factors, and management (Table 2-13).

TABLE 2-13   Other Central Nervous Sysytem Infections

DISEASE (INFECTIOUS ORGANISM)	RISK FACTORS	SIGNS AND SYMPTOMS	DIAGNOSTICS	MANAGEMENT
Leprosy (*Mycobacterium leprae*)	• Recent immigrant from Africa, South America, or Asia • Armadillo exposure in United States • Transmission via respiratory droplets	• Loss of sensation in extremities due to invasion of peripheral nerves (organism prefers cooler environment) • Leonine facies • Hairless skin • Symptoms occur secondary to robust immune response against the organism	• Clinical and biopsy—acid-fast bacillus	• Dapsone, rifampin, +/- clofazimine (used in more extensive lepromatous form)
Epidural abscess (*Staphylococcus aureus*)	• Intravenous drug abuse • Hematogenous spread • Recent neurosurgery (laminectomy) or intervention (lumbar puncture, epidural anesthesia) • Vertebral osteomyelitis	• Back pain with point tenderness to palpation • Fever • Acute neurologic deficits (motor and sensory deficits, bladder, and bowel dysfunction)	• Magnetic resonance imaging (MRI)	• Abscess drainage and surgical decompression to prevent complications of cord compression or cauda equina syndrome • Antistaphylococcus antibiotics (oxacillin, dicloxacillin, nafcillin) • MRSA coverage (vancomycin or linezolid) • Steroids for acute neurologic deficits
Botulism (*Clostridium botulinum*)	• Unpasteurized honey in newborns • Canned foods (creates environments that is ideal for spore germination) • Aged seafood • Wound contamination • All risk factors are associated with ingestion of preformed toxin	• Initial symptoms are gastrointestinal related • Dilated pupils and other cranial neuropathies • Symmetric, descending flaccid paralysis • Repetitive nerve stimulation shows incremental increase in muscle contraction on electromyography • Pathophysiology: inability to release acetylcholine from the presynaptic terminal	• Serology or stool for presence of neurotoxin	• Supportive care and horse-derived antitoxin • Clean wound and administer penicillin
Lyme disease (*Borrelia burgdorferi*)	• Camping and outdoors in northeastern United States • Other locations include Midwest and West Coast • Transmitted by Ixodes tick (same tick also transmits babesiosis)	• Neurologic: cranial nerve neuropathies (commonly occurs bilaterally involving CN VII), aseptic meningitis, encephalitis, radiculopathy, transverse myelitis • Dermatologic: targetoid rash with area of central clearing (bull's-eye; erythema migrans) • Rheumatologic: chronic migrating polyarthritis • Cardiac: atrioventricular block, myocarditis, arrhythmias, pericarditis	• Clinical if classic targetoid rash with central clearing is identified • Serology, ELISA, Western blot, polymerase chain reaction (PCR) • Lumbar puncture	• Doxycycline • Amoxicillin: children <8yr old, pregnant women • Intravenous ceftriaxone: cardiac and neurologic manifestations

TABLE 2-13   Other Central Nervous Sysytem Infections

DISEASE (INFECTIOUS ORGANISM)	RISK FACTORS	SIGNS AND SYMPTOMS	DIAGNOSTICS	MANAGEMENT
Neurosyphilis (*Treponema pallidum*)	• Unprotected sex	• Primary syphilis: painless genital ulcer and adenopathy • Secondary syphilis: rash involving palms and soles, alopecia areata • Tertiary syphilis: neurosyphilis, tabes dorsalis, meningitis, vasculitis, Argyll Robertson pupils • Cardiac manifestations (part of tertiary syphilis): aortic regurgitation, thoracic aortic aneurysm • Gummas	• Sensitive: VDRL, RPR (maybe negative in early primary syphilis) • Specific: FTA-ABS	• Intramuscular penicillin for primary and secondary syphilis; oral doxycycline for penicillin-allergic patients • Intravenous penicillin for tertiary syphilis • Desensitization for penicillin-allergic tertiary syphilis and pregnant women • Jarisch Herxheimer reaction: fevers, chills, joint pain due to the release of inflammatory and antigenic components caused by the death of syphilis during treatment
Rabies (rhabdovirus)	• Animal bite: dog (most common in developing countries), raccoon, bats	• Long incubation period • Nonspecific: fever, chills, malaise, headache • Hydrophobia, laryngospasm, encephalitis, hyperactivity, coma, and death	• PCR from saliva • Antibodies • Autopsy: Negri bodies	• Determine if postexposure prophylaxis (PEP) is necessary: initiate only if bitten by high-risk wild animal or pet that is unavailable for quarantine • If pet is available for quarantine, observe for 10 days for signs of rabies • PEP: thoroughly clean the wound, 4 doses of rabies vaccine at days 0, 3, 7 and 14; human rabies immunoglobulin
Neurocysticercosis (*Taenia solium*)	• Ingestion of undercooked pork • Contaminated water • Pig farmers • Immigrants from Mexico or South America	• Chronic headache, vomiting • Papilledema • Seizures	• MRI: enhancing and nonenhancing calcified lesions in the brain with edema, Swiss-cheese appearance, hydrocephalus	• Albendazole +/- steroids • Antiepileptics in cases of seizure
Prion	• Cannibalism (kuru) • Family history and familial forms • Ingestion of beef (mad cow disease) • Most case are sporadic; however, some are hereditary or iatrogenic (contaminated transplant and surgical instruments)	• Rapidly progressive dementia, personality changes, startle myoclonus • Extrapyramidal symptoms (dystonia, rigidity, chorea, athetosis) • Pathophysiology: misfolded protein induces misfolding of other proteins into beta pleated sheets	• Cerebrospinal fluid: elevated 14-3-3 protein • Electroencephalogram: biphasic and triphasic spike wave complexes • MRI: cortical ribbon sign (also seen in anoxic injury); however, imaging is mostly normal • Genetic testing: prion protein gene (PRNP) • Biopsy: spongiform encephalopathy	• No cure available, only symptomatic • Death within 1yr of symptoms

ELISA, Enzyme-linke immunosorbent assay; *FTA-ABS*, fluorescent treponemal antibody absorption; *MRSA*, methicillin-resistant *Staphylococcus aureus*; *RPR*, rapid plasma reagin; *VDRL*, Venereal Disease Research Laboratory.

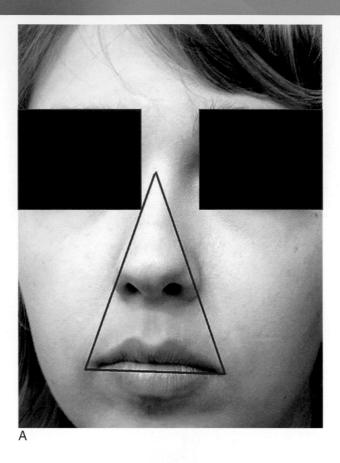

A

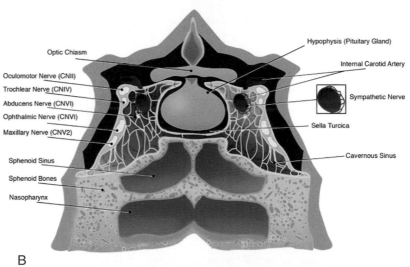

B

Figure 2-21: Cavernous sinus is a common site for spread of infection involving (A) the danger triangle of the face and sinuses. (B) Spread of infection may result in inflammation and thrombosis of the cavernous sinus with associated cranial nerve palsies (III, IV, V1, V2, VI). (Images courtesy of Kuybu O, Dossani RH; CC BY-SA [https://creativecommons.org/licenses/by-sa/3.0])

Many CNS infections originate extracranially such as infections involving the danger triangle, which have the potential to spread into the cavernous sinus (Fig. 2-21).

XVI. **Brain Tumors**
   A. Key principles of brain tumors
      1. Signs and symptoms
         a. Chronic worsening headache that wakes patient up at night
         b. Vomiting
         c. Visual disturbances
         d. Seizures, papilledema

TABLE 2-14   Types of Brain Tumors

TYPE OF MALIGNANCY	LOCATION	KEY FEATURES
Astrocytoma	Cerebral hemisphere (glioblastoma multiforme)	Glioblastoma multiforme: • Crosses corpus callosum ("butterfly" lesion) • GFAP positive Graded from 1–4 based on WHO classification: • Grade I: pilocytic astrocytoma • Grade II: low-grade astrocytoma • Grade III: anaplastic astrocytoma • Grade IV: glioblastoma multiforme
Oligodendroglioma	Frontal lobe	• Present as calcification on imaging • Tumor of cells that myelinate neurons in the central nervous system
Ependymomata	Cauda equina	• Overgrowth of cells lining the ventricles results in signs and symptoms of obstructive hydrocephalus • Common cause of spinal cancer resulting in extramedullary spinal compression
Meningioma	Dural reflection of cerebral hemisphere and parasagittal region	• Tumor that arises from arachnoid cells • Often have dural attachment ("dural tail"), which connects the tumor to the meninges • Benign, slow-growing lesion that tends to recur after excision • Symptoms related to compression of the cortex • Commonly seen in women
Schwannoma	Cerebellopontine angle	• Peripheral nerve sheath tumor • Associated with neurofibromatosis type II: will have bilateral CN VIII schwannomas
Pituitary adenoma	Sella turcica	• Bitemporal hemianopia due to compression of the optic chiasm • Endocrine dysfunction: hyperprolactinemia, hypopituitarism

GFAP, Glial fibrillary acidic protein; WHO, World Health Organization.

    e. Altered mental status
    f. Gait disturbances
    g. More specific signs and symptoms related to location of the tumor
  2. Risk factors
    a. Family history
    b. Li-Fraumeni
    c. Neurofibromatosis
    d. Ionizing radiation
    e. Presence of primary malignancy (lung, renal, breast, melanoma) as metastasis is the most common cause of brain malignancy
      • Metastases can be nonhemorrhagic, hemorrhagic, dural, epidural, or meningeal
      • Present as well-circumscribed masses along the grey-white junction
  3. Location: supratentorial in adults, infratentorial in children (Table 2-14)
  4. Diagnostics: neuroimaging (CT or MRI) and biopsy
  5. Management: depends on stage and location +/− chemoradiation
    a. Low grade: surgical resection with serial imaging
    b. High grade or unresectable: chemoradiation
  6. Prognosis: depends on type of malignancy
    a. Glioblastoma has the worst prognosis
    b. Pilocytic astrocytoma has the best prognosis
XVII. **Sleep**
  A. Definitions
    1. Alterations in sleep physiology (Table 2-15) secondary to lack of sleep, drugs, or alterations in neurotransmitters result in abnormalities in sleep and/or REM latency
    2. REM latency: defined as the time it takes to fall asleep and enter REM sleep; normally takes 90 minutes, but is shorter in depression and narcolepsy
    3. Sleep latency: defined as the time it takes to fall asleep; normally takes 15 minutes, but is longer in insomnia and shorter in narcolepsy
  B. Insomnia
    1. Definition
      a. Inability to initiate or stay asleep resulting in significant social or occupational impairment

TABLE 2-15   Sleep Physiology

STAGES OF SLEEP	FEATURES	WAVEFORM PATTERNS ON ELECTROENCEPHALOGRAPHY
Awake	• Alert, active state	Beta waves: low voltage, high frequency
Drowsy	• Similar state of mind seen in meditation	Alpha waves
Stage I	• Light sleep	Fast theta waves
Stage II	• Intermediate sleep • Most of sleep is spent in stage II (40–50%) • Increased by use of benzodiazepines • Associated pathology: bruxism	Sleep spindles and K complexes Image courtesy of Stage2sleep.svg: User:Neocadre.Jjustam at en.wikipediaderivative work: Neocadre [Public domain]
Stage III	• Deep sleep • Decreased in the elderly resulting in feeling less refreshed after a night sleep • Decreased by use of benzodiazepines • Associated pathology: nocturnal enuresis, night terrors, sleepwalking	Slow delta waves Images courtesy of MrSandman at English Wikipedia [Public domain]
Rapid eye movement	• Occurs every 90–120 min • "Brain is awake, body asleep." In other stages of sleep the "brain is asleep, body is awake." • Predominates in the second half of the night • Dreams are present during this stage of sleep • Associated pathology: narcolepsy, dream enactment	Similar waveform pattern as being in the awake state: low-voltage, high-frequency sawtooth waves

b. Patients also note early-morning awakenings and nonrestorative sleep
c. Can be acute (jet lag, before an important exam or job interview) or chronic (psychiatric or medical disorder)
d. Most cases of insomnia are secondary to underlying pathology
e. Primary insomnia makes up only 10% of cases
2. Causes
a. Psychiatric disorders
- Major depressive disorder
- Anxiety
- Fibromyalgia
- Chronic fatigue syndrome
b. Medications
- Stimulants
- Atypical antidepressants (tricyclic antidepressants [TCAs], bupropion)
- Beta blockers
- Withdrawal from sedative drugs
c. Medical disorders
- Hyperthyroidism
- CNS pathology
- Chronic obstructive pulmonary disease
- Congestive heart failure (CHF)
- Renal failure
d. Diagnostics
- Clinical after ruling out reversible causes of insomnia; primary insomnia is a diagnosis of exclusion
- Insomnia disorder requires insomnia for >3 nights/week for three months
e. Management: first-line treatment is behavior modification targeted at improving sleep hygiene
- Dark room with no lights, television, clocks, or computers
- Dissociate bedroom, all activities except for sleeping—avoid eating, working, or watching television in the bed
- Avoid daytime naps
- Maintain regular sleep schedule
- Ensure optimal sleeping environment with comfortable clothes and room temperature
- Avoid eating large meals, caffeine, alcohol, and stimulating activities (exercise) before sleep
- Address maladaptive thoughts regarding sleep and expectations ("I must have 8 hours of sleep")
- Pharmacologic treatment should be limited to short-term use (Table 2-16)
C. Narcolepsy
1. Definition: REM-related sleep disorder resulting in decreased REM latency and extension of REM sleep physiology into the awake state

TABLE 2-16 **Sleeping Aids**

FEATURES	EFFECT ON SLEEP AND ADVERSE EFFECTS
Benzodiazepines	- Increases stage II sleep, decreases stage III and rapid eye movement sleep - Similar effect on sleep physiology as alcohol and barbiturates - Avoid in elderly due to fall risk and paradoxic benzodiazepine effect - Risk of dependence and respiratory depression
Ramelteon	- Melatonin agonist - Nonaddictive; safer in the elderly
Antihistamines	- Decreases onset to sleep - Does not simulate normal sleep physiology - Easy access for patients due to being over the counter - Avoid in elderly due to anticholinergic side effects
Nonbenzodiazepine hypnotics (zolpidem, zaleplon, eszopiclone)	- Primarily used for insomnia - Decreased dependence risk compared to benzodiazepines
Sedating antidepressants (tricyclic antidepressants [TCAs], trazodone)	- Require high doses compared to antidepressant effect - Trazodone can cause priapism; TCAs can result in anticholinergic effects

2. Epidemiology
   a. Onset occurs during adolescence and early adulthood
   b. Increased incidence in families
3. Pathophysiology: decreased hypocretin (orexin) production from the lateral hypothalamus
4. Signs and symptoms
   a. Excessive daytime sleepiness
   b. Cataplexy: sudden loss of muscle tone following stimulus (laughter, stress, loud sounds, flashing lights)
   c. Hypnogogic hallucinations: visual or auditory hallucinations before sleep
   d. Hypnopompic hallucinations: visual or auditory hallucinations before awakening
   e. Sleep paralysis: inability to move upon awakening due to extended REM sleep (brain is awake, but body is asleep)
   f. Vivid dreams
5. Diagnostics
   a. Daytime multiple sleep latency test
      • Test that measures the amount of time to onset of sleep during five 20-minute daytime napping episodes
      • Shortened sleep latency (<8 minutes to fall asleep) and at least two REM episodes during the five naps
      • Symptoms must be present for >3 months
   b. Overnight polysomnography: usually normal, but may reveal sleep fragmentation
6. Management: behavioral modification plus pharmacologic
   a. Behavior modification
      • Maintain good sleep hygiene
      • Scheduled naps: helps prevent sleep attacks
      • Sufficient sleep duration
   b. Pharmacologic
      • Modafinil (dopamine agonist), armodafinil: first line
      • Other stimulants
         ▪ Amphetamines
         ▪ Methylphenidate
         ▪ Pemoline
      • Cataplexy prophylaxis: TCAs, sodium oxybate

D. Obstructive sleep apnea (OSA)
   1. Definition: periodic episodes of hypopnea (decreased airflow by >50% associated with arousal or >4% desaturation) or apnea (cessation of airflow >10 seconds) that occur when patient is sleeping
   2. Risk factors
      a. Age: airways become increasingly floppy and easily collapse when lying down
      b. Obese
      c. Middle-aged males
      d. Family history
   3. Pathophysiology: obstruction of the upper airway (usually at the level of the oropharynx) during sleep due to thick neck, enlarged adenoids, and other anatomic abnormalities (short mandible, excessive soft tissue, deviated septum) (Fig. 2-22)
   4. Signs and symptoms
      a. Daytime sleepiness: secondary to multiple nighttime awakenings that may or may not be apparent to the patient
      b. Nonrestorative sleep
      c. Morning headache: secondary to mild respiratory acidosis (will have compensatory metabolic alkalosis)
      d. Hypertension: systemic (release of catecholamines) and pulmonary hypertension (chronic hypoxia)
      e. Thick neck
      f. Loud snoring
      g. Nighttime awakenings: secondary to hypoxia
      h. Cognitive dysfunction: memory impairment, difficulty concentrating
      i. Erectile dysfunction
   5. Diagnostics
      a. Polysomnography
         • Airflow cessation despite continued respiratory effort

- During episodes of hypoxemia there will be muscle retraction as patient is trying to wake up
        b. Apnea-hypopnea index: number of episodes of apnea and hypopnea per hour
            - Diagnosis of OSA requires at least five episodes per hour
            - Severe OSA characterized by >30 episodes per hour
    6. Management
        a. Weight loss
        b. Continuous positive airway pressure (CPAP): keeps airway open using forceful positive pressure
        c. Sleep in nonsupine position
        d. Avoidance of sedatives (alcohol, benzodiazepines)
        e. Surgical: uvulopalatopharyngoplasty (surgical widening of the airway by removing redundant soft tissue)
        f. Oral appliances: helps avoid tongue obstruction
    7. Complications
        a. Polycythemia: release of erythropoietin due to chronic hypoxia
        b. Cardiac arrhythmias, sudden cardiac death, CHF
        c. Pulmonary hypertension: chronic pulmonary vascular vasoconstriction secondary to hypoxia
        d. Insulin resistance
E. Central sleep apnea
    1. Definition: neurologic disorder localized to the brainstem (stroke, genetics, drugs) resulting in irregular respiratory efforts (Fig. 2-23)
        a. Rather than breathing at a constant 12–20 breaths per minute patient will have decreased respiratory rate occurring at irregular intervals
        b. Lack of respiration results in decreased oxygen saturation providing stimulus to breathe
    2. Management: targeted at increasing respiratory rate and maintaining oxygen saturation
        a. CPAP or supplemental oxygen
        b. Acetazolamide: induces metabolic acidosis with compensatory respiratory alkalosis
        c. Avoidance of sedatives

Other causes of sleep apnea include Prader-Willi syndrome, acromegaly, and amyotrophic lateral sclerosis.

F. Other causes of sleep apnea include Prader-Willi syndrome, acromegaly, and amyotrophic lateral sclerosis.
G. Other sleep-related disorders/circadian rhythm disorders
    1. Delayed sleep phase syndrome
        a. Circadian rhythm disorder, which results in sleep onset insomnia and excessive early-morning sleepiness

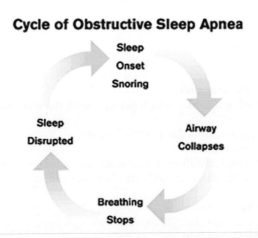

Cycle of Obstructive Sleep Apnea

Sleep
Onset
Snoring

Airway
Collapses

Breathing
Stops

Sleep
Disrupted

Figure 2-22: The cycles of obstructive sleep apnea. Initiation of continuous positive airway pressure prevents airway collapse through positive pressure and prevents breathing cessation and sleep disruption. (Image courtesy of Timt775.)

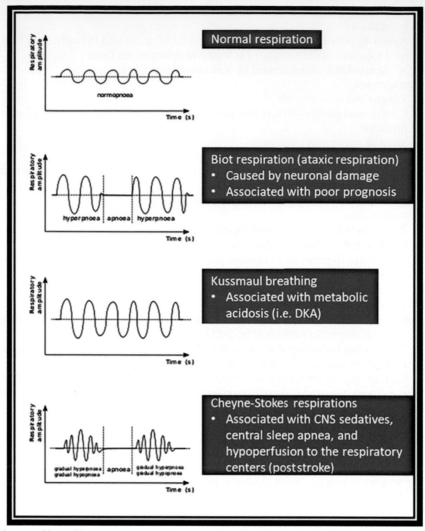

Figure 2-23: Abnormal breathing patterns and their associated conditions. *CNS,* Central nervous system; *DKA,* diabetic ketoacidosis. (Modified Image courtesy of Sav vas; CC BY-SA [https://creativecommons.org/licenses/by-sa/3.0])

    b. Commonly referred to as "night owls"
    c. Able to achieve restorative sleep if patient can set own schedule
    d. Treatment involves light or behavioral therapy

Lamotrigine is also used in bipolar depression and seizures.

  2. Advanced sleep phase disorder
    a. Circadian rhythm disorder, which presents with the inability to stay awake in the evening
    b. Early-morning insomnia due to early bedtime
  3. Shift work sleep disorder
    a. Sleep disorder due to shift work that is incompatible with a normal circadian rhythm
    b. Patients have difficulty initiating, maintaining sleep, and daytime sleepiness
XVIII. Miscellaneous
  A. Trigeminal neuralgia
    1. Causes
      a. Idiopathic: most common
      b. Multiple sclerosis (may present bilaterally)
      c. Dilation or aneurysm of the superior cerebellar artery, cerebellopontine angle tumor: results in compression of the trigeminal nerve

2. Signs and symptoms
   a. Extremely painful electrical shocklike pains with light touch (brushing teeth, combing hair, wind)
   b. Recurrent painful episodes last seconds to minutes
   c. Normal neurologic exam
3. Diagnostics
   a. Clinical
   b. Neuroimaging to rule out structural causes such as tumor of the cerebellopontine angle and multiple sclerosis
4. Management: most cases resolve spontaneously
   a. Pharmacologic
      • Carbamazepine
      • Oxcarbazepine
      • Baclofen: GABA agonist also used as muscle relaxant
      • Lamotrigine
   b. Surgical: after failure of pharmacologic therapy
      • Surgical gangliolysis
      • Suboccipital craniectomy: decompression of the trigeminal nerve
      • Gamma knife surgery

B. Restless leg syndrome

Carbamazepine is also used for bipolar disorder and seizures. Side effects include blood dyscrasias, Stevens-Johnson syndrome, and neural tube defects.

1. Epidemiology: affects 5%–15% of adults
2. Cause: no known etiology; however, associated with many conditions
3. Associations
   a. Iron deficiency anemia
   b. Chronic kidney disease (uremia)
   c. Diabetes mellitus
   d. MS, essential tremor, Parkinson disease
   e. Pregnancy
   f. Drugs (antidepressants, dopamine antagonists)
4. Signs and symptoms
   a. Uncomfortable crawling, tingling, pulling sensation of the lower extremities
   b. Occurs primarily at night or at sleep onset
   c. Relieved by moving legs
   d. Worse in the evening or at rest
   e. Insomnia
5. Diagnostics: clinical
6. Management: nonpharmacologic plus treatment of associated condition
   a. Nonpharmacologic
      • Supportive management: leg massage, heating pads
      • Behavioral changes
        ▪ Avoid aggravating factors such as lack of sleep and drugs
        ▪ Distracting activities during periods of rest
        ▪ Exercise
        ▪ Decreased caffeine intake
7. Pharmacologic: both classes are equally effective, therefore choose drug based on side effect profile and other comorbidities
   a. Dopamine agonists (pramipexole, ropinirole)
   b. Alpha-2 delta calcium channel ligands (gabapentin, pregabalin)

Head, Eyes, Ears, Nose, and Throat

HEAD

Sinusitis

– Pathophysiology: upper respiratory infection (URI) → inflammation, edema, and blockage of nasal passages → impaired clearance of bacteria
– Causes
  • Viruses: most common
  • Bacterial (*Streptococcus pneumonia, Haemophilus influenzae, Moraxella*)
  • Nasal blockage
    ▪ Nasal polyps
    ▪ Foreign body
    ▪ Wegener granulomatosis
  • Nasal irritation (allergies, cigarette smoke)
  • Genetic syndromes (primary ciliary dyskinesia, cystic fibrosis)
  • Immunodeficiencies
– Signs and symptoms
  • Fever
  • Cough
  • Rhinorrhea
  • Decreased transillumination
  • Facial tenderness
– Diagnostics
  • Clinical
  • Computed tomography (CT) scan
    ▪ If presentation is unclear or to look for anatomic abnormalities causing recurrent sinusitis
    ▪ Mucosal thickening, opacification, air fluid levels
  • Biopsy/aspiration for recurrent sinusitis or nonresponsive to multiple antibiotics
– Management
  • Initially symptomatic treatment only
  • Indications for antibiotics (amoxicillin-clavulanate)
    ▪ Persistent symptoms lasting >10 days
    ▪ Worsening symptoms
    ▪ Severe fever (>102 °F)
    ▪ Copious purulent rhinorrhea
  • ENT referral for anatomic abnormality
– Complications
  • Meningitis, brain abscess
  • Cavernous sinus thrombosis: contiguous spread through the bone or venous channels
  • Orbital cellulitis: most commonly from ethmoid sinusitis
  • Osteomyelitis of facial bones

Maxillary sinus is most commonly affected in sinusitis. *Staphylococcus aureus* is seen in cases of chronic sinusitis. *Pseudomonas* is seen in cases of nosocomial sinusitis.

Sinus development (from earliest to latest): maxillary and ethmoid sinus are present at birth, sphenoid at age five, frontal begins development at age eight and continues into adolescence.

Cervicofacial Actinomyces
- Risk factors
  - Dental infection/extraction
  - Immunosuppression
  - Diabetes mellitus
- Signs and symptoms
  - Enlarging nontender indurated mass of the mandible
  - Draining sinus tracts connecting to the skin
  - Yellow sulfur granules
- Diagnostics
  - Fine-needle aspiration
  - Culture: branching filamentous nonacid-fast gram-positive rods
- Management
  - Long-term penicillin
  - Surgery in severe cases

Head and Neck Cancer
- Risk factors
  - Smoking, alcohol
  - Radiation
  - Betel nut chewing
  - Viral infection
    - Human papillomavirus (oropharyngeal carcinoma)
    - Ebstein-Barr virus (EBV) (nasopharyngeal carcinoma)
  - Immunodeficiency (human immunodeficiency virus [HIV], solid organ transplant)
- Types: five anatomic locations; most commonly squamous cell carcinoma
  - Oral cavity
  - Pharynx
  - Larynx
  - Nasal cavity
  - Salivary glands
- Signs and symptoms
  - Asymptomatic: results in late detection and poor prognosis
  - Nontender cervical/submandibular lymphadenopathy
  - Weight loss
  - Dysphasia
  - Neck mass
  - Hoarseness
  - Leukoplakia, erythroplakia
- Diagnostics
  - Panendoscopy (laryngoscopy, bronchoscopy, esophagoscopy) and biopsy
  - CT/magnetic resonance imaging (MRI)/positron-emission tomography scan for staging
- Management: surgery +/− chemoradiation

EYES
Infection and Inflammation
Basic anatomic structures (Fig. 3-1) of the eye are important to note as they may be involved in inflammatory or infectious pathologies such as the iris, ciliary body, retina, optic nerve, and sclera. The cornea, lens, and choroid are often involved in traumatic circumstances. The anterior and posterior cavities are key in understanding glaucoma.

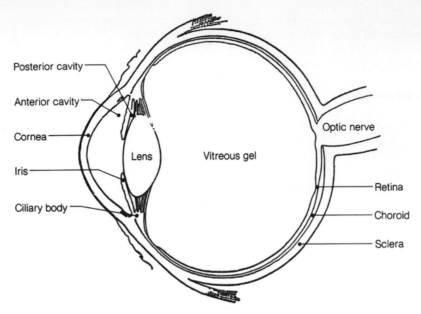

Figure 3-1: Eye anatomy, sagittal section (Image courtesy of the National Cancer Institute.)

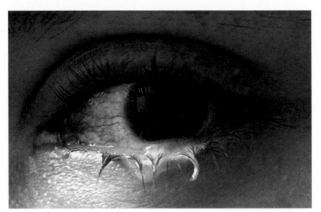

Figure 3-2: Bacterial conjunctivitis showing purulent discharge and conjunctival erythema. (Image courtesy of CNX OpenStax.)

Conjunctivitis can be caused by bacteria (Fig. 3-2), viruses, or allergies. These are often diagnosed clinically and treated based on the most likely causative etiology, patient risk factors, and epidemiology (Table 3-1).

Uveitis
– Definition: inflammation of the iris, ciliary body, and choroid
– Causes
  • Idiopathic: most common cause
  • Systemic inflammatory diseases
  • Sympathetic ophthalmia (autoimmune uveitis)
  • Collagen vascular disease (systemic lupus erythematosus, rheumatoid arthritis, scleroderma, polyarteritis nodosa, dermatomyositis, Behcet)
  • Seronegative spondyloarthropathies
  • Infections (tuberculosis, Lyme disease, cytomegalovirus [CMV], Toxoplasma, syphilis)
– Signs and symptoms
  • Pain (absent with posterior uveitis)
  • Erythema
  • Photophobia
  • Abnormal pupillary response due to involvement of iris and ciliary body
  • Hypopyon
  • Synechiae: adhesions of the iris to the lens
  • Iris nodules
  • Keratic precipitates (mutton fat)

TABLE 3-1   Types of Conjunctivitis

	BACTERIAL	VIRAL	ALLERGIC
Causes	Poor contact lens hygiene: *Staphylococcus* or *Streptococcus* Sexually active or newborns of infected mothers: *Chlamydia* or *Gonococcal*	Preceding upper respiratory tract infection Most common cause is adenovirus Other less common viruses include varicella zoster virus (VZV) and herpes simplex virus (HSV)	Atopy, eczema
Signs and symptoms	Unilateral purulent discharge causing eyelids to be stuck together upon waking up Less itching compared to viral conjunctivitis May have preauricular adenopathy Chlamydia conjunctivitis is the most common cause of blindness worldwide	Starts initially in one eye and spreads to the contralateral eye Watery discharge Itchy and erythematous Herpes zoster ophthalmicus: shingles of cranial nerve V with associated fever and papular rash	Bilateral erythematous, itchy eyes Little to no discharge May present with other atopic symptoms such as allergic rhinitis and asthma
Diagnostics	Clinical		
Treatment	Saline lavage if *Staphylococcus* or *Streptococcus* is suspected +/− fluoroquinolones ophthalmic antibiotics If gonorrhea or chlamydia suspected: azithromycin (or doxycycline) plus ceftriaxone	Supportive management as most cases are self-limited If the VZV or HSV is suspected: acyclovir	Avoidance of allergen Symptomatic management with topical antihistamine (levocabastine, emedastine) and topical nonsteroidal antiinflammatory drugs (ketorolac)

For all cases of conjunctivitis there is normal pupillary reaction, intraocular pressure, and no impairment of visual acuity.

- Diagnostics: slit-lamp examination
- Management
  - Steroids
  - Pain control in cases of anterior uveitis (cyclopentolate, tropicamide, atropine)
    - Mydriatic component of these drugs dilates the pupils and breaks the synechiae providing pain relief
  - Treatment of the underlying disease

Preseptal/Orbital Cellulitis
- Microbiology: URI organisms
  - *S. pneumonia*
  - *H. influenzae*
  - *Neisseria meningitidis*
  - *Staphylococcus aureus*
- Pathophysiology
  - Infection of the orbital septum differentiates preseptal from orbital cellulitis
  - Infection anterior to orbital septum is preseptal cellulitis; infection posterior to orbital septum is orbital cellulitis
  - Often preceded by URI, sinusitis, dacryocystitis, blepharitis, or dental infection
  - Less commonly hematogenous spread
- Signs and symptoms
  - Unilateral tenderness, edema, and erythema around the orbit (Fig. 3-3)
  - Conjunctival injection
  - Ophthalmoplegia, pain with extraocular movements, proptosis, and visual deficits
    - These symptoms are only present in orbital cellulitis indicating spread of infection posterior to the orbital septum
- Diagnostics: clinical
  - Normal ocular exam is suggestive of preseptal cellulitis
  - Limited or abnormal ocular exam is suggestive of orbital cellulitis
  - Can be confirmed with orbital CT
- Management
  - Preseptal cellulitis: oral antibiotics targeting upper respiratory organisms
    - Clindamycin
    - TMP-SMX plus amoxicillin-clavulanate

- Orbital cellulitis: broad-spectrum IV antibiotics (vancomycin plus piperacillin-tazobactam) as this is a medical emergency
- Complications
  - Blindness
  - Meningitis
  - Cavernous sinus thrombosis
  - Brain or subperiosteal abscess

Keratitis is defined as inflammation of the cornea with a wide range of ideologies, including bacterial, viral, fungal, and ultraviolet (UV) related. Regardless of etiology, they have similar signs and symptoms and are differentiated based on their fluorescein staining pattern (Table 3-2).

Scleritis/Episcleritis
- Definition: inflammatory disease of the sclera (scleritis) or outer sclera (episcleritis)
- Signs and symptoms

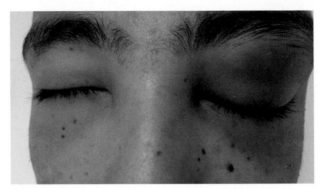

Figure 3-3: Patient with left preseptal orbital cellulitis.

TABLE 3-2   Types of Keratitis

	BACTERIAL	VIRAL	FUNGAL	PHOTOKERATITIS
Causes	• *Pseudomonas, Staphylococcus, Streptococcus* • Most common cause of keratitis • Seen in frequent contact lens users	• Herpes simplex virus • Most common cause of corneal blindness in the United States	• *Candida, Aspergillus, Fusarium* • Risk factors: immunodeficiency, topical steroids	• Exposure to ultraviolet (UV) radiation • Risk factors: snow sports, tanning beds, welders • Snow reflects 80% of UV radiation resulting in significant UV exposure in skiers and snowboarders who do not wear sunglasses
Signs and symptoms	Eye pain, photophobia Discharge, blurry vision Erythema, hypopyon Foreign body sensation			
Diagnostics	Fluorescein staining showing denudement of the squamous epithelium with different patterns for different etiologies: Bacterial: abrasion or ulcer Viral: lesions formed in a dendritic pattern Interstitial: no defect present on staining as squamous epithelium remains intact Fungal: poorly delineated borders of the ulcer Photokeratitis: superficial punctate			
Management	Ophthalmic moxifloxacin or cefazolin plus tobramycin	Often self-limited; however, treatment reduces duration of symptoms Oral: acyclovir, ganciclovir Ophthalmic eyedrops: trifluridine, vidarabine	Ophthalmic natamycin or voriconazole Oral amphotericin B or voriconazole in severe cases	Oral nonsteroidal antiinflammatory drugs and other analgesics Topical antibiotic ointments may be helpful: erythromycin, bacitracin Patient education on the importance of using eye protection against UV radiation

- Mild to moderate eye pain, erythema, watery discharge
- Symptoms tend to be more severe in scleritis with photophobia and decreased visual acuity
- Associations
  - Rheumatoid arthritis
  - Inflammatory bowel disease
- Diagnostics: infusion of epinephrine into the affected eye
  - In episcleritis, the epinephrine will cause vasoconstriction and the blanching of the eye causing it to appear more white
  - In scleritis, there will be no response to epinephrine infusion
- Management: symptomatic
  - Most cases are self-limiting and can be managed with nonsteroidal antiinflammatory drugs (NSAIDs)
  - Corticosteroids, immunosuppressive in severe cases of scleritis

Sympathetic Ophthalmia
- Definition: granulomatous uveitis that occurs secondary to trauma in the contralateral eye
- Pathophysiology
  - Antigens in the eye are normally protected from the immune system
  - Trauma to the contralateral eye results in exposure to hidden ocular antigens into the systemic circulation and formation of an autoimmune response
  - Formation of autoantibodies results in cell-mediated damage to the contralateral eye
- Signs and symptoms
  - Anterior uveitis
  - Papilledema
  - Blindness
- Diagnostics: clinical
- Management: corticosteroids and/or immunomodulators

Elderly Eyes
Cataracts
- Risk factors
  - Elderly, diabetic
  - Smoking
  - UV exposure
- Associations: commonly a disease of the elderly, however, may be a manifestation of other diseases
  - Prematurity: disappears within a few weeks
  - Late manifestation of electrical burns
  - Congenital: TORCH infection (rubella, varicella), chromosomal abnormalities
  - Systemic disease
    - Galactosemia (bilateral)
    - Myotonic dystrophy
    - Wilson disease
  - Drugs: steroids, quetiapine
- Pathophysiology: oxidative damage of the lens resulting in opacification
- Signs and symptoms
  - Painless blurry vision, often bilateral (one eye may initially be affected before the other) (Figs. 3-4 and 3-5)
  - Glares and halos associated with nighttime driving
  - Loss of red reflex late in disease
  - Second sight phenomenon: improvement of presbyopia due to myopic shift, which increases the convergence power of the lens (patients will note they no longer require their reading glasses)
- Diagnostics: slit-lamp examination
- Management: surgical lens extraction and implantation of artificial lens

Age-Related Macular Degeneration (ARMD)
- Epidemiology: most common cause of blindness in the elderly
- Risk factors
  - Age (60+)
  - Smoking
  - UV exposure
- Pathophysiology: atrophy and degeneration of the outer retina and retinal pigment epithelium
- Types
  - Atrophic/nonexudative ("dry"): accounts for 90% of cases
  - Exudative ("wet")

Eye with Cataract

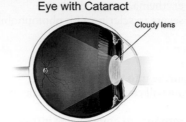

Cloudy lens, or cataract, causes blurry vision

Figure 3-4: Illustration of patient with cataracts. (Image courtesy of Bruce Blaus.)

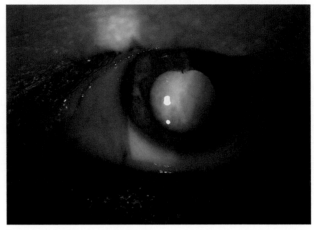

Figure 3-5: Patient with advanced cataracts showing presence of cloudy lens. (Image courtesy of Levai Lehar.)

- Signs and symptoms
  - Chronic central vision loss with preservation of peripheral vision
    - Acute onset seen in exudative type due to neovascularization
  - Drusen deposits: accumulation of yellow granular cholesterol exudates
    - Common finding seen in the eyes of the elderly, even those without ARMD
  - Scotoma
  - Retinal detachment (seen more commonly in wet-type macular degeneration)
    - Abnormal blood vessel growth in the subretinal space resulting in accumulation of fluid and retinal detachment
  - Metamorphopsia: straight lines appear curvy
- Diagnostics
  - Dilated eye exam
    - Atrophic: drusens in the macular region
    - Exudative: neovascularization
  - Amsler grid: grid with horizontal and vertical lines, which patient will perceive as curvy (Figs. 3-6 and 3-7)
  - Fluorescein angiography for exudative type
- Management
  - Atrophic: no effective treatment
    - Lifestyle modifications to compensate for decreased visual acuity (color-coded pill bottles, talking glucometer, magnification devices, well-lit environment)
  - Exudative
    - VEGF inhibitors (bevacizumab, ranibizumab, pegaptanib, zivaflibercept) to inhibit angiogenesis
    - Antioxidants (vitamins C and E), zinc, copper, beta-carotene
    - Laser photocoagulation

Macula: central portion of the eye that contains cone cells and involved in fine visual acuity. Therefore, some of the activities to be first affected in ARMD are driving and reading.

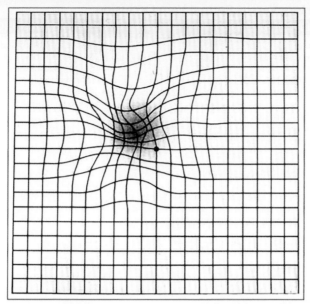

Figure 3-6: Amsler grid in patient with age-related macular degeneration. (Image courtesy of National Eye Institute.)

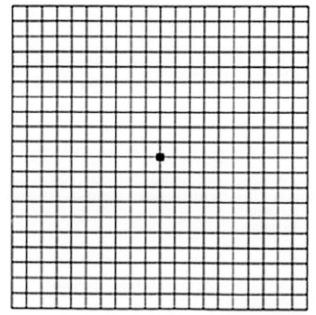

Figure 3-7: Amsler grid in patient with normal vision. (Image courtesy of National Eye Institute.)

Disorders of the Retina

Vascular disease of the retina can affect both the retinal artery and vein. They are primarily differentiated based on their fundoscopic findings (Table 3-3). Early recognition of these entities is important as it can potentially lead to permenant blindness.

Retinal Detachment
– Risk factors
  • Trauma, ocular surgery
  • Exudative ARMD
  • Diabetic retinopathy
  • Connective tissue disorders (Marfan syndrome, Ehlers-Danlos)
  • Myopia
  • Retinopathy of prematurity
  • Retinitis

TABLE 3-3 Retinal Artery Versus Retinal Vein Occlusion

	RETINAL ARTERY OCCLUSION	RETINAL VEIN OCCLUSION
Causes	• Vascular risk factors: • Hypertension • Diabetes • Hyperlipidemia • Carotid artery stenosis, transient ischemic attack • Giant cell arteritis • Cardioembolic • Thrombophilia (consider if seen in younger patients)	• Similar risk factors as retinal artery occlusion • Most commonly caused by mechanical compression of retinal vein by a thickened retinal artery from systemic hypertension • Other risk factors include coagulopathy, glaucoma, alcohol, trauma
Signs and symptoms	• Painless sudden loss of vision • Drastic decrease in visual acuity • Branch retinal artery occlusion will present with limited loss of vision confined to the area supplied by the occluded artery	• Similar signs and symptoms as retinal artery occlusion; however, vision loss is not as acute as seen in retinal artery occlusion • May have pain, photophobia, erythema, watery discharge • May be complicated by neovascularization or macular edema
Diagnostics	• Fundoscopy: • Retinal pallor (due to lack of blood supply) • Cherry red macula (due to receiving blood supply from choriocapillaries) • Boxcar arrangement of blood in the retinal veins	• Fundoscopy: • Swelling of the optic disc • Scattered diffuse hemorrhage ("blood and thunder") • Dilation and tortuosity of the retinal veins • Cotton-wool spots • Fluorescein angiography
Management	• Ocular massage: dislodges the thrombus further down the circulation to limit the degree of decreased visual acuity and improve retinal perfusion • Hyperbaric oxygen: maximizes oxygenation • IV acetazolamide, mannitol, anterior chamber paracentesis: reduces intraocular pressure • Treat underlying cause	• Conservative management if there is absence of macular edema and neovascularization • Intravitreal VEGF inhibitors: reduces macular edema • Photocoagulation: reduces neovascularization • May have partial recovery of vision within months • Treat underlying cause

- Pathophysiology
  - Accumulation of fluid in the subretinal space → separation of the sensory retina from the retinal pigment epithelium
  - Neurosensory layer of the retina contains photoreceptors with the rods and cones, which degenerate upon separation from the retinal pigment epithelium → loss of vision
  - Tractional forces on the retina
  - Posterior vitreous detachment
- Signs and symptoms
  - Flashing lights
  - Floaters
  - Painless unilateral sudden loss of vision (retina lacks pain receptors)
  - "Red veil" or "curtain coming down"
  - Leukocoria
- Diagnostics
  - Fundoscopy
    - Vitreous debris
    - Elevated and detached retina
    - Weiss ring: white fibrous ring signifying the point of attachment between the posterior vitreous and the round optic nerve
    - Tobacco dust cells: retinal pigment epithelial cells that have floated into the vitreous humor
  - Ophthalmic ultrasound
    - Vitreous hemorrhage
    - Retinal elevation
- Management
  - Conservative management if retinal detachment is due to posterior vitreous detachment as symptoms of floaters will self-resolve
  - Surgical
    - Retinopexy (pneumatic, laser, or cryoretinopexy)
    - Scleral buckle

Retinal detachment is an ophthalmologic emergency.

Retinopathy
– Causes
  - Systemic disease (hypertension, diabetes)
  - Prematurity (further discussed in the pediatric section)
  - Infections (HIV)
  - Genetic disease (sickle cell, Alport syndrome)
  - Drugs (chloroquine, hydroxychloroquine)
– Signs and symptoms
  - May be asymptomatic
  - Chronic progressively worsening visual deficits
  - Floaters
  - Blindness at end-stage disease: diabetic retinopathy is the most common cause of blindness in US adults
– Diagnostics: differentiated based on characteristic appearances on the fundoscopy
  - Hypertensive retinopathy
    - Cotton-wool spots
    - Flame and dot-blot hemorrhages
    - Papilledema
    - Uniform narrowing of arterioles
    - Complications
      - Retinal detachment
      - Optic neuropathy
  - Chronic hypertensive retinopathy
    - Arterial venule (A-V) nicking and crossing: atherosclerosis reduces the radius of the arteries, which compensate by expanding and as a result compress the veins
    - Copper and silver wiring: represent narrowing of the vessel lumen
    - Macular star: seen in advanced stages
    - Complications
      - Retinal vein occlusion (secondary to A-V nicking)
      - Retinal detachment
      - Optic nerve atrophy
  - Diabetic retinopathy
    - Nonproliferative retinopathy
      - Microaneurysms
      - Tiny hemorrhages
      - Hard exudates
      - Retinal edema
    - Proliferative retinopathy
      - Angiogenic factors are secreted in response to ischemia
      - Neovascularization results in newly formed vessels that are fragile and prone to rupture
      - Vitreous hemorrhage
      - Glaucoma
      - Macular edema: primary cause of visual impairment
– Management
  - Optimization of underlying etiology
  - Management of complications
    - Nonproliferative diabetic retinopathy: observation or panretinal photocoagulation (in severe cases)
    - Proliferative diabetic retinopathy
      - Panretinal photocoagulation
      - VEGF inhibitors (also used for macular edema)
    - Vitreous hemorrhage: early vitrectomy

Retinitis Pigmentosa
– Definition: genetic progressive dystrophy and degeneration of photoreceptors (death of rods, followed by cones)
– Causes: group of genetic disorders inherited in a variety of patterns (dominant, recessive, X linked). Can occur secondary to genetic syndromes and acquired causes; however, most cases present solely with ophthalmic symptoms

- Drugs (phenothiazine, thioridazine)
- Genetic syndromes (Waardenburg syndrome, Refsum disease, Bardet-Biedl syndrome, abetalipoproteinemia)
- Infectious (tertiary syphilis, toxoplasmosis, herpes)
- Trauma
    - Signs and symptoms
        - Nyctalopia: difficulty with night vision
        - Peripheral vision deficits
        - Photopsia
        - Visual acuity maintained until late in disease
        - Macular edema and cataracts
    - Diagnostics
        - Fundoscopy
            - Attenuated retinal blood vessels
            - Optic disc pallor
            - Retinal pigmentation in a bony spiculum pattern
        - Electroretinogram: decreased signal of rods and cones
    - Management: no present cure, only symptomatic treatment targeted at slowing the rate of photoreceptor degeneration and treatment of complications
        - Vitamin and nutritional supplementation
        - Macular edema: carbonic anhydrase inhibitor reduces intraocular pressure
        - Cataracts: extraction

Rods: function to improve night vision, differentiation of corners and edges
Cones: function to visualize details and colors

Refractive Errors
Refractive errors: occur due to the inability to focus images on the retina (Fig. 3-8; Table 3-4). Most cases can be treated with corrective lenses.

Miscellaneous
Glaucoma
- Risk factors
    - Blacks, Asians
    - Family history
    - Diabetics
- Causes
    - In most cases of open-angle glaucoma, cause is unknown
    - Drugs (anticholinergic, tricyclic antidepressant, steroids)
- Pathophysiology: excess production or decrease the drainage of aqueous humor → elevated intraocular pressure → compression of the retina and optic nerve head → blindness

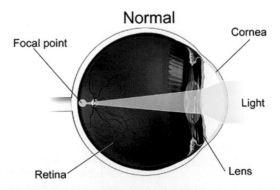

Figure 3-8: Diagram of normal refraction demonstrating light passing through the eye and converges at the focal point to allow for optimal visual dexterity and depth perception. Refractive errors occur due to the inability to focus images on the retina. Most cases can be treated with corrective lenses. (Image courtesy of Blausen Medical Communications.)

TABLE 3-4   Comparing Types of Refractive Errors

REFRACTIVE ERRORS	FEATURES	ILLUSTRATION
Hyperopia	• Weakness in refractive power of the eye due to shorter than normal anteroposterior (AP) axis or excessively concave refractive system resulting in image being projected posterior to the retina • Treat with convex (converging) corrective lenses • Distant objects appear more clearly than near objects • Associated with amblyopia, glaucoma	
Myopia	• Excessive refractive power in the eye due to a longer than normal AP axis or increased convexity of the refractive system resulting in the image being projected anterior to the retina • Treat with concave (diverging) corrective lenses • Near objects appear more clearly than distant objects • Associated with Marfan, Ehlers-Danlos, amblyopia, glaucoma, retinal detachment, retinopathy of prematurity	
Astigmatism	• Abnormal curvature of the refractive system (cornea is not perfectly spheric) resulting in irregular projections of the image along the vertical and horizontal axes • Occurs in combination with hyperopia and myopia • Treat with cylindric lenses • Associated with keratotorus and keratoconus	 **Astigmatism** Focal point Astigmatic cornea *Astigmatic cornea distorts the focal point of light in front of and/or behind the retina*
Presbyopia	• Inability to focus on near objects due to decreased elasticity of the lens and strength of the ciliary muscles. Loss of accommodation on the lens • Incidence increases in age Treat with reading glasses	 **Presbyopia** Focal point Less flexible lens *The lens ages and stiffens, bringing the focal point behind the retina and causing blurry vision*

– Types
  • Acute angle-closure glaucoma
  • Chronic angle-closure glaucoma
  • Open angle glaucoma: accounts for 90% of cases
– Signs and symptoms: acuity of symptoms and gonioscopy differentiate the types of glaucoma

Acetazolamide also used in benign intracranial hypertension, altitude sickness. Adverse effects include metabolic acidosis. Latanoprost may result in browning of the iris. Pilocarpine adverse effects include miosis and cyclospasm.

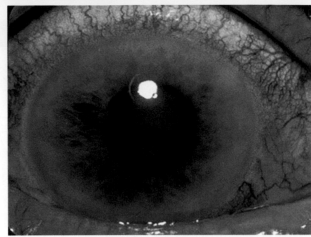

Figure 3-9: Acute angle-closure glaucoma with fixed, nonreactive middilated pupil. (Image courtesy of Jonathan Trobe, MD.)

- Red, painful, rock-hard eye
- Fixed, nonreactive, middilated pupil (Fig. 3-9)
- Decreased visual acuity
- Mild visual deficits (loss of peripheral vision)
- Occasional halos
- Blindness: seen in cases of acute angle-closure glaucoma or chronic open angle glaucoma
- Diagnostics
  - Fundoscopic exam: increased cup-to-disc ratio and cupping of the optic disc; normal ratio <0.5
  - Tonometry: increased intraocular pressure; normal pressure 12–20 mm Hg
  - Gonioscopy: measures angle of the anterior chamber
- Management
  - Pharmacologic
    - Acetazolamide (carbonic anhydrase inhibitor): decreases production of aqueous humor
    - Timolol (topical beta blocker): decreases aqueous humor production
    - Latanoprost (prostaglandin analog): increases outflow of aqueous humor
    - Pilocarpine (cholinergic analogue): opens canal of Schlemm allowing passage of aqueous humor from posterior chamber to anterior chamber of the eye
    - Mannitol (osmotic diuretic)
  - Surgical
    - Laser trabeculoplasty
    - Iridotomy: burns hole in the iris to facilitate flow of aqueous humor

Aqueous humor: produced from the ciliary body. Flows out from the posterior chamber to the anterior chamber and is eventually reabsorbed by a trabecular meshwork and the canal of Schlemm. Its flow becomes obstructed from the posterior to anterior chamber due to a lens that is anatomically more forward.

Acute angle-closure glaucoma: ophthalmologic emergency due to sudden worsening of chronic angle-closure glaucoma. Precipitated by extrinsic factor that causes pupillary dilation (stress, dark room, anticholinergic, sympathomimetic, decongestants). Must be treated emergently with IV acetazolamide and mannitol due to risk of blindness.

Other Ophthalmologic Entities
- Chalazion (lid nodule)
  - Painless noninfectious granulomatous swelling of the eyelids due to obstruction of sebaceous glands from poor hygiene, chronic blepharitis, or skin conditions (rosacea)
  - Treat with eyelid hygiene therapy such as warm compresses and eyelid cleaners
  - Hordeolum (stye)
  - Painful infectious (most commonly *S. aureus*) granulomatous swelling of the eyelid due to obstruction of sebaceous glands

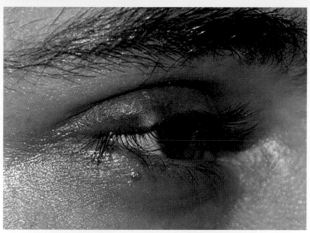

Figure 3-10: Upper eyelid stye. (From Andre Riemann / Public domain.)

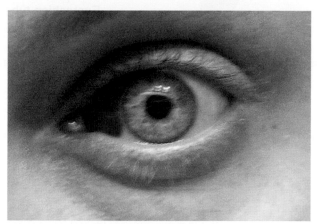

Figure 3-11: Subconjunctival hemorrhage. (From Standardissue at en.wikipedia; CC BY-SA [https://creativecommons.org/licenses/by-sa/3.0])

- May start off as chalazion that develops into a localized abscess (Fig. 3-10)
- Similar risk factors as chalazion
- Treat with eyelid hygiene therapy +/− antibiotics in advanced cases
- Subconjunctival hemorrhage
  - Caused by trauma or Valsalva
  - May appear scary to the patient; however, most cases are benign and will self-resolve (Fig. 3-11)
  - No treatment necessary
- Corneal abrasion
  - Caused by trauma, contact lens, or foreign body
  - Diagnose with fluorescein staining on the cornea
  - Treat with topical antibiotics and provide pain control

EARS
Otitis Media
- Risk factors
  - Small eustachian tube
  - Recent URI (Fig. 3-12)
  - Immunodeficiency (consider if patient has multiple episodes of otitis media with associated complications)
- Microbiology
  - *S. pneumonia*
  - *H. influenzae*
  - *Moraxella catarrhalis*

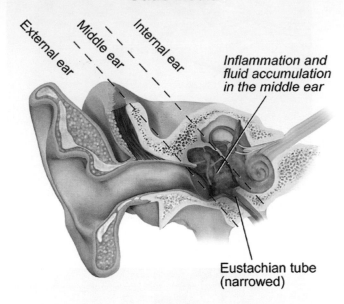

Figure 3-12: Anatomy and pathophysiology of otitis media. (Image courtesy of Bruce Blaus.)

- Signs and symptoms
  - Ear pain and tugging
  - Fever, erythema
  - Purulent otorrhea
- Diagnostics: clinical
  - Fundoscopy
    - Fullness and bulging of the tympanic membrane
    - Lack of light reflex
    - Middle ear effusion
    - Tympanic membrane retraction
  - Pneumatic otoscopy
    - Puff of air into the middle ear and the tympanic membrane does not move
    - Lack of mobility is most sensitive and specific for otitis media
- Management: antibiotics
  - Amoxicillin
  - Azithromycin if penicillin allergic
  - Second-line treatment or if unresponsive to initial antibiotic treatment
    - Amoxicillin-clavulanate (covers beta-lactamase–resistant organisms)
    - Cefuroxime
    - IM ceftriaxone
- Complications
  - Brain abscess, meningitis
  - Mastoiditis, conductive hearing loss
  - Tympanic membrane perforation
  - Labyrinthitis
  - Cholesteatoma, tympanosclerosis
  - Orbital cellulitis
  - Retropharyngeal abscess

Otitis Externa (Swimmer's Ear)

- Risk factors
  - Excessive wetness of the ear canal
  - Trauma
- Microbiology
  - Pseudomonas: most common cause
  - *S. aureus*: second most common cause

- Diphtheroides, viridans streptococci
- Signs and symptoms
  - Ear pain with manipulation of the outer ear
  - Conductive hearing loss
  - Edema, erythema, otorrhea
  - Preauricular lymphadenopathy
- Diagnostics
  - Clinical
  - May require CT scan if there is suspicion of temporal bone invasion
- Management: mostly symptomatic treatment; however, may use topical otic antibiotics and analgesics
  - Antibiotics
    - Fluoroquinolones: first line
    - Alternatives: side effects in parentheses
      - Aminoglycosides (ototoxicity)
      - Neomycin (contact dermatitis)
  - Analgesics: NSAIDs
  - Prevention: alcohol wipes after getting wet, earplugs
- Complications: malignant otitis externa

Malignant Otitis Externa
- Signs and symptoms
  - Invasion into temporal or mastoid bone resulting with associated cranial nerve abnormalities (facial, vestibular)
  - Conductive hearing loss
  - Severe unrelenting ear pain
  - Osteomyelitis of the skull base and temporomandibular joint
- Diagnostics: otoscopy (granulation tissue, edema of the external auditory canal)
  - Management: IV antipseudomonal antibiotics (piperacillin, ticarcillin)

Mastoiditis
- Risk factors
  - Acute or chronic otitis media: extension of infection into air cells
  - Wegener granulomatosis

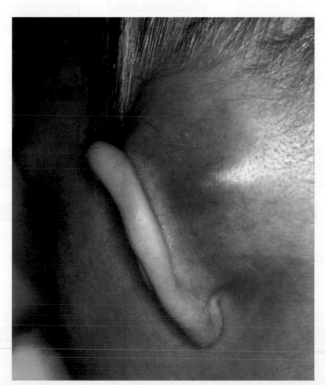

Figure 3-13: Erythema and tenderness of the mastoid bone consistent with mastoiditis. (Image courtesy of B. Welleschik.)

- Signs and symptoms
  - Tenderness and erythema of the mastoid bone (Fig. 3-13)
  - Anterior and inferior displacement of the pinna
- Diagnostics
  - Clinical
  - Temporal bone CT scan: evaluates for bony invasion, which will appear as loss of trabecular bone
- Management
  - IV antibiotics targeting upper respiratory tract organisms
  - Myringotomy
  - Mastoidectomy if there is presence of bony destruction

Cholesteatoma
- Causes
  - Acquired (chronic otitis media, tympanostomy tubes)
  - Congenital
- Pathophysiology: overgrowth of keratin debris (squamous epithelium) within the middle ear
- Signs and symptoms
  - Conductive hearing loss (Fig. 3-14; Table 3-5): erosion of the ossicles
  - Chronic malodorous otorrhea
  - Otalgia
  - Vertigo, tinnitus
- Diagnostics
  - Otoscopy
    - White plaque on the tympanic membrane
    - Retraction pocket behind the tympanic membrane with granulation tissue and skin debris
  - CT/MRI: determines extent of extracranial and intracranial involvement
- Management: tympanomastoid surgery with ossicular reconstruction

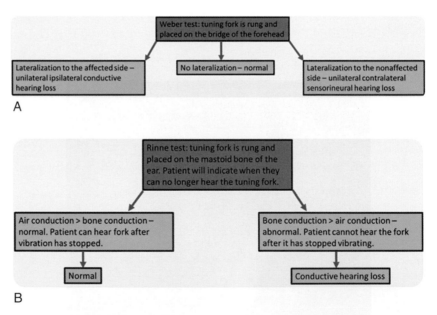

Figure 3-14: Evaluation of hearing loss using (A) Weber and (B) Rinne tests.

TABLE 3-5   Interpretation of Tuning Fork Results in Evaluation of Hearing Loss

TEST	NORMAL	CONDUCTIVE HEARING LOSS	SENSORINEURAL HEARING LOSS
Weber	No lateralization	Lateralization to affectessd ear	Lateralization to the nonaffected ear
Rinne	Air conduction > bone conduction	Bone conduction > air conduction	Air conduction > bone conduction

- Complications
  - Meningitis, brain abscess
  - Cranial nerve palsies
  - Intracranial expansion and erosion

Presbycusis
- Epidemiology: most common cause of sensorineural hearing loss
- Definition: age-related sensorineural hearing loss
- Causes: these result in presbycusis occurring at an earlier age
  - Exposure to loud noises
  - Chronic otitis media
  - Ototoxic medications
  - Genetics
- Pathophysiology: degeneration of hair cells at the cochlear base results in decreased high-frequency hearing; low-frequency hearing is maintained
- Signs and symptoms
  - Chronic, decreased, symmetric hearing loss bilaterally
  - Increased volume of appliances (television, radio) noted by family members
  - Tinnitus, vertigo
  - Difficulty hearing in loud environments due to competing background noise
  - Maintain good hearing in quiet one-on-one environment
- Diagnostics
  - Clinical
  - Confirmed with audiometry
- Management: hearing aids

Ramsay Hunt Syndrome
- Pathophysiology: varicella-zoster virus (VZV) reactivation infection of the ear
- Signs and symptoms
  - Vesicles along the auditory canal
  - Ipsilateral facial nerve palsy
  - Otalgia
  - Balance, taste, hearing, and lacrimation may be affected with involvement of other cranial nerves (CN V, VII, or X)
- Diagnostics: clinical
  - Management: valacyclovir plus prednisone

Bullous myringitis: postinfectious (acute otitis media) bullous and vesicle formation on the tympanic membrane. Most commonly caused by *Mycoplasma*. Treat with macrolides and topical analgesics.

NOSE
Nasal Septal Perforation
- Causes
  - Drugs
    - Cocaine, methamphetamine
    - Decongestants
    - Intranasal corticosteroids
  - Wegener granulomatosis
  - Trauma (piercings, digital trauma)
  - Iatrogenic (postrhinoplasty)
- Signs and symptoms (Fig. 3-15)
  - Whistling noise during respiration
  - Crusting, epistaxis
  - Nasal pressure and discomfort
  - Sensation of nasal obstruction: due to turbulent airflow through nasal passages
- Diagnostics
  - Clinical
  - Biopsy of perforated margin to rule out malignancy
- Management
  - Nasal packing
  - Surgery in severe cases

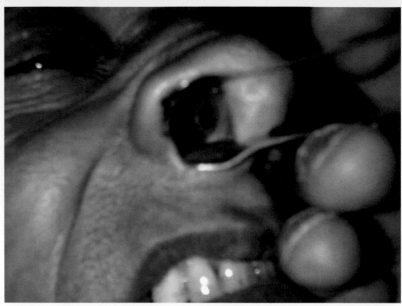

Figure 3-15: Patient with nasal septal perforation. (Image courtesy of Dr. J.S. Bhandari, India.)

Nasal septum has poor regenerative capacity due to inadequate blood supply to the nasal cartilage. It primarily receives its blood supply and nutrients via diffusion through the overlying mucosa.

Nasal Polyps
- Causes
  - Aspirin sensitivity (aspirin-exacerbated respiratory disease)
  - Cystic fibrosis
  - Atopy: asthma, chronic sinusitis, allergic rhinitis
- Signs and symptoms
  - Asymptomatic
  - Dyspnea on nasal breathing
  - Nasal airway obstruction
  - Postnasal drip
  - Rhinorrhea
  - Snoring, anosmia with larger polyps
- Diagnostics
  - Clinical: glistening gray mass in the nasal cavity
  - Biopsy if etiology of nasal polyp is unknown or suspicious for malignancy
- Management
  - Topical nasal steroids (mometasone, fluticasone, budesonide)
  - Surgical resection: polyps tend to recur if not followed up by medical management

Nasopharyngeal Carcinoma
- Risk factors
  - EBV infection
  - Smoking
  - Genetics (Asian descent)
  - Salt-cured foods
- Signs and symptoms
  - Epistaxis
  - Rhinorrhea
  - Headaches
  - Cranial nerve palsies
  - Serous otitis media
  - Cervical lymphadenopathy
- Diagnostics: biopsy
- Management: surgical excision +/− chemoradiation

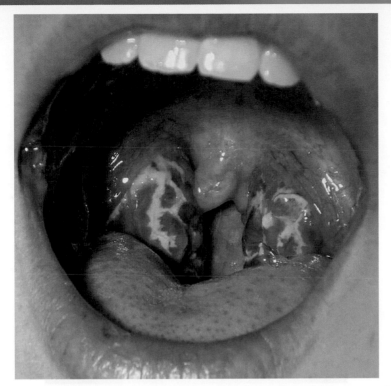

Figure 3-16: Streptococcal pharyngitis with erythematous pharynx, tonsillar enlargement, and exudates. (Image courtesy of Dr. James.)

THROAT

Pharyngitis

- Microbiology
  - Viruses
    - Adenovirus
    - Coxsackie
    - CMV
  - Bacteria: group A streptococcus
- Signs and symptoms
  - Rapid-onset fever and sore throat
  - Erythematous pharynx
  - Tonsillar enlargement and exudates (Fig. 3-16)
  - Palate petechiae
  - Enlarged and tender cervical lymph nodes
  - Cough, rhinorrhea, and conjunctivitis tend to suggest a viral etiology
- Diagnostics
  - Clinical
  - Rapid strep test; if negative, follow up with throat cultures
- Management: antibiotics to prevent acute rheumatic fever
  - Penicillin or amoxicillin
  - Tonsillectomy for multiple recurrent infections within the past year
- Complications
  - Retropharyngeal abscess
  - Peritonsillar abscess

Retropharyngeal Abscess

- Definition: infection between the posterior pharyngeal wall and prevertebral fascia
- Signs and symptoms
  - Neck pain and stiffness
  - Odynophagia/dysphagia
  - Muffled voice
  - Enlargement of posterior pharyngeal wall
- Diagnostics
  - Neck x-ray: widening of the prevertebral stripe (Fig. 3-17)

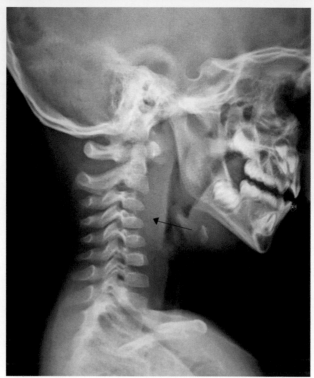

Figure 3-17: Widening of the prevertebral strip secondary to prevertebral soft tissue swelling in a patient with a retropharyngeal abscess. (From James Heilman, MD; CC BY-SA [https://creativecommons.org/licenses/by-sa/3.0])

- CT scan
  - Ring enhancement with central lucency
  - Anterior airway displacement
- Management
  - Incision and drainage
  - IV antibiotics
    - Third-generation cephalosporin plus ampicillin-sulbactam

OR

    - Clindamycin
- Complications
  - Airway compromise
  - Posterior mediastinitis, aspiration pneumonia
  - Sepsis, thrombophlebitis
  - Erosion through the carotid sheath, vertebral osteomyelitis

Peritonsillar Abscess
- Signs and symptoms
  - Dysphasia
  - Trismus: painful spastic contractions of the jaw
  - Asymmetric tonsillar enlargement with associated displacement of the uvula away from the affected side (Fig. 3-18)
  - "Hot potato" voice
  - Pooling of saliva
- Diagnostics: clinical
- Management
  - Incision and drainage
  - Antibiotics covering for group A streptococcus and respiratory anaerobes

Lemierre syndrome: septic thrombophlebitis of the internal jugular vein, which commonly occurs as a complication of oropharyngeal abscesses. Can result in septic emboli being thrown into the lungs. Diagnose with Doppler of the internal jugular vein. Treat with IV antibiotics and anticoagulation.

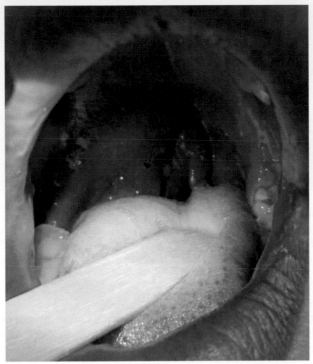

Figure 3-18: Patient with right-sided peritonsillar abscess. (From James Heilman, MD; CC BY-SA [https://creative-commons.org/licenses/by-sa/3.0])

Laryngitis
- Causes
  - Viral infection
  - Gastroesophageal reflux disease
- Signs and symptoms
  - Cough
  - Hoarseness
  - Nasal congestion
  - URI symptoms
- Diagnostics: clinical
- Management
  - Self-resolving
  - Voice rest to prevent formation of vocal nodules

CHAPTER 4 Pulmonology

LUNG ANATOMY AND PHYSIOLOGY
Lung anatomy (Fig. 4-1) and physiology (Figs. 4-2 and 4-3) are essential to understanding common pathologies because the lung functions as a site of gas exchange and pH homeostasis (Fig. 4-4). When the lung is compromised it can lead to a downstream effect that can affect other organs such as the cardiovascular and renal systems.

PHYSICAL EXAM
A thorough physicial exam (Table 4-1) in a patient with shortness of breath not only involves ausculation but also evaluation of the digits (Fig. 4-5) to determine acuity of the dyspnea. Nonpulmonary causes can also present as shortness of breath, and focused physical exams for these systems should also be performed.

ALTITUDE SICKNESS
Altitude Sickness
- Pathophysiology
  - At higher altitudes there is decreased FiO_2 → decreased alveolar O_2 → decreased arterial O_2
  - In response, individuals must hyperventilate to maintain arterial oxygen
  - Hyperventilation results in respiratory alkalosis and metabolic compensation (via excretion of bicarbonate)
  - Process of metabolic compensation can take several days resulting in a temporary increase in pH while the body compensates for the respiratory alkalosis
  - Hypoxemia results in vasoconstriction of the pulmonary vasculature → increased capillary pressure → pulmonary edema
  - Loss of cerebral autoregulation (due to profound hypoxemia) and increased cerebral vascular permeability result in cerebral edema
- Signs and symptoms
  - Central nervous system (CNS)
    - Confusion: secondary to cerebral edema
    - Impaired mentation
    - Light-headedness
  - Pulmonary
    - Crackles on auscultation: secondary to pulmonary edema
    - Dyspnea on exertion
  - Gastrointestinal (GI)
    - Nausea, vomiting
    - Anorexia
- Diagnostics: clinical
- Management
  - Supplemental oxygen
  - Acetazolamide (carbonic anhydrase inhibitor): accelerates acclimatization to high altitude
    - Induces a metabolic acidosis with respiratory compensation (increases respiratory rate)
    - Improves pulmonary edema through its diuretic effect
  - Dexamethasone: improves symptoms without accelerating acclimatization
- Prevention: gradual ascent, preacclimatization (hypobaric hypoxia)

GENETIC PULMONARY SYNDROMES
Cystic Fibrosis
- Epidemiology
  - Autosomal recessive genetic disorder

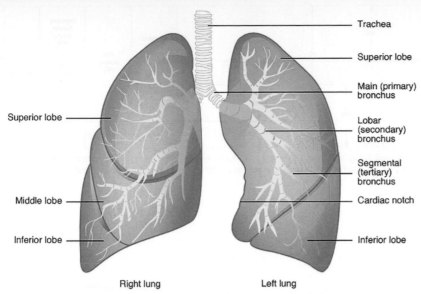

Figure 4-1: Basic lung and tracheobronchial anatomy. Air enters the lung through a broad segmenting airway system that starts centrally and branches peripherally starting with the trachea. This is further subdivided into the main bronchi, lobar bronchi, segmental bronchus, bronchioles, and terminal bronchioles, which make up the conducting zone. Further, smaller and more distal subdivisions into the respiratory bronchioles, alveolar ducts, and alveoli make up the respiratory zone. (Image courtesy of Anatomy & Physiology, Connexions Website, OpenStax College.)

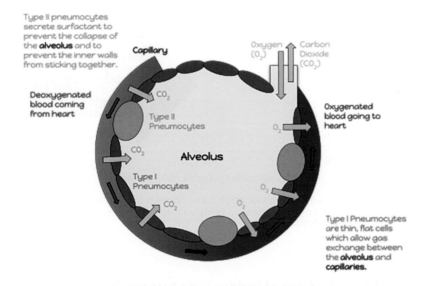

Figure 4-2: Basic anatomy and physiology of gas exchange at the alveoli. Deoxygenated blood comes from the periphery, to the right side of the heart, and eventually the pulmonary capillaries where carbon dioxide is exchanged at the alveolar capillary interface. (Image courtesy of Katherine Butler.)

- Commonly affects whites
– Pathophysiology
  - Defective chloride channels prevent movement of chloride ions across membranes resulting in thick secretions
  - Deletion of phenylalanine at the 508 position
– Signs and symptoms
  - Pulmonary
    - Recurrent pneumonia with Staphylococcus aureus (<20 years old) and Pseudomonas (>20 years old)

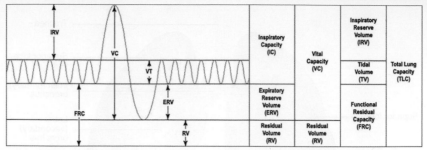

Figure 4-3: Diagram of lung volumes. Changes in lung volume can provide information regarding obstructive versus restrictive lung disease. Differences between obstructive and restrictive lung disease are discussed in the chapter.

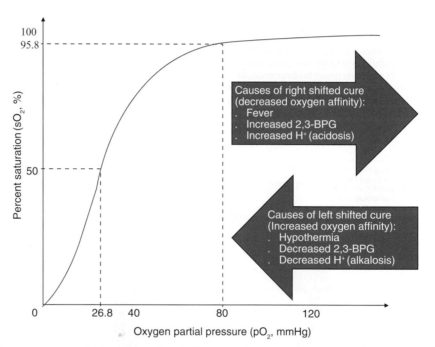

Figure 4-4: Diagram of hemoglobin oxygen dissociation curve. Various causes can result in shifts of the hemoglobin oxygen dissociation curve allowing for increased or decreased oxygen unloading to peripheral tissues. 2,3-BPG, = 2,3-Bisphosphoglyceric acid; H±, = hydrogen ions.

TABLE 4-1   Physical Exam Findings of Various Lung Pathologies

DISEASE	AUSCULTATION	TACTILE FREMITUS	PERCUSSION	ADDITIONAL NOTES
Atelectasis (collapse of alveoli)	Decreased breath sounds	Decreased	Dullness	Ipsilateral tracheal deviation
Pneumonia	Crackles, egophony, bronchophony	Increased	Dullness	
Pneumothorax	Decreased breath sounds	Decreased	Hyperresonance	Contralateral tracheal deviation
Pleural effusion	Decreased breath sounds	Decreased	Dullness	Contralateral tracheal deviation in very large effusions
Asthma	Wheezing	Decreased		

In addition to imaging and laboratory findings, key physical exam features can help differentiate the various pulmonary causes of shortness of breath.

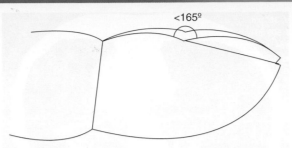

Figure 4-5: Digital clubbing with associated increased Lovibond angle (angle between the nail bed and proximal nailfold), a sign of chronic heart or lung disease.

- Bronchiectasis, chronic bronchitis
- Allergic bronchopulmonary aspergillosis (ABPA)
- Nasal polyps
- GI
  - Recurrent pancreatitis, steatorrhea, fat-soluble vitamin deficiencies (A, D, E, K)
  - Meconium ileus in newborns, rectal prolapse
  - Jaundice, biliary cirrhosis
  - Failure to thrive
- Genitourinary
  - Decreased fertility in females (thick cervical mucus)
  - Infertility in males (absence of vas deferens)
- Diagnostics: clinical and genetic testing
  - Increased sweat chloride concentration
  - Newborn screen: increased immunoreactive trypsinogen
  - Abnormal nasal potential difference
- Management: mostly symptomatic, no present cure
  - Pneumonia: antibiotics covering S. aureus and Pseudomonas
  - Pancreatic insufficiency, steatorrhea: pancreatic enzyme replacement
  - Pulmonary secretions
    - Chest physiotherapy
    - Albuterol/saline
    - Mucolytics (N-acetylcysteine), DNase
  - Ivacaftor: CFTR modulator that treats cystic fibrosis patients with G551D mutation by restoring function of the defective protein

Alpha-1 Antitrypsin Deficiency
- Epidemiology
  - Codominance inherited disorder affecting the lungs and liver in young patients
  - Minimal to nonexistent smoking or alcohol history
- Pathophysiology
  - Alpha-1 antitrypsin normally prevents breakdown of elastin by elastase in the lungs
  - Deficiency of alpha-1 antitrypsin results in unopposed elastase activity in the alveoli
  - Alpha-1 antitrypsin proteins build up in the liver resulting in hepatocellular dysfunction
- Signs and symptoms
  - Pulmonary
    - Dyspnea, cough, wheezing
    - Chronic obstructive pulmonary disease (COPD)
    - Panacinar emphysema affecting predominantly the lower lobes
  - GI
    - Jaundice (hyperbilirubinemia)
    - Cirrhosis, hepatocellular carcinoma
- Diagnostics
  - Serology: alpha-1 antitrypsin levels
  - Periodic acid-Schiff–positive and diastase-resistant globules in the liver
  - Computed tomography (CT) thorax (Fig. 4-6)
- Management
  - Avoid smoking and occupational exposure
  - Enzyme replacement in severe cases
  - Liver/lung transplant

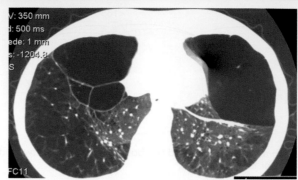

Figure 4-6: Computed tomography thorax demonstrating predominantly lower lobe emphysema and bullae in a patient with alpha-1 antitrypsin.

Primary Ciliary Dyskinesia (Kartagener Syndrome)

Smoking increases the number of inflammatory cells (polymorphonuclear neutrophils, macrophages) that release elastase, accelerating the loss of elastin in the alveoli. In addition, smoking inhibits alpha-1 antitrypsin.

- Epidemiology: autosomal recessive disorder affecting the lungs, heart, genitourinary system, and other organ systems that rely on cilia for proper function
- Pathophysiology: dynein arms defect resulting in immotile cilia
- Signs and symptoms
  - Pulmonary: impaired clearance of secretions
    - Recurrent pneumonia, sinusitis, otitis media
    - Bronchiectasis
    - Nasal polyps
  - Cardiac: impaired cardiac looping during embryonic phase
    - Dextrocardia (part of situs inversus)
    - Transposition of the great vessels
  - Genitourinary: impaired beating cilia resulting in decreased fertility
    - Males
      - Immotile sperm prevent sperm from reaching egg
      - Epispadias
    - Females: increased risk of ectopic pregnancy as egg is less able to travel down the fallopian tube, and therefore more likely to be fertilized in the fallopian tubes
  - GI: pyloric stenosis
- Diagnostics
  - Screening: low nasal nitric oxide level
  - Definitive: visualization of ciliary defects with transmission electron microscopy after nasal or bronchial biopsy
  - Imaging: situs inversus (reversal of normal organ anatomy) (Fig. 4-7), dextrocardia (heart points toward the right) (Fig. 4-8)
- Management: symptomatic, most patients have a normal active life and life span

Respiratory Infections
Acute Bronchitis
- Microbiology
  - Viral upper respiratory infection (URI)
  - URI organisms (*Streptococcus pneumoniae, Haemophilus influenzae, Moraxella*)
- Signs and symptoms
  - Productive cough
  - Mild hemoptysis
  - Dyspnea, chest discomfort
  - Wheezes, crackles
- Diagnostics: clinical
  - Chest x-ray to rule out pneumonia: may have mild congestive changes; however, no opacities or consolidation

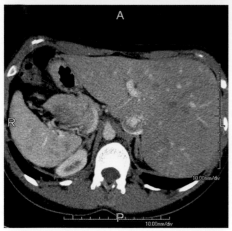

Figure 4-7: Situs inversus in a patient with Kartagener syndrome. (From John S. To, MD.)

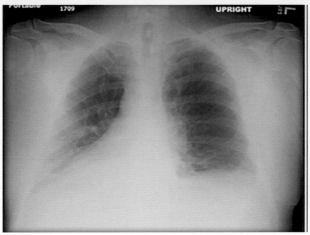

Figure 4-8: Dextricardia in a patient with Kartagener syndrome. (From John S. To, MD.)

– Management
  • Supportive management
    ▪ Nonprescription analgesics
    ▪ Cough suppressant (dextromethorphan, guaifenesin)
    ▪ Bronchodilators
  • Antibiotics: generally, not recommended; if required in special circumstances (pertussis, limit spread of infection), macrolides are first line

Chronic bronchitis is an obstructive lung disorder, while acute bronchitis is an infectious disorder. However, acute exacerbations of chronic bronchitis are generally treated similarly to acute bronchitis.

Common Cold
– Microbiology
  • Viral infection (most commonly rhinovirus): >100 antigenic serotypes, therefore reinfection is very common
  • Less common causes
    ▪ Coronavirus
    ▪ Adenovirus
    ▪ Parainfluenza, respiratory syncytial virus (RSV)
    ▪ Coxsackievirus
– Signs and symptoms
  • Low-grade fever
  • Nonproductive cough
  • Rhinorrhea
  • Headache
  • Sore throat
  • History of sick contacts
– Diagnostics: clinical
– Management: supportive management
  • Rehydration
  • Analgesics, cough suppressants, decongestants, antihistamines
  • Prevention with proper hand hygiene (handwashing)
– Complications: superimposed bacterial infection
Influenza
– Risk factors
  • Close contacts: transmission via respiratory droplets
  • Lack of vaccination
  • Primary lung disease (COPD, chronic bronchitis, interstitial lung disease): these risk factors also increase the risk of complications
  • Elderly, young children
  • Poor hand hygiene

– Signs and symptoms
  - Sudden-onset fever
  - Headache
  - Myalgias
– Diagnostics
  - Clinical
  - May be confirmed with influenza polymerase chain reaction (PCR)
– Management: antivirals vs symptomatic management depending on duration of symptoms upon presentation
  - <48 hours after onset: neuraminidase inhibitors (oseltamivir, zanamivir)
  - >48 hours after onset: symptomatic management
– Complications
  - Superimposed bacterial infection: commonly caused by methicillin-resistant S. aureus (MRSA)
  - Myositis, rhabdomyolysis
  - Myocarditis, pericarditis
  - Encephalitis, transverse myelitis

Pneumonia
Pneumonia
– Definition: infection of the lung parenchyma extending into the alveoli
– Microbiology
  - *S. pneumoniae* (most common cause)
  - Other bacterial causes: commonly associated with specific exposures (Table 4-2)
    - *Mycoplasma*
    - *Klebsiella*

TABLE 4-2   Key Pneumonia Associations and Treatment

ORGANISM	ASSOCIATION	TREATMENT
Mycoplasma	• Interstitial "walking" pneumonia • Breakouts in crowded areas such as dormitories and prisons • IgM cold agglutinins: hemolytic anemia • Bullous myringitis • Erythema multiforme	• Macrolides • Fluoroquinolone • Doxycycline
Klebsiella	• Alcoholics, diabetics, aspiration • Currant jelly sputum	• Carbapenems (cover for extended spectrum beta-lactamase organisms)
Pseudomonas	• Cystic fibrosis • Ecthyma gangrenosum	• Piperacillin-tazobactam • Ticarcillin-clavulanate • Carbapenems • Ceftazidime, cefepime • Aminoglycosides • Aztreonam • Fluoroquinolones
Legionella	• Air conditioners, showers, water aerosols • Gastrointestinal and central nervous system (CNS) symptoms • Hyponatremia • Detected with urinary antigen	• Macrolides • Fluoroquinolones
Pneumocystis pneumonia	• Human immunodeficiency virus (HIV) with CD4 <200 • Bilateral interstitial pneumonia • Increased lactate dehydrogenase, A-a gradient	• TMP-SMX
Chlamydia psittaci	• Parrots	• Tetracyclines • Macrolides
Chlamydia pneumonia	• Hoarseness	• Tetracyclines • Macrolides
Haemophilus influenzae	• Chronic obstructive pulmonary disease exacerbation	• Amoxicillin-clavulanate
Coxiella burnetii	• Cattle/sheep amniotic fluid • Culture-negative endocarditis	• Doxycycline
Nocardia	• Branching filaments, weakly acid fast: mimics tuberculosis • Immunocompromised (HIV, organ transplant recipients, chronic glucocorticoid use) • Cutaneous and CNS spread (brain abscess)	• TMP-SMX • Add carbapenems for CNS spread

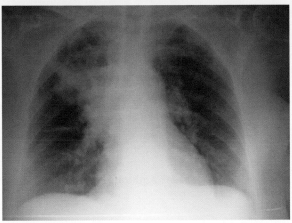

Figure 4-9: Right upper lobe consolidation consistent with pneumonia. (Image courtesy of Benjamín Herreros, Isabel Plaza, Rebeca García, Marta Chichón, Carmen Guerrero, and Emilio Pintor.)

- *Pseudomonas*
- *Legionella*
- *Pneumocystis carinii*
- *Chlamydia pneumonia/psittaci*
- *H. influenzae*
- *Coxiella burnetii*
- Viral causes
  - Influenza
  - RSV, parainfluenza
  - Adenovirus
  - Herpes simplex virus
  - Paramyxovirus
- Signs and symptoms
  - Sudden-onset fever
  - Productive cough
  - Pleuritic chest pain
  - Dyspnea on exertion
  - Crackles on auscultation
  - Dullness to percussion
- Diagnostics: clinical plus chest imaging
  - Chest x-ray (Fig. 4-9)
    - Consolidation
    - Infiltrate
    - Opacity
  - Chest CT: better for visualizing lung anatomy and lower lobes
- Management: antibiotics (CURB-65 criteria to determine whether to treat inpatient vs outpatient)
  - Outpatient: younger, healthier patients with no comorbidities, no recent antibiotic use, and stable vital signs
    - Macrolides (azithromycin, clarithromycin)

OR

  - Respiratory fluoroquinolone (levofloxacin)
  - Inpatient: older, multiple comorbidities, unstable vital signs, high risk of outpatient treatment failure
    - Antipneumococcal beta-lactam + macrolide/doxycycline (e.g., ceftriaxone + azithromycin)
    - Cover for multidrug-resistant organisms (MRSA +/− Pseudomonas) if hospital-acquired pneumonia is suspected
      - Vancomycin OR linezolid +/− antipseudomonal penicillins (piperacillin-tazobactam)
  - Intensive care unit (ICU): respiratory distress requiring mechanical ventilation, septic shock
    - Similar to inpatient treatment with coverage for multidrug-resistant organisms such as MRSA +/− Pseudomonas
- Complications
  - Parapneumonic effusion
  - Empyema

- Prevention: vaccination
  - Influenza vaccine: annually for all >6 months of age
  - Pneumococcal vaccine
    - Increased risk for invasive pneumococcal disease
    - >65 years of age

Summary of diagnostics and treatment of inpatient pneumonia:
- Blood cultures, sputum culture, urinary antigen *(S. pneumoniae, Legionella)*, polymerase chain reaction
- Pulse oximetry, arterial blood gas
- Ceftriaxone covers typical organisms *(S. pneumoniae. H. influenzae);* azithromycin covers atypical *(Mycoplasma, Klebsiella, Legionella)*

Other notes regarding pneumonia:
- Beta-lactam + macrolide can also be used for outpatient treatment in cases of major comorbidities, recent antibiotic use, and residing in areas of high-resistance *S. pneumoniae.*
- Other antipneumococcal beta-lactams include cefotaxime, ceftazidime, ertapenem, ampicillin-sulbactam.
- Other antipseudomonal antibiotics include imipenem, meropenem, cefepime, ceftazidime.
- Watch for QT prolonging effects of fluoroquinolones and macrolides.
- Chest x-ray patterns (lobar, bronchopneumonia, interstitial) do not help distinguish between the different infectious etiologies.

CURB-65 criteria: receive 1 point for each of the following signs or symptoms. Score of >2 is an indication for inpatient treatment.
- **C**onfusion
- **U**remia (blood urea nitrogen >19 mg/dL)
- **R**espiratory rate (>30)
- **B**lood pressure (<90 systolic or <60 diastolic)
- Age >**65**

Hospital-acquired pneumonia: development of pneumonia after 48 hours of hospitalization.
  Guidelines no longer include patients coming from community settings such as nursing homes, dialysis centers, and other outpatient clinics as evidence suggests that these patients are not as high risk for multidrug-resistant pathogens as previously thought. Therefore the treatment of these patients as hospital acquired vs community acquired should be done on a case-by-case basis.

Aspiration Pneumonia
- Risk factors
  - Vomiting
  - Alcoholics, altered mental status
  - Elderly, debilitated
  - Epilepsy
  - Dysphasia, ineffective gag reflex
  - Zenker diverticulum
  - Gastroesophageal reflux disease (GERD)
  - Intubation, feeding tubes
- Symptoms
  - Cough, fever, malaise
  - Foul-smelling sputum
  - Pleuritic chest pain
  - Respiratory distress
  - Wheezing
- Diagnostics: chest x-ray
  - Infiltrates involving right lower lobe (sitting up) or posterior segment of right upper lobe (supine)

- Infiltrates will take a few days to develop (vs aspiration pneumonitis where infiltrates develop within hours)
- Air fluid levels, cavitation
– Management: antibiotics to prevent development of lung abscess
- Ampicillin-sulbactam
- Amoxicillin-clavulanate
- Clindamycin
– Complications: lung abscess

Bronchial anatomy favors objects (foreign bodies) or contents (oropharyngeal secretions) entering the right lung as the right mainstem bronchus has a greater vertical orientation compared to the left main stem bronchus.

Aspiration Pneumonitis
– Aspiration of gastric contents resulting in lung injury
– Rapid development of respiratory distress and cyanosis
– Chest x-ray shows infiltrates involving one or multiple lobes within 2 hours
– Rapid clinical recovery within 24–36 hours; radiographic resolution within 4–7 days
– Management with respiratory support; antimicrobials are not indicated once diagnosis has been confirmed

Mycobacterium Tuberculosis
– Risk factors
- Recent immigrants from Africa or Asia
- Immunodeficiency
- Prisons, shelters
- IV drug abuse, alcohol abuse
- Silicosis
– Signs and symptoms: depending on stage of tuberculosis (TB)
- Primary TB: mostly asymptomatic
  - May have mild respiratory symptoms such as cough, low-grade fever that self-resolves within a week
- Secondary TB (reactivation): decrease in immune function (human immunodeficiency virus [HIV], elderly, immunomodulators) allows previously walled-off Mycobacterium to spread throughout the lungs and extrapulmonary (miliary TB)
  - Fever, weight loss, night sweats
  - Chronic productive cough
  - Hemoptysis
– Diagnostics
- Chest x-ray
  - Primary TB: often normal. May have nonspecific infiltrate, hilar adenopathy
  - Secondary reactivation
    ○ Apical opacity/infiltrate/cavity
    ○ Pleural effusion
    ○ Bronchiectasis
    ○ Miliary TB: multiple 2- to 4-mm millet seed–like lesions throughout the entire lung field (Fig. 4-10)
- Purified protein derivative (PPD): area of induration
  - Inject area of skin and follow-up in 48–72 hours
  - Only used to diagnose latent TB
  - Two-step PPD should be done for patients who have never had a PPD skin test
- Interferon (IFN)–gamma release assay
  - Direct measurement of *Mycobacterium* activity since IFN-gamma is released by cell-mediated immune response to contain the acid-fast bacilli
  - No cross reactivity with Bacille Calmette-Guérin vaccine
  - Unable to distinguish between latent vs active TB
- Acid-fast bacilli smear
- Sputum culture: obtain three morning sputum specimens for culture
- Nucleic acid amplification test
– Management: multidrug regimens to prevent development of drug resistance
- RIPE plus negative pressure isolation (Table 4-3)
  - **R**ifampin
  - **I**soniazid

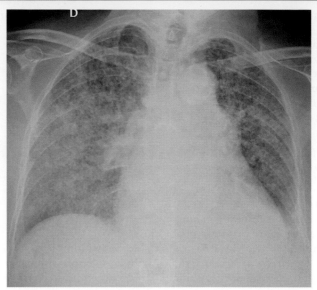

Figure 4-10: Chest radiograph of miliary tuberculosis showing bilateral reticulonodular opacities. (Image courtesy of Benjamín Herreros, Isabel Plaza, Rebeca García, Marta Chichón, Carmen Guerrero, and Emilio Pintor.)

TABLE 4-3   Tuberculosis Drugs and Their Side Effects

DRUG	MECHANISM	SIDE EFFECT
Rifampin	RNA polymerase inhibitor	• Red-orange body fluids • Cytochrome p450 inducer
Isoniazid	Inhibits enzyme involved in the synthesis of mycolic acid (component in *Mycobacterium* cell wall)	• Hepatotoxicity • Drug-induced lupus • Peripheral neuropathy (prevent with concurrent vitamin B6 administration)
Pyrazinamide	Unknown mechanism	• Hyperuricemia: increases risk of gout exacerbation
Ethambutol	Arabinosyltransferase inhibitor: decreases carbohydrate polymerization of cell wall	• Optic neuropathy: red-green color blindness

- ▪ **P**yrazinamide
- ▪ **E**thambutol
- Type and duration of treatment depends upon stage of TB (latent, primary pulmonary, extrapulmonary)
  - ▪ Latent (only positive PPD, negative chest x-ray): isoniazid ×9 months
  - ▪ Primary pulmonary: RIPE ×2 months (intensive phase), followed by rifampin plus isoniazid ×4 months (continuation phase)
  - ▪ Extrapulmonary: same as primary pulmonary with addition of corticosteroids in cases of meningitis, miliary TB, pericardial and pleural effusions

Check for glucose-6-phosphate dehydrogenase deficiency before administering dapsone or primaquine.

- – Complications: extrapulmonary TB
  - Meningitis, intracerebral tuberculoma
  - Miliary TB (hematogenous or lymphatic spread): bone, meninges, liver, spleen, pericardium, intestine, genitourinary
  - Pott disease: TB involving vertebral bodies
  - Pericarditis (most common cause of constrictive pericarditis in developing world)
  - Pleural effusion
  - Adrenal insufficiency (MCC in developing world)
  - Fibrosing mediastinitis

- Screening: PPD (area of induration and risk factors determine positivity; lower threshold for those at higher risk of false negatives)
  - >5 mm
    - Known exposure to TB
    - HIV
    - Organ transplant recipients
    - Radiographic findings consistent with previously healed TB
  - >10 mm: high-risk populations
    - Recent immigrants <5 years from TB endemic areas
    - IV drug abusers
    - High-risk environments (TB lab personnel, hospitals, prisons, nursing homes, shelters)
    - Children <4 years old
    - High risk for reactivation (long-term corticosteroid use, leukemia, end-stage renal disease, diabetes, malabsorption syndromes)
  - >15 mm: low-risk populations
    - Healthy individuals with no risk factors

Additional notes regarding tuberculosis (TB):
- Bacille Calmette-Guérin vaccine decreases the incidence of invasive TB
- Streptomycin used as second-line treatment for resistant cases of TB
- TB prefers the lung apices due to high oxygen tension (increased V/Q mismatch)

PCP Pneumonia
- Risk factors
  - HIV with CD4 <200 (AIDS-defining lesion)
  - Organ transplant recipients
  - T-cell immunodeficiency
  - Long-term glucocorticoid use
  - Severe malnutrition
- Sign and symptoms
  - Dry cough
  - Fever
  - Hypoxia
  - Tachypnea, dyspnea
- Diagnostics
  - Chest x-ray: diffuse bilateral ground glass opacities
  - Elevated lactate dehydrogenase (LDH): highly sensitive for PCP
  - Bronchoalveolar lavage: microscopic identification of PCP (methenamine silver stain)
  - Sputum stain
- Management
  - TMP-SMX: first line for treatment and prophylaxis
  - Alternatives: used in cases of sulfa allergy or TMP-SMX toxicity (bone marrow suppression, rash)
    - IV pentamidine
    - Clindamycin + primaquine
    - TMP + dapsone
    - Dapsone or atovaquone: prophylaxis only
  - Corticosteroids: improves mortality in severe cases of hypoxia
    - <92% O_2 pulse oximetry, PaO_2 <70 mm Hg
    - Arterial-alveolar gradient >35 mm Hg
  - HAART (highly active antiretroviral therapy)

Systemic mycoses: Fungal infection that is most commonly asymptomatic. If patients become symptomatic, they present with cough, fever, dyspnea, weight loss, malaise, myalgias. Chest x-ray will show calcified nodules, granuloma, cavitation. Differentiated based on extrapulmonary findings and geography (Table 4-4). Most cases are self-resolving without hosts being aware that they have inhaled and cleared the fungal infection.

Aspergillosis
- Risk factors
  - Immunocompromised (prolonged neutropenia, chronic glucocorticoids, organ transplant recipients)
  - Preexisting lung cavity (common after TB infection)

TABLE 4-4   Differentiating Systemic Mycoses

FUNGUS	LOCATION	EXTRAPULMONARY MANIFESTATIONS	DIAGNOSTICS	MANAGEMENT
Histoplasmosis	• Ohio and Mississippi river valleys, Midwest • Bat (spelunking) or bird droppings • Decayed wood	• Erythema nodosum • Erythema multiforme • Fibrosing mediastinitis • Arthralgias • Pancytopenia (bone marrow infiltration) • Hepatosplenomegaly (involvement of the reticuloendothelial system)	• Urine/serum antigen • Narrow-based budding yeasts	• Itraconazole or fluconazole • Amphotericin B for disseminated disease
Blastomycosis	• East and central United States, Wisconsin, Great Lakes • Inhalation of spores • Contact with soil or rotting wood	• Ulcerated skin lesions: verrucous heaped up skin lesions with irregular borders (mimics squamous cell carcinoma) • Lytic bone lesions • Genitourinary: prostatitis, epididymal orchitis	• Culture • Broad-based buds on microscopy	
Coccidiomycosis (San Joaquin fever; valley fever)	• US Southwest • Inhalation of spores	• Erythema nodosum/multiforme • Arthralgias (desert rheumatism) • Skin and bone lesions • Maculopapular rash	• Sputum culture • Polymerase chain reaction	
Paracoccidiomycosis	• Central and South America • Inhalation of spores	• Dissemination to reticuloendothelial system (hepatosplenomegaly, anemia)	• Culture	

- • Chronic granulomatous disease (due to catalase-positive activity neutralizing hydrogen peroxide byproducts)
  • Sarcoidosis
  • Histoplasmosis
  • Bronchial cysts, bronchiectasis
  • Lung neoplasia
- – Associated syndromes
  • ABPA: discussed in obstructive lung disorders
  • Pulmonary aspergilloma

Crescent sign: fungal ball is smaller than the cavity in which it resides. Fungus ball changes in position in the larger cavity resulting in air fluid levels.

- • Invasive aspergillosis
  • Mycotoxicosis
- – Signs and symptoms
  • Pulmonary aspergilloma: most commonly asymptomatic
  • Invasive aspergillosis: triad of worsening fever, hemoptysis, pleuritic chest pain due to erosion of lung parenchyma
- – Diagnostics
  • Chest x-ray/CT
    ▪ Invasive aspergillosis
      ○ Bilateral pulmonary infiltrates, mediastinal adenopathy
      ○ Ground-glass opacity
      ○ Lung abscess
    ▪ Aspergilloma (mycetoma): solid halolike mass lesion with "crescent sign"
  • Elevated beta-D-glucan (component of many fungal cell wall)
  • Culture, biopsy
- – Management

- Invasive aspergillosis
  - Voriconazole or itraconazole
  - Echinocandins (anidulafungin, caspofungin, micafungin): used in combination with voriconazole/itraconazole for severe cases of invasive aspergillosis
  - Aspergilloma: surgical resection
- Complications: invasive aspergillosis
  - Hematogenous spread to CNS
  - Pulmonary vasculature invasion → thrombosis and infarct

PLEURAL DISORDERS

The pleural space is a thin space between the visceral and parietal pleura that provides lubrication for the lung as it moves up and down with inspiration and expiration (Fig. 4-11).

Pneumothorax

- Definition: air in the pleural space
- Types
  - Spontaneous pneumothorax
  - Tension pneumothorax
- Risk factors
  - Underlying lung pathology (emphysema, interstitial lung disease, pneumonia, asthma, bronchiectasis)
  - Smoking
  - Marfanoid habitus (tall, young healthy males with apical blebs)
  - Trauma (rib fracture, penetrating wound)
  - Iatrogenic (central line placement, mechanical ventilation, lung biopsy)
  - Lymphangioleiomyomatosis
- Signs and symptoms
  - Sudden-onset acute shortness of breath
  - Chest pain
  - Decreased breath sounds
  - Hemodynamic instability: seen only with tension pneumothorax

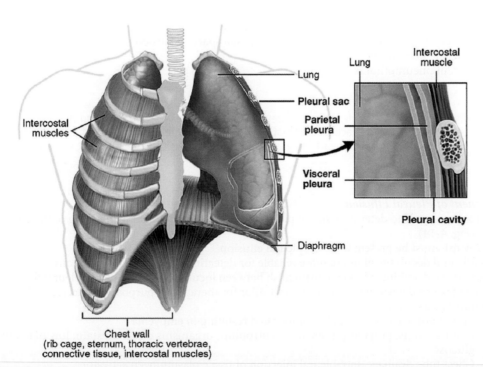

Figure 4-11: Illustrating normal pleural anatomy. The lung is surrounded by a visceral pleural, and the chest wall is covered in a parietal pleura; the space between these two is referred to as the pleural cavity and the site of air (pneumothorax) or fluid (pleural effusion) accumulation when there is pleural pathology. (Image courtesy of OpenStax College.)

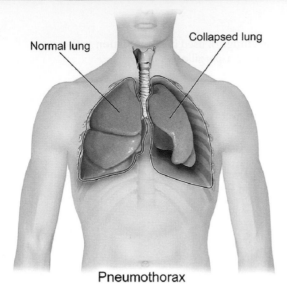

Figure 4-12: Diagram depicting development of left-sided pneumothorax. (Image courtesy of Blausen Medical.)

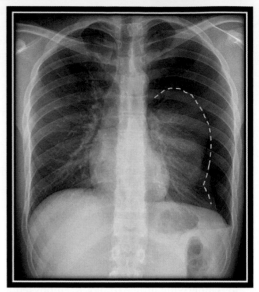

Figure 4-13: Chest x-ray in patient with left-sided pneumothorax. (Image courtesy of Hellerhoff.)

- Diagnostics: clinical plus chest x-ray
  - Chest x-ray (Figs. 4-12 and 4-13)
    - Visceral pleural line
    - Decreased lung markings
    - Contralateral tracheal and mediastinal deviation; ipsilateral flattening of hemidiaphragm; seen only with tension pneumothorax
- Management: depends on size of pneumothorax, comorbidities, and acuity of symptoms
  - Small, simple pneumothorax in healthy adults with mild symptoms: supplemental oxygen, observation
  - Large to moderate pneumothorax: chest tube placement
  - Tension pneumothorax: immediate needle decompression into the second intercostal space midclavicular line followed by chest tube placement
    - Placement of needle into the second intercostal space in tension pneumothorax converts it into a simple pneumothorax
  - Recurrent pneumothorax: pleurodesis

Tension pneumothorax pathophysiology: air in the pleural space prevents lung from fully expanding, and this worsens with each inspiratory breath as air enters the pleural space but is unable to exit creating a ball valve mechanism → tracheal deviation, compression of the mediastinal structures (heart, great vessels) → restriction of cardiac output → hemodynamic instability

Management of Pleural Effusions
- Chest x-ray is used to determine size of pleural effusion; will demonstrate blunting of the costophrenic angle (Fig. 4-14)
  - >250 mL must be present to detect pleural effusion
  - Left lateral decubitus films are more reliable for detecting smaller pleural effusions
  - Left lateral decubitus films can distinguish between loculated vs free-flowing pleural fluid
- Thoracentesis to determine etiology (Table 4-5) or for therapeutic purposes (to decrease chest discomfort and dyspnea)
  - Parapneumonic effusions can be complicated resulting in empyema
    - Fluid analysis: polymorphonuclear neutrophils, organisms on Gram stain, low pH, low glucose
    - Chest tube drainage, intrapleural injection of tissue plasminogen activator
    - Broad-spectrum antibiotics covering anaerobes
- Pleurodesis for recurrent refractory pleural effusion
- Pulmonary embolism (PE) causes both transudative and exudative effusions

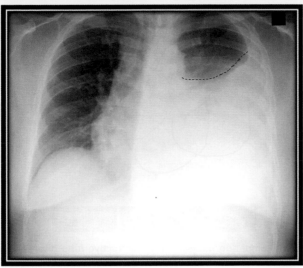

Figure 4-14: Large left pleural effusion with mediastinal shift and meniscus sign. The meniscus sign is a good indicator of a layering pleural effusion.

TABLE 4-5   Comparing Types and Causes of Pleural Effusions

	TRANSUDATE	EXUDATE	CHYLOTHORAX
Appearance	• Clear	• Cloudy	• Milky
Etiologies	• Increased hydrostatic pressure: congestive heart failure • Decreased oncotic pressure: nephrotic syndrome, cirrhosis • Hepatic hydrothorax (right-sided pleural effusions due to increased permeability of the right hemidiaphragm)	• Infectious (parapneumonic effusion if it occurs secondary to pneumonia) • Inflammatory (collagen vascular diseases), acute pancreatitis • Malignancy (lung, breast, lymphoma) • Esophageal rupture (Boerhaave syndrome): left-sided pleural effusions	• Ruptured thoracic duct
Fluid analysis	• Low protein content • None of Light criteria are met	• High protein content • Elevated amylase (due to saliva, release of pancreatic enzymes): esophageal rupture, acute pancreatitis • >1 of Light criteria are met	• Elevated triglycerides

Table courtesy of OpenStax College.

Light criteria: used to differentiate transudate vs exudate. Need only one of three criteria to characterize effusion as exudative:
• Pleural effusion protein to serum ratio >0.5
• Pleural effusion lactate dehydrogenase (LDH) to serum ratio >0.6
• Pleural effusion LDH >2/3 upper limit of normal

Tests for pleural fluid:
• Protein
• Lactate dehydrogenase
• Cytology
• Amylase
• pH
• Microbiology
• Cell count with differential

Asbestosis
– Risk factors: occupational exposure
   • Roofing
   • Shipbuilding
   • Plumbing

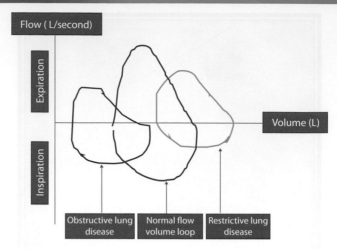

Figure 4-15: Flow volume loop comparing patients with obstructive lung disease, normal, and restrictive lung disease. Flattening of the expiratory curve in obstructive lung disease due to inability to expel carbon dioxide. Restrictive lung disease results in similar volume curve as a normal patient, except with smaller lung volumes due to impaired entry of air into the lungs. *ICS*, Inhaled corticosteroids; *LABA*, long-acting beta agonist.

- • Pipe fitting
- • Insulators
- – Signs and symptoms: >20-year latency from exposure to development of symptoms
  - • Chronic worsening cough, dyspnea, wheezing
  - • Cyanosis
  - • Clubbing
  - • Rales
- – Diagnostics
  - • Chest x-ray
    - ▪ Pleural plaques and thickening
    - ▪ Reticulonodular infiltrates primarily affecting the lower lobes
  - • CT chest: honeycombing in advanced cases
  - • Pulmonary function tests (PFTs): restrictive lung disease
  - • Biopsy: ferruginous bodies (iron-containing bodies resembling dumbbells visualized on Prussian blue staining)
- – Management: symptomatic
  - • Bronchodilators
  - • Supplemental oxygen
- – Complications
  - • Bronchogenic carcinoma (most common malignancy associated with asbestosis)
    - ▪ Smoking combined with asbestosis exposure increases the risk of bronchogenic carcinoma exponentially
  - • Mesothelioma (very high association with asbestosis exposure)
  - • Increased risk of malignancy of the larynx, oropharynx, esophagus, biliary system, and kidneys

Mesothelioma
- – Very poor prognosis
- – Presents with hemorrhagic plural effusion, cough, weight loss
- – Strongly associated with asbestos exposure
- – Benign mesothelioma is unrelated to asbestos exposures and has a very good prognosis

OBSTRUCTIVE LUNG DISEASE
Asthma
- – Definition: airway hyperreactivity resulting in bronchoconstriction (Fig. 4-15) and obstructive lung disease (Fig. 4-16)
- – Risk factors
  - • Family history, males
  - • Allergies, atopy
  - • Lack of breast milk

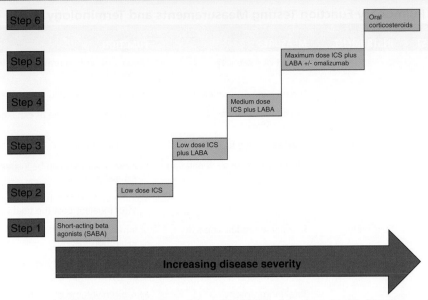

Figure 4-16: Summary of asthma step-up therapy with each additional treatment added to the previous step.

Pulse paradoxus: decrease in systolic blood pressure >10 mm Hg during inspiration.

- Triggers
  - GERD (nighttime asthma)
  - URI
  - Pollen, dander
  - Drugs: aspirin, beta blockers, smoking
  - Cold weather, exercise
- Signs and symptoms
  - Wheezing, dyspnea, tachypnea
  - Cough, chest pain
  - Improvement of symptoms with bronchodilators
  - Pulses paradoxus, absent breath sounds and wheezing, cyanosis: seen in severe cases
- Diagnostics
  - Clinical: severity determined based on the frequency of symptoms (intermittent, mild, moderate, severe), presence of nighttime symptoms, and effect on daily activities
  - PFTs (Table 4-6)
    - Obstructive lung pattern
      - Reversible airway obstruction with improvement of forced expiratory volume in 1 second (FEV1) >12% upon administration of bronchodilators; differentiates asthma from COPD
    - Methacholine challenge: used to diagnose patients who describe history of asthma with normal PFTs and currently asymptomatic
      - Decrease of FEV1 >20% upon administration is diagnostic
  - Arterial blood gas (ABG)
    - Respiratory alkalosis
    - Normal pH or respiratory acidosis may be indicative of respiratory fatigue and worsening asthma exacerbation
  - Peak expiratory flow (PEF): used to determine severity of asthma exacerbation and how far patient is from baseline; home device allows patient to self-triage (home vs emergency department [ED]) based on present symptoms
- Management
  - Avoid exacerbating factors
  - Pharmacologic: step-up management with each treatment added on to the previous treatment regimen
    - Step 1: short-acting beta agonists (SABA): albuterol, levalbuterol
      - Used for acute exacerbations and patients with intermittent asthma

TABLE 4-6   Pulmonary Function Testing Measurements and Terminology

PULMONARY FUNCTION TEST	INSTRUMENT	MEASURES	FUNCTION
Spirometry	Spirometer	Forced vital capacity	Volume of air that is exhaled after maximum inhalation
		Forced expiratory volume	Volume of air exhaled in one breath
		Forced expiratory flow, 25–75%	Air flow in the middle of exhalation
		Peak expiratory flow	Rate of exhalation
		Maximum voluntary ventilation	Volume of air that can be inspired and expired in 1 min
		Slow vital capacity	Volume of air that can be slowly exhaled after inhaling past the tidal volume
		Functional residual capacity	Volume of air left in the lungs after normal expiration
		Residual volume	Volume of air in the lungs after maximum exhalation
		Total lung capacity	Maximum volume of air that the lungs can hold
		Expiratory reserve volume	The volume of air that can be exhaled beyond normal exhalation
Gas diffusion	Blood gas analyzer	Arterial blood gases	Concentration of oxygen and carbon dioxide in the blood

- Step 2: low-dose inhaled corticosteroids (fluticasone, budesonide)
  - First-line treatment for chronic asthma
  - Side effects: oral thrush (rinse mouth after use)
- Step 3: low dose of inhaled corticosteroids (ICS) plus long-acting beta agonists (LABA: salmeterol, formoterol) or medium dose ICS monotherapy
- Step 4: medium dose of inhaled corticosteroid plus LABA
- Step 5: maximum dose of inhaled corticosteroids plus LABA
  - Consider omalizumab (E monoclonal antibody) in patients with high levels of immunoglobulin E (IgE)
- Step 6: oral corticosteroids
  - If patient is not responding to step-up management; ensure that patient is administering medication in the proper manner
- Alternatives
  - Leukotriene antagonists: montelukast, zafirlukast
  - Theophylline
    - Phosphodiesterase inhibitor with narrow therapeutic index
    - Side effects: arrhythmias, neurotoxicity
  - Zileuton
  - Cromolyn sodium: prevents mast cell degranulation
  - Magnesium sulfate: used in severe asthma exacerbations in the ED in patients unresponsive to initial treatment
- Thermoplasty: removes smooth muscle hyperplasia in bronchial airways
– Complications: ABPA

Long-acting beta agonist side effects: tremors, arrhythmias

Management of acute asthma exacerbation
– Severity determined based on difference of PEF from patient to baseline and ABG
– Administer SABA, corticosteroids, O_2
– Monitor response to treatments based on PEF, pulse oximetry, and presence of wheezing

- Never use LABA in acute exacerbations as it increases mortality
- Decision whether to admit patient from the ED with asthma exacerbation is dependent on degree of response
  - Good response: discharge from the ED
  - Poor or worsening response: admit to the floors or ICU
  - Consider mechanical ventilation or noninvasive positive pressure ventilation (bilevel positive airway pressure [BiPAP]) in patients who develop respiratory fatigue, normalizing pH, altered mental status, "silent chest" with absent wheezing and breath sounds
    - Additional considerations and notes when managing chronic asthmatics
    - Consider referring patient to pulmonologist at step 3 or 4
    - Most patient's asthma symptoms will significantly decrease or resolve by adolescence
    - Avoid use of beta blockers (especially nonspecific beta blockers) unless necessary in patients with chronic asthma
    - Ensure vaccination against pneumococcal and influenza

Aspirin-induced asthma/respiratory disease: aspirin inhibits cyclooxygenase, which results in shunting of the arachidonic acid system down the leukotriene pathway increasing leukotriene levels, which have bronchoconstrictive effects.

Allergic Bronchopulmonary Aspergillosis
- Risk factors
  - Asthma
  - Cystic fibrosis
- Pathophysiology: hypersensitivity reaction to fungal antigens that colonize the bronchopulmonary tree
- Signs and symptoms
  - Recurrent refractory asthma exacerbations
  - Fever, malaise
  - Expectoration brownish sputum and mucous plug
  - Rhinosinusitis
- Diagnostics: no single definitive test; combination of signs and symptoms meeting diagnostic criteria
  - Chest x-ray: central bronchiectasis (recurrent fleeting pulmonary infiltrates)
  - Eosinophilia
  - Elevated serum IgE
  - IgE and IgG antibodies against *Aspergillus*
- Management
  - Avoidance of aspergillus antigen (mold, basements)
  - Itraconazole + systemic glucocorticoids

Bronchiectasis
- Definition: permanent abnormal chronic dilation of large to midsize airways
- Risk factors
  - Cystic fibrosis, primary ciliary dyskinesia (Kartagener syndrome)
  - Chronic infection (TB, *Aspergillus*): results in focal bronchiectasis
  - Collagen vascular disease (rheumatoid arthritis, Sjögren syndrome)
  - Smoking
  - Neoplasia, foreign body
  - Common variable immunodeficiency
  - Recurrent aspiration
- Signs and symptoms
  - High volume, chronic productive cough
  - Hemoptysis
  - Dyspnea, wheezing
  - Chest pain
- Diagnostics: chest imaging
  - Chest x-ray: initial test
  - CT scan: bronchial wall thickening and dilation, lack of airway tapering (Figs. 4-17 and 4-18)
- Management: dilation of airway is irreversible; treatment is directed at the underlying cause to prevent further airway dilation
  - Acute exacerbations: antibiotics based on prior sputum cultures and sensitivities
  - Prophylactic macrolides for recurrent exacerbations
  - Long-term chest physiotherapy
  - Focal resection in cases of focal bronchiectasis

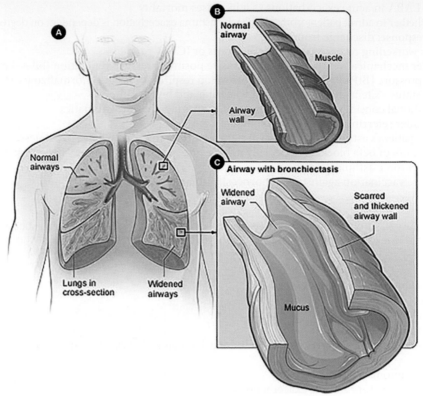

Figure 4-17: Illustration of normal airway versus bronchiectasis. (Image courtesy of National Heart Lung and Blood Institute.)

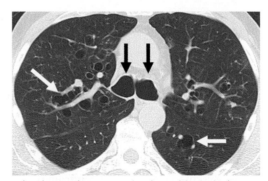

Figure 4-18: Computed tomography thorax demonstrating bronchiectasis. (Image courtesy of Mcgfowler / CC BY-SA [https://creativecommons.org/licenses/by-sa/3.0])

- Complications: severe hemoptysis

Chronic Obstructive Pulmonary Disease
- Definition: classification of disorders that includes chronic bronchitis and emphysema
- Risk factors: smoking
- Signs and symptoms
  - Chronic productive cough lasting >3 months for 2 consecutive years: chronic bronchitis
  - Wheezing, hyperresonance on percussion, distant heart sounds
  - Dyspnea on exertion, tachypnea, pursed lip breathing
  - Chest pain/discomfort, barrel-shaped chest (increased anteroposterior diameter)
- Diagnostics: clinical plus imaging
  - Chest x-ray (Figs. 4-19 and 4-20):
    - Hyperinflation and flattening of diaphragms
    - Visualization of >10 posterior ribs
    - Increased retrosternal space (on lateral radiographs)
  - CT scan: centriacinar emphysema involving the upper lobes, cysts/bulla
  - PFTs: obstructive lung disease (FEV1/forced vital capacity [FVC] <70% + FEV1 <80%) with incomplete airflow limitation after administration of bronchodilators

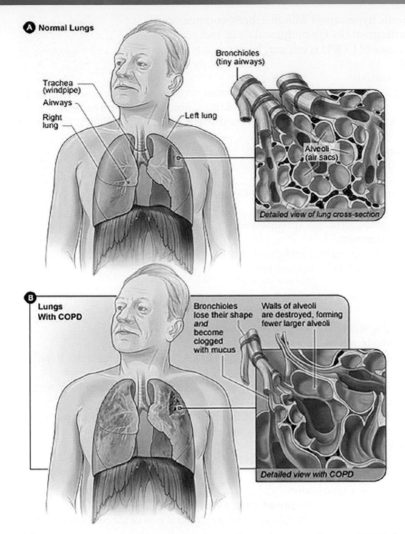

Figure 4-19: Normal lung versus patient with chronic obstructive pulmonary disease *(COPD)*. (Image courtesy of National Heart Lung and Blood Institute.)

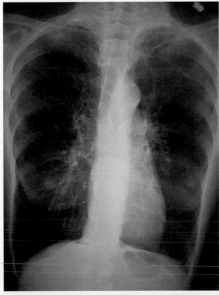

Figure 4-20: Chest x-ray in patient with severe chronic obstructive pulmonary disease showing increased lung volumes with diaphragmatic flattening, and small heart size. (Image courtesy of James Heilman, MD.)

- ABG: chronic hypercapnia with metabolic compensation
- Electrocardiogram (ECG): multifocal atrial tachycardia
- Biopsy if cause of COPD is unclear; however, it is rarely needed
- Management
  - Smoking cessation
  - GOLD staging (group A, B, C, D) to determine severity of disease based on several factors: FEV1, severity of symptoms, presence of comorbidities, number of exacerbations
    - Group A has lowest risk and less severe disease; group D has highest risk and most severe disease
  - Acute exacerbation
    - SABA (albuterol, levalbuterol)
    +
    - Short-acting muscarinic antagonist (ipratropium)
    +
    - Systemic glucocorticoids (prednisone)
  - Chronic management
    - Long-acting muscarinic antagonist (tiotropium, aclidinium, umeclidinium, glycopyrrolate): first line for chronic COPD management
    +/−
    - LABA (salmeterol, indacaterol, olodaterol, vilanterol)
    +/−
    - Inhaled glucocorticoids (fluticasone, budesonide)
    - Other considerations
      ○ Severe disease will require the addition of LABA and in some cases triple therapy (LAMA-LABA-glucocorticoid)
      ○ Long-term oxygen for chronic hypoxemia: PaO_2 <55 mm Hg or O_2 saturation <88%: mortality benefit
      ○ Roflumilast (phosphodiesterase-4 inhibitor): refractory COPD patients with multiple exacerbations (>2) requiring hospitalization per year
      ○ Pulmonary rehabilitation
      ○ Pneumococcal and influenza vaccination
- Complications
  - Acute-on-chronic exacerbation
    - Worsening cough, sputum production, dyspnea
      ○ Add antibiotics to acute exacerbation regimen if two of three abovementioned symptoms are present
    - Respiratory failure requiring mechanical ventilation
  - Cor pulmonale

Emphysema is a pathologic diagnosis defined as enlargement and destruction of air spaces distal to the terminal bronchioles.

Restrictive Lung Disease
Interstitial Lung Disease
- Definition: inflammation of the alveolar walls resulting in pulmonary fibrosis and impaired gas exchange
- Causes (Table 4-7)
  - Idiopathic
  - Pneumoconiosis (exposure to nonorganic dust matter) (Table 4-8)
    - Coalmining
    - Silicosis
    - Asbestosis
    - Berylliosis
  - Hypersensitivity pneumonitis (exposure to organic dust matter)
  - Infectious
    - TB
    - Systemic mycoses
  - Drugs
    - Smoking
    - Methotrexate

TABLE 4-7 Causes of Interstitial Lung Diseases

CAUSES	KEY FEATURES
Hypersensitivity pneumonitis	• Inhalation of organic antigen: mold, bird droppings, air conditioner • Present similarly to pneumonia with fevers, chills, pulmonary infiltrates. Improvement of symptoms after removal of causative antigen • Combination of type III (immune complex deposition) and type IV hypersensitivity reaction (T-cell mediated) • Serology: IgG and IgA against inhaled antigen
Goodpasture syndrome	• Type II hypersensitivity reaction with antibodies against glomerular basement membranes (alveoli, glomeruli) • Presents with pulmonary (cough, dyspnea, hemoptysis) and renal (hematuria, renal failure, glomerulonephritis) symptoms • Serology: anti-GBM antibodies • Treat with plasmapheresis, in addition to glucocorticoids and immunosuppressants
Langerhans histiocytosis	• Common in cigarette smokers • Presents with "punched-out" lytic bone lesions, brownish purple papules, lymphadenopathy, hepatosplenomegaly, pneumothorax, diabetes insipidus, and other endocrinopathies • Treat with steroids +/− other chemotherapeutic agents
Pulmonary alveolar proteinosis	• Accumulation of proteinaceous surfactant material in the alveoli due to decreased clearance secondary to disruption of granulocyte-macrophage colony-stimulating factor (GM-CSF) signaling • Cough with "gelatinous" chunky sputum, dyspnea on exertion, fever, weight loss • Chest x-ray: bilateral alveolar opacities in a "bat wing" distribution • Treat with lung lavage plus GM-CSF; avoid use of glucocorticoids
Radiation	• Occurs postthoracic radiation (especially lung, breast, thyroid cancer) • Risk factors for development include volume of irradiated lung, dose radiation, and method • Acute symptoms develop within 4–12 wk, while late-stage symptoms develop up to 1 yr later • Chest x-ray: straight line effect, which does not follow normal anatomic boundaries and instead follows the outline of the radiation port, is diagnostic

Other causes of interstitial lung disease will be discussed separately in their appropriate organ system sections.

TABLE 4-8 Comparing Types of Pneumoconiosis

EXPOSURE	KEY FEATURES
Asbestosis	• Risk factors: shipyard workers, plumbers, insulators, pipe fitting • Primarily affects lower lung lobes • Pleural plaques • Ferruginous bodies: asbestos fibers that resemble dumbbells • Increased risk of bronchogenic carcinoma in mesothelioma
Coal worker's pneumoconiosis (CWP)	• Risk factors: coal miner • Simple CWP: multiple small lung nodules involving the upper lobes • Complicated CWP: multiple coalesce lung nodules >1 cm, progressive massive fibrosis • Caplan syndrome: rheumatoid arthritis with interstitial lung disease
Silicosis	• Risk factors: sandblasting, quarry miners • Eggshell calcifications and lung nodules primarily involving upper lobes • Increased risk of pulmonary tuberculosis due to interference with macrophage phagocytosis
Berylliosis	• Risk factors: manufacturing (aerospace, electronics, ceramics, fluorescent bulbs, dental) • Chest x-ray: hilar adenopathy similar to sarcoidosis • Biopsy: noncaseating granulomas • Good response to steroids

These are a group of restrictive lung diseases associated with occupational exposures.

- ▪ Bleomycin, busulfan
- ▪ Amiodarone
- ▪ Nitrofurantoin
- Autoimmune
- Granulomatous-associated
- Pulmonary alveolar proteinosis
- Radiation
- Smoke inhalation, gastric aspiration

- Signs and symptoms
  - Chronic worsening dyspnea
  - Persistent nonproductive cough
  - Tachypnea, cyanosis, clubbing
  - Crackles, "velcro rales"
- Diagnosis: diagnosis of exclusion
  - High-resolution CT pattern +/− biopsy to determine specific cause
  - PFTs
    - Restrictive lung disease pattern
    - Low DLCO
- Management: symptomatic; often presents in late-stage disease with poor prognosis
  - Removal of causative agent
  - Glucocorticoids +/− immunosuppressants (azathioprine, mycophenolate)
  - Antifibrotic agents (pirfenidone): early results shown to slow disease progression by downregulating production of growth factors and procollagen
  - Lung transplant

Sarcoidosis

- Risk factors
  - Females
  - 20–40 years old
  - Blacks
- Signs and symptoms
  - Asymptomatic
  - Pulmonary
    - Dyspnea on exertion
    - Fine rales, respiratory distress
  - Extrapulmonary
    - HEENT
      ○ Parotid enlargement
      ○ Uveitis, iritis
    - Neurologic
      ○ Facial nerve palsy
      ○ Hydrocephalus, lymphocytic meningitis
      ○ Guillain-Barré syndrome
    - Dermatologic
      ○ Lupus pernio (reddish purple cutaneous lesion involving cheeks, nose, lips, and ears)
      ○ Erythema nodosum
    - Cardiac
      ○ Arrhythmias (complete atrioventricular block)
      ○ Restrictive cardiomyopathy
      ○ Valvular dysfunction
    - GI: hepatosplenomegaly
    - Musculoskeletal: arthritis
    - Renal
      ○ Interstitial nephritis
      ○ Nephrolithiasis (secondary to hypercalcemia from vitamin D–producing macrophages)
    - Endocrine (secondary to granulomatous infiltration)
      ○ Hypopituitarism
      ○ Adrenal insufficiency
- Associated syndromes
  - Heerfordt syndrome (uveoparotid fever): parotid enlargement and uveitis
  - Lofgren syndrome (acute sarcoidosis): arthritis, erythema nodosum, hilar adenopathy
- Diagnostics
  - Chest x-ray: bilateral hilar adenopathy (Fig. 4-21)
  - Supporting features
    - Pulmonary hypertension
    - Elevated angiotensin-converting enzyme levels
  - Biopsy: noncaseating granulomas
- Management: prednisone

Obesity Hypoventilation Syndrome

- Pathophysiology: massively obese individuals → restrictive lung disease type picture secondary to excessive weight on the thorax → prevents full lung expansion and impaired ability to expel CO_2

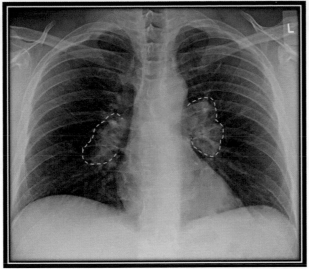

Figure 4-21: Bilateral hilar adenopathy in a patient with sarcoidosis. (Modified image courtesy of James Heilman, MD.)

- Signs and symptoms
  - Respiratory distress
  - Decreased breath sounds
  - Dyspnea on exertion and immobility
- Diagnostics
  - ABG: chronic hypercapnia with metabolic compensation
  - PFTs: restrictive lung disease
    - This differentiates it from COPD patients who also present with chronic hypercapnia with metabolic compensation; however, COPD patients have spirometry consistent with obstructive lung disease
- Management: weight loss +/− bariatric surgery

PULMONARY VASCULAR DISORDERS
Venous Thromboembolism
- Definition: disease spectrum in which venous clots originate from the veins of the lower extremities (legs, pelvis) and lodge themselves into the pulmonary or systemic (right to left shunt) vasculature
- Risk factors
  - Immobility, trauma
  - Inherited coagulopathies (factor V Leiden, antiphospholipid syndrome)
  - Acquired coagulopathies (nephrotic syndrome)
  - Drugs (smoking, oral contraceptive pills)
  - Malignancy (especially pancreatic cancer)
- Signs and symptoms
  - Deep vein thrombosis (DVT) (Table 4-9)
    - Leg circumference discrepancy
    - Unilateral leg pain, erythema
    - Positive Homan sign (pain upon forceful dorsiflexion of the foot)
  - PE (Table 4-10)
    - Cough, shortness of breath, hemoptysis
    - Pleuritic chest pain
    - Tachycardia, hypotension, elevated jugular venous pressure
- Diagnostics
  - Chest x-ray: usually normal; however, may occasionally have some peculiar findings
    - Atelectasis
    - Wedge-shaped infarction: uncommon due to lung's dual blood supply
    - Hampton hump: pleural-based lesion
    - Westermark sign: oligemia of lung lobe
  - CT pulmonary angiogram: filling defect (Fig. 4-22)
  - Lower extremity ultrasound: noncompressible lower extremity veins

TABLE 4-9   Wells Criteria Deep Vein Thrombosis Score Interpretation

PROBABILITY	SCORE	MANAGEMENT
High	3–8 points	Immediate anticoagulation plus lower-extremity Doppler ultrasound
Moderate	1–2 points	Lower-extremity Doppler ultrasound
Low	-2–0 points	D-dimer

TABLE 4-10   Wells Criteria Pulmonary Embolism (PE) Score Interpretation

PROBABILITY	SCORE	MANAGEMENT
PE unlikely	<4	D-dimer
PE likely	>5	Computed tomography angiogram

Three-tier model is also used to divide patients into low risk (<2 points), moderate risk (2–6 points), high risk (>6 points).

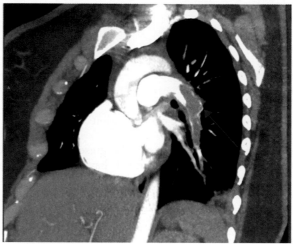

Figure 4-22: Filling defect in the pulmonary artery secondary to pulmonary embolism on computed tomography pulmonary angiogram. (Image courtesy of James Heilman, MD.)

- ECG: sinus tachycardia, nonspecific ST-T wave changes, S1Q3T3, right ventricular (RV) dysfunction (right axis deviation, right bundle branch block)
- Echocardiogram: used to evaluate degree of right heart dysfunction
    - RV dilation/hypokinesis
    - Tricuspid regurgitation
    - Flattening of the interventricular septum and subsequent impaired LV filling
- ABG: respiratory alkalosis, hypoxia
- Management: anticoagulation
    - Prevention
        - Early ambulation postsurgery
        - Subcutaneous heparin
        - Cessation of causative drugs
    - Acute management: low-molecular-weight heparin
        - Heparin should be discontinued once therapeutic International Normalized Ratio (2–2.5) has been achieved and switched to chronic management (warfarin, direct oral anticoagulants [DOACs])
        - Heparin is administered before diagnostic tests are done if there is high suspicion of venous thromboembolism; it can later be discontinued if diagnostic tests come back negative
        - Unfractionated heparin is preferred for patients with severe renal failure
        - Other indications of heparin as anticoagulant of choice include pregnancy and malignancy
    - Chronic management
        - Warfarin for 6 months

- o Epoxide reductase inhibitor preventing synthesis of the vitamin K–dependent clotting factors (2, 7, 9, 10, protein C&S)
  - o Monotherapy in acute PE management can result in warfarin-induced skin necrosis
  - o Protein C has the shortest half-life of all vitamin K–dependent factors and functions as an anticoagulant. Therefore when warfarin is administered as monotherapy, protein C levels are the first to decrease resulting in a temporary prothrombotic state
  - ▪ DOACs
    - o Only direct anticoagulants can be administered without heparin pretreatment
    - o Examples
- Direct thrombin inhibitors (dabigatran, argatroban)
- Xa inhibitors (rivaroxaban, apixaban)
  - ▪ Advantage: do not require injections or monitoring
  - ▪ Disadvantage: reversal agents are not readily available
- Idarucizumab: direct thrombin reversal agent
- Andexanet: Xa inhibitor reversal agent
- Thrombolytics: used in certain clinical settings
  - ▪ Massive PE with unstable vitals
  - ▪ Acute RV dysfunction
- Embolectomy: if there is contraindication or failure of thrombolysis
- Inferior vena cava filters
  - ▪ Contraindications to anticoagulant use
  - ▪ Failure of anticoagulation on therapeutic levels
  - ▪ Severe RV dysfunction: the next PE can potentially be fatal

Wells criteria deep vein thrombosis (DVT) probability: used to stratify patients based on their symptoms and risk factors to determine most appropriate step in management
- -2 points: alternative diagnosis is more likely than DVT
- 1 point:
  - o Lower-extremity paralysis/paresthesia
  - o Recent surgery or mobility
  - o Lower-extremity tenderness
  - o Swelling of entire leg
  - o Lower extremity circumference discrepancy >3 cm
  - o Greater pitting edema in the symptomatic leg
  - o Collateral non-varicose superficial veins
  - o Active or recent cancer (treated with the last six months)

Other tests use to evaluate and diagnose DVT/PE

Wells criteria pulmonary embolism probability:
- 3 points:
  - o Signs and symptoms of DVT or pulmonary embolism (PE) is most likely diagnosis
- 1.5 points:
  - o Heart rate >100
  - o >3 days of mobilization
  - o Surgery within the last 4 weeks
  - o Previous PE or DVT
- 1 point:
  - o Hemoptysis
  - o Malignancy

- D-dimer
  - Highly sensitive rule-out test using patients with low suspicion of DVT/PE. Negative tests (D-dimer <500) requires no further workup, positive test should prompt CT pulmonary angiogram and/or lower extremity Doppler ultrasound
  - May be falsely elevated by infection, inflammation, age >50
  - Ensure adjusted D-dimer calculator is used for patients age >50
- Ventilation/perfusion (V/Q) scan
  - Used where CT angiogram chest is contraindicated

- Nuclear medicine scan that attempts to determine presence of V/Q mismatch
- Less useful in patients with poor lung function (smokers, COPD) as these patients are unable to fully ventilate their lungs with the inhaled tracer
- Results classified as normal, low, moderate, or high probability of PE; only high-probability scan confirms PE

The decision to anticoagulate patients with subsegmental PEs remains controversial.

Other material aside from thrombus can embolize to the heart and lungs resulting in cardiopulmonary compromise. These present under certain clinical circumstances and may have additional extrapulmonary manifestations (Table 4-11).

Pulmonary Hypertension
- Definition: >25/8 mm Hg mean arterial pressure in the pulmonary arteries
- Causes: divided by World Health Organization into five categories based on the etiology
  - Type I: idiopathic pulmonary arterial hypertension (BMPR2 mutation, connective tissue disorders)
  - Type II (most common cause): pulmonary hypertension due to left heart disease (LV dysfunction)
  - Type III: pulmonary hypertension due to primary lung disease (COPD, interstitial lung disease, obstructive sleep apnea) or hypoxia
  - Type IV: pulmonary hypertension due to chronic thromboembolic disease
  - Type V: miscellaneous (glycogen storage disease, myeloproliferative disorder, sarcoidosis, Langerhans histiocytosis, vasculitis)
- Signs and symptoms
  - Angina, dyspnea
  - Syncope
  - Elevated jugular vein distention (JVD), loud S2, RV heave
  - Pitting edema
  - Ascites
  - Hepatomegaly, splenomegaly: secondary to elevated right heart pressures transmitted to the portal venous system
  - Tricuspid regurgitation (systolic murmur at left sternal border that increases with inspiration)
- Diagnostics
  - Chest imaging: enlarged/dilated proximal pulmonary arteries and narrowing of distal vessels
  - ECG: right ventricular hypertrophy, right axis deviation
  - Echocardiogram
  - Right heart or Swan-Ganz catheter: direct measurement of pulmonary pressures
  - V/Q scan (may show chronic thromboembolic disease)
- Management: treat underlying etiology
  - Idiopathic pulmonary hypertension
    - Endothelin receptor antagonists (bosentan, ambrisentan, macitentan)

TABLE 4-11   Other Types of Emboli

TYPE OF EMBOLI	ASSOCIATIONS
Air	- Most commonly due to venous access (central venous, Swan-Ganz catheter, pacemaker), trauma, neurosurgical or otolaryngologic procedures, or barotrauma from mechanical ventilation - Suspect in cases of sudden-onset respiratory distress with known risk factors - Management: supplemental oxygen, left lateral decubitus with head-down position
Fat	- Fractures involving the long bones (humerus, femur) - Other causes include orthopedic surgery and pancreatitis - Triad of respiratory distress, neurologic impairment, petechial rash - Supportive management with most patients making full recovery
Paradoxic	- Connection between the right and left heart (atrial septal defect, ventricular septal defect) results in deep vein thrombosis (DVT) entering the systemic circulation - Consider in patients with DVT presenting with stroke, splenic/renal infarction
Amniotic fluid	- Amniotic fluid enters the maternal systemic circulation during labor and delivery - Presents with sudden onset cardiorespiratory arrest, hemorrhage from disseminated intravascular coagulation, neurologic dysfunction (seizures) - Supportive management with poor outcomes

- Phosphodiesterase inhibitors (sildenafil, tadalafil)
  - Prolongs vasodilatory effect of nitric oxide
  - Also used to treat erectile dysfunction
  - Contraindicated with nitrates
- Prostacyclin analogs (epoprostenol, iloprost, selexipag)
- Guanylate cyclase stimulants (riociguat)
- Diuresis
- Supplemental oxygen
- Lung transplantation
- Complications: cor pulmonale

NEOPLASIA
Lung nodule principles
- Common incidental finding on lung imaging while working up other pathologies
- It is important stratify lung nodules (Table 4-12) to determine further management based on patient risk factors, size, appearance, and previous imaging
- This will determine whether patient will require early intervention, repeat imaging, or no further workup (Table 4-13)
- When lung nodule is detected, the most appropriate next step is to examine previous imaging

Lung Cancer
- Risk factors
  - Smoking
  - Occupational exposure (asbestos)
  - Previous thoracic radiation
- Key manifestations
  - Cough, fever, weight loss
  - Chest pain, dyspnea
  - Wheezing, tachypnea
  - Pleural effusion, postobstructive pneumonia
  - Phrenic nerve, recurrent laryngeal nerve palsy
  - Pancoast tumor: squamous cell carcinoma of the superior sulcus
    - Horner syndrome: triad of ptosis, miosis, and anhidrosis due to invasion of superior cervical ganglion
    - Brachial plexus palsies

TABLE 4-12   Comparing High-Risk and Low-Risk Lung Nodules

	HIGH-RISK FEATURES	LOW-RISK FEATURES
Patient risk factors	• Heavy smoker (>30 pack-yr history) • Previous thoracic radiation (breast cancer, Hodgkin lymphoma, thyroid carcinoma) • >40 yr old	• Non-smoker • No previous radiation • <35 yr old
Appearance	• Sparse calcification • Spiculated surface • Subsolid	• Dense calcification • Smooth surface • Solid
Size	• >2 cm	• <9 mm
Previous imaging	• Previously not present or enlarging nodule	• Present but unchanged over several years

TABLE 4-13   Management is Based on Whether Nodule is Low, Moderate, or High Risk of Being Malignant

TYPE OF NODULE	MANAGEMENT
High risk	• Video-assisted thoracic surgery excisional biopsy • Nonsurgical biopsy if patient is a poor surgical candidate

Intermediate risk	• Noncontrast surveillance computed tomography chest
	• Nonsurgical biopsy
	  • Bronchoscopy: centrally located lesions
	  • Transthoracic needle biopsy: smaller peripherally located lesions

Low risk	• No further workup

Other causes of superior vena cava syndrome: fibrosing mediastinitis (tuberculosis or histoplasmosis infection), upper extremity deep vein thrombosis, lymphoma

- • Superior vena cava (SVC) syndrome: carcinoma obstructing the SVC and impeding venous return of blood from head, neck, and arms
  - ▪ Facial plethora
  - ▪ Ipsilateral neck vein distention
  - ▪ JVD
- • Metastases: bone, adrenal, brain
- – Types/location
  - • Central
    - ▪ Small cell lung cancer: all other cancers are considered non–small cell lung cancer
    - ▪ Squamous cell carcinoma
  - • Peripheral
    - ▪ Adenocarcinoma
    - ▪ Large cell carcinoma
    - ▪ Bronchoalveolar carcinoma
- – Paraneoplastic syndromes
  - • Small cell lung cancer
    - ▪ Lambert-Eaton syndrome (antibodies against presynaptic voltage-gated calcium channels)
    - ▪ Syndrome of inappropriate antidiuretic hormone
    - ▪ Ectopic adrenocorticotropic hormone (Cushing)
    - ▪ Cerebellar degeneration (anti-Yo antibodies), encephalomyelitis (anti-hU antibodies)
  - • Squamous cell carcinoma: parathyroid hormone–related peptide (hypercalcemia)
  - • Adenocarcinoma: hypertrophic pulmonary osteoarthropathy (digital clubbing)
  - • Large cell carcinoma: beta-human chorionic gonadotropin (gynecomastia, galactorrhea)
  - • Other paraneoplastic syndromes: polymyositis, dermatomyositis, hypercoagulability (Trousseau syndrome, DVT)
- – Diagnostics
  - • Chest imaging: lung mass with high-risk features (Figs. 4-23 and 4-24)
    - ▪ Squamous cell carcinoma: central cavitation and necrosis
    - ▪ Bronchoalveolar carcinoma: mimics pneumonia
  - • Sputum cytology
  - • Fluorodeoxyglucose positron emission tomography scan

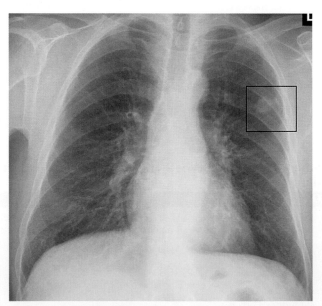

Figure 4-23: Lung nodule on chest x-ray in the left upper lobe. (Image courtesy of Hellerhoff.)

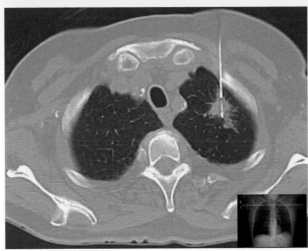

Figure 4-24: Computed tomography–guided lung biopsy of left lung mass, highly suspicious for cancer. (Image courtesy of Hellerhoff.)

- Biopsy: important to differentiate the different subtypes of lung cancer as this will determine whether patient will require surgery vs chemoradiation
  - Staging: CT chest/abdomen/pelvis; magnetic resonance imaging brain
- Management: overall poor prognosis due to late-stage detection
  - Small cell lung cancer: chemoradiation
  - Non–small cell lung cancer: surgical excision
    - Obtain PFTs before surgery to determine if patient has the necessary lung reserve to tolerate a pneumonectomy/lobectomy
    - Minimum FEV1 of 800 mL postsurgery is required
- Screening: annual low-dose chest CT
  - Criteria: must meet all three to qualify
    - 55–80 years old
    - >30 pack-year smoking history
    - <15 years smoking free

Adenocarcinoma is the most common cause of lung cancer in females and nonsmokers.

ACUTE RESPIRATORY DISTRESS SYNDROME (ARDS)
- Pathophysiology: severe lung injury that results in leaky capillaries and accumulation of fluid in the alveoli
- Causes
  - Sepsis
  - Aspiration
  - Pneumonia
  - Trauma, pulmonary contusion
  - Burns
  - Pancreatitis
- Signs and symptoms
  - Dyspnea
  - Hypoxia, hypercapnia
  - Crackles, rhonchi
- Diagnostics
  - Clinical
  - Chest x-ray: complete "white out" with bilateral infiltrates (Fig. 4-25)
  - PO_2/FiO_2 ratio <300
  - ABG: low PaO_2, high $PaCO_2$
  - Brain natriuretic peptide: normal

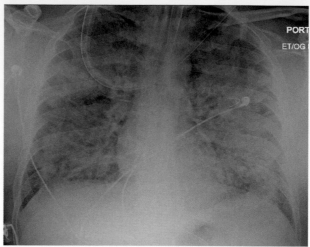

Figure 4-25: Complete whiteout of the lungs in a patient with acute respiratory distress syndrome. (Image courtesy of James Heilman, MD.)

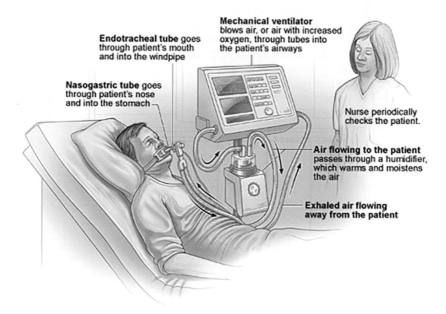

Figure 4-26: Diagram depicting various aspects of a typical mechanically ventilated patient in the intensive care unit. (Image courtesy of National Heart Lung and Blood Institute.)

- • Swan-Ganz catheter: normal pulmonary capillary wedge pressure (PCWP); differentiates it from congestive heart failure (CHF), which has an elevated PCWP
- – Management: respiratory support with mechanical ventilation
  - • Low tidal volume ventilation: mild hypercapnic respiratory acidosis is expected and tolerated
  - • Lowest FiO_2 necessary to maintain oxygenation due to risk of oxygen toxicity

Ventilators
Noninvasive Ventilation
- – Definition: ventilation that does not require use of an artificial airway (i.e., endotracheal tube) (Fig. 4-26)
- – Types
  - • Continuous positive airway pressure
  - • BiPAP

– Indications: respiratory failure unresponsive to less aggressive forms of supplemental oxygen (high-flow oxygen, nasal cannula) and prior to attempting mechanical ventilation
  • Hypercapnic respiratory failure in COPD exacerbation
  • Cardiogenic pulmonary edema
  • Acute hypoxemic respiratory failure
– Contraindications
  • Impaired mental status, inability to cooperate
  • Vomiting
  • Need for emergent intubation
  • Facial surgery

Mechanical Ventilation

– Definition: ventilation that involves direct access to the trachea via an artificial airway
– Types of airways
  • Orotracheal: most common
  • Nasotracheal
  • Tracheostomy
– Indications for intubation
  • Altered mental status (Glasgow Coma Scale <8): most common
  • Severe hypoxemia/hypercarbia (e.g., COPD exacerbation, CHF exacerbation, pneumonia) unresponsive to noninvasive ventilation
  • Airway protection: hematemesis, hemoptysis
– Goals
  • Oxygenation: increase FiO_2 and/or positive end-expiratory pressure
  • Ventilation: increase respiratory rate and/or tidal volume
  • Airway protection
– Indications for extubating: underlying reason for intubation has been treated
  • Improved mentation
  • Improved oxygenation and ventilation

Approach to ABG Interpretation

ABG interpretation requires a stepwise approach (Fig. 4-27) by first determining whether the pH is within the normal or abnormal range (Table 4-14). Subsequently, once it has been determined to be

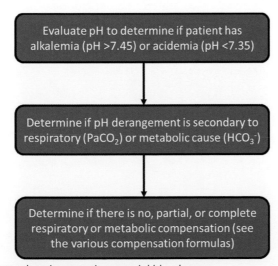

Figure 4-27: Algorithmic approach to interpreting arterial blood gases.

TABLE 4-14   Normal Arterial Blood Gas Values

PARAMETER	NORMAL VALUES
pH	7.35–7.45
HCO_3^-	22–28 mEq/L
$PaCO_2$	35–45 mm Hg
PaO_2	80–100 mm Hg

TABLE 4-15   Formulas for Primary Respiratory and Metabolic Disorders

PRIMARY DISORDER	COMPENSATORY FORMULA
Metabolic acidosis	$PaCO_2 = 1.5 \times [HCO_3^-] + 8 \pm 2$
Metabolic alkalosis	$PaCO_2 = 0.7 \times [HCO_3^-] + 20 \pm 5$
Respiratory acidosis	Every 10-mm Hg increase in $PaCO_2$, $[HCO_3^-]$ should increase by 1 mmol/L acutely and 4 mmol/L chronically
Respiratory alkalosis	Every 10-mm Hg decrease in $PaCO_2$, $[HCO_3^-]$ should decrease by 2 mmol/L acutely, and 5 mmol/L chronically

In addition, pH decreases by 0.08 acutely and 0.03 chronically in respiratory acidosis. The reverse is true in respiratory alkalosis, as pH increases by 0.08 acutely and 0.03 chronically.

abnormal, the source can be determined based on ABG findings. Lastly, compensatory formulas can determine whether the patient is responding appropriately to maintain the pH within a normal range (Table 4-15).

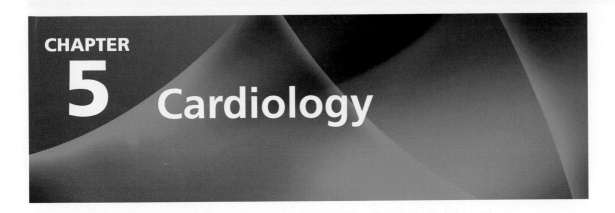

CORONARY ARTERY DISEASE

Coronary Artery Disease
- Risk factors
  - Hypertension
  - Diabetes
  - Dyslipidemia (elevated low-density lipoprotein [LDL], decreased high-density lipoprotein [HDL])
  - Autoimmune (systemic lupus erythematosus [SLE], rheumatoid arthritis)
  - Family history
  - Drugs (cocaine, smoking)
- Pathophysiology: deposition of atherosclerotic plaques along the lumen of the coronary vessels (Fig. 5-1), which results in progressive narrowing and ischemia to the distal myocardium without infarction
- Signs and symptoms: substernal chest pain
  - Worsened by exertion
  - Improved by nitroglycerin or rest
- Diagnostics (Table 5-1)
  - Intensity of diagnostic testing dependent upon risk stratification (TIMI score)
    - Low risk: no diagnostic testing indicated
    - Intermediate risk: cardiac stress test
    - High risk: cardiac catheterization
  - Electrocardiogram (ECG): evaluate for ST elevation, T-wave inversions, new left bundle branch block (LBBB)
  - Troponins: sensitive for myocardial damage
  - Calcium scoring: look for evidence of calcium deposition in the coronary arteries; higher calcium score indicates greater coronary artery disease
- Management: risk factor modification
  - Lifestyle modifications
    - Weight loss
    - DASH diet (low salt, low fat, high fiber)
    - Smoking cessation
    - Exercise (30 min/day, 5×/week)
  - Antihypertensive with goal <140/90: thiazides, calcium channel blockers, angiotensin-converting enzyme (ACE)/angiotensin-receptor blocker (ARB) are all considered first line
  - Antianginal
    - Beta blockers (metoprolol)
    - Calcium channel blockers (verapamil, diltiazem)
    - Sublingual nitrate: used for acute angina
    - Ranolazine: used for refractory angina
  - Antiplatelets: aspirin or clopidogrel (if aspirin intolerant)
  - Strict glycemic control with goal HbA1c <7%
  - Medium to high-intensity statin (atorvastatin, rosuvastatin) with goal LDL <100

Maximal heart rate = 220 minus patient's age

MYOCARDIAL INFARCTION (MI)

ST elevation myocardial infarction (STEMI)
- Risk factors: same as coronary artery disease

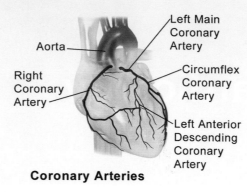

Figure 5-1: Coronary artery anatomy. (Image courtesy of Blausen Medical.)

TABLE 5-1   Diagnostic testing for coronary artery disease

TEST	FEATURES
ECG	• Quick, cheap, noninvasive test • Screens for ST-T wave abnormalities
Troponin	• Highly sensitive test used to screen for evidence of myocardial damage • Positive within 3–6 hr, peaks at 24 hr, remains positive for up to 2 wk
CK-MB	• Enzyme used to detect myocardial damage, not as sensitive as troponin • May be used to detect reinfarction as levels return to normal within 36–48 hr

Stress test	• ECG stress test: first-line stress test if patient has normal baseline ECG, able to exercise (increase heart rate >85% maximum); provides good prognostic information
	  • Positive test: ST segment depression, chest pain, hypotension, lightheadedness/dizziness
	• Nuclear myocardial perfusion: use in patients who cannot exercise
	  • Positive test: decreased uptake of nuclear tracer at increased heart rate with normal uptake at rest; this indicates evidence of reversible ischemia and myocardial tissue that may benefit from revascularization
	• Dobutamine stress echocardiogram: use in patients who cannot exercise; equivalent to myocardial perfusion scan; dobutamine is a beta-1 agonist that increases heart rate and myocardial oxygen demand
	  • Positive test: wall motion abnormalities (dyskinesis, hypokinesis) at increased heart rates

CT calcium score	• Alternative for patients with intermediate risk and unable to exercise; detects calcification of coronary arteries • Calcium score >100 indicates increased likelihood of cardiac event • Lack of coronary artery calcification has high negative predictive value for cardiac event
Coronary angiography	• Invasive test that directly visualizes coronary arteries; catheter inserted through radial or femoral artery and contrast dye is injected into the coronary arteries to visualize coronary artery anatomy • Ideal test for high-risk patient with high likelihood of coronary artery disease, NSTEMI/STEMI • Allows for intervention with stent placement and revascularization • Risks include development of hematoma or pseudoaneurysm at catheter insertion point (less common with radial artery insertion), atheroembolic disease (livedo reticularis, acute interstitial nephritis with urine eosinophilia, pancreatitis)

ECG, Electrocardiography; *NSTEMI,* non-ST elevation myocardial infarction; *STEMI,* ST elevation myocardial infarction.

TABLE 5-2   Differentiating angina, NSTEMI, and STEMI

	CHEST PAIN	TROPONIN	ST ELEVATION
Stable angina	Only on exertion	Negative	Negative
Unstable angina	Worsening of previous chest pain, presence of chest pain with less exertion compared to previously	Negative	Negative
NSTEMI	Persistent, unrelenting, unrelieved by rest or nitroglycerin	Positive	Negative
STEMI	Persistent, unrelenting, unrelieved by rest nitroglycerin	Positive	Positive

NSTEMI, non-ST elevation myocardial infarction; *STEMI,* ST elevation myocardial infarction.

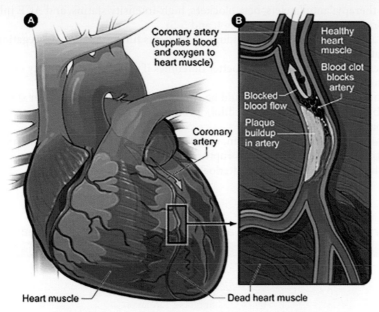

Figure 5-2: Pathophysiology of myocardial infarction.

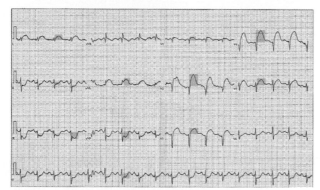

Figure 5-3: Example electrocardiography tracings showing anterior myocardial infarction with reciprocal changes and the inferior leads.

- Pathophysiology: rupture of atherosclerotic plaque resulting in 100% occlusion of coronary artery and infarction of myocardial tissue (Fig. 5-2)
- Sign and symptoms (Table 5-2)
  - Substernal, pressure-like chest pain with radiation to the neck and left arm
  - Pain lasting >20 minutes, unrelieved by rest or nitroglycerin
  - Diaphoresis
  - Sensation of doom
  - Nausea, vomiting
  - Shortness of breath, jugular vein distention (JVD), crackles on auscultation
  - Atypical signs and symptoms seen in elderly, women, diabetics
- Diagnostics
  - Elevated troponin, CK-MB
  - ECG: ST elevation in contiguous leads and distributions; new LBBB (Fig. 5-3)
    - Lead II, III, aVF: right coronary artery (RCA) occlusion, inferior/posterior wall infarction +/− right ventricle infarction
    - Lead I, aVL, V5, V6: left circumflex occlusion, lateral wall infarction
    - V1, V2: left anterior descending (LAD) septal branches, septal infarction
    - V3, V4: distal LAD, anterior wall infarction (worst prognosis)
  - Cardiac catheterization
- Management
  - Revascularization via percutaneous coronary intervention (PCI)
    - Door to balloon time of <90 minutes at PCI-capable facility
    - Door to balloon time of <120 minutes at a non–PCI-capable facility
    - Antifibrinolytics: tissue plasminogen activator if PCI cannot be performed within the appropriate time windows

- Medical therapy: antiplatelets, beta blockers, high-intensity statins, and ACE inhibitors/ARBs have mortality benefits (Tables 5-3, 5-4, and 5-5)
  - Dual antiplatelet (aspirin + clopidogrel): prevents further platelet aggregation and thrombus formation
    - Ticagrelor or prasugrel have better outcomes if coronary angioplasty or stenting is planned
    - Dual antiplatelet therapy should be continued for 6–12 months after stent placement
  - Beta blockers (metoprolol, carvedilol): prolongs diastole allowing for increased time for coronary perfusion
  - High-intensity statin (atorvastatin, rosuvastatin): decreases LDL cholesterol, stabilizes endothelial plaque, and prevents rupture
  - ACE inhibitor/ARB: decreases afterload, improves systolic function

TABLE 5-3 Pharmacology of coronary artery disease and congestive heart failure

	MORTALITY BENEFIT	MECHANISM OF ACTION	SIDE EFFECT
Aspirin	Yes	• Cyclooxygenase inhibitor preventing platelet aggregation and thrombus formation	• Bleeding, gastritis
Beta blockers (metoprolol, carvedilol, bisoprolol)	Yes	• Decreases heart rate, prolongs diastole to allow coronary artery perfusion • Decreases myocardial oxygen demand	• Bradycardia, hypotension, • Exacerbation of asthma or COPD • Sexual dysfunction
ACE inhibitor, angiotensin receptor blockers	Yes	• Prevents deleterious effects of RAAS and ventricular remodeling • ACE inhibitors: efferent arteriole vasodilator decreasing glomerular hyperfiltration	• Cough, angioedema • Hyperkalemia • Mild renal dysfunction (tolerate up to >30% increase in creatinine after initiation) • If patient develops cough on ACE inhibitor, switch to angiotensin receptor blocker
Statins (atorvastatin, rosuvastatin)	Yes	• Decreases LDL cholesterol • Stabilize endothelial plaques preventing rupture due to antioxidant effect	• Transaminitis, myositis • Myositis worsened when combined with fibrate (gemfibrozil)
Hydralazine/nitrates	Yes, particularly in black patients	• Combination of arterial and venous vasodilator • Decreases afterload; decreases preload, which decreases myocardial oxygen demand	• Hypotension • Flushing • Reflex tachycardia
Mineralocorticoid receptor antagonists (spironolactone, eplerenone)	Yes, only in select cases: NYHA class III/IV, ejection fraction <35%, ejection fraction <40% after STEMI	• Aldosterone receptor antagonist • Prevents deleterious effects of RAAS and ventricular remodeling	• Hyperkalemia • Antiandrogenic → gynecomastia (only with spironolactone) • If patient develops gynecomastia on spironolactone, switch to eplerenone
Digoxin	No; however, decreases length of hospital stay	• Sodium-potassium ATPase inhibitor resulting in increased intracellular calcium and myocardial contractility • AV nodal blocker	• Digoxin toxicity: nausea, vomiting, anorexia, visual disturbances (halos), atrial tachycardia, AV block • Increased risk of toxicity in hypokalemia and renal dysfunction
Loop diuretics (furosemide)	No; first line for symptomatic pulmonary edema	• Inhibits sodium-potassium to chloride channel at the loop of Henle	• Electrolyte abnormalities: hypokalemia, hypomagnesemia, hypocalcemia • If there is allergic reaction to sulfur component, switch to ethacrynic acid

ACE, Angiotensin-converting enzyme; *AV,* atrioventricular; *COPD,* chronic obstructive pulmonary disease; *LDL,* low-density lipoprotein; *NYHA,* New York Heart Association; *RAAS,* renin-angiotensin-aldosterone system; *STEMI,* ST elevation myocardial infarction.

TABLE 5-4 Other medications used in coronary artery disease

	USES	MECHANISM OF ACTION	SIDE EFFECT
Clopidigrel	• Part of dual antiplatelet therapy during acute myocardial infarction • Aspirin intolerant in any condition where aspirin is commonly used (strokes, peripheral artery disease) • 6–12 mo poststenting to reduce risk of drug-eluting stent thrombosis	• Adenosine diphosphate (ADP) receptor antagonist preventing platelet aggregation	• Bleeding • Rarely associated with thrombotic thrombocytopenic purpura (TTP)
Ticagrelor, prasugrel, ticlopidine	• Prasugrel/ticagrelor best for angioplasty and stenting in combination with aspirin	• ADP receptor antagonist preventing platelet aggregation	• Ticlopidine: associated with neutropenia, TTP • Bleeding
Heparin	• Non-ST segment myocardial infarction (NSTEMI), unstable angina	• Increases potency of antithrombin III	• Bleeding • Heparin-induced thrombocytopenia: increases risk of thrombosis; switch to direct thrombin inhibitors (dabigatran, bivalirudin)
Abciximab, tirofiban, eptifibatide	• NSTEMI (produces mortality benefit), percutaneous coronary intervention, and stenting	• Inhibit platelet aggregation by blocking glycoprotein IIb/IIIa	• Bleeding

TABLE 5-5 Antihyperlipidemics

	MECHANISM OF ACTION	SIDE EFFECTS
Fibrates	• Inhibits lipoprotein lipase reducing triglycerides	• Elevated LFTs • Increased risk of myopathy when combined with statins • Cholesterol gallstones
Niacin	• Increases HDL	• Flushing, pruritus (due to release of histamine, prostaglandins); relieved by taking NSAIDs prior to medication • Hyperuricemia, hyperglycemia
Ezetimibe	• Blocks LDL reabsorption via the intestinal border	• Diarrhea
Cholestyramine	• Bile acid sequestrants preventing reabsorption of bile acids via enterohepatic circulation → forces liver to use cholesterol to replace lost bile acids	• Bloating, flatus, diarrhea • Fat-soluble vitamin deficiencies • Drug interactions • Binds to *Clostridium difficile* toxin

HDL, High-density lipoprotein; *LDL*, low-density lipoprotein; *LFTs*, liver function tests; *NSAIDs*, nonsteroidal antiinflammatory drugs.

- Complications
  - Arrhythmias
    - Ventricular fibrillation
      - Most common cause of death post-MI
      - Occur within the first 24 hours
      - Treat with defibrillation and amiodarone
    - Bradycardia
      - Sinus node infarction secondary to RCA occlusion
      - Treat with atropine or cardiac pacing
  - Hypotension
    - Occurs after right ventricular infarction (ST elevation in RV4)
    - Will present with hypotension, JVD, clear lungs; avoid nitrates if suspected
    - Treat with aggressive IV fluids to increase preload; may use inotropic agents (dobutamine, dopamine, milrinone) if unresponsive to fluids

- Pericarditis
  - Acute pericarditis
    - Transmural infarction results in adjacent inflammation of the pericardium; develops within 2–5 days
    - Presents with pain that improves when sitting up and worse when lying down
    - Presence of pericardial friction rub, diffuse ST elevation on ECG
    - Treat with acetaminophen/aspirin; avoid other nonsteroidal antiinflammatory drugs (NSAIDs) the first 7–10 days after MI
  - Dressler syndrome
    - Post-MI autoimmune syndrome; develops weeks after myocardial infarction
    - Pericardial antigens are released into the blood post-MI resulting in development of immune response and antibodies against antigens
    - Treat with NSAIDs +/− colchicine
- Mechanical: develops within 3–7 days after MI
  - Septal rupture
    - Results in formation of ventricular septal defect; new holosystolic murmur at left sternal border
    - Step up in oxygenation from right atrium to right ventricle
    - Urgent repair required
  - Papillary muscle rupture
    - Most commonly involves the mitral valve resulting in acute mitral regurgitation and pulmonary edema
    - New-onset systolic murmur heard at the cardiac apex with radiation to the axilla
    - Urgent repair required
  - Free wall rupture
    - Infarcted myocardium is weakened making it prone to free wall rupture
    - Treat with emergency pericardiocentesis and surgical repair

CONGESTIVE HEART FAILURE
Congestive Heart Failure (CHF)
- Risk factors: same as coronary artery disease
- Causes
  - Coronary artery disease
  - Infections
    - Viral myocarditis
    - Parasites (*Trypanosoma cruzi* infection: Chagas disease)
  - Chemotherapy
    - Doxorubicin (irreversible cardiotoxicity)
    - Trastuzumab (reversible cardiotoxicity)
  - Alcohol, thiamine deficiency
- Types
  - Systolic (decreased ejection fraction)
  - Diastolic (preserved ejection fraction)
- Signs and symptoms
  - Dyspnea on exertion
  - Orthopnea, paroxysmal nocturnal dyspnea
  - Displaced apical impulse
  - Chest pain, palpitations
  - Increased JVD
  - Pitting lower extremity edema
- Diagnostics
  - Echocardiogram
  - Chest x-ray (Fig. 5-4)
- Management: see pharmacotherapy table (see Table 5-3)

Pharmacotherapy in the Treatment of Coronary Artery Disease and Congestive Heart Failure
   Other Causes of Chest Pain
Prinzmetal Angina (Vasospastic Angina)
- Pathophysiology: transient vasospasm of coronary arteries resulting in ST elevation without troponin elevation
- Risk factors
  - Lack typical coronary artery disease risk factors
  - Associated with other vasospastic disorders (smoking, migraines, esophageal spasm)

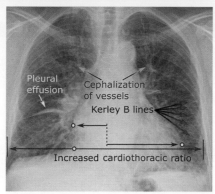

Figure 5-4: Radiographic signs of pulmonary edema in a patient with congestive heart failure. (Image courtesy of Mikael Häggström.)

- Signs and symptoms: unpredictable cardiac chest pain occurring at rest/night, in women and younger patients
- Diagnostics
  - Ambulatory ECG
    - Ventricular arrythmias
    - Transient ST elevation during episodes of chest pain
  - Coronary angiography to rule out coronary artery disease
  - Vasospastic episodes may be induced by intracoronary acetylcholine/ergonovine and may aid in diagnosis
- Management
  - Vasodilators: calcium channel blockers, sublingual nitrates
  - Caution with triptans, propranolol, aspirin (inhibits prostaglandin) as these medications may worsen vasospasm

Takotsubo Cardiomyopathy (Stress-Induced Cardiomyopathy)
- Epidemiology: postmenopausal woman
- Pathophysiology: overwhelming, highly stressful life-threatening event (physical, emotional) resulting in excessive release of catecholamines (epinephrine, norepinephrine) and transient systolic dysfunction
- Signs and symptoms: similar to acute MI
  - Chest pain
  - Shortness of breath
  - Diaphoresis
  - Nausea, vomiting
- Diagnostics: same as coronary artery disease/MI
  - ECG: ST elevation
  - Elevated troponins
  - Echocardiogram: left ventricular apical ballooning
  - Cardiac catheterization: normal coronary angiography
- Management: most cases are self-resolving once acute stressor subsides
- Complications
  - Heart failure
  - Cardiogenic shock

Anomalous Coronary Arteries
- Coronary arteries that pass between the great vessels
- During increased activity, great vessels dilate causing compression of the coronary arteries resulting in chest pain, syncope, or sudden death
- Detected by computed tomography (CT) angiogram

Cardiovascular abnormalities are just one of the many organ systems that present with chest pain. Other organ systems can similarly present with chest pain and must be thoroughly evaluated due to life-threatening potential (Table 5-6).

Hypertension

Essential Hypertension
- Risk factors
  - Elderly
  - Blacks

TABLE 5-6   Noncardiac causes of chest pain

ORGAN SYSTEM	ETIOLOGIES
Dermatologic	• Herpes zoster
Musculoskeletal	• Costochondritis • Rib fracture
Pulmonary	• Pleurisy/pleuritis • Pneumonia • Pulmonary embolism • Pneumothorax
Gastrointestinal	• Gastroesophageal reflux disease • Esophageal rupture (Boerhaave syndrome)
Psychiatric	• Panic attack

- • Western diet (high salt, high fat)
- • Smoking, obesity, alcohol
- • Family history
- – Signs and symptoms: asymptomatic unless patient has a hypertensive emergency (severe hypertension with end-organ damage)
- – Diagnostics
  - • Two separate blood pressure readings done 2 weeks apart >140/90
  - • Ambulatory blood pressure readings if office readings are significantly elevated compared to patient's home blood pressure readings; may be indicative of white coat hypertension
- – Management
  - • Lifestyle modification
    - • Weight loss
    - • Dietary modification
    - • Smoking/alcohol cessation
  - • Medical management: thiazide diuretics, calcium channel blockers, ACE/ARBs (Table 5-7)
    - • All three classes are equivalent for management of primary hypertension
    - • Thiazides and calcium channel blockers are preferred in blacks
    - • ACE/ARBs are preferred in diabetics and chronic kidney disease
- – Complications
  - • Related to longstanding chronic hypertension (Fig. 5-5)
  - • Hypertensive urgency: blood pressure >180/110 without evidence of end-organ damage
  - • Hypertensive emergency: blood pressure >180/110 with evidence of end-organ damage (headache, visual disturbances, MI, stroke, aortic dissection, pulmonary edema, transaminitis, acute kidney injury); these are often seen in the patients with secondary causes of hypertension (Table 5-8)

Management of hypertensive urgency/emergency
- – Treat with gradual lowering of blood pressure, 25% decrease in mean arterial pressure over first 24 hours to avoid ischemic injury (MI, stroke)
- – Management: all the following are good options to lower blood pressure, and the choice should be based on the patient's comorbidities and side effect profile
  - • Labetalol
  - • Hydralazine
  - • Nicardipine, clevidipine
  - • Fenoldopam (dopamine agonists)
  - • Enalapril
  - • Nitroprusside (increases release of nitric oxide; monitor for cyanide toxicity during prolonged infusion and renal insufficiency)

Cyanide toxicity: elevated anion gap acidosis (lactic acidosis), flushing (cherry red) respiratory distress, arrhythmias, almond breath, altered mental status, seizures, coma. Treat with sodium nitrite, sodium thiosulfate, or hydroxocobalamin

Medications causing drug-induced lupus: sulfasalazine, hydralazine, isoniazid, phenytoin, procainamide, etanercept

TABLE 5-7 Pharmacotherapy of hypertension

MEDICATION	MECHANISM OF ACTION	SIDE EFFECTS	OTHER USES
Thiazide diuretics	• Inhibits NaCl channel in distal convoluted tubule	• Hyperglycemia, hyperlipidemia, hyperuricemia (gout), hypercalcemia, hyponatremia, hypokalemia, hypomagnesemia • Allergic reaction (sulfa drug) • Associated with causing acute pancreatitis, allergic interstitial nephritis	• Hypertension with concurrent osteoporosis • Recurrent nephrolithiasis secondary to hypercalciuria • Nephrogenic diabetes insipidus
Calcium channel blockers (amlodipine, nifedipine)	• Inhibits calcium from entering smooth muscle arterioles resulting in vasodilation	• Flushing headache, peripheral edema (dilation of precapillary vessels); lower risk when combined with ACE inhibitors, which cause postcapillary venodilation and normalize capillary hydrostatic pressure • Constipation • Gingival hyperplasia • Hyperprolactinemia (verapamil) • AV block	• Stable angina • Dihydropyridine calcium channel blockers (diltiazem, verapamil) used for rate control in atrial fibrillation • Nimodipine to prevent cerebral vasospasm post–subarachnoid hemorrhage
ACE inhibitors (-pril), ARBs (-sartan)	• ACE inhibitors: inhibit conversion of angiotensin I to angiotensin II • ARBs: inhibit effects of angiotensin II on vasculature	• Dry cough (more common with ACE inhibitors → switch to ARBs; occurs due to increased bradykinin and bronchial irritation) • Hyperkalemia, angioedema, teratogenic • Renal insufficiency, especially in the presence of renal artery stenosis • ACE inhibitors associated with drug-induced pemphigus vulgaris	• CHF, post-MI • Diabetic nephropathy
Beta blockers (metoprolol, carvedilol, labetalol)	• AV nodal blocker resulting in decreased heart rate and prolonged diastole	• Bradycardia, hypotension • Sexual dysfunction • Sleepiness, sedation • Worsening asthma/COPD (more common in nonselective beta blockers)	• CHF, post-MI, stable angina, aortic dissection • Migraine prophylaxis • Atrial fibrillation, SVT • Glaucoma (topical beta blockers [timolol]) • Propranolol, nadalol: esophageal variceal prophylaxis (decreases portal pressures) • Propranolol: thyroid storm (decreases adrenergic symptoms), performance anxiety, essential tremors
Hydralazine	• Arterial vasodilator	• Reflex tachycardia • Drug induced lupus (antihistone antibodies)	• Safe to use during pregnancy • Combined with isosorbide dinitrate to treat heart failure in black patients
Alpha blockers (doxazosin, prazosin)	• Blocks alpha receptors on vasculature resulting in vasodilation	• Orthostatic hypotension • Priapism	• Benign prostatic hyperplasia • Prazosin for PTSD nightmares
Clonidine	• Alpha-2 receptor agonist resulting in decreased sympathetic outflow	• Rebound hypertension • CNS depression	• Opiate withdrawal • ADHD • Tourette syndrome
Minoxidil	• Arterial vasodilator, opens potassium channels	• Hypertrichosis	• Topically administer in androgenic alopecia

Hypertensive medication safe in pregnancy: hydralazine, beta blockers, methyldopa, calcium channel blockers.
ACE, Angiotensin-converting enzyme; *ADHD*, attention-deficit/hyperactivity disorder; *ARB*, angiotensin-receptor blocker; *AV*, atrioventricular; *CHF*, congestive heart failure; *CNS*, central nervous system; *COPD*, chronic obstructive pulmonary disease; *MI*, myocardial infarction; *PTSD*, posttraumatic stress disorder; *SVT*, supraventricular tachycardia.

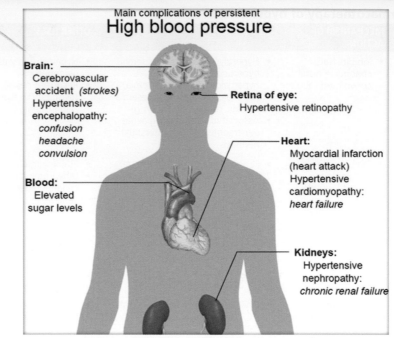

Figure 5-5: Complications of long-standing hypertension involving the brain, eyes, heart, kidneys, and blood. (Image courtesy of Mikael Häggström.)

Aortic Pathologies
Aortic Dissection
- Risk factors
  - Hypertension
  - Connective tissue disorders (cystic medial necrosis): Marfan, Ehlers-Danlos
  - Congenital anomalies: bicuspid aortic valve, aortic coarctation
  - Trauma
  - Cocaine
  - Large vessel vasculitis (giant cell, Takayasu)
- Signs and symptoms
  - Chest pain with radiation to the back
  - Blood pressure differential in upper extremities: uncommon and cannot be used to rule out aortic dissection
- Diagnostics
  - Chest x-ray: widened mediastinum
  - Confirm with CT angiography (normal renal function) (Fig. 5-6), magnetic resonance (MR) angiography (nonemergency) or transesophageal echocardiography (TEE) (abnormal renal function, hemodynamic instability)
- Management
  - Medical
    - Blood pressure control with beta blockers (labetalol, propranolol, metoprolol) to decrease shearing forces in descending aortic dissection
    - Avoid antiplatelet medication if suspicious due to increased risk of bleeding into false lumen
  - Surgical
    - Indicated for ascending aortic dissections (Stanford type A) (Figs. 5-7 and 5-8)
    - May be indicated for descending dissection (Stanford type B) (see Figs. 5-7 and 5-8) dissection that continues to expand or occludes major arteries downstream (renal, iliac)
    - Typically avoided in descending dissections due to risk of injuring spinal arteries branching off the descending aorta
- Complications
  - Proximal extension of dissection
    - Aortic regurgitation
    - Pericardial effusion/tamponade
    - Inferior wall MI (right coronary artery)
    - Stroke (carotid artery)
    - Horner syndrome (superior cervical ganglion)

TABLE 5-8   Causes of secondary hypertension

ETIOLOGY	FEATURES
Renovascular	• Decreased renal perfusion secondary to fibromuscular dysplasia (young female) or atherosclerotic deposition in renal arteries (elderly male) resulting in functional renal artery stenosis and activation of renin-angiotensin-aldosterone system • Abdominal bruit, recurrent flash pulmonary edema, atrophic kidney • Elevated renin and aldosterone (secondary hyperaldosteronism), elevated creatinine (>30%) after initiation of ACE inhibitor or ARB • Diagnose with CT/MR angiography, duplex ultrasound, or renal arteriogram • Fibromuscular dysplasia may involve carotid and vertebral arteries (TIA, stroke, headache, tinnitus, dizziness); treat with antihypertensive and revascularization (percutaneous transluminal angioplasty) • Renovascular hypertension due to atherosclerotic deposition is managed medically with antihypertensive and risk factor modification; no benefit for revascularization
Hyperthyroidism	• Tachycardia, atrial fibrillation, weight loss, irritability, anxiety, heat intolerance, hypertension • Low TSH, increased free T4
Hyperaldosteronism	• May be due to solitary adenoma (most common) or bilateral hyperplasia • Mild hypernatremia, hypokalemia, metabolic alkalosis. No peripheral edema due to aldosterone escape induced diuresis • Easily induced hypokalemia after use of loop/thiazide diuretics, elevated aldosterone after high salt diet, aldosterone-renin ratio >20 • Surgically resect solitary adenoma; medically manage bilateral hyperplasia with aldosterone antagonists (spironolactone, eplerenone)
Hypercortisolism (Cushing disease/ syndrome)	• Weight gain, buffalo hump, hyperglycemia, central obesity, osteoporosis, easy bruising, abdominal striae, CNS disturbances (depression, mania, psychosis), leukocytosis, myopathy, cataracts, glaucoma, peptic ulcers • May have some aldosterone-like effect due to intrinsic mineralocorticoid activity (hypokalemia, metabolic alkalosis) • May be ACTH dependent (pituitary or ectopic tumor) or independent (adrenal adenoma) or iatrogenic (high-dose glucocorticoids) • Cause established using 24-hr urine cortisol, late night salivary cortisol, or dexamethasone suppression test • Treat by stopping the offending agent (glucocorticoids) or surgical resection (pituitary tumor, adrenal adenoma)
Pheochromocytoma	• Adrenal medullary tumor producing excessive catecholamines • Paroxysms of headache, severe hypertension, palpitations, diaphoresis, tremors, panic attack • Control blood pressure with nonselective alpha blockers (phenoxybenzamine, phentolamine) • Avoid use of beta blockers if suspected due to potential unopposed alpha vasoconstriction and development of severe life-threatening hypertension • Elevated urinary and serum metanephrine • Rule of 10s: 10% bilateral, 10% in children, 10% familial (associated with MEN 2 A/2B syndromes, von Hippel-Lindau disease), 10% extraadrenal (organ of Zuckerkandl located at aortic bifurcation), 10% recur, 10% malignant • Treat with surgical resection after optimizing blood pressure control
Coarctation of the aorta	• Elevated blood pressure in upper extremities, low blood pressure in lower extremities (diminished femoral pulses) • Lower extremity claudication, continuous murmur along the left interscapular region, headaches, epistaxis, headaches, visual disturbances, aortic dissection • Associated with Turner syndrome, bicuspid aortic valve, septal defects; may be acquired due to Takayasu arteritis vasculitis • Chest x-ray with evidence of rib notching (enlarged intercostal arteries), "3" sign (aortic indentation) • Diagnose with echocardiogram; treat with balloon angioplasty/stenting
Preeclampsia/eclampsia	• Severe uncontrolled hypertension during pregnancy • Associated with grand mal seizures (eclampsia), proteinuria, renal insufficiency, visual disturbances, headaches, pulmonary edema, HELLP syndrome (hemolysis, elevated liver enzymes, low platelets) • Increased risk of peripartum cardiomyopathy • Treat with blood pressure control (hydralazine, labetalol), delivery, and magnesium
Pain/anxiety	• Release of stress hormones (cortisone, catecholamines) results in elevated blood pressure • Treat underlying etiology

Consider secondary hypertension in any patient with new-onset hypertension who is young (<35), old (>55), or with difficult to control hypertension.
ACE, Angiotensin-converting enzyme; ACTH, adrenocorticotropic hormone; ARB, angiotensin-receptor blocker; CNS, central nervous system; CT/MR, computed tomography/magnetic resonance; TIA, transient ischemic attack; TSH, thyroid-stimulating hormone.

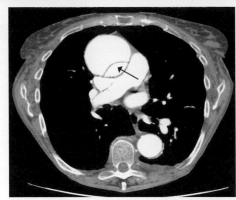

Figure 5-6: Aortic dissection on axial computed tomography chest. (Image courtesy of James Heilman, MD.)

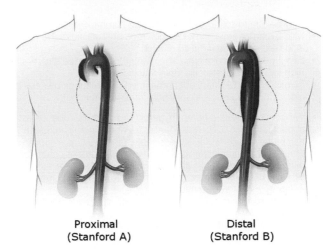

Proximal
(Stanford A)

Distal
(Stanford B)

Figure 5-7: Classification of aortic dissection using the Stanford classification.

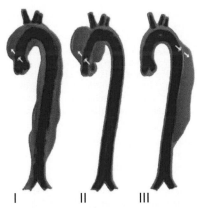

I   II   III

Figure 5-8: Classification of aortic dissection using the DeBakey system. Type I dissections originate in the ascending aorta and extend to involve the aortic arch. Type II tears are confined to the ascending aorta only. Type III tears occur in the descending aorta and extend proximally or distally, however, do not involve the left subclavian artery.

- Distal extension of dissection
  - Renal failure (renal artery)
  - Lower extremity ischemia/claudication (iliac/spinal arteries)
  - Hemothorax

Aortic Aneurysm
  - Definition: dilation of aorta >3 cm
  - Risk factors
    - Smoking
    - Atherosclerosis
    - Hypertension

- Family history, polycystic kidney disease, whites
- Connective tissue disorders (Marfan, Ehlers-Danlos)
- Tertiary syphilis (endarteritis obliterans)
- Trauma
- Medium/large vessel vasculitis (giant cell arteritis, Takayasu, Behcet syndrome)
- Rheumatologic: spondyloarthropathies, rheumatoid arthritis
- Signs and symptoms: depends on location of aneurysm (thoracic vs abdominal)
  - Abdominal aortic aneurysm
    - Asymptomatic (most common)
    - Abdominal/back/flank pain
    - Pulsatile midline abdominal mass
    - Ecchymoses
    - Hypotension, syncope: indicative of impending rupture
  - Thoracic aortic aneurysm
    - Chest pain, shortness of breath
    - Aortic regurgitation murmur
- Diagnostic: typically found on imaging done for other purposes
  - Abdominal ultrasound
  - MR imaging/CT angiogram
- Management: close monitoring ± repair depending on size and rate of expansion
  - Medical management
    - Risk factor modification (blood pressure control, smoking cessation, statin + aspirin)
    - Follow-up ultrasound every 6–12 months
  - Surgical management
    - Indications
      - Aneurysm >5-5 cm
      - Rapidly expanding aneurysm (>1 cm/year)
      - Compressive/erosive complications (esophagus, major artery, intestine)
      - Rupture (emergent repair)
    - May be repaired via endovascular or open surgery; both have similar outcomes, choice depends on anatomy and risk of perioperative complications
- Complications
  - Rupture
  - Atheroembolic disease
  - Fistulas (arteriovenous, aortoduodenal)
- Screening: one-time abdominal ultrasound for males aged 65–75 with current or previous smoking history

Abdominal aortic aneurysm is considered a coronary artery disease equivalent.

Peripheral Artery Disease
- Risk factors
  - Same as coronary artery disease as it is a coronary artery disease equivalent
  - Thromboangiitis obliterans (Buerger disease)
- Signs and symptoms (Fig. 5-9)
  - Commonly affects lower extremities (buttocks, thighs, calf, foot) depending on peripheral artery involved
  - Intermittent claudication worsened by exertion
  - Lower extremity ulcerations involving distal toes
  - Decrease peripheral pulses
  - Atrophied, smooth, shiny skin, poor wound healing, toe ulcerations
  - Limb ischemia, rest pain: severe cases
- Diagnostics
  - Ankle-brachial index (ABI)
    - <0.9 indicative of peripheral artery disease
    - Lower ABI indicates increase disease severity
    - >1.3 indicative of vascular calcification common in diabetics and is nondiagnostic for PAD
  - Toe brachial index: used when ABI is nondiagnostic
  - Arterial angiogram: done prior to surgical intervention to determine severity and location of lesion

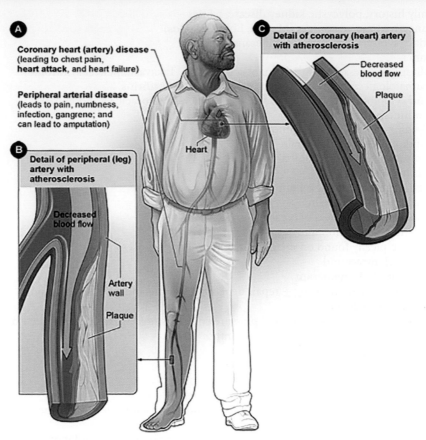

Figure 5-9: Anatomy, pathophysiology, and complications of peripheral artery disease. Buildup of atherosclerotic plaque results in partial obstruction of blood flow, which results in ischemia and exertional pain due to inadequate supply to meet demand. (Image courtesy of the National Heart Lung and Blood Institute.)

- Management
  - Medical
    - Lifestyle modifications
      - Smoking cessation, strict glycemic control
      - Graded exercise regimen: increases collaterals to improve walking distance and quality of life
    - Pharmacotherapy
      - Antiplatelet (aspirin, clopidogrel), statin: first line
      - Cilostazol: second line
  - Surgical: only if patient has failed medical management
    - Percutaneous revascularization
    - Surgical bypass
    - Thrombectomy if patient develops acute arterial occlusion with threatening limb ischemia

Leriche syndrome (aortoiliac disease, peripheral arterial disease subtype): buttock pain/atrophy, erectile dysfunction, decreased femoral pulses

CARDIOMYOPATHY

Cardiomyopathy is an insult to the heart, which may be acquired or genetic resulting in abnormal heart function and changes in the heart morphology (Fig. 5-10). Different insults result in different subtypes of cardiomyopathies and therefore different treatments to treat the underlying cause (Table 5-9).

Athlete's heart: symmetric left ventricular hypertrophy secondary to prolonged intense exercise. Benign entity, however, must be distinguished from hypertrophic obstructive cardiomyopathy.

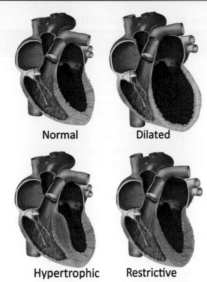

Figure 5-10: Visual representation of the various types of cardiomyopathy and their effects on the ventricular wall thickness. Dilated cardiomyopathy results in a thin-walled left ventricle. Hypertrophic cardiomyopathy results in asymmetric hypertrophy of the ventricular septum. Restrictive cardiomyopathy results in diffuse left ventricular hypertrophy. (Image courtesy of Blausen Medical.)

VALVULAR HEART DISEASE

Left-sided valvular heart disease is far more common than right-sided valvular heart disease. As valvular heart disease progresses in severity it develops characteristic ausculatory findings (Fig. 5-11; Table 5-10), and combined with patient risk factors a particular valvular heart disease diagnosis can be made. Echocardiogram is also essential in evaluating the heart morphology, function, and other associated abnormalities that can ultimately guide treatment and determine whether medical or surgical management is needed (Table 5-11).

Patients with severe valvular disease undergoing cardiac surgery for other indications should have concomitant valvular surgery.

Right-Sided Valvular Disease
- Tricuspid regurgitation
  - Associations
    - IV drug users
    - Pulmonary hypertension
    - Systemic carcinoid (may also cause tricuspid/pulmonic stenosis)
    - Complications of pacemaker placement
  - Auscultation: holosystolic murmur at left sternal border, increased with deep inspiration
  - Management: treat underlying disorders, surgical repair
- Pulmonic stenosis
  - Associations
    - Congenital disorders (congenital rubella infection, tetralogy of Fallot, Noonan syndrome)
    - Systemic carcinoid
  - Auscultation
    - Systolic murmur at the upper left sternal border
    - Increase with deep inspiration
    - Wide splitting S2
    - Pulmonic ejection sound
  - Management: balloon valvuloplasty

All nonbioprosthetic valve replacements will require long-term anticoagulation, and prosthetic valves require preprocedural antibiotic prophylaxis (see Table 5-11).

Mitral Valve Prolapse (MVP)
- Definition: myxomatous degeneration of the mitral valve with associated elongation and redundancy of the chordae tendineae

TABLE 5-9   Differentiating types of cardiomyopathy

	DILATED	RESTRICTIVE	HYPERTROPHIC OBSTRUCTIVE (HOCM)
Causes	• Ischemia/infarction • Long-standing hypertension • Tachyarrhythmias • Drugs: alcohol, cocaine • Medications: daunorubicin, trastuzumab • Infections: viral (coxsackie, adenovirus), parasitic (*Trypanosoma cruzi* [Chagas disease]) • Radiation • Pregnancy related (peripartum cardiomyopathy) • Systemic disorders: connective tissue disorders, hemochromatosis • Vitamin/mineral deficiencies: B1, selenium	• Systemic infiltrative disorders (sarcoidosis, amyloidosis, hemochromatosis, scleroderma) • Endomyocardial fibrosis (children/teens in the tropics, hypereosinophilia) • Fabry disease • Radiation	• Genetically inherited disorder (sarcomere mutation)
Signs and symptoms	• Pulmonary edema • Lower extremity edema • Congestive hepatopathy, ascites • Elevated jugular vein distention (JVD) • Displaced apical impulse	• Similar to dilated cardiomyopathy with evidence of more right heart failure symptoms (JVD, pulmonary hypertension, congestive hepatopathy, ascites) • Kussmaul sign: increased JVD on inspiration (noncompliant right heart cannot accommodate increased venous return) • Extracardiac manifestations secondary to underlying systemic disorder	• Syncope, lightheadedness • Chest pain • Ventricular dysrhythmias • Sudden death in young athletes • Murmur similar to aortic stenosis (quieter murmur with increased left ventricular volume: squatting, handgrip, leg raising) • Crescendo-decrescendo murmur heard along the left sternal border without carotid radiation
Diagnostics	• Echocardiogram: four-chamber cardiac enlargement, thin walls	• Echocardiogram: prominently enlarged bilateral atria, normal ventricles, rapid diastolic filling • S4 murmur	• Echocardiogram: asymmetrically thickened interventricular septum, aortic valve obstruction, systolic anterior motion of the mitral valve
Management	• Same as congestive heart failure (CHF) (see CHF pharmacotherapy section)	• Treat underlying etiology • Similar to dilated cardiomyopathy	• Avoid dehydration and increasing heart rate (strenuous activities, diuretics) • Prolong diastole: beta-1 blockers (metoprolol, atenolol), dihydropyridine calcium channel blockers (diltiazem, verapamil) • For patients at increased risk of sudden death: defibrillator, surgical or alcohol ablation of asymmetrically enlarged interventricular septum • Genetic testing; if confirmed test all first-degree relatives for mutation

Many of the systemic disorders causing restrictive cardiomyopathy may also cause dilated cardiomyopathy.

- Signs and symptoms
  - Asymptomatic (most common)
  - Midsystolic click murmur heard in mitral region; may be associated with mitral regurgitation murmur
  - MVP syndrome: palpitations, atypical chest pain, panic attacks
  - Rare: arrhythmias, sudden cardiac death, transient ischemic attack (TIA)/stroke

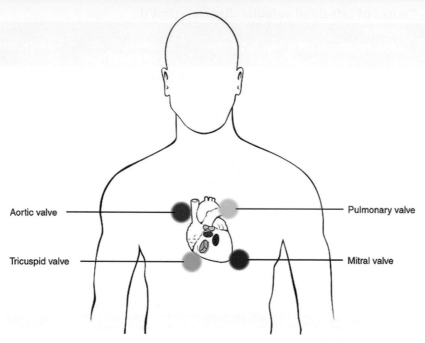

Figure 5-11: Locations for listening to heart murmurs. Aortic valve: right second intercostal space; pulmonary valve: left upper sternal border; tricuspid valve: left sternal border; mitral valve: left fifth intercostal space mid-clavicular line. The heart murmurs can be accentuated using different maneuvers (Table 5-13). (Image courtesy of OpenStax College.)

TABLE 5-10   Causes of left-sided valvular disease

	DIASTOLIC		SYSTOLIC	
	AORTIC REGURGITATION	**MITRAL STENOSIS**	**MITRAL REGURGITATION**	**AORTIC STENOSIS**
Risk factors	• Tertiary syphilis • Ankylosing spondylitis • Aortic dissection • Giant cell arteritis • Endocarditis • Trauma	• Rheumatic heart disease	• Hypertension • Ischemia (papillary muscle rupture) • Mitral valve prolapse	• Elderly • Bicuspid aortic valve (early calcification) • Rheumatic heart disease
Auscultatory location	• Diastolic decrescendo murmur heard at left lower sternal border	• Rumbling diastolic murmur heard in the fifth intercostal space midclavicular line associated with opening snap	• Systolic murmur heard in the fifth intercostal space midclavicular line with radiation to the axilla	• Crescendo-decrescendo systolic murmur heard in the right second intercostal space with radiation to the carotids
Signs and symptoms	• Waterhammer pulse • De Musset sign: head bobbing • Quinke sign: nail bed pulsations • Muller sign: oscillating uvula • Traube sign: systolic/ diastolic murmur heard over the femoral arteries • Biphasic pulse	• Atrial fibrillation • High-intensity S1 sound • Left atrial dilation: chest x-ray (straightening left heart border, elevated left main bronchus), esophageal compression (dysphagia), recurrent laryngeal nerve compression (hoarseness)	• Acute: dyspnea, pulmonary edema • Chronic: symptoms related to left atrial dilation	• Syncope, angina, dyspnea • Displaced apical impulse • Pulsus parvus et tardus • Paradoxic splitting with closure of pulmonic valve prior to aortic valve in severe cases • Concomitant angiodysplasia and acquired von Willebrand factor deficiency

Continued

TABLE 5-10   Causes of left-sided valvular disease—cont'd

| | DIASTOLIC | | SYSTOLIC | |
	AORTIC REGURGITATION	MITRAL STENOSIS	MITRAL REGURGITATION	AORTIC STENOSIS
Management	• Medical management: decrease afterload with vasodilators • Surgical indications: symptomatic severe aortic regurgitation, asymptomatic severe aortic regurgitation with ejection fraction <50%	• Medical management only for symptomatic treatment • Surgical indications: severe mitral stenosis (<1.5 cm²), severely symptomatic	• Medical management only for symptomatic treatment • Surgical indications: severe primary mitral regurgitation with ejection fraction <30%, asymptomatic severe primary mitral regurgitation with ejection fraction 30–60% and/or left ventricular end-systolic diameter >40 mm	• Surgical indications (valve replacement): development of symptoms, decreased valve area (<1 cm²), ejection fraction <50% • Cardiac catheterization prior to surgical repair for possible concurrent coronary artery bypass graft and exclude coronary artery disease as cause of symptoms • Transcatheter aortic valve replacement for poor surgical candidates

TABLE 5-11   Indications for antibiotic prophylaxis in valvular heart disease

HIGH-RISK PROCEDURE	HIGH-RISK VALVULAR LESION
• Dental procedures with gingival manipulation • Respiratory tract procedures involving incision are biopsy of respiratory mucosa • Gastrointestinal/genitourinary procedure with ongoing infection • Procedure on infected skin	• Prosthetic heart valves or prosthetic material in cardiac valve repair • Prior history of infective endocarditis • Unrepaired cyanotic congenital heart disease • Repaired congenital heart disease with residual defect

Prophylaxis requires the presence of both a high-risk procedure in a high risk of valvular lesion. Prophylaxis with amoxicillin.

TABLE 5-12   Duke criteria (two major, one major with three minor, or five minor to diagnose endocarditis)

Major criteria	• Positive blood cultures with typical microorganisms • Endocardial involvement (vegetation on echocardiogram, new murmur)
Minor criteria	• Risk factors (high-risk cardiac lesion, high-risk behavior) • Fever • Immunologic phenomena: glomerulonephritis, Osler nodes, Roth spots, positive rheumatoid factor • Vascular phenomena: emboli, mycotic aneurysm, intracranial hemorrhage, Janeway lesions, conjunctival hemorrhages, septic pulmonary infarcts • Positive blood cultures that do not meet major criteria

  – Diagnostics: echocardiogram
  – Management: none

Mitral valve prolapse common in patients with connective tissue disorders (Marfan, Ehlers-Danlos), autosomal dominant polycystic kidney disease, muscular dystrophies.

Endocarditis
  – Definition: infection and seeding of the heart valves or device
  – Risk factors
    • Valvular heart disease
    • Prosthetic valve
    • Bacteremia
    • IV drug abuse *(Staphylococcus aureus)*
    • Colon cancer, inflammatory bowel disease *(Streptococcus Gallolyticus, Clostridium septicum)*
    • Dental cleaning/infection/cavities *(Viridans streptococci)*
    • Gastrointestinal/genitourinary infection with manipulation *(Enterococci)*
  – Signs and symptoms
    • Fever, malaise
    • New murmur or worsening of preexisting murmur
  – Diagnostics (Duke criteria) (Table 5-12)
    • Blood cultures
    • Transthoracic echocardiography (TTE), followed by TEE if necessary

- Management
  - Long term (4–6 weeks) antibiotics pending culture sensitivity
  - Surgical indications
    - Valve rupture, congestive heart failure
    - Fungal endocarditis
    - Recurrent emboli
    - Abscess formation
- Complications
  - Embolism: infarct, invasion, or abscess formation of end organ (lung, brain, spleen, kidney, bone, joint)
  - Perivalvular abscess
    - Worsening murmur in patient with preexisting endocarditis
    - ECG changes (atrioventricular [AV] block)
    - New fevers

Culture-negative endocarditis: Coxiella, Bartonella, HACEK (Haemophilus, Actinobacillus, Cardiobacterium, Eikenella, and Kingella)

Pericardial Disease
Pericarditis
- Causes
  - Infectious
    - Viral (coxsackie, adenovirus)
    - Lyme disease
  - Rheumatologic/vasculitic
    - SLE
    - Rheumatoid arthritis
    - Antineutrophil cytoplasmic antibody + vasculitis
  - Iatrogenic
    - Postcardiac surgery
    - Radiation
  - Metastatic disease
  - Uremia
  - Trauma
- Signs and symptoms
  - Chest pain worse when lying flat, relieved when sitting forward
  - Friction rub on auscultation
- Diagnostics
  - Chest x-ray (Fig. 5-12)
  - ECG: diffuse ST elevation, PR depression
  - Echocardiogram: assess for complications such as effusion/tamponade
- Management
  - Idiopathic/viral: NSAIDs plus colchicine (prevents recurrence)
  - Uremia: dialysis

TABLE 5-13   Maneuvers and murmurs

MURMUR	MANEUVER	HEMODYNAMIC RESPONSE	EFFECT
Aortic/mitral/tricuspid/ pulmonic stenosis or regurgitation	Leg raise	Increases venous return and preload	Louder murmur
	Squatting	Increases afterload Increases venous return and preload	Louder murmur
	Standing/Valsalva	Decreases venous return and preload	Softer murmur
	Handgrip	Increases afterload	Louder murmur except with aortic stenosis
HOCM/MVP	Same maneuvers as above	Same hemodynamic response as above	Softer murmur with leg raise, squatting, handgrip Louder murmur with standing, Valsalva

In general, increasing the blood in the heart worsens most murmurs except hypertrophic obstructive cardiomyopathy (HOCM) and mitral valve prolapse (MVP).

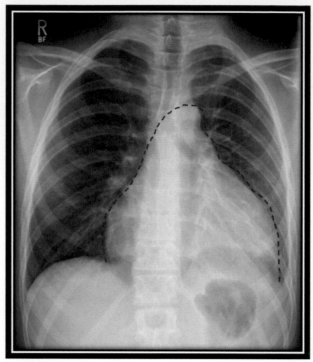

Figure 5-12: Chest radiograph demonstrating globular, water bottle–shaped heart secondary to pericardial effusion. (Image courtesy of Hellerhoff.)

- Complications: pericardial effusion/tamponade

Pericardial Effusion
- Complication of pericarditis
- Presents with increased JVD, distant heart sounds, pulsus paradoxus
- ECG: electrical alternans (alternating low amplitude of P-QRS)
- Chest x-ray: globular, "water bottle" heart
- Pericardiocentesis if there is evidence of hemodynamic compromise

---

Postmyocardial infarction pericarditis: two types
- 2–5 days postinfarction: transmural infarction results in adjacent inflammation of the pericardium; treat with aspirin
- Weeks to months postinfarction (Dressler syndrome): exposure of hidden pericardial antigens results in development of autoantibodies; treat with nonsteroidal antiinflammatories

---

Constrictive Pericarditis
- Causes
  - Tuberculosis
  - Iatrogenic: cardiac surgery, radiation
- Signs and symptoms
  - Elevated jugular venous pressure
  - Kussmaul sign: increase JVD on inspiration
  - Pulses paradoxus: decrease in systolic blood pressure >10 mm Hg upon inspiration
  - Pericardial knock
  - Signs of right heart failure (hepatomegaly, peripheral edema, ascites)
- Diagnostics
  - ECG: low-voltage QRS
  - CT chest: rimlike calcification around the heart
  - Echocardiogram: equalization of diastolic pressures
- Management
  - Glucocorticoids to decrease the risk of constrictive pericarditis in tuberculosis
  - Pericardiectomy

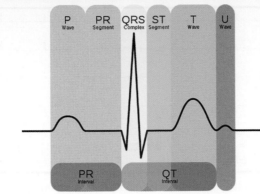

Figure 5-13: Normal electrocardiography intervals.

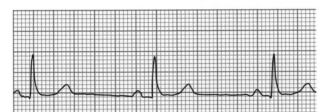

Figure 5-14: Sinus bradycardia. Electrocardiography characteristics: sinus rhythm, narrow-complex QRS complex, heart rate <60. Associations: well-trained athletes, medications (beta blockers, calcium channel blocker, digoxin). Management: avoid causative agents; typically asymptomatic and not treated; may require pacemaker if symptomatic.

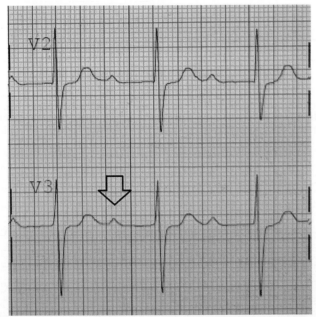

Figure 5-15: First-degree atrioventricular (AV) block. Electrocardiography characteristics: prolonged PR interval (>0.20), delayed conduction through the AV node. Management: none, asymptomatic.

ARRHYTHMIAS

Normal ECG parameters:
- Heart rate: 60–100
- PR interval: 0.12–0.2 sec
- QRS duration: <0.12 sec
- QT interval: >0.45 sec in males, 0.47 sec in females

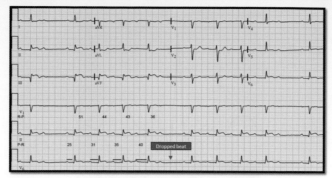

Figure 5-16: Second-degree atrioventricular (AV) block type I. Electrocardiography characteristics: gradually prolonging PR interval with eventual dropped beat. Management: benign; similar to first-degree AV block.

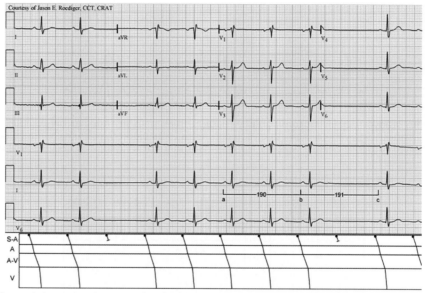

Figure 5-17: Second-degree atrioventricular (AV) block type II. Electrocardiography characteristics: fixed prolonged PR interval with dropped beats *(blue arrow).* Associations: pathology is distal to the AV node in the bundle of His. Management: high risk to progress to third-degree AV block and therefore requires pacemaker.

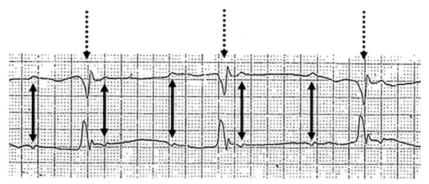

Figure 5-18: Third-degree atrioventricular (AV) block. Electrocardiography characteristics: dyssynchrony between P waves *(solid arrows)* and QRS *(dotted arrows);* AV dissociation. Management: pacemaker. (Image courtesy of Gregory Marcus, MD, MAS, FACC.)

6.1 Bradyarrhythmia

Definition: abnormally slow heart rhythm (Figs. 5-13 to 5-18)

Sick Sinus Syndrome

- ECG characteristics: alternating bradycardia tachycardia (tachy-brady syndrome)
- Associations: degeneration/fibrosis of the sinoatrial node commonly seen in elderly; presents with fatigue, light-headedness, dizziness, palpitations, syncope
- Management: pacemaker for symptomatic cases

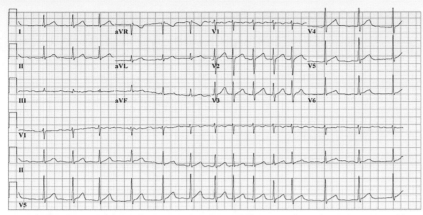

Figure 5-19: Electrocardiography characteristics of atrial fibrillation: no P waves, irregularly irregular QRS complexes. (Image courtesy of CardioNetworks.)

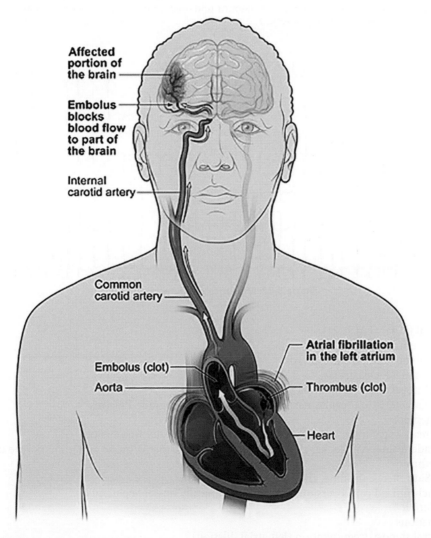

Figure 5-20: Pathophysiology of atrial fibrillation cardioembolic phenomenon. (Image courtesy of National Heart Lung and Blood Institute.)

6.2 Tachyarrhythmias

Supraventricular Tachycardia (SVT)
  – Definition: tachycardia occurring above the bundle of His
  – Types
    • Atrial fibrillation (Fig. 5-19, 5-20)

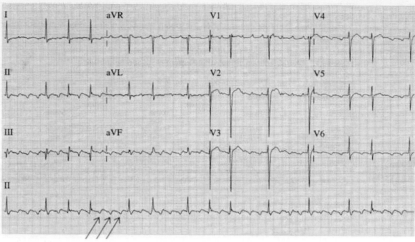

Figure 5-21: Atrial flutter with alternating 2:1 and 3:1 block. Electrocardiography characteristics include saw-tooth pattern of multiple atrial contractions, narrow-complex QRS; >3 different P-wave morphologies. Associations: primary pulmonary disease. Management: treatment of underlying pulmonary disease. No indication for antiarrhythmics. (Image courtesy of CardioNetworks.)

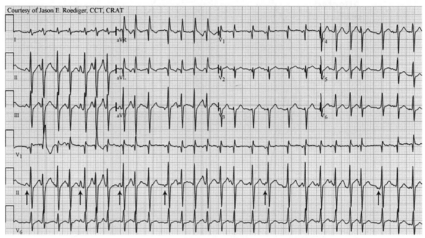

Figure 5-22: Multifocal atrial tachycardia.

- Atrial flutter (Fig. 5-21)
- AV reentrant tachycardia
- AV nodal reentrant tachycardia
- Junctional tachycardia
- Multifocal atrial tachycardia (Fig. 5-22)
  - ECG characteristics: regular narrow complex QRS, retrograde P waves
  - Management
    - Increase vagal tone: Valsalva, carotid massage, cold water immersion
    - IV adenosine: AV blocker that slows conduction via the AV node and unmasks the underlying rhythm
      - Side effects: flushing, chest pain, bronchospasm
    - Synchronized cardioversion: for hemodynamically unstable patients

Atrial Fibrillation
- Associations
  - Mitral stenosis/regurgitation (left atrial dilation)
  - Hyperthyroidism
  - Alcohol toxicity (holiday heart syndrome)
  - Hypertension, ischemic heart disease
  - Postcardiac surgery
  - Sick sinus syndrome
  - Sepsis
  - Wolff-Parkinson-White

TABLE 5-14 CHA$_2$DS$_2$VASc score

RISK FACTOR	SCORE
Congestive heart failure	1
Hypertension	1
Age >75	2
Diabetes mellitus	1
Stroke, transient ischemic attack	2
Prior vascular disease (myocardial infarction, peripheral artery disease)	1
Age 65–74	1
Sex (female)	1

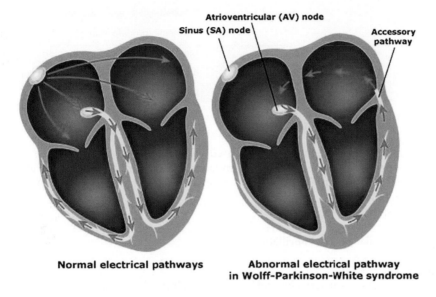

Figure 5-23: Pathophysiology of Wolff-Parkinson-White. Accessory pathway is a direct connection from the atrium to the ventricle bypassing the atrioventricular node. Electrical impulse passes through the myocardium resulting in prolonged duration (>0.12 seconds) of electrical impulse.

- Management
  - Rate or rhythm control: both approaches are equivalent
    - Rate control
      - Beta blockers (metoprolol, atenolol) or calcium channel blockers (verapamil, diltiazem): first line
      - Digoxin for patients with decompensated heart failure and unable to tolerate beta blocker or calcium channel blocker
    - Rhythm control
      - Class IC antiarrhythmics (flecainide, propafenone)
      - Class III antiarrhythmics (amiodarone, sotalol)
  - Anticoagulation: prevent cardioembolic disease
    - Indication calculated using CHA$_2$DS$_2$VASc score; score >2 is indication for anticoagulation (Table 5-14)
    - Valvular atrial fibrillation: warfarin only
    - Nonvalvular atrial fibrillation
      - Warfarin, direct thrombin inhibitors (dabigatran), or Xa inhibitors (apixaban, rivaroxaban)
  - Cardioversion
    - Patients who have known atrial fibrillation for <48 hours
    - Patients with atrial fibrillation >48 hours will require pre- and postcardioversion anticoagulation
    - Hemodynamically unstable

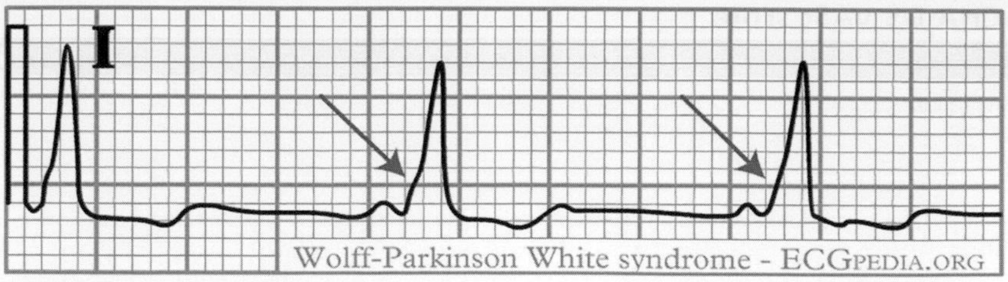

Figure 5-24: Wolff-Parkinson-White electrocardiography characteristics: delta wave (slurring of the wide-complex QRS), short PR interval (<0.12 seconds).

TABLE 5-15   Antiarrhythmics pharmacotherapy

MEDICATION CLASS	MECHANISM OF ACTION	EXAMPLES
Class IA	Sodium channel blocker	Disopyramide, quinidine, procainamide
Class IB		Mexiletine, lidocaine, phenytoin
Class IC		Flecainide, propafenone
Class II	Beta blocker	Metoprolol, atenolol, propranolol, esmolol
Class III	Potassium channel blocker	Amiodarone, sotalol, dofetilide, ibutilide, dronedarone
Class IV	Calcium channel blocker	Verapamil, diltiazem

- Ablation
  - Patients unresponsive to medication, used as last resort
  - Ectopy originates at the site of the pulmonary vein entering the left atrium as the muscular tissue around the pulmonary vein has different electrical properties compared to the rest of the atrial myocytes
- Complications: thromboembolism

Atrial Flutter
- Associations: similar to atrial fibrillation
- Management
  - Rate control
    - Beta blockers or calcium channel blockers: first line
    - Digoxin
  - +/− anticoagulation: lone atrial flutter is typically not treated with anticoagulation; however, due to the high likelihood of concurrent atrial fibrillation, anticoagulation is often indicated
  - Radiofrequency ablation: used more often in atrial flutter compared to atrial fibrillation due to its higher success rate and preventing recurrence; ablation of reentrant circuit located around the tricuspid annulus

Wolff-Parkinson-White
- Associations
  - May initially present as SVT and unmasked with AV-nodal blocking agent with degeneration of SVT into atrial/ventricular fibrillation (Figs. 5-23 and 5-24)
  - Congenital abnormality
- Management: treat only if symptomatic
  - Class IA (procainamide) or 1 C antiarrhythmics (flecainide); class III antiarrhythmics may also be considered (Table 5-15)
  - Ablation of accessory pathway
  - Avoid AV nodal blocking agents as this promotes conduction through the accessory pathway (bundle of Kent)

Ventricular Tachycardia
- Associations
  - Ischemic heart disease
  - Electrolyte abnormalities
    - Hypokalemia
    - Hypomagnesemia
    - Hypocalcemia
  - Prolonged QT
  - Drugs (tricyclic antidepressants [TCAs], anticholinergics)
- Management
  - Acute: determine stability

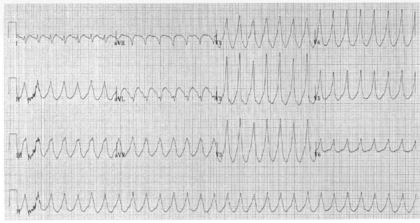

Figure 5-25: Ventricle tachycardia electrocardiography characteristics: wide-complex QRS tachycardia.

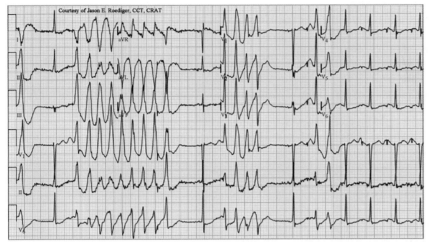

Figure 5-26: Torsades de pointes. Electrocardiography characteristics: varying amplitude QRS (polymorphic ventricular tachycardia). Associations: prolonged QT interval (antiarrhythmics, antipsychotics, antidepressants, macrolides, fluoroquinolones, tricyclic antidepressants, antiemetics), hypomagnesemia. Management: IV magnesium, defibrillation.

- Stable
  - Nonsustained ventricular tachycardia
- No treatment
- Workup for underlying etiology
  - Sustained ventricular tachycardia (Figs. 5-25 and 5-26)
- Antiarrhythmics (amiodarone, lidocaine, procainamide)
  - Unstable (hemodynamic instability): synchronized cardioversion
  - Pulseless: unsynchronized cardioversion, treat as cardiac arrest
- Chronic
  - Optimize treatment of underlying etiology
  - Antiarrhythmics (see Table 5-15)
  - Implantable cardioverter-defibrillator placement: secondary prevention of cardiac arrest if no reversible cause is identified
  - Radiofrequency ablation

CARDIAC ARREST
Code Blue
- Definition: cardiac rhythm that requires cardiopulmonary resuscitation (CPR)
- Indications for chest compressions only
  - Asystole
  - Pulseless electrical activity
- Indications for chest compression plus unsynchronized cardioversion ("shock")
  - Ventricular fibrillation

TABLE 5-16 Asystole or pulseless electrical activity is caused by the six *H*s and six *T*s

H	T
Hypoxia	Tension pneumothorax
Hypovolemia	Tamponade (cardiac)
Hydrogen ions (acidosis)	Thrombosis (cardiac)
Hyperkalemia	Thrombosis (pulmonary)
Hypokalemia	Toxins
Hypothermia	Trauma

- Pulseless ventricular tachycardia
  - During CPR, one of the team members should be assigned to look through the patient's chart and determine a potential cause for the cardiac arrest (Table 5-16)

Code blue step-by-step
1. No pulse
2. Begin CPR with chest compressions
3. Determine rhythm
   a. Ventricular fibrillation or pulseless ventral tachycardia → shock plus epinephrine
   b. Asystole or pulseless electrical activity → epinephrine only
4. Continue chest compressions
5. Recheck rhythm and repeat step 3. Continue until non-CPR rhythm is obtained or pulse is palpated

Additional points
- Chest compressions involve doing 30 compressions at a rate of 100–120 beats/minute followed by two breaths over 2-minute cycles followed by a pulse check to determine whether CPR should be continued
- Epinephrine should be given every 3–5 minutes during CPR
- An advanced airway is often used, and when present compressions may be administered continuously without stopping to provide the two breaths after 30 compressions. Instead, the provider who is managing the airway will use a bag valve mask to give the patient a breath every 5–6 seconds

CARDIAC NEOPLASMS

Myxoma
- Epidemiology
  - Most common primary cardiac tumors
  - Benign gelatinous growth most commonly located in the left atrial appendage
- Signs and symptoms
  - Nonspecific constitutional symptoms (release of interleukin-6):
    - Fever, malaise
    - Weight loss, weakness
    - Raynaud
  - Valvular dysfunction
    - Diastolic murmur in mitral valve area, "diastolic plop" secondary to transit obstruction through the mitral valve; murmur quality changes with position
  - Invasion
    - Myocardium (arrhythmias, heart block)
    - Pericardium (pericardial effusion)
    - Lung (dyspnea, mimics bronchogenic carcinoma)
  - Embolization
    - TIA/stroke
    - Symptoms related to organ infarct (spleen, kidney, colon)
- Diagnostics: visualization of tumor on TTE or TEE
- Management: surgical resection

Rhabdomyoma
- Most common pediatric cardiac tumor
- Associated with tuberous sclerosis
- Most cases spontaneously regress; surgical resection if symptomatic (arrhythmias, outflow obstruction)

Metastatic
- Most common cause of cardiac tumor
- Commonly originate from primary melanoma, lung, breast, esophageal, renal cancer, or leukemia/lymphoma

CHAPTER 6 Gastroenterology

ORAL AND SALIVARY GLANDS

Calculous Sialolithiasis/Sialadenitis
- Definition: formation of stones and obstruction within the salivary ducts (Fig. 6-1)
- Signs and symptoms
  - Localized, unilateral painful swelling at the angle of the mandible or in front of the ear
  - Intermittent pain and swelling
  - Palpable calculous
  - Fever if infection occurs secondary to obstruction
- Diagnostics
  - Plain films: will visualize most cases of sialolithiasis as most stones are radiopaque
  - Sonogram
  - Sialography: gold standard
- Management
  - Manual compression and manipulation
  - Sialagogues
  - Shockwave lithotripsy
  - Sialoendoscopy

Acute Parotitis
- Causes
  - Infectious (*Staphylococcus aureus*, mumps virus)
  - Chronic vomiting (anorexia, bulimia)
  - Dehydration, poor oral hygiene, xerostomia
  - Debilitated (elderly, postoperative)
- Signs and symptoms
  - Painful, unilateral parotid enlargement
  - Bilateral enlargement may be indication of systemic process (Sjögren syndrome, bulimia, mumps)
  - Edema, erythema
  - Fever
  - Purulent discharge from Wharton or Stenson duct
- Diagnostics: clinical
  - Sonogram
  - Radiographs/sialography to rule out calculous sialadenitis
- Management
  - Sialagogues (lemon wedges, hard candy): increase salivation to facilitate expectoration of pus and infectious contents
  - Rehydration
  - Antibiotics covering methicillin-resistant *S. aureus* (MRSA; vancomycin, linezolid)

Tumors in smaller salivary glands such as sublingual or submandibular are more likely to be malignant; however, overall, most salivary gland tumors are benign.

Parotid Neoplasia
- Risk factors
  - Smoking
  - Radiation exposure
  - Sjögren syndrome

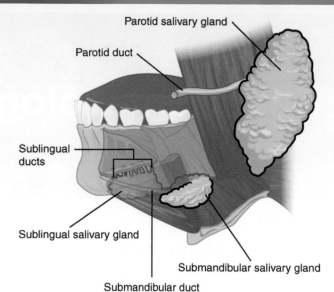

Figure 6-1: Normal anatomy of the salivary gland. (Image courtesy of OpenStax College.)

- Types
  - Pleomorphic adenoma (mixed tumor): most common benign and overall salivary gland tumor; small potential for malignant degeneration
  - Other benign tumors
    - Wharton tumor (more common in men)
    - Oncocytoma
    - Benign lymphoepithelial cysts
  - Mucoepidermoid carcinoma: most common malignant salivary gland tumor
  - Other malignant tumors
    - Adenoid cystic carcinoma
    - Acinic cell carcinoma
  - Lymphoma: develops as a complication of long-standing Sjögren syndrome
- Signs and symptoms
  - Painless unilateral enlargement at the angle of the mandible
  - Facial pain/paralysis: indicative of malignant tumor infiltrating cranial nerve VII
  - Local lymphadenopathy
- Diagnostics
  - Fine-needle aspiration
  - Computed tomography (CT)/magnetic resonance imaging (MRI): determine extent of tumor growth and aid with presurgical planning
- Management
  - Benign: superficial parotidectomy with wide margins due to high recurrence rate with incomplete excision
  - Malignant: total parotidectomy with excision of facial nerve

Frey syndrome: postoperative complication following parotidectomy presenting as gustatory sweating due to aberrant parasympathetic innervation of sweat glands that are divided during surgery

Esophagus
Zenker Diverticulum
- Definition: true diverticulum (involvement of mucosa, submucosa, and muscularis externa) of the proximal esophagus seen in elderly males
- Pathophysiology: weakness in the cricopharyngeal muscle results in posterior herniation of the proximal esophagus between the muscle fibers
- Signs and symptoms
  - Dysphagia
  - Sensation of food stuck in the throat
  - Regurgitation, halitosis

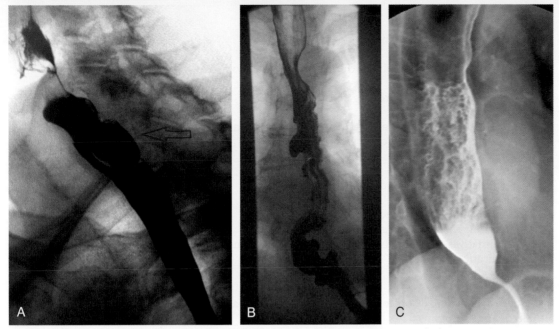

Figure 6-2: Differentiating (A) Zenker diverticulum. (Image courtesy of James Heilman, MD.), (B) esophageal spasm. (Image courtesy of Hellerhoff.), and (C) achalasia on barium esophagram. (Image courtesy of Hellerhoff.)

- • Neck mass
- • Chest discomfort
- – Diagnostics
  - • Barium esophagram (Fig. 6-2)
  - • Avoid esophagogastroduodenoscopy (EGD) if Zenker diverticulum is suspected due to high risk of perforation
- – Management: surgery
  - • Open/endoscopic
  - • Cricopharyngeal myotomy
- – Complications: aspiration

Other types of esophageal diverticula
- – Traction diverticula
  - • Located in midesophagus
  - • Caused by mediastinal adenopathy (pulmonary tuberculosis) and inflammation
  - • No treatment necessary
- – Epiphrenic diverticula
  - • Located in lower esophagus
  - • Caused by achalasia or esophageal spasms
  - • Treat underlying cause

Achalasia
- – Definition: esophageal motility disorder characterized by incomplete relaxation of the lower esophageal sphincter (LES)
- – Causes
  - • Idiopathic
  - • Adenocarcinoma of the lower esophagus or proximal stomach: pseudoachalasia
  - • Chagas disease
  - • Scleroderma
  - • Nissen fundoplication: iatrogenic cause of achalasia
- – Pathophysiology: acquired loss of motor neurons in the myenteric plexus of the LES
- – Signs and symptoms
  - • Dysphasia to both solids and liquids
  - • Sensation of food stuck in the throat

- Weight loss
- Regurgitation
- Heartburn, chest discomfort
- Diagnostics
  - Barium esophagram: "bird's beak" appearance due to narrowing at the distal esophagus (see Fig. 6-2)
  - Manometry: increased resting pressure at the LES
  - EGD with biopsy
    - Loss of motor neurons in the myenteric plexus on pathology
    - Rules out malignant etiologies (pseudoachalasia)
- Management
  - Pharmacologic
    - Calcium channel blockers
    - Nitrates
    - Botulinum toxin injection
  - Surgical: pneumatic dilation, myotomy
  - Alternatives: avoid meals before bed, remain in the upright position while eating
- Complications: aspiration

Esophageal Spasm
- Causes: idiopathic disorder characterized by painful spasms of the esophagus
- Signs and symptoms
  - Presents similarly to acute coronary syndrome (ACS) with severe crushing substernal chest pain unrelated to exertion and relieved by nitrates
  - Dysphagia, odynophagia
  - Worsened by hot or cold food
- Diagnostics
  - Rule out ACS: check electrocardiography (ECG), cardiac enzymes
  - Barium esophagram: "rosary bead" or "corkscrew" appearance during episodes of contraction (see Fig. 6-2)
  - Manometry: diffuse, random, high-amplitude contractions of the esophagus
  - Endoscopy: normal
- Management: no effective treatment
  - Calcium channel blockers (diltiazem)
  - Nitrates
  - Tricyclic antidepressants (TCAs; imipramine)
  - Phosphodiesterase inhibitor (sildenafil)

Gastroesophageal Reflux Disease (GERD)
- Causes
  - Sliding hiatal hernia (herniation of the GE junction above the diaphragm)
  - Gastric outlet obstruction
  - Gastric dysmotility
- Pathophysiology: excessive relaxation of the LES resulting in retrograde flow of stomach acid into the esophagus (Fig. 6-3)
- Signs and symptoms
  - Heartburn, dyspepsia usually after meals
  - Metallic taste in the mouth
  - Nausea, vomiting, early satiety
  - Chest discomfort
  - Belching, regurgitation
  - Nocturnal asthma
  - Chronic cough, hoarseness
- Diagnostics: additional testing only done in unresponsive or atypical cases
  - Clinical: retrospective diagnosis of GERD if patient responds to proton pump inhibitors (PPIs)
  - 24-hour pH monitoring: most sensitive and specific, used in specific cases
    - Prior to Nissen fundoplication
    - Patients unresponsive to PPIs
  - Endoscopy with biopsy
    - Assess for changes to esophageal mucosa (Barrett esophagus)
    - Presence of alarming symptoms such as weight loss, gastrointestinal (GI) bleeding, anemia, elderly, signs of obstruction, persistent vomiting

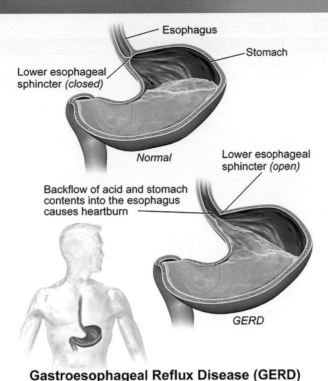

Gastroesophageal Reflux Disease (GERD)

Figure 6-3: Pathophysiology of gastroesophageal reflux disease. (Image courtesy of Blaus Medical.)

- Management
  - Behavioral modification
    - Avoid spicy, fatty foods, chocolates, peppermints, alcohol, large meals before bedtime
    - Sleep with torso elevated
    - Weight loss
  - Pharmacologic:
    - PPIs
    - H2 blockers, antacids
  - Surgical: for cases unresponsive to behavioral and pharmacologic management
    - Nissen fundoplication: procedure that wraps the GE junction around the LES
- Complications
  - Barrett esophagus: metaplasia of the LES from normal stratified squamous epithelium to columnar epithelium; precursor to adenocarcinoma
  - Esophageal strictures/spasms
  - Aspiration pneumonia
  - Erosive esophagitis
  - Dental erosion
  - Laryngitis

Paraesophageal hernias: herniation of the gastric fundus through the diaphragm resulting in increased risk of strangulation and ulceration; may require surgical repair

Esophagitis can be due to infection or be pill induced (Table 6-1). A thorough history and medicine reconciliation is essential to determine the etiology as pill-induced esophagitis will require the cessation of the medication, while infectious esophagitis will need antimicrobials.

Esophageal Rings/Web

- Definition
  - Ring: circumferential protrusion of the esophageal mucosa into the lumen
  - Web: partial protrusion of the esophageal mucosa into the lumen
- Causes: unknown, hypothesized to be from chronic GERD
- Signs and symptoms
  - Intermittent dysphagia to solids
  - Sensation of food stuck in throat
  - Dyspepsia

TABLE 6-1   **Infectious versus pill-induced esophagitis**

	INFECTIOUS	PILL INDUCED
Causes	• Herpes simplex virus (HSV) • Cytomegalovirus (CMV) • Candida	• Bisphosphonates • Nonenteric-coated NSAIDs • Potassium chloride • Iron • Tetracyclines
Signs and symptoms	• History of immunocompromised (infectious) • Dysphagia • Odynophagia • Retrosternal chest pain • Oral thrush (candida) • Upper gastrointestinal bleeding	

Diagnostics	• Endoscopy with biopsy:
	  • Candida: white plaques
	  • HSV: round ovoid ulcers
	  • CMV: large linear ulcers
		• History plus visualization on endoscopy

Management	• HSV: acyclovir • CMV: ganciclovir • Candida: fluconazole	• Removal of pill • Symptomatic management and monitoring for signs of esophageal perforation

NSAIDs, Nonsteroidal antiinflammatory drugs.

- Associations
  - Rings
    - Hiatal hernia
    - Eosinophilic esophagitis
  - Webs
    - Plummer Vinson syndrome: triad of esophageal web, iron deficiency anemia, and increased risk of squamous cell carcinoma
  - Both: autoimmune dermatologic conditions (bullous pemphigoid, pemphigus vulgaris)
- Diagnostics: barium esophagram
- Management
  - Thoroughly chew food
  - Pneumatic dilation: can be complicated by esophageal perforation (Table 6-2)
  - Long-term PPIs

Esophageal Cancer
- Risk factors
  - Squamous cell carcinoma
    - Smoking
    - Alcohol
    - Elderly
    - Nitrate-containing foods
    - Vitamin/mineral deficiencies (beta-carotene, B1, zinc, selenium)
    - Hereditary
      - Peutz-Jeghers syndrome
      - Cowden syndrome (PTEN tumor suppressor gene mutation)
  - Adenocarcinoma
    - Long-standing GERD (Barrett esophagus)
    - Smoking
    - Obesity
    - High calorie and fat intake
- Signs and symptoms
  - Progressive dysphagia to solids > liquids
  - Weight loss
  - GI bleed
  - Chest discomfort, dyspepsia
  - Cough, hoarseness
  - Vomiting, regurgitation
- Diagnostics
  - Initial test: barium esophagram (asymmetric narrowing of the esophageal lumen)
  - Biopsy
  - Integrated positron emission tomography (PET)/CT for staging

TABLE 6-2 Differentiating mallory-weiss tear versus boerhaave syndrome

	MALLORY-WEISS TEAR	BOERHAAVE SYNDROME
Definition	• Longitudinal submucosal laceration of the distal esophagus or proximal stomach	• Transmural laceration of the esophagus
Causes	• Severe vomiting and retching (due to sudden increase in intraabdominal pressure)	• Severe vomiting and retching • Other causes of esophageal perforation: recent EGD, penetrating trauma
Signs and symptoms	• Self-resolving hematemesis • Epigastric or back pain	• Acute retrosternal chest pain • Subcutaneous emphysema • Crepitus in the suprasternal notch • Odynophagia, dysphagia • Fever, septic shock
Diagnostics	• Clinical: if patient describes appropriate story and is no longer symptomatic at time of presentation • EGD: longitudinal submucosal laceration	• Gastrografin esophagram: extravasation of contrast through the transmural tear • Computed tomography thorax • Chest x-ray: pneumomediastinum, left-sided pleural effusion (due to rupture of left posterolateral distal esophagus) • Thoracentesis plus pleural fluid analysis: elevated amylase (due to saliva in the esophageal contents)
Management	• Majority of cases self-resolve requiring no treatment • Persistent bleeding: epinephrine, electrocautery, IV PPIs or antiemetics	• Surgical repair • Alternative for surgical repair: drainage, endoscopic stent placement, esophagectomy (last resort)

Barium swallow is generally avoided if transmural tear is suspected as extravasation into the mediastinum can result in mediastinitis.
EGD, Esophagogastroduodenoscopy; *PPI*, proton pump inhibitor.

TABLE 6-3 Acute versus chronic gastritis

	ACUTE	CHRONIC
Causes	• Alcohol • NSAIDs • Burns • Trauma	• *Helicobacter pylori* infection • Pernicious anemia
Signs and symptoms	• Epigastric pain • Hematemesis, melena	
Diagnostics	• Clinical • EGD: inflammation and erosion of the gastric mucosa	• *H. pylori*: urease breath test, stool antigen • Pernicious anemia: antiintrinsic factor antibodies, antiparietal cell antibodies, low vitamin B12 levels (MCV >100)
Management	• PPIs and removal of causative agent	• *H. pylori*: triple therapy • Pernicious anemia: B12 replacement

EGD, Esophagogastroduodenoscopy; *MCV*, mean corpuscular volume; *NSIADs*, nonsteroidal antiinflammatory drugs; *PPI*, proton pump inhibitor.

   – Management
   • Localized disease: surgical resection
   • Metastatic disease: chemoradiation, palliative stent placement

STOMACH
Gastritis can be acute or chronic in this differential, which is important as the etiologies and ultimately management are different (Table 6-3).
Peptic Ulcer Disease (PUD)
   – Causes
   • *Helicobacter pylori* infection
   • Nonsteroidal antiinflammatory drugs (NSAIDs), steroids, cholinomimetics
   • Gastrinoma (Zollinger-Ellison syndrome)
   • Burns (Cushing ulcer)
   • Head trauma (Curling ulcer)

- Signs and symptoms
    - Gnawing epigastric pain immediately (gastric ulcer) or hours (duodenal ulcer) after meals
    - Nausea, vomiting, belching
    - Hematemesis, black stools
    - Early satiety
- Diagnostics
    - *H. pylori* testing: urea breath test, stool assay
    - EGD: most commonly located on lesser curvature stomach
    - Gastric ulcer should be biopsied to rule out malignancy and followed up with repeat endoscopy to document resolution/improvement in select high-risk cases
- Management
    - Avoid causative agents
    - *H. pylori* eradication
        - Triple therapy: amoxicillin, clarithromycin, PPI
        - Quadruple therapy: metronidazole, tetracycline, bismuth, PPI
    - Refractive: selective vagotomy
- Complications
    - Perforation
    - Gastric outlet obstruction
    - Malignancy
    - GI bleed

Gastric versus duodenal ulcer symptoms:
- Gastric ulcer: symptoms worsen after meals due to stimulation of acid production in the stomach resulting in increased damage to preexisting ulcer
- Duodenal ulcer: pain of ulcer improves after meals as secretion of bicarbonate increases from Brunner glands located into the duodenum as it prepares for incoming acidic load from the stomach

Gastroparesis
- Causes
    - Idiopathic: most common cause
    - Long-standing uncontrolled diabetes (vagus nerve neuropathy)
    - Medications
        - Opioids
        - TCAs
        - Muscarinic cholinergic antagonists
- Signs and symptoms
    - Nausea, vomiting
    - Colicky abdominal pain and distention
    - Early satiety
    - Anorexia
    - Hypoglycemia after meals: longer gastric emptying time results in less carbohydrate absorption into the blood and insulin functioning in a carbohydrate depleted environment
    - Constipation
- Diagnostics
    - Clinical
    - Gastric emptying scintigraphy: nuclear medicine study that examines percentage of gastric contents remaining 4 hours after meal
        - Mild: 10%–15%
        - Moderate: 15%–35%
        - Severe: >35%
    - Rule out mechanical obstruction
- Management
    - Acute
        - IV fluid resuscitation
        - IV antiemetics: ondansetron, granisetron
        - IV erythromycin (motilin receptor agonist; limited long-term viability due to tachyphylaxis)

Substitute metronidazole for amoxicillin for penicillin-allergic patients.

- Chronic
  - Dietary modifications: small, frequent low-fat meals
  - Metoclopramide (D2 receptor antagonist)
  - Domperidone
  - Glucose control
- Complications: secondary to chronic vomiting
  - Mallory-Weiss
  - Boerhaave syndrome
  - Metabolic derangements (hypokalemia, metabolic alkalosis)

Malignancy Related
Pernicious Anemia
- Risk factors
  - Family history
  - Personal history of other autoimmune disease
- Pathophysiology
  - Chronic gastritis results in atrophy of parietal cells and decreased production of intrinsic factor
  - Antibodies against intrinsic factor preventing vitamin B12 absorption
- Signs and symptoms
  - Fatigue (secondary to megaloblastic anemia)
  - Weight loss, epigastric discomfort, glossitis
  - Neuropsychiatric (secondary to B12 deficiency): memory deficits, confusion, altered mental status

Strict vegans and postgastric bypass surgery can also result in B12 deficiency.

- Diagnostics
  - Serology
    - Antiintrinsic factor antibody
    - Antiparietal cell antibodies
    - Decreased B12 levels
    - Elevated methylmalonic acid levels (obtained if B12 levels are unequivocal)
  - Peripheral smear: hypersegmented neutrophils (Fig. 6-4)
- Management: B12 replacement
- Complications

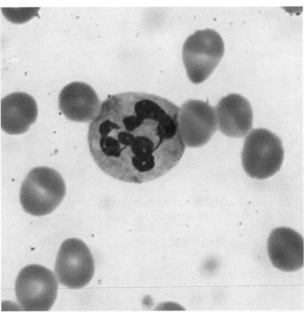

Figure 6-4: Hypersegmented neutrophils in the setting of megaloblastic anemia in a patient with pernicious anemia. (Image courtesy of Ed Uthman from Houston, TX, USA.)

- Gastric cancer
- Gastric carcinoid

Ménétrier Disease (Protein-Losing Hypertrophic Gastropathy)
- Signs and symptoms
  - Epigastric pain
  - Anorexia
  - Weight loss
  - Nausea, vomiting
- Diagnostics
  - EGD: large gastric mucosal folds (extreme foveolar hyperplasia with glandular atrophy)
  - Supporting labs
    - Hypoalbuminemia
    - Achlorhydria
- Management
  - Supportive management with high protein diet
  - Treatment of *H. pylori* or cytomegalovirus (CMV) infection if present
  - Pharmacologic: may or may not help
    - PPIs
    - Somatostatin analogues (octreotide)
    - Cetuximab (epidermal growth factor receptor monoclonal antibody)
- Complications: gastric cancer

Zollinger-Ellison Syndrome (Gastrinoma)
- Pathophysiology: gastrin producing tumor resulting in stimulation of parietal cells to produce excessive hydrochloric acid
- Signs and symptoms
  - Epigastric/abdominal pain
  - Chronic fatty diarrhea (gastrin breaks down pancreatic enzymes preventing absorption of fats)
  - Nausea, vomiting, belching
  - Refractory PUD (unresponsive to high-dose PPIs)
  - Upper GI bleed (melena, anemia)
- Diagnostics
  - Elevated gastrin levels (>1000): ensure patient is off PPIs or H2 blockers before measuring gastrin levels as this may cause gastrin to be falsely elevated
  - Secretin stimulation test: secretin should normally inhibit gastrin; however, failure for gastrin levels to decrease is confirmatory for gastrinoma
  - Calcium infusion study: if secretin test is negative but suspicion for gastrinoma remains high; calcium infusion should result in increased gastrin levels in gastrinoma
  - EGD: multiple, larger virulent ulcers extending into the duodenum and jejunum
  - Somatostatin receptor scintigraphy (nuclear octreotide skin): localizes location of all gastrinoma-producing cells
  - CT scan
  - Somatostatin receptor scintigraphy

Evaluate for metastatic disease.

- Management
  - Localized disease
    - Surgical resection
    - Most commonly located in the gastrinoma triangle (confluence of the cystic and common bile duct, second and third part of the duodenum, neck, and body of the pancreas)
  - Medical management
    - Octreotide (somatostatin analog)
    - PPIs
  - Chemotherapy for advanced cases
- Complications
  - Gastric cancer
  - Perforation
  - Other MEN1-associated malignancies (pituitary, parathyroid)

Gastric Adenocarcinoma
- Risk factors
  - Alcohol
  - Tobacco
  - Preserved foods
  - Chronic atrophic gastritis with intestinal metaplasia (pernicious anemia, *H. pylori*)
  - Adenomatous gastric polyps
  - Ménétrier disease
  - Blood type A
- Signs and symptoms
  - Nausea, vomiting (nonbilious)
  - Succussion splash: sloshing sound heard when stethoscope is placed on patient's abdomen and is rocked back and forth
  - Weight loss, early satiety
  - GI bleed
  - Heartburn
- Diagnostics
  - EGD with biopsy
    - Ulcerating heaped-up lesions
    - Linitis plastica (involvement of all layers of stomach, decreased stomach elasticity): poor prognosis
  - CT abdomen/pelvis for staging
- **Metastatic associations**
  - Virchow nodes: left supraclavicular lymph node
  - Sister Mary Joseph nodules: periumbilical lymph nodes
  - Krukenberg tumor: ovaries
  - Blumer shelf tumor: rectum
  - Irish node: left axillary lymph node
- Management: most cases present in advanced disease due to vague nonspecific symptoms
  - Localized disease: surgical resection (gastrectomy)
  - Metastatic disease: chemoradiation, palliative

SMALL INTESTINE
Carcinoid
- Pathophysiology
  - Serotonin-producing tumor
  - Localized disease is asymptomatic as serotonin is metabolized in the liver to 5-hydroxyindoleacetic acid (5-HIAA)
  - Metastatic disease (especially to the liver) allows serotonin to bypass liver metabolism and enter the systemic circulation
- Signs and symptoms (only seen in metastatic disease)
  - Episodic flushing
  - Wheezing
  - Diarrhea
  - Telangiectasias
  - Tricuspid regurgitation/stenosis (monoamine oxidase enzyme in pulmonary circulation metabolizes serotonin and prevents left-sided valvular involvement)
  - Niacin deficiency causing pellagra (diarrhea, dementia, dermatitis)

Carcinoid tumors secrete other products in addition to serotonin such as histamine, tachykinins, prostaglandins, kallikrein.

- Diagnostics
  - Elevated 24-hour urine 5-HIAA
  - CT or MRI abdomen/pelvis scan for staging (liver metastases most common)
  - PET imaging with radiolabeled somatostatin analogues
  - Endoscopy with biopsy
- Management
  - Localized disease
    - Observation if tumor is <2 cm
    - Surgical resection if tumor is >2 cm; lower threshold if tumor is in the ileum due to high risk of malignancy
    - Most commonly located in the appendix
  - Metastatic disease: somatostatin analogues (octreotide, lanreotide)

Pellagra in carcinoid syndrome occurs secondary to depletion of tryptophan in the production of excessive serotonin. Tryptophan is also the precursor in the production of niacin.

Malabsorption Syndromes

Lactose Intolerance
- Epidemiology
  - Africans, Asians, Latinos, Natives
  - Most common cause of diarrhea
- Pathophysiology
  - Primary: lactase enzyme deficiency along the intestinal brush border whose concentration steadily declines as we age
  - Secondary: postinfectious gastroenteritis, which destroys the intestinal brush border resulting in temporary lactose intolerance until intestinal villi and lactase enzyme are regenerated
- Signs and symptoms: occur only after ingestion of lactose containing products
  - Abdominal discomfort/cramping
  - Bloating
  - Watery diarrhea
  - Flatulence
  - No systemic symptoms or lab abnormalities
- Diagnosis
  - Clinical
  - Lactose hydrogen breath test: increased levels after ingestion of lactose
  - Elevated stool osmolar gap in otherwise healthy patient with diarrhea
- Management
  - Avoidance of lactose-containing foods (milk, ice cream, cheese)
  - Lactase supplements before lactose ingestion

Whipple Disease
- Epidemiology: white males, 40–60 years old
- Microbiology: infection with *Tropheryma whippelii* (nonacid-fast gram-positive bacilli)
- Signs and symptoms
  - Chronic diarrhea, steatorrhea, bloating, weight loss
  - Fever
  - Lymphadenopathy
  - Congestive heart failure, valvular regurgitation
  - Migratory arthralgias
  - Visual (supranuclear ophthalmoplegia) and neurologic deficits (dementia, seizures)
- Diagnostics
  - Biopsy: periodic acid-Schiff–positive foamy macrophages in the lamina propria of the small intestine
  - Polymerase chain reaction (PCR) of cerebrospinal fluid if neurologic involvement is present
- Management
  - Long-term antibiotics: IV ceftriaxone followed by TMP-SMX for 12 months

LARGE INTESTINE

Diverticulosis
- Epidemiology: most common cause of lower GI bleed in the elderly (>50 years old)
- Definition: colonic outpouchings that occur secondary to chronic constipation and meat-based Western diet (high protein, low fiber)
- Sign and symptoms
  - Asymptomatic (most common)
  - Chronic constipation
  - Painless hematochezia: outpouchings of the colonic wall cause weakness and result in bleeding in the associated arterial supply
- Diagnostics
  - Colonoscopy (often incidental finding on colonoscopy done for other reasons)
  - CT abdomen and pelvis
  - Barium enema

- Associations: polycystic kidney disease
- Management
  - Most cases resolve spontaneously
  - Endoscopic or surgical intervention for refractory cases
  - Prevention of complications with a high-fiber diet
- Complications: diverticulitis

Diverticulitis
- Pathophysiology: obstruction and inflammation of a diverticula due to cancer or fecalith
- Signs and symptoms
  - Left lower-quadrant abdominal pain
  - Fevers, chills
  - Nausea, vomiting
  - Constipation, diarrhea
  - Increased urgency, dysuria (bladder irritation from inflamed sigmoid colon)
  - Palpable mass in some cases
- Diagnostics
  - CT abdomen pelvis with oral and IV contrast: bowel wall thickening, pericolic fluid collections
  - Upright plain film to rule out perforation
  - Colonoscopy to determine cause of diverticulitis should be done 4–6 weeks after resolution due to increased risk of perforation in the acute setting
- Management: may be treated inpatient or outpatient depending on severity, patient comorbidities, age, and presence of complications
  - Medical
    - IV fluids, bowel rest (nil per os)
    - Antibiotics: cover gram negatives and anaerobes
      - Ciprofloxacin plus metronidazole
      - TMP-SMX plus metronidazole
      - Amoxicillin-clavulanate
      - Piperacillin-tazobactam
      - Moxifloxacin
  - Surgical
    - If unresponsive to medical therapy
    - Development of complications such as perforation, abscess, obstruction, fistula (colovesical), toxic megacolon
    - Multiple recurrences

Diarrhea
- Causes
  - Malabsorption: chronic pancreatitis, lactose intolerance, celiac disease (Table 6-4; Fig. 6-5), Whipple disease
  - Infectious: bacterial, viral, parasitic (Table 6-5)
  - Medications: antibiotics
  - Inflammatory: ulcerative colitis, Crohn disease (Table 6-6; Fig. 6-6)
  - Psychiatric: irritable bowel syndrome
- Signs and symptoms
  - Increased frequency or decreased consistency of bowel movement
  - Watery, bloody, floating
  - Dehydration, anemia, hemoconcentration
- Diagnostics
  - Clinical
  - Electrolyte derangements: hypokalemic, nonanion gap metabolic acidosis
- Management: fluid resuscitation and treat underlying etiology

Angiodysplasia
- Epidemiology: common cause of lower GI bleed in >60 years old
- Pathophysiology: abnormally formed dilated veins in the colonic submucosa
- Signs and symptoms
  - Diarrhea
  - Melena
  - Anemia
  - Hematochezia in severe cases

TABLE 6-4   Celiac disease versus tropical sprue

	CELIAC DISEASE	TROPICAL SPRUE
Signs and symptoms	• Chronic diarrhea, weight loss • Iron deficiency anemia, fat-soluble vitamin deficiencies • Dermatitis herpetiformis (subepidermal microabscesses at the tip of the dermal papillae) on extensor surfaces such as elbows, knees, and buttocks: specific for celiac disease • D-xylose test: lower urinary and venous D-xylose levels • Less common: elevated transaminases, arthritis, neurologic symptoms	
Diagnostics	• Serology: immunoglobulin A (IgA) antiendomysial, IgA antitransglutaminase antibodies • Serology may be falsely negative in patients with IgA deficiency, in these cases check for IgG • EGD with biopsy: atrophy and effacement of small intestinal villi	• EGD with biopsy: blunted villi with increased inflammatory cells in the lamina propria
Management	• Gluten-free diet • Dapsone for dermatitis herpatiformis	• Tetracycline plus folic acid for 3–6 mo
Complications	• Increased risk for T-cell lymphoma	• None

EGD, Esophagogastroduodenoscopy.

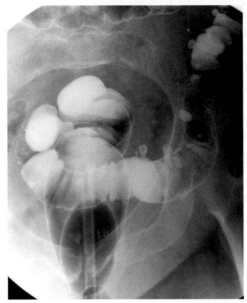

Figure 6-5: Colonic outpouchings in a patient with diverticulosis on barium enema examination.

- – Associations
  - Aortic stenosis
  - Von Willebrand factor deficiency
  - Advanced renal disease
- – Diagnostics
  - Colonoscopy: most commonly bleeding from the right colon
  - Angiography if colonoscopy cannot be performed
- – Management
  - Coagulation of the lesion
  - Hemicolectomy for persistent life-threatening bleeds

Irritable Bowel Syndrome
- – Causes
  - Idiopathic: possible psychiatric component
  - Diagnosis of exclusion
- – Signs and symptoms
  - Alternating diarrhea and constipation
  - Chronic abdominal pain (may be improved after bowel movement)
- – Associations: other psychomotor conditions (fibromyalgia, chronic fatigue syndrome, migraines)

TABLE 6-5   Causes of infectious diarrhea and their associations

ETIOLOGY	ASSOCIATIONS	MANAGEMENT
Bacillus cereus	• Fried rice • Acute onset • Vomiting	• Supportive
Staphylococcus aureus	• Potato salad, mayonnaise • Acute onset • Vomiting	
Shigella	• Uncooked beef • Hemolytic uremic syndrome	
Giardia	• Campers, hikers	• Metronidazole
Clostridium difficile	• Recent antibiotic use • Pseudomembranous colitis	• Oral vancomycin (first line) or fidaxomicin • Metronidazole
C. botulinum	• Unpasteurized honey (infants) • Canned foods • Flaccid paralysis	• Antitoxin
Vibrio vulnificus	• Seashells, oysters • Severe infections in hemochromatosis, liver disease, blood transfusions due to high affinity for iron • Sepsis, hemorrhagic bullae	• Tetracycline plus third-generation cephalosporin
Campylobacter	• Guillain-Barré syndrome • Pseudoappendicitis • Chickens, turtles	• Supportive • Fluoroquinolones in severe cases or if patient is immunocompromised
Salmonella	• Chickens, raw eggs • Gallbladder colonization	
Cryptosporidium	• Immunocompromised (AIDS <100 CD4 cells) • Chronic watery diarrhea	• Nitazoxanide, paromomycin
Entamoeba histolytica	• Travel to Africa, South America, Southeast Asian • Bloody diarrhea • Liver abscess	• Metronidazole, paromomycin
Trichinella	• Undercooked pork • Myalgias, periorbital edema, eosinophilia	• Albendazole, mebendazole
Tenia solium	• Undercooked pork • Cysts in muscles (cysticercosis) or brain (neurocysticercosis)	• Praziquantel • Albendazole plus steroids for central nervous system infection

Other iron-loving organisms: *Yersinia, Listeria, Vibrio.*
AIDS, Acquired immunodeficiency virus.

- Diagnostics
  - Normal labs, imaging, and colonoscopy
  - Rome criteria: recurrent abdominal pain for at least 1 day/week in the last 3 months with two of the following
    - Symptoms related to defecation
    - Change in stool frequency
    - Change in stool form
- Management: symptomatic
  - Initially attempt lifestyle and dietary modification (avoidance of gas-producing foods, lactose, gluten)
  - Diarrhea
    - Loperamide
    - Bile acid sequestrants: cholestyramine, colestipol
    - 5-HT3 antagonist (alesetron)
  - Constipation
    - Psyllium
    - Polyethylene glycol
    - Magnesium citrate
    - Lubiprostone, linaclotide
  - Cramping/spasms
    - Dicyclomine
    - Hyoscyamine

Both vitamin B12 and bile acids are reabsorbed in the terminal ileum resulting in B12 deficiency in Crohn disease when there is terminal ileum involvement. Loss of bile acids results in increased concentration of bilirubin conjugates and total calcium in the gallbladder. This alters the hepatic bile composition resulting in cholesterol supersaturation and formation of gallstones.

TABLE 6-6 Differentiating inflammatory bowel disease; ulcerative colitis versus crohn disease

	ULCERATIVE COLITIS	CROHN DISEASE
Epidemiology	• Bimodal distribution: age 15–40, age 50–80	• Second and third decades of life
Signs and symptoms	• Chronic bloody diarrhea, rectal pain, tenesmus, incontinence • Serology: ANCA positive, elevated inflammatory markers, leukocytosis, anemia	• Chronic watery diarrhea, abdominal pain, nausea, vomiting • Serology: ASCA positive, elevated inflammatory markers, leukocytosis, anemia
Colonoscopy	• Continuous mucosal inflammation starting in the rectum and extending proximally • Pseudopolyps	• Skip lesions: areas of transmural inflammation separated by normal intestine • May involve any part of the gastrointestinal tract; most commonly involves terminal ileum
Biopsy	• Crypt abscesses	• Transmural granulomas
Complications	• Toxic megacolon	• Fistulas (enteroenteric, enterocystic, intravaginal) • Abscesses • Obstruction
Extraintestinal manifestations	• *Erythema nodosum* • *Pyoderma gangrenosum* • Primary sclerosing cholangitis • Arthritis, uveitis, spondyloarthritis	• Nephrolithiasis (increased oxalate absorption) • Subacute combined degeneration (B12 deficiency, terminal ileitis) • Gallstones (lack of bile acid reabsorption and cholesterol supersaturation) • Arthritis, uveitis, spondyloarthritis
Treatment	• Acute exacerbation: steroids • Maintenance therapy: mesalamine, sulfasalazine • Surgery is curative and indicated for disease refractory to medical management	• Acute exacerbation: steroids • Maintenance therapy: anti-TNF agents (infliximab, etanercept), immunomodulators (azathioprine, mercaptopurine) • Surgery for the management of complications such as fistulas, strictures, bowel obstruction
Risk of colon cancer	• Increased after 8–10 years of colonic involvement • Follow-up with colonoscopy every 1–3 yr after having ulcerative colitis for 8–10 yr • Presence of primary sclerosing cholangitis further increases risk	• Increased risk only if there is colonic involvement

ANCA, Antineutrophil cytoplasmic antibody; *ASCA*, anti-*Saccharomyces cerevisiae* antibodies; *TNF*, tumor necrosis factor.

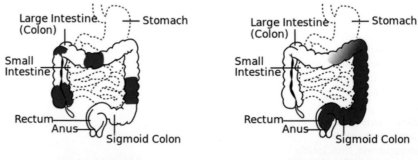

Crohn Disease   Colitis Ulcerosa

Figure 6-6: Colonic distribution of Crohn disease *(left)* and ulcerative colitis *(right)*. Skip lesions seen in Crohn disease vs diffuse colonic involvement starting from the rectum in ulcerative colitis. (Image courtesy of Samir.)

Toxic Megacolon
- Causes
  - *Clostridium difficile*
  - Ulcerative colitis
  - Ischemic colitis
  - Volvulus
  - Diverticulitis
- Signs and symptoms
  - Peritoneal signs (severe ileus, guarding, rigidity, rebound tenderness)
  - Worsening fever (>38°C), abdominal distention
  - Hemodynamic instability
  - Altered mental status

Avoid barium contrast enema if toxic is megacolon suspected due to high risk of perforation.

- Diagnostics
  - Abdominal x-ray: initial test
    - Right colonic dilation >6 cm
    - Haustral folds that do not extend across entire lumen
    - Multiple air fluid levels in the colon
  - CT abdomen and pelvis
- Supporting labs
  - Leukocytosis >10,500
  - Lactate >2.2
- Management: medical emergency due to risk of perforation
  - Medical
    - IV fluids, nasogastric tube, bowel rest
    - IV corticosteroids for inflammatory bowel disease (IBD)–induced toxic megacolon
    - Antibiotics
      - Third-generation cephalosporin (ceftriaxone) plus metronidazole
      - *C. diff* colitis related: oral vancomycin plus IV metronidazole
  - Surgical: for patients unresponsive to medical management or those who have perforated
    - Subtotal colectomy with end ileostomy

Colon Cancer
- Risk factors
  - Age >50 years
  - Family history
  - IBD (ulcerative colitis)
  - High-fat, low-fiber diet
  - Genetic mutations
    - Hereditary nonpolyposis colorectal cancer (HNPCC)
    - Familial adenomatous polyposis (FAP)
    - Peutz-Jeghers syndrome
- Key manifestations
  - Iron deficiency anemia
  - Weight loss
  - Constipation
  - Change in stool diameter ("pencil-thin" stools)
  - Bowel obstruction
  - Melena, hematochezia
- Associated polyposis syndromes
  - Gardner syndrome
    - FAP variant
    - APC gene mutation
    - Thousands of polyps
    - Colon cancer plus soft tissue tumors (desmoid, lipomas, osteomas, fibromas, sebaceous or epidermoid cysts)
  - Turcot syndrome
    - FAP variant
    - APC gene mutation
    - Thousands of polyps
    - Colon cancer plus CNS neoplasms (medulloblastoma, glioblastoma)

- Peutz-Jeghers syndrome
  - Mucocutaneous pigmentation (lips, perioral, buccal mucosa)
  - Hamartomatous polyps (small intestine): may present as intussusception or small bowel obstruction
  - Increased risk of other cancers (breast, stomach, small intestine, pancreas)
- Hereditary nonpolyposis colorectal cancer (Lynch syndrome)
  - DNA mismatch repair gene mutation
  - Colon cancer without the development of polyps
  - Increased risk for multiple other cancers (endometrial, ovarian, gastric, pancreatic, urothelial, skin)
- Diagnostics
  - Barium enema: apple-core lesion
  - CT abdomen and pelvis
  - Colonoscopy: definitive diagnosis
- Management
  - Surgical resection for localized disease
  - Chemoradiation for advanced disease
- Screening: dependent on presence of risk factors
  - No risk factors: colonoscopy starting at age 50
  - First-degree relative diagnosed before age 60: colonoscopy starting at age 40 or 10 years before diagnosis, whichever start screening earlier
  - FAP: colonoscopy starting at 10–12 years old with plan for early colectomy before inevitable progression to colon cancer
  - Peutz-Jeghers: colonoscopy starting at age 12
  - HNPCC: colonoscopy starting at 20–25 years old

ANORECTAL

Hemorrhoids occur due to engorgement of the arteriovenous connections of the anal canal and may be painful or painless depending on their location above or below the dentate line; however, regardless of their location the treatment is similar (Table 6-7).

Anal Cancer
- Epidemiology: most commonly squamous cell carcinoma; rarely adenocarcinoma
- Risk factors
  - Human papillomavirus (HPV) serotypes 16, 18, 31, 33
  - Anal intercourse
  - Smoking
  - Human immunodeficiency virus

TABLE 6-7   Internal versus external hemorrhoids

	INTERNAL HEMORRHOIDS	EXTERNAL HEMORRHOIDS
Definition	Engorgement of arteriovenous connections in the anal canal	
Causes	• Low-fiber diet • Constipation • Increased portal pressures (cirrhosis, obesity, pregnancy)	
Signs and symptoms	• Usually painless (visceral innervation) • Bright red blood per rectum • Classified from grade I (no prolapse) to IV (irreducible) based on degree of prolapse • Sensation of perianal fullness	• Extremely painful (somatic innervation), especially if thrombosed • Bright red blood per rectum or on toilet paper • Itchy, mucous discharge
Location	• Above the dentate line (lined by columnar epithelium)	• Below the dentate line (lined by squamous epithelium)
Diagnosis	• Anoscopy • Proctoscopy	

Treatment	• Medical
	  • High-fiber diet
	  • Topical analgesics and steroids: hydrocortisone/lidocaine
	  • Antispasmodics: topical nitroglycerin, nifedipine
	  • Sitz bath: warm bath used to alleviate anal sphincter spasms; used for acute flares
	• Surgical
	  • Rubber band ligation
	  • Sclerotherapy
	  • Excision for severe unresponsive cases	

- Signs and symptoms
  - Anal pain/mass
  - Rectal fullness
  - Constipation
- Diagnostics: biopsy
- Management: Nigro protocol chemoradiation (5-fluorouracil + mitomycin) preferred over surgery due to preservation of anal sphincter
- Prevention
  - HPV vaccine
  - Barrier contraceptives (chronic)
  - Smoking cessation

HEPATOBILIARY

There are several viral hepatitides with the most common being hepatitis A through E. Hepatitis A and E are acute viruses; hepatitis B and C are chronic and potentially lead to cirrhosis if untreated (Table 6-8). Thorough understanding of hepatitis B serology can allow for differentiation between acute infection, chronic infection, and prior vaccination (Table 6-9). Hepatitis B and C will often require pharmacotherapy to prevent chronic hepatitis and subsequent cirrhosis; however, this pharmacotherapy comes with side effects (Table 6-10). Lastly, hepatitis can also be caused by noninfectious etiologies such as drug, malignancy, vascular, and autoimmune disorders (Table 6-11).

TABLE 6-8   Differentiating viral hepatitides

	HEPATITIS A/E	HEPATITIS B	HEPATITIS C
Risk factors	• Fecal-oral transmission • Travel to endemic areas (Africa, Latin America, Asia)	• Unprotected intercourse • Needlestick • Vertical transmission (infected mother to baby): results in chronic infection of the baby 90% of time	• IV drug abuse
Signs and symptoms	Abdominal pain, jaundice, malaise, fatigue, fever		
Diagnostics	• IgM antibody	• See table below	• Hepatitis C IgG, PCR
Management	• Supportive care	• Acute infection: supportive care • Chronic infection (positive serology after 6 mo): tenofovir, entecavir, adefovir, lamivudine, interferon	• Dependent upon genotype (most common type genotype 1) • Ledipasvir-sofosbuvir • Ribavirin, interferon
Complications	• Acute liver failure in 1–2% • Increased mortality in pregnant women: hepatitis E	• Superinfection when coinfected with hepatitis D (on its own hepatitis D lacks the virulence factors to be infectious)	• Chronic infection: cirrhosis, hepatocellular carcinoma
Associations	• None	• Serum sickness reaction with acute infections: fever, joint pain, rash, lymphadenopathy • Polyarteritis nodosa • Membranous glomerulonephritis	• Porphyria cutanea tarda • Lichen planus • Cryoglobulinemia • Membranoproliferative glomerulonephritis

Ig, Immunoglobulin; *PCR*, polymerase chain reaction.

TABLE 6-9   Hepatitis B serology

	SURFACE ANTIGEN (HBS)	SURFACE ANTIBODY (HBAB)	CORE ANTIBODY (HBC)
Acute infection	+	−	+ IgM
Acute infection with resolution	−	+	+ IgG
Chronic infection	+	+	+ IgG
Vaccination	−	+	−
Window phase	−	−	+ IgM

Ig, Immunoglobulin.

TABLE 6-10   Side effects of hepatitis treatments

Tenofovir	• Renal insufficiency • Osteoporosis
Adefovir	• Hematuria
Interferon	• Fever, malaise, arthralgias, myalgias • Leukopenia, thrombocytopenia • Depression
Ribavirin	• Hemolytic anemia • Teratogenic

Many treatments for hepatitis B can result in acute hepatitis exacerbation upon discontinuation of therapy with associated hepatomegaly and lactic acidosis.

TABLE 6-11   Differentiating noninfectious hepatitis

Drugs	• Alcohol, acetaminophen • Statins • Methotrexate • Oral contraceptive pills, anabolic steroids • Antiarrhythmics (amiodarone) • Anticonvulsants (valproic acid, carbamazepine) • Antibiotics: macrolides, amoxicillin-clavulanate, tuberculosis drugs (rifampin, isoniazid), antifungal (-*azoles*)
Vascular	• Shock liver: hypotension resulting in ischemic liver and markedly elevated AST/ALT >1000 • Portal/hepatic vein thrombosis: paroxysmal nocturnal hemoglobinuria, hypercoagulability, malignant invasion, pregnancy, myeloproliferative disorders (polycythemia vera), chronic inflammatory states
Malignancy	• Commonly metastatic from colon, pancreas, lung, breast: presence of multiple irregular nodules on imaging (CT/MRI) • Less commonly primary malignancy resulting in solitary nodule; elevated AFP
Nonalcoholic steatohepatitis	• Diagnosis of exclusion • Seen commonly in patients with metabolic syndrome (elevated triglycerides, low HDL, increased waist circumference, elevated blood pressure) • Treatment is weight loss and avoidance of hepatotoxic agents
Autoimmune	• Seen in middle-aged women with chronic progressive hepatitis and other autoimmune diseases (type I diabetes, primary sclerosing cholangitis) • Antibodies: ANA, antismooth muscle, antiliver kidney microsomal type 1/2 • Wide range of liver manifestations from mild asymptomatic transaminitis to acute liver failure and cirrhosis • Treatment is oral glucocorticoids, avoidance of hepatotoxic agents

AFP, Alpha-fetoprotein; *ANA*, antinuclear antibody; *AST/ALT*, aspartate transaminase/alanine aminotransferase; *CT/MRI*, computed tomography/magnetic resonance imaging; *HDL*, high-density lipoprotein.

Other Infectious Viral Hepatitides
- Epstein-Barr virus (EBV)
  - Epidemiology: adolescence, young adults
  - Signs and symptoms
    - Fever, malaise
    - Jaundice, splenomegaly
    - Tonsillar exudates
  - Diagnostics: heterophile antibody positive
  - Management
    - Supportive
    - Steroids only if impending airway obstruction from tonsillar enlargement
  - Complications
    - Airway obstruction secondary to tonsillar enlargement
    - Increased risk of splenic rupture from contact sports
- CMV
  - Similar presentation to EBV
  - Heterophile antibody negative
- Dengue fever
  - Epidemiology
    - Endemic to South America, Africa, Southeast Asia
    - Transmitted by mosquito bite

- Signs and symptoms
  - Fever, headache
  - Retroorbital pain
  - Breakbone fever: severe myalgias, arthralgias
  - Maculopapular rash
  - Hemorrhage from mucosal surfaces (epistaxis, hematochezia, melena, hematuria)
- Supporting labs
  - Leukopenia
  - Thrombocytopenia
  - Transaminitis
  - Reverse transcriptase PCR, viral antigen nonstructural protein 1
  - Dengue immunoglobulin M (IgM)
  - Positive tourniquet test: presence of petechiae upon inflation of blood pressure cuff
- – Management: supportive care

Cirrhosis
- – Definition: loss of synthetic and metabolic function of the liver secondary to chronic consult resulting in fibrosis and destruction of the liver architecture
- – Causes
  - Alcohol (most common cause)
  - Chronic hepatitis B/C
  - Others
    - Autoimmune
    - Drug induced
    - Infectious
    - Metabolic
    - Cardiac (right heart failure resulting in congestive hepatopathy)
    - Nonalcoholic steatohepatitis
- – Signs and symptoms
  - Chronic abdominal pain/distention, ascites
  - Hyperestrinism (spider angiomas, telangiectasia, gynecomastia, palmar erythema, testicular atrophy)
  - Portal hypertension (gastric/esophageal varices, hemorrhoids, caput medusa)
  - Asterixis
  - Splenomegaly (thrombocytopenia secondary to splenic sequestration)
  - Jaundice (hyperbilirubinemia)
- – Diagnostics
  - Liver biopsy: definitive diagnosis (destruction and loss of liver architecture associated with collagen deposition and fibrosis)
  - Supporting labs
    - Synthetic dysfunction
      - Elevated International Normalized Ratio (decrease production of vitamin K–dependent coagulation factors)
      - Hypoalbuminemia
    - Metabolic dysfunction
      - Hyperammonemia
      - Hyperbilirubinemia
      - Hyperestrinism
    - Portal hypertension
      - Esophageal varices
      - Rectal hemorrhoids
      - Caput medusa
- – Management
  - Treat underlying cause
  - Avoidance of hepatotoxic agents
  - Prevention and management of complications
  - Definitive treatment with liver transplant
- – Complications
- – Portal hypertension (Fig. 6-7)
  - Esophageal variceal hemorrhage
    - Definition: life-threatening complication of portal hypertension as elevated portal pressure results in dilated submucosal esophageal veins that are predisposed to rupturing and presenting with massive hematemesis, melena, and altered mental status

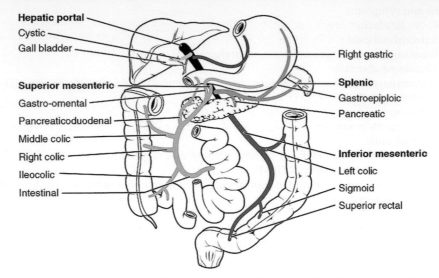

Figure 6-7: Normal portal venous drainage. The gastrointestinal tract is primarily drained by the inferior mesenteric, superior mesenteric, and splenic veins. The superior mesenteric and splenic veins join to form the portal vein, which supplies most oxygen and nutrients to the liver. In addition, toxins and other metabolites are drained through the portal system to be metabolized by the liver before this blood reenters the systemic circulation via the hepatic vein and inferior vena cava. (Image courtesy of OpenStax College.)

- Management
  - Aggressive fluid resuscitation, airway protection (consider intubation)
  - Prophylactic antibiotic (ceftriaxone or ciprofloxacin or TMP-SMX) for possible concurrent bacterial peritonitis
  - IV octreotide (splanchnic vasoconstriction and reduction of portal pressures)
  - Emergent endoscopy after stabilization (sclerotherapy, variceal ligation)
  - Less effective alternatives
- Balloon tamponade (temporary)
- Transjugular intrahepatic portosystemic shunt (TIPS; potentially worsens hepatic encephalopathy as it allows ammonia to bypass liver metabolism and enter the systemic circulation)
  - Prevention: nonselective beta blockers (propranolol, nadalol) to reduce portal pressures
- Rectal hemorrhoids
  - Bright red blood per rectum on the surface of the stool
  - Diagnosed by visual inspection or anoscopy
  - Treat with sitz bath, topical nitroglycerin/nifedipine, rubber band ligation
- Ascites
  - Definition: accumulation of fluid within the peritoneal space secondary to elevated portal pressures (portal hypertension) and decreased oncotic pressure (hypoalbuminemia)
  - May be caused by other etiologies
    - Congestive heart failure
    - Malignancy (ovarian peritoneal carcinomatosis)
    - Tuberculosis
    - Nephrotic syndrome
  - Diagnostics
    - Etiology of ascites determined by serum albumin and ascites gradient (SAAG) from paracentesis
- SAAG >1.1: portal hypertension
- SAAG <1.1: infectious, malignancy
  - Management: focused on reduction of portal pressures
    - Paracentesis if excess fluid is causing discomfort
    - Furosemide plus spironolactone
- Spontaneous bacterial peritonitis (SBP)
  - Definition: infection involving the peritoneal cavity often occurring with ascites
  - Signs and symptoms
    - Worsening abdominal pain/distention
    - Unexplained leukocytosis, renal failure
    - Altered mental status

- Diagnosis
  - >250 polymorphonuclear lymphocytes on paracentesis
  - Most commonly caused by *Escherichia coli, Klebsiella;* may also be caused by *Staphylococcus, Streptococcus*
- Management
  - Third-generation cephalosporin (cefotaxime, ceftriaxone) or fluoroquinolone (levofloxacin) if allergic to cephalosporin
  - Prophylaxis (indicated for patients at high risk for developing recurrent SBP): TMP-SMX or fluoroquinolone (ciprofloxacin, norfloxacin)
- Hepatic encephalopathy
  - Definition: worsening neuropsychiatric symptoms in the setting of cirrhosis
  - Signs and symptoms
    - Confusion, headache, altered mental status
    - Sleep disturbances (diurnal variation), mood changes
    - Asterixis, myoclonus, hyperreflexia
    - Fetor hepaticus (musty breath odor)
    - Cerebral edema, seizures, coma: in severe cases
  - Diagnostics
    - Clinical: presence of symptoms plus precipitating factors (GI bleeding, infection, hypovolemia, alkalosis, hypokalemia, sedatives)
    - Hyperammonemia: degree of hyperammonemia not strongly correlated to severity of hepatic encephalopathy
  - Management: reduction of systemic ammonia
    - Lactulose
      - Acidification of gut lumen resulting in increased conversion of ammonia to ammonium, which cannot be readily absorbed from the gut and excreted via the feces
      - Reduces bacterial colonic load due to cathartic affects → decreased GI transit time → decreased time for ammonia absorption
    - Rifaximin (used in combination with lactulose): antibiotic that reduces number of ammonia-producing bacteria

---

Most common cause of liver cancer is metastasis (most commonly from colon cancer).

- Hepatorenal syndrome
  - Definition: oliguric renal failure in the setting of cirrhosis secondary to renal vasoconstriction (decreased perfusion) and excess vasodilatory substances (nitric oxide)
  - Triggers
    - Decreased intravascular volume (diarrhea, vomiting, sepsis, diuresis, hemorrhage, SBP)
    - Decreased glomerular filtration rate (GFR) (NSAIDs, angiotensin-converting enzyme inhibitor)
  - Classification: regardless of subtype most patients commonly die from infection, hemorrhage, or dialysis complications
    - Type I: rapidly progressive, death within weeks
    - Type II: less progressive; however, death within 3–6 months
  - Diagnostics: renal studies consistent with prerenal azotemia (decreased GFR, low urine sodium, FeNa <1%, elevated blood urea nitrogen/creatinine ratio); however, unresponsive to IV fluids
  - Management: supportive care until patient can receive liver transplant
    - Octreotide
    - Midodrine: alpha agonist that increases blood pressure
    - Low-dose dopamine (increases renal vasodilation)
    - TIPS
- Hepatopulmonary syndrome
  - Definition: hypoxia secondary to liver failure and portal hypertension
  - Pathophysiology: thought to be secondary to intrapulmonary vascular dilation as cirrhotic liver cannot metabolize vasodilators such as nitric oxide → ventilation-perfusion mismatch and possible development of intrapulmonary shunts

- Signs and symptoms
  - Liver failure
  - Orthodeoxia (hypoxia when sitting upright)
  - Platypnea (dyspnea in upright position, relieved when supine)
- Management: supportive care until patient can receive a liver transplant with supplemental oxygen
- Hepatocellular carcinoma

Hepatocellular Carcinoma

Additional notes regarding cirrhosis:
- Severity of liver disease classified by Child-Pugh score (class A, B, C): scoring system considers the following: ascites, bilirubin, encephalopathy, Internaltion Normalized Ratio (INR), albumin
- Candidacy for liver transplant classified using Model for End Stage Liver Disease (MELD) score: more of a quantitative approach compared to Child-Pugh taking into account creatinine, bilirubin, INR, sodium
- Patients with cirrhosis should be monitored periodically with alpha-fetoprotein monitoring for the development of hepatocellular carcinoma

- Risk factors
  - Any cause of cirrhosis
  - Occasionally hepatitis B can cause hepatocellular carcinoma without evidence of cirrhosis
  - Toxins (aflatoxin, vinyl chloride)
  - Hepatic adenoma
  - Infectious (schistosomiasis)
  - Metabolic (alpha-1 antitrypsin, Wilson disease, hemochromatosis)
- Signs and symptoms
  - Abdominal pain, weight loss
  - Worsening hepatomegaly in a patient with known cirrhosis
- Paraneoplastic syndromes
  - Hypoglycemia
  - Polycythemia
- Diagnostics
  - Elevated alpha-fetoprotein
  - Contrast-enhanced CT/MRI: lesion >1 cm, nonrim arterial phase hyperenhancement relative to liver parenchyma
  - Liver biopsy: only if atypical imaging appearance
- Management
  - Localized disease
    - Surgical resection; however, most patients are high-risk surgical candidates due to liver failure
    - Nonsurgical alternatives: thermal ablation, embolization
  - Extensive disease: chemotherapy
    - Alpha-fetoprotein also elevated in germ cell tumors and genetic abnormalities during pregnancy (neural tube defects, aneuploidy, abdominal wall defects)
    - Sorafenib/regorafenib (tyrosine kinase, vascular endothelial growth factor inhibitors)

Wilson Disease (Hepatolenticular Degeneration)
- Epidemiology

Alpha-fetoprotein also elevated in germ cell tumors and genetic abnormalities during pregnancy (neural tube defects, aneuploidy, abdominal wall defects).

- Autosomal recessive disorder
- Early adolescents or adulthood
- Pathophysiology: disorder of copper metabolism with decreased levels of ceruloplasmin (copper transporter) → elevated free copper levels deposited in various organs (liver, basal ganglia) → oxidative damage
- Signs and symptoms
  - Neuropsychiatric
    - Tremors, ataxia, dysarthria
    - Delirium, hallucinations (auditory/visual)
  - Seizures

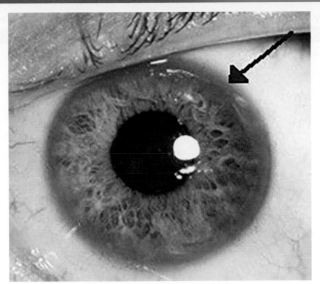

Figure 6-8: Kaiser-Fleischer ring in patient with Wilson disease. (Image courtesy of Herbert L. Fred, MD, Hendrik A. van Dijk.)

- GI
  - Abdominal pain
  - Hepatomegaly, jaundice
- Musculoskeletal
  - Pseudogout
  - Calcium pyrophosphate deposition disease (CPPD)
- Hematological: Coombs negative hemolytic anemia
- Renal
  - Type 2 renal tubular acidosis, nephrolithiasis
  - Fanconi syndrome
- Eyes
  - Kayser-Fleischer rings (greenish brown rings around the cornea representing copper deposition in Descemet membrane) (Fig. 6-8)
  - Cataracts

Consider Wilson disease in any young patient presenting with tremors and ataxia.

- Diagnosis
  - Slit-lamp examination
  - Decreased ceruloplasmin levels (may be decreased due to underlying liver dysfunction caused by primary disease process)
  - Increased urinary copper after administration of penicillamine
  - Liver biopsy: increased hepatic copper (>250 µg per gram dry weight)
- Management: copper excretion
  - Copper chelators: penicillamine, trientine
  - Zinc (interferes with intestinal absorption)
- Complications
  - Cirrhosis
  - Hepatocellular carcinoma

Neuropsychiatric symptoms of Wilson's may present similarly to schizophrenia and must be ruled out before diagnosing a patient with schizophrenia.

Disease progression of primary sclerosing cholangitis (see Table 6-12) is not affected by colectomy done for inflammatory bowel disease.

TABLE 6-12   Primary biliary cirrhosis (pbc) versus primary sclerosing cholangitis (PSC)

	PBC	PSC
Epidemiology	• Middle-aged women	• Middle-aged men
Signs and symptoms	• Jaundice • Pruritus (increased bile acids deposited in skin) • Abdominal pain • Malabsorption of fat-soluble vitamin (inability to excrete bile acids into the small intestine) • Xanthelasma/xanthomas (hyperlipidemia)	• Jaundice • Pruritus • Abdominal pain • Malabsorption of fat-soluble vitamins
Associations	• Other autoimmune diseases: Sjögren syndrome, rheumatoid arthritis, CREST syndrome, Hashimoto, Addison disease	• Inflammatory bowel disease
Diagnostics	• Elevated alkaline phosphatase with normal to slightly elevated bilirubin • Serology: antimitochondrial antibody, elevated IgM, ANA • MRCP: dilated intrahepatic ducts	• Elevated alkaline phosphatase with normal to slightly elevated bilirubin • Serology: p-ANCA • MRCP: dilated intra- and extrahepatic ducts, "beads on a string"
Treatment	• Ursodeoxycholic acid (delays disease progression) • Cholestyramine (pruritus) • Calcium, vitamin D, bisphosphonates for osteoporosis • Liver transplantation	• Ursodeoxycholic acid, cholestyramine • Endoscopic stenting of strictures • Liver transplantation
Complications	• Biliary cirrhosis • Osteoporosis	• Biliary cirrhosis • Cholangiocarcinoma • Gallbladder cancer • Colon cancer (increased risk independent of IBD)

Use of ursodeoxycholic acid in primary sclerosing cholangitis has not been proven to be as beneficial in delaying disease progression as seen in primary biliary cirrhosis.

ANA, Antinuclear antibody; *IBD,* inflammatory bowel disease; *Ig,* immunoglobulin; *MRCP,* magnetic resonance cholangiopancreatography; *p-ANCA,* perinuclear antineutrophil cytoplasmic antibody.

Cholangiocarcinoma
 – Definition: malignancy of the intra- or extrahepatic biliary ducts
 – Risk factors
   • Primary sclerosing cholangitis (Table 6-12)
   • Ulcerative colitis
   • Clonorchis sinensis (liver fluke infection associated with undercooked fish; treated with praziquantel)
   • Choledochal (biliary) cyst
 – Signs and symptoms
   • Abdominal pain, palpable abdominal mass
   • Obstructive jaundice (light-colored stools, dark-colored urine, pruritus)
   • Weight loss
 – Diagnosis
   • Elevated CA-19-9
   • Endoscopic retrograde cholangiopancreatography (ERCP) with biopsy
   • Percutaneous transhepatic cholangiography
 – Management
   • Extremely poor prognosis (<1-year survival after diagnosis) as most tumors are unresectable
   • Palliative stenting for biliary obstruction

Klatzkin tumor: cholangiocarcinoma involving proximal third of common bile duct at the union of the right and left hepatic ducts.

Pancreas

Acute Pancreatitis
 – Causes
   • Alcohol, gallstones
   • Hypertriglyceridemia (>1000)

- Drugs
  - Diuretics (thiazides, furosemide)
  - Valproate
  - Azathioprine
  - Didanosine
  - Pentamidine, metronidazole, tetracycline
  - GLP-1 analogues
- Infectious (CMV, mumps, legionella)
- Iatrogenic (ERCP, cholesterol emboli postcardiac catheterization)
- Trauma

Imipenem should be avoided in those with seizure disorders as it lowers the seizure threshold.

- Signs and symptoms
  - Epigastric pain radiating to the back
  - Nausea, vomiting, anorexia
  - Severe cases
    - Fever, tachycardia, hypotension
    - Hypoxia, tachypnea
    - Cullen sign (periumbilical discoloration: hemoperitoneum)
    - Grey Turner sign (flank discoloration: retroperitoneal bleed)
    - Hypocalcemia (saponification)
- Diagnostics
  - Two of three criteria required to make the diagnosis
    - Epigastric pain radiating to the back, worsened by food
    - Amylase/lipase >3 times the upper limit of normal
    - CT abdomen/pelvis (pancreatic inflammation, peripancreatic fluid and fat stranding) (Fig. 6-9)
  - Abdominal ultrasound or ERCP to diagnose etiology (gallstones)
- Management
  - IV fluid resuscitation
  - Advanced diet as tolerated
  - Pain control often requiring narcotics
  - Laparoscopic cholecystectomy during same hospital admission if gallstones are determined to be the etiology on abdominal ultrasound
- Complications: secondary to the release of pancreatic enzymes, cytokines, and other inflammatory markers resulting in inflammation and organ dysfunction

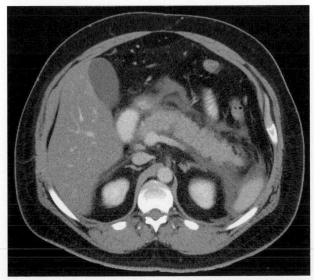

Figure 6-9: Computed tomography abdomen and pelvis in a patient with acute pancreatitis showing pancreatic enlargement, edema, and peripancreatic fluid. (Image courtesy of Hellerhoff.)

- Adult respiratory distress syndrome (massive inflammatory response results in widespread vasodilation and leakage of capillaries)
- Necrotizing pancreatitis (visualized on repeat imaging in patient who continues to worsen and have sepsis physiology)
  - Requires biopsy-proven evidence of infection before starting antibiotics
  - Antibiotics
  - Carbapenem monotherapy (meropenem, imipenem)
    OR
  - Cefepime/fluoroquinolone plus metronidazole
  - May require necrosectomy
- Pseudocyst: rule of 6 s
  - Develop within 6 weeks
  - Observe if <6 cm in size
  - Drain if >6 cm in size or if symptomatic
- Hypotension, acute renal failure (secondary to excessive loss of intravascular volume)
- GI bleed, ileus

Multiple scoring systems (Ranson criteria, APACHE II, BISAP score) exist as prognostic indicators; however, none have been reported to predict disease severity. There is some utility in triaging patients to determine appropriate level of care.

Chronic Pancreatitis
  - Causes
    - Repeated episodes of acute pancreatitis resulting in chronic inflammation → fibrosis → loss of pancreatic exocrine (digestive enzymes) and endocrine (insulin secretion) function
    - Cystic fibrosis
  - Signs and symptoms
    - Weight loss, anorexia
    - Chronic epigastric abdominal pain, worsened by meals
    - Malabsorption (fat-soluble vitamin deficiencies), loose greasy stools
    - Hyperglycemia (lack of insulin)
  - Diagnostics
    - Clinical
    - Imaging: pancreatic calcifications on abdominal CT/x-ray
    - Secretin stimulation test: secretin stimulates the release of bicarbonate-rich fluid; however, in chronic pancreatitis this response will be lacking
    - Normal amylase/lipase
    - Low fecal elastase, increased stool fat
    - Carbohydrate deficient transferrin: biomarker of chronic alcohol intake
  - Management
    - Pancreatic enzyme supplementation (should be taken with PPI or H2 blocker to prevent breakdown of pancreatic enzymes by gastric acid)
    - Alcohol cessation
    - Pain control
  - Complications
    - Vitamin deficiencies
      - Vitamin A: blindness, cataracts, dry eyes
      - Vitamin D: osteoporosis, hypocalcemia
      - Vitamin E: spinocerebellar ataxia, hemolytic anemia
      - Vitamin K: bleeding, easy bruising
      - B12 deficiency: macrocytic megaloblastic anemia, corticospinal/spinocerebellar tract dysfunction, dementia
        - Pancreatic lipase is required to separate R-binder from B12 and allow B12 to combine with intrinsic factor to be absorbed at the terminal ileum
    - Splenic vein thrombosis: splenic vein runs along the posterior aspect of the pancreas; chronic inflammation can result in thrombosis and development of gastric varices
    - Pancreatic cancer
    - Narcotic addiction

Pancreatic Cancer
- Risk factors
  - Smoking, alcohol
  - Chronic pancreatitis
  - Obesity
  - Genetics (BRCA, Peutz-Jeghers, family history)
- Signs and symptoms
  - Weight loss, anorexia, steatorrhea
  - Chronic gnawing abdominal pain, worse at night
  - Courvoisier sign: palpable jaundice (cancer involving head of the pancreas resulting in common bile duct obstruction)
  - Migratory superficial thrombophlebitis
  - New-onset diabetes in older patient without risk factors
- Diagnostics
  - CT/MRI abdomen and pelvis (also used for staging)
  - Biopsy
- Management: dismal prognosis as most cancers have metastasized upon diagnosis
  - Surgery: Whipple procedure (pancreaticoduodenectomy along with removal of common bile duct, gallbladder, and partial gastrectomy)
  - Palliative chemotherapy

CHAPTER 7
Nephrology

NEPHROLOGY BASICS

Nephrology requires a thorough understanding of the basic nephron anatomy and physiology as various ions and electrolytes are absorbed in specific parts of the nephron (Fig. 7-1). Additionally, different medications and congenital anomalies block channels in certain parts of the nephron producing characteristic urinalysis (Table 7-1), acid-base (Figs. 7-2 to 7-5; Tables 7-2 to 7-5), and electrolyte (Table 7-6) abnormalities.

Urinalysis
Interpreting Acid-Base Disorders

Urine anion gap = sodium − chloride
- If positive → renal tubular acidosis
- If negative → diarrhea

Congenital Nephron Disorders

Fanconi Syndrome
- Pathophysiology: hereditary or acquired defective proximal tubular bicarbonate reabsorption (type II renal tubular acidosis [RTA])
- Key manifestations
  - Growth delay, muscle weakness
  - Hypovolemia
  - Rickets, osteomalacia
- Diagnostics
  - Urinalysis
    - Aminoaciduria, phosphaturia
    - Proteinuria
    - Glucosuria
  - Administer bicarbonate and test urine pH, which will be elevated due to defective ability to reabsorb bicarbonate
- Management: same as type II RTA
  - Fluid resuscitation
  - High-dose bicarbonate
  - Thiazide diuretics: volume depletion, resulting in enhanced bicarbonate reabsorption
  - Electrolyte repletion

Bartter Syndrome
- Defective sodium-potassium-chloride channel at the thick ascending limb
- Similar physiology to taking loop diuretics
- Electrolyte derangements: hypokalemia, hypomagnesemia, hypocalcemia
- Urinalysis: hyperkaluria, hypermagnesuria, hypercalciuria

Gitelman Syndrome
- Defective sodium chloride channel at the distal convoluted tubules
- Similar physiology to taking thiazide diuretics
- Electrolyte derangements: hypercalcemia, hypokalemia
- Urinalysis: hyperchloruria, hyperkaluria

Liddle Syndrome
- Overactive epithelial sodium channel in the collecting duct
- Triad of hypertension, hypokalemia, metabolic alkalosis
- Treat with potassium-sparing diuretics (amiloride, triamterene)

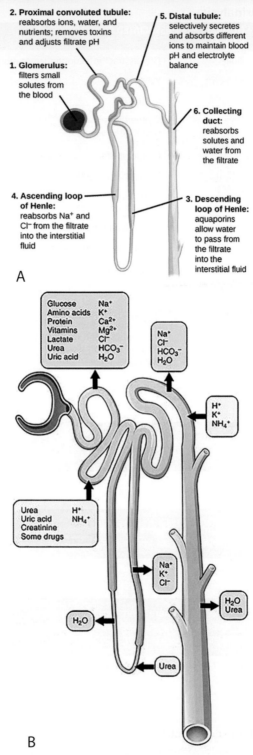

2. Proximal convoluted tubule: reabsorbs ions, water, and nutrients; removes toxins and adjusts filtrate pH

1. Glomerulus: filters small solutes from the blood

5. Distal tubule: selectively secretes and absorbs different ions to maintain blood pH and electrolyte balance

6. Collecting duct: reabsorbs solutes and water from the filtrate

4. Ascending loop of Henle: reabsorbs Na^+ and Cl^- from the filtrate into the interstitial fluid

3. Descending loop of Henle: aquaporins allow water to pass from the filtrate into the interstitial fluid

A

Glucose	Na^+
Amino acids	K^+
Protein	Ca^{2+}
Vitamins	Mg^{2+}
Lactate	Cl^-
Urea	HCO_3^-
Uric acid	H_2O

Na^+
Cl^-
HCO_3^-
H_2O

H^+
K^+
NH_4^+

Urea	H^+
Uric acid	NH_4^+
Creatinine	
Some drugs	

Na^+
K^+
Cl^-

H_2O
Urea

H_2O

Urea

B

Figure 7-1: Nephron anatomy and physiology. Diagrams show the function of the various parts of the nephron (A) and the ions and molecules that are absorbed and secreted (B). (Images courtesy of OpenStax College.)

ELECTROLYTE DERANGEMENTS

Hypernatremia
- Causes: differentiated based on volume status
  - Hypovolemic
    - Sweating, burns
    - Decreased free water intake
    - Diarrhea, diuretics
    - Diabetes insipidus (if thirst drive absent)

TABLE 7-1   Interpreting Urinalysis

COMPONENTS OF URINALYSIS	NORMAL RANGES	ASSOCIATED PATHOLOGIES
WBCs	None	• Urinary tract infection/inflammation
Leukocyte esterase	Negative	• Pyuria
Nitrites	Negative	• Bacteriuria
Red blood cells (RBCs)	None	• Glomerulonephritis • Nephrolithiasis • Cystitis • Coagulopathy
Protein	<30 mg/dL	• Multiple etiologies
Ketones	None	• Starvation • Diabetic ketoacidosis
Bilirubin	None	• Hepatobiliary pathology; direct hyperbilirubinemia
Specific gravity	1.010	• <1.010: loss of free water (psychogenic polydipsia, diabetes insipidus) • >1.010: increased reabsorption of free water (dehydration, SIADH)
pH	5.5–8	• Varies based on acid-base status
Casts (white blood cells [WBCs], RBCs, eosinophil, hyaline, "muddy-brown")	None	• WBCs: pyelonephritis, interstitial nephritis • RBCs: glomerulonephritis • Eosinophils: allergic interstitial nephritis • Hyaline: dehydration • Granular: acute tubular necrosis

SIADH, Syndrome of inappropriate antidiuretic hormone.

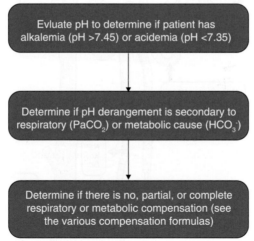

Figure 7-2: Approach to acid-base derangements.

- Euvolemic
  - Diabetes insipidus (if thirst drive intact)
  - Hyperventilation
- Hypervolemic
  - Hypercortisolism
  - Hyperaldosteronism
- Key manifestations: symptom severity correlated with change in absolute sodium or change in sodium over time
  - Headaches, visual disturbances
  - Confusion, altered mental status
  - Cerebral edema, seizures, coma
- Diagnostics: serum sodium >145 mmol/L
- Management: gradual correction of sodium, no more than 0.5 mEq/L/hour
  - Treat underlying etiology; correct volume status before correcting hypernatremia

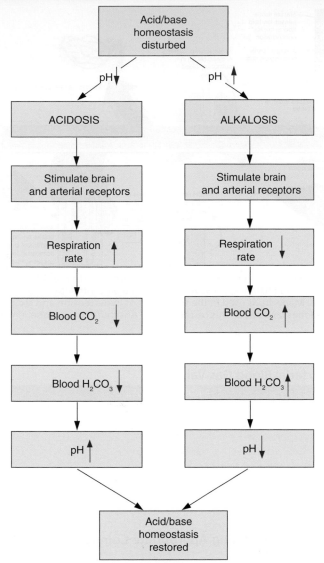

Figure 7-3: Summary of the body's response to pH derangements. (Image courtesy of OpenStax College.)

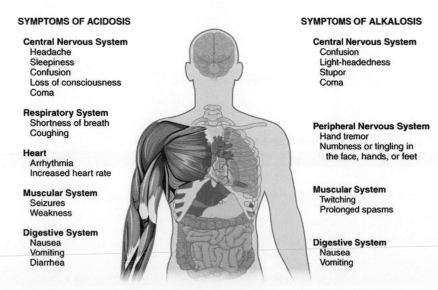

Figure 7-4: Signs and symptoms of acidosis and alkalosis. (Image courtesy of OpenStax College.)

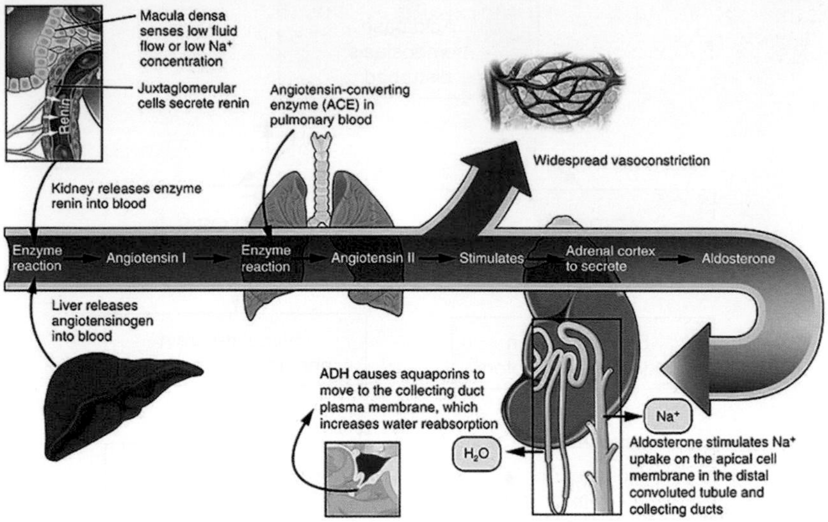

Figure 7-5: Normal physiology of the renin-angiotensin-aldosterone system (RAAS). Functions to maintain adequate blood pressure and sodium balance; however, this may be a detrimental response in certain disorders such as congestive heart failure. Many drugs used in the treatment of hypertension and congestive heart failure aim to inhibit enzymes and hormones involved in this cascade. *ADH*, Antidiuretic hormone. (Image courtesy of OpenStax College.)

TABLE 7-2   Normal Arterial Blood Gas Values

PARAMETER	NORMAL VALUES
pH	7.35–7.45
HCO_3^-	22–28 mEq/L
$PaCO_2$	35–45 mm Hg
PaO_2	80–100 mm Hg

TABLE 7-3   Formulas for Determining Appropriate Compensation in Acute and Chronic Settings

ACID-BASE ABNORMALITIES	COMPENSATORY RESPONSE
Respiratory acidosis	Acute: 10 mm Hg increase in $PaCO_2$ results in 1 mEq/L increase in bicarbonate Chronic: 10 mm Hg increase in $PaCO_2$ results in 3.5 mEq/L increase in bicarbonate
Respiratory alkalosis	Acute: 10 mm Hg decrease in $PaCO_2$ results in 2 mEq/L decrease in bicarbonate Chronic: 10 mm Hg decrease in $PaCO_2$ results in 5 mEq/L decrease in bicarbonate
Metabolic acidosis	$PaCO_2 = 1.5$ (serum bicarbonate) $+8 \pm 2$
Metabolic alkalosis	1 mEq/L increase in bicarbonate results in 0.7 mm Hg increase in $PaCO_2$

TABLE 7-4   Causes of High Anion Gap Metabolic Acidosis

ETIOLOGIES	MANAGEMENT
Lactic acidosis	IV fluids
Diabetic ketoacidosis	IV fluids, insulin, potassium
Methanol, ethylene glycol	Fomepizole (alcohol dehydrogenase inhibitor) +/− dialysis
Uremia	Dialysis
Iron toxicity	Deferoxamine, deferasirox
Salicylates	Sodium bicarbonate (alkalinizes urine) +/− dialysis

Elevated anion gap occurs secondary to the presence of unmeasured acids. Normal anion gap is 10–14, assuming normal albumin.

TABLE 7-5   Causes of Nonanion Gap Metabolic Acidosis

SOURCE	ETIOLOGIES	TREATMENT
Renal	Renal tubular acidosis	Bicarbonate replacement
	Carbonic anhydrase inhibitors	Discontinue medications
Gastrointestinal	Diarrhea	Fluid resuscitation

Differentiate between renal vs gastrointestinal loss of bicarbonate using urine anion gap.

TABLE 7-6   Normal Electrolytes Ranges

Sodium	135–145 mEq/L
Potassium	3.5–5 mEq/L
Chloride	95–110 mEq/L
Bicarbonate	22–28 mEq/L
Blood urea nitrogen	8–20 mg/dL
Creatinine	0.6–1.2 mg/dL
Glucose	80–120 mg/dL
Calcium	8.5–10.5 mg/dL
Magnesium	1.5–2 mEq/L
Phosphorus	3–4.5 mg/dL

- • Severe, hypovolemic hypernatremia: 0.9% normal saline
- • Mild, asymptomatic hypernatremia: oral free water +/− 5% dextrose in water (D5W)
- – Complications: cerebral edema after rapid overcorrection

Hyponatremia
- – Causes
  - • Pseudohyponatremia
    - ▪ Hyperglycemia
    - ▪ Paraproteinemia
  - • Hypovolemic
    - ▪ Decreased free water intake
    - ▪ Insensible losses (sweating, burns, fever)
    - ▪ Diarrhea
    - ▪ Thiazide diuretics
  - • Euvolemic
    - ▪ Syndrome of inappropriate antidiuretic hormone (SIADH)
    - ▪ Hypothyroidism
    - ▪ Hypocortisolism
    - ▪ Thiazide diuretics
    - ▪ Excessive free water intake (psychogenic polydipsia)
    - ▪ Legionnaire disease
    - ▪ Beer drinkers potomania
  - • Hypervolemic
    - ▪ Congestive heart failure (CHF)
    - ▪ Nephrotic syndrome
    - ▪ Cirrhosis
- – Signs and symptoms: same as hypernatremia
- – Diagnostics (Fig. 7-6; Table 7-7)
  - • Serum sodium, serum osmolality
  - • Urine sodium, urine osmolality
  - • Thyroid-stimulating hormone, cortisol
- – Management
  - • General principles
    - ▪ Slow, gradual correction of sodium (no greater than 0.5 mEq/L/hour)
    - ▪ Treat underlying etiology

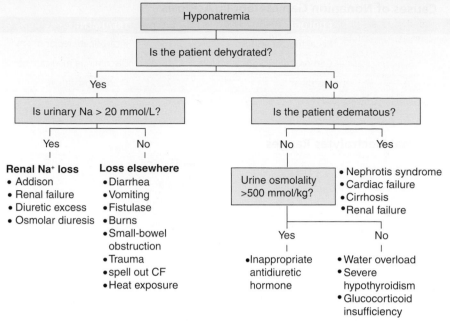

Figure 7-6: Algorithm for approach to hyponatremia.

TABLE 7-7 Interpreting Urine Studies in Hyponatremia

Urine sodium	Elevated (>20 mEq/L) → renal losses of sodium (thiazide diuretics, cerebral salt wasting, adrenal insufficiency)
	Decreased (<20 mEq/L) → excessive free water reabsorption in response to hypovolemia
Urine osmolality	Less than the serum osmolality → psychogenic polydipsia, beer drinker potomania
	Greater than serum osmolality → syndrome of inappropriate antidiuretic hormone

- Consider antidiuretic hormone (ADH) antagonist (tolvaptan, conivaptan) if standard therapy fails
- Hypertonic saline if severely symptomatic (seizures, coma)
  - Specific treatments
    - Hypovolemic hyponatremia: fluid resuscitation
    - SIADH: fluid restriction +/− salt tablets +/− loop diuretic
    - Hypothyroidism, hypercortisolism: hormone replacement
    - CHF: diuresis
- Complications: central pontine myelinolysis after rapid overcorrection

SIADH
- Pathophysiology: autonomous secretion of ADH
- Causes
  - Drugs
    - Selective serotonin reuptake inhibitors
    - Desmopressin
    - Sulfonylurea
    - Oxytocin
  - Pulmonary
    - Small cell lung cancer
    - Pneumonia
    - Positive pressure ventilation
  - Central nervous system
    - Head trauma
    - Infection
    - Stroke
  - Miscellaneous: postoperative anesthesia, pain

- Signs and symptoms: similar to hypernatremia/hyponatremia
- Diagnostics: diagnosis of exclusion
  - Urine osmolality (inappropriately concentrated) > serum osmolality
  - Low blood urea nitrogen (BUN)/creatinine and uric acid
- Management
  - Mild, asymptomatic: fluid restriction
  - Severe, symptomatic: hypertonic saline +/− ADH antagonist
  - May consider loop diuretics

Hyperkalemia
- Causes
  - Decreased excretion
    - Acute kidney injury
    - Drugs
      - Angiotensin-converting enzyme (ACE) inhibitors, angiotensin receptor blockers (ARBs)
      - Potassium-sparing diuretics (amiloride, triamterene)
      - Mineralocorticoid antagonists (spironolactone, eplerenone)
    - Primary adrenal insufficiency
  - Increased production
    - Rhabdomyolysis
    - Hemolysis
  - Transcellular shifts
    - Hypoinsulinemia (diabetic ketoacidosis [DKA])
    - Beta blockers
    - Digoxin (sodium-potassium ATPase inhibitor)
    - Acidosis
  - Pseudohyperkalemia (hemolyzed sample)
- Signs and symptoms
  - Muscle aches, weakness
  - Numbness, paresthesia
  - Palpitations, arrhythmias
- Diagnostics
  - Elevated serum potassium >5.5; repeat potassium levels if elevated to ensure true hyperkalemia and rule out pseudohyperkalemia
  - Electrocardiology (ECG) (Fig. 7-7)
    - Peaked T waves
    - Prolonged PR interval
    - Widening QRS complex
- Management: rapidly reduce levels to prevent the fatal cardiac arrhythmias
  - Mild, asymptomatic, no ECG changes: furosemide or kayexalate

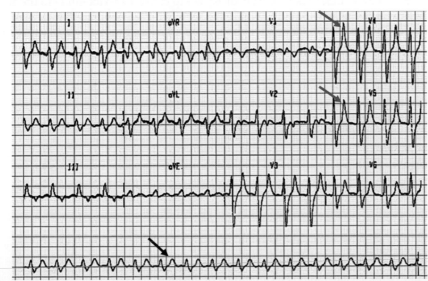

Figure 7-7: Electrocardiography in patient with hyperkalemia showing small or absent P waves; wide QRS; shortened or absent ST segment; wide, tall, and tented T waves *(blue arrows)*, and ventricular fibrillation *(black arrow)*. (Modified Image courtesy of Michael Rosengarten BEng, MD.)

- Severe, symptomatic, ECG changes
  - Calcium gluconate (first line): stabilize cardiac membranes to prevent fatal arrhythmias
  - Drive potassium intracellularly: insulin plus glucose; sodium bicarbonate
  - Potassium excretion
    - Renal excretion: furosemide (renal excretion)
    - Intestinal excretion (block sodium-potassium exchange preventing potassium reabsorption): kayexalate or patiromer
  - Hemodialysis

Hypokalemia
- Causes
  - Renal losses
    - Loop/thiazide diuretic
    - Hyperaldosteronism
    - Hypomagnesemia (refractory hypokalemia secondary to increased urinary loss)
    - Bartter syndrome
    - Hypercortisolism
  - Gastrointestinal (GI) losses
    - Diarrhea, laxative abuse
    - Vomiting, nasogastric suction: metabolic alkalosis compensation by hypokalemia
    - Intestinal fistulas
  - Other causes: beta agonists, insulin administration
- Signs and symptoms
  - Weakness, muscle cramps
  - Paralysis, decreased deep tendon reflexes (DTRs)
  - Ileus
  - Palpitations, arrhythmias
- Diagnostics
  - Serum potassium <3.3
  - ECG: flattening T waves, U waves
- Management: oral or IV potassium repletion

Hypokalemia increases risk of digoxin toxicity.

Calcium Metabolism
- Regulation and calcium homeostasis achieved through the kidneys, bone, and GI tract; hormonally regulated via parathyroid hormone and vitamin D (Fig. 7-8)
- Renal
  - Parathyroid hormone acts on the distal convoluted tubule to increase calcium reabsorption and phosphate excretion
  - Parathyroid hormone stimulates 1-alpha hydroxylase to convert 25-vitamin D to the active form (1,25-vitamin D)
- Bone: parathyroid hormone stimulates osteoblasts → osteoblasts stimulate osteoclasts to increase bone resorption → increase serum calcium and phosphate
- GI tract: vitamin D increases reabsorption of calcium and phosphate

Hypercalcemia
- Causes
  - Endocrinopathies
    - Hyperparathyroidism (most commonly parathyroid adenoma)
    - Hyperthyroidism (stimulates osteoclasts and bone breakdown)
  - Medications related
    - Thiazide diuretics
    - Hypervitaminosis D
    - Milk alkali syndrome (excessive antacid intake)
    - Lithium (increases parathyroid hormone [PTH] levels)
    - Foscarnet
  - Malignancies
    - Bone metastases
    - Multiple myeloma (releases osteoclast-activating factor)
    - PTH-like peptide (squamous cell carcinoma of the lung)
    - Lymphoma (macrophages in granulomas/lymphomas convert 25-vitamin D to 1,25-vitamin D due to presence of 1-alpha hydroxylase)

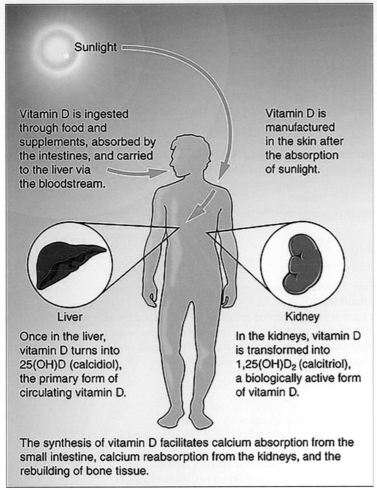

Figure 7-8: Vitamin D synthesis and its role in the calcium homeostasis. (Image courtesy of OpenStax College.)

- Sarcoidosis (same mechanism as lymphoma)
- Immobilization
- Familial hypocalciuric hypercalcemia (FHH)
- Key manifestations
  - Renal
    - Nephrolithiasis
    - Nephrogenic diabetes insipidus
  - Musculoskeletal
    - Bone pain, osteoporosis, pathologic fractures
    - Arthralgias
    - Muscle weakness
    - Osteitis fibrosa cystica ("brown tumors of the bone")
    - Gout/pseudogout
  - GI
    - Abdominal pain, constipation
    - Pancreatitis
    - Peptic ulcer disease (calcium stimulates gastrin secretion)
  - Neurologic
    - Headache, confusion
    - Seizures
  - Cardiovascular: hypertension, shortened QT interval
- Diagnostics
  - Elevated serum calcium
  - PTH levels, serum phosphate
  - Other testing pending suspicion of other disease
    - Malignancy: PTH-related peptide, protein electrophoresis, skeletal survey, or bone scan

- Sarcoidosis, lymphoma: imaging (positron emission tomography/computed tomography [CT]) to locate biopsy accessible site
      - Hypervitaminosis D: elevated 1,25 vitamin D levels
      - FHH: decreased urine calcium excretion (measured with the following ratio formula: urine calcium ÷ creatinine clearance)
        - <0.01 in FHH
        - >0.02 in primary hyperparathyroidism
      - Parathyroid adenoma: sestamibi scintigraphy, neck ultrasound
  - Management
    - IV fluids
    - Osteoclast inhibitors (bisphosphonates +/− calcitonin)
    - Glucocorticoids: granulomatous/lymphoma–related hypercalcemia
    - Loop diuretics: concurrent heart failure
    - Hemodialysis as last resort
    - Other treatments pending specific disease discussed elsewhere

Calcium correction factor: calcium + 0.8*(4 − albumin)

Familial Hypocalciuric Hypercalcemia
- Autosomal dominant inheritance
- Mutation of calcium-sensing receptor resulting in decreased parathyroid sensitivity to hypercalcemia; therefore higher than normal levels of calcium are required to suppress PTH
- Differentiated from primary hyperparathyroidism based on urine calcium excretion; decreased in FHH, increased in primary hyperparathyroidism

Hypocalcemia
- Causes
  - Electrolyte
    - Hyperphosphatemia (precipitate with calcium)
    - Hypomagnesemia (decreased release of PTH, increased PTH resistance)
  - Hormonal
    - Hypoparathyroidism (post–thyroid surgery): most common cause of hypocalcemia
    - Pseudohypoparathyroidism (end-organ resistance to PTH)
  - Renal
    - Loop diuretics
    - Chronic kidney disease (inability to convert 25-vitamin D to 1,25 vitamin D)
  - Other causes
    - Acute pancreatitis (secondary to saponification)
    - DiGeorge syndrome (congenital lack of parathyroid glands)
    - Massive blood transfusion (citrate in blood chelates calcium)
    - Calcitonin
- Key manifestations
  - Neuromuscular
    - Perioral numbness and tingling
    - Chvostek sign (facial nerve paresthesias)
    - Trousseau sign (carpopedal spasms upon inflation of blood pressure cuff)
  - Neurologic
    - Confusion, altered mental status
    - Seizure
    - Basal ganglia calcifications
  - Cardiovascular: prolonged QT interval
- Diagnostics
  - Serum calcium <8.5 mg/dL
  - PTH, vitamin D levels
  - Albumin and/or ionized calcium to ensure true hypocalcemia
- Management: IV or oral calcium repletion

Hypermagnesemia
- Causes
  - Iatrogenic (magnesium infusion to treat torsades du pointes, preeclampsia/eclampsia)
  - Chronic kidney disease
  - Magnesium enemas/laxative

- Signs and symptoms
  - Nausea, headache
  - Decreased DTRs, paralysis
  - Apnea, pulmonary edema, respiratory failure
  - Arrhythmias, cardiac arrest
- Diagnostics: serum magnesium
- Management
  - IV fluids plus furosemide
  - IV calcium in severe cases to treat neuromuscular and cardiac manifestations

Hypomagnesemia
- Causes
  - Foscarnet, amphotericin B
  - Cyclosporine
  - Loop/thiazide diuretics
  - Alcoholism, malnutrition
  - Diarrhea, malabsorption syndromes
- Signs and symptoms
  - Muscle aches, cramps
  - Paresthesia, tetany, hyperreflexia
  - Seizures
  - Arrhythmias
- Diagnostics
  - Serum magnesium
  - Check calcium, phosphorus, and potassium levels due to increased risk of hypocalcemia, hypophosphatemia, and hypokalemia
- Management: magnesium replacement

Phosphate Metabolism
- Homeostasis maintained via the kidneys, bones, and GI tract
- Vitamin D increases reabsorption of calcium and phosphorus from the GI tract
- PTH stimulates osteoclast-induced bone resorption and releases phosphate from bones
- PTH causes urinary phosphate excretion

Hyperphosphatemia
- Causes
  - Chronic kidney disease: secondary hyperparathyroidism with decreased ability to excrete excess phosphate
  - Pseudohypoparathyroidism
  - Hypoparathyroidism, hypervitaminosis D
  - Rhabdomyolysis, tumor lysis syndrome: release of intracellular phosphate
  - Foscarnet
- Diagnostics
  - Serum phosphate
  - Serum calcium (phosphate binds to calcium causing hypocalcemia) and PTH levels (secondary to hypocalcemia)
- Management
  - Dietary restrictions of phosphate
  - Phosphate binders (sevelamer, lanthanum)
  - Antacids (calcium carbonate/acetate)

Hypophosphatemia
- Causes
  - Primary hyperparathyroidism
  - Refeeding syndrome (rapid depletion of extracellular phosphorus secondary to increased intracellular uptake for the use for adenosine triphosphate synthesis)
  - Vitamin D deficiency
  - Phosphate binders, cyclosporine, milk alkali syndrome
  - Malabsorption syndromes, alcohol
- Key manifestations
  - Muscle weakness, myalgias, rhabdomyolysis, osteomalacia
  - Numbness, paresthesias, confusion
  - Arrhythmias, cardiomyopathy
  - Hemolysis, red blood cell (RBC)/white blood cell (WBC) dysfunction
- Diagnostics: serum phosphate
- Management: phosphate repletion

ACUTE KIDNEY INJURY

There are several definitions of acute kidney injury based on a rise in creatinine over a particular time frame; however, the underlying theme is an abrupt loss of renal function often secondary to an acute pathology that does not allow the kidneys enough time to compensate (Table 7-8). Identifying this pathology is important as it guides the management of acute kidney injury (Table 7-9).

TABLE 7-8   Differentiating Prerenal Versus Intrarenal Versus Postrenal Azotemia

	PRERENAL	INTRARENAL	POSTRENAL
Pathophysiology	• Low intravascular volume, hypoperfusion state	• Direct tubular injury	• Obstruction resulting in hydronephrosis and pressure atrophy
Etiologies	• Systolic congestive heart failure • Anaphylaxis, sepsis • Renal artery stenosis, fibromuscular dysplasia • Severe diarrhea, hemorrhage • Hypoalbuminemia (protein-losing enteropathy, cirrhosis, nephrotic syndrome, malnutrition)	• Prolonged prerenal azotemia, ischemia • Drugs: aminoglycosides, vancomycin, NSAIDs, ACE inhibitors, ARBs, cyclosporin, cisplatin, amphotericin B, methanol • Iodine contrast • Glomerulonephritides • Bence-Jones proteins • Tumor lysis syndrome • Rhabdomyolysis, hemoglobinuria	• Neurogenic bladder (uncontrolled diabetes, multiple sclerosis) • Bilateral nephrolithiasis • Urethral stricture • Cervical, prostate, or bladder cancer • Benign prostatic hyperplasia
Diagnostics	• BUN/creatinine ratio >20 • Fractional excretion of sodium <1%	• BUN/creatinine ratio <20 • Muddy brown granular cast (acute tubular necrosis) • Fractional excretion of sodium >1%	• BUN/creatinine ratio <20 • Fractional excretion of sodium >1% • Renal ultrasound showing hydronephrosis

ACE, Angiotensin-converting enzyme; *ARB*, angiotensin receptor blocker; *BUN*, blood urea nitrogen; *NSAID*, nonsteroidal antiinflammatory drug.

TABLE 7-9   Management of Acute Kidney Injury

	ETIOLOGY OF ACUTE KIDNEY INJURY	MANAGEMENT
Prerenal	• Systolic congestive heart failure	• Inotropes, ACE inhibitors, ARBs, beta blockers
	• Anaphylaxis	• IM epinephrine
	• Sepsis, severe diarrhea	• IV fluids
	• Hemorrhage	• Blood transfusion
	• Renal artery stenosis, fibromuscular dysplasia	• Percutaneous revascularization
	• Hypoalbuminemia	• IV albumin, increase enteral nutrition
Intrinsic renal	• Aminoglycosides, vancomycin, NSAIDs, ACE inhibitors, ARBs, cyclosporin, cisplatin, amphotericin B, methanol	• Stop causative agent and use less nephrotoxic alternative
	• Iodine contrast	• IV fluids pre- and postcontrast administration +/– N-acetylcysteine
	• Glomerulonephritides	• Treat underlying etiology
	• Bence-Jones proteins	• Treat underlying multiple myeloma
	• Tumor lysis syndrome	• Prophylactic allopurinol, rasburicase
	• Rhabdomyolysis, hemoglobinuria	• IV fluids
Postrenal	• Neurogenic bladder	• Bladder decompression with Foley
	• Bilateral nephrolithiasis	• IV fluids, ureteroscopy with stent placement
	• Benign prostatic hyperplasia	• Bladder decompression with Foley, alpha agonist (tamsulosin, doxazosin), 5-alpha reductase inhibitor (finasteride)

ACE, Angiotensin-converting enzyme; *ARB*, angiotensin receptor blocker; *NSAID*, nonsteroidal antiinflammatory drug.

Chronic Kidney Disease
Chronic Kidney Disease
- Causes
  - Diabetes mellitus
  - Hypertension
  - Polycystic kidney disease
  - Glomerulonephritis
  - Chronic ascending urinary tract infections (UTIs)
- Signs and symptoms: most commonly asymptomatic; symptoms related to electrolyte and hormonal derangements
  - Hyperkalemia: paralysis, arrhythmias
  - Hyperuricemia: gout
  - Hyperphosphatemia: soft tissue calcifications; associated hypocalcemia
  - Hypermagnesemia: decreased DTRs, apnea, arrhythmias
  - Anemia: fatigue, palpitations
- Management: focused on treating underlying etiology to prevent progression to end stage renal disease (ESRD)
- Complications: ESRD
  - Defined as severe renal dysfunction resulting in life-threatening uremic-, volume-, and electrolyte-related complications that cannot be managed through alternative medical means (Table 7-10, Table 7-11)
  - Treated with dialysis as a temporizing measure
  - Definitive treatment is renal transplant

> Hyperphosphatemia and hypermagnesemia occur due to inability to renally excrete excess electrolytes.

> "AEIOU" indications for dialysis:
> - Refractory, life-threatening acidosis (decreased ability to excrete H+ ions)
> - Refractory, life-threatening electrolyte derangements (hyperkalemia)
> - *I*ntoxications: salicylates, lithium, methanol, ethylene glycol
> - Refractory volume overload
> - *U*remic encephalopathy, pericarditis, bleeding diathesis

Renovascular Disorders
The two most common renovascular disorders, fibromuscular dysplasia and renal artery stenosis, result in narrowing of the vessel caliber. The two pathologies are easily distinguished based on the patient population with renal artery stenosis affecting elderly male and fibromuscular dysplasia affecting young females (Table 7-12).

GLOMERULOPATHY
Glomerulonephritis: inflammation of the glomeruli secondary to an abnormal immune response, deposition, and infiltration of immune complexes resulting in dysfunction of the glomerular basement membrane. May be primary or secondary glomerulopathy (Table 7-13).

Many present as nephritic or nephrotic syndrome (Tables 7-14 and 7-15).

Renal Tubular Acidosis
RTA is common cause of nonanion gap metabolic acidosis. It occurs secondary to a disease process resulting in damage to various parts of the nephron and is differentiated from other causes of nonanion gap metabolic acidosis using urine anion gap (Table 7-16).

TABLE 7-10   Stages of Chronic Kidney Disease Differentiated Based on Glomerular Filtration Rate (GFR) and Albuminuria

STAGES OF CHRONIC KIDNEY DISEASE	GFR (ML/MIN/1.73M2)	ALBUMINURIA (MG/DAY)
Stage I	>90	<30
Stage II	60–89	30–300
Stage III	30–59	>300
Stage IV	15–29	-
Stage V	<15	-

TABLE 7-11   Organ System Complications of End Stage Renal Disease (esRD)

ORGAN SYSTEM	COMPLICATIONS	PATHOPHYSIOLOGY	MANAGEMENT
Neurology	Encephalopathy	Uremia	Dialysis
Cardiac	Coronary artery disease (most common cause of death in ESRD)	Accelerated atherosclerosis (increased oxidant stress), coronary artery calcification, inhibition of nitric oxide	Optimization of coronary artery disease risk factors (smoking cessation, antihypertensives, exercise, antihyperglycemic)
	Pericarditis	Uremia	Dialysis
Pulmonary	Pulmonary edema	Volume overload secondary to oliguria and sodium retention	Dialysis
Gastrointestinal	Nausea, vomiting, anorexia	Uremia	Symptomatic management
Musculoskeletal	Renal osteodystrophy, osteitis fibrosa cystica, osteomalacia	Secondary hyperparathyroidism in response to hypocalcemia and hypovitaminosis D	Cinacalcet
Hematology	Normocytic normochromic anemia	Erythropoietin deficiency	Erythropoietin stimulating agents
	Bleeding, infections	Uremic-induced platelet and neutrophil dysfunction (inability to degranulate)	Dialysis
Dermatology	Calciphylaxis	Calcium phosphate precipitates result in vascular calcifications and skin necrosis	Symptomatic management, wound care
	Pruritus	Uremia	Symptomatic management (topical emollients, antihistamines, gabapentin, ultraviolet light)
Endocrine	Hypoglycemia (palpitations, diaphoresis, altered mental status)	Decreased insulin excretion	Insulin dose adjustment
	Hypocalcemia (tetany, paresthesias)	Decreased conversion of 25-vitamin D to 1,25-vitamin D	Calcium, vitamin D supplementation

TABLE 7-12   Renal Artery Stenosis Versus Fibromuscular Dysplasia

	RENAL ARTERY STENOSIS	FIBROMUSCULAR DYSPLASIA
Pathophysiology	• Atherosclerotic deposition resulting in circumferential narrowing of renal vasculature	• Abnormal vessel development resulting in formation of aneurysm and functional narrowing of involved vasculature
Signs and symptoms	• Elderly male, severe resistant hypertension • Diffuse atherosclerotic disease (transient ischemic attack [TIA], angina, peripheral artery disease) • Systolic-diastolic abdominal bruit • Recurrent flash pulmonary edema • +/− Renal atrophy • Rise in creatinine (>30%) upon initiation of ACE inhibitor or ARB • Elevated renin and aldosterone levels (secondary hyperaldosteronism)	• Young female, severe resistant hypertension • Carotid (TIA, amaurosis fugax), vertebral (headache, tinnitus, visual disturbances)
Diagnostics	• Renal duplex Doppler ultrasound • Computed tomography/magnetic resonance angiography	
Treatment	• Risk factor modification: smoking cessation, statins, aspirin, anti-hypertensives (ACE inhibitor or ARB)	• Antihypertensives (ACE inhibitor or ARB) followed by revascularization (percutaneous transluminal angioplasty)

ACE, Angiotensin-converting enzyme; *ARB,* angiotensin receptor blocker.

TABLE 7-13 Causes of Glomerulonephritis

	GLOMERULONEPHRITIDES	KEY FEATURES
Nephrotic syndrome	Membranous glomerulonephritis	• Associations: hepatitis B/C, syphilis, systemic lupus erythematosus (SLE), rheumatoid arthritis, solid organ malignancies (lung, breast, colon), gold, penicillamine, coagulopathy (renal vein thrombosis)
	Membranoproliferative glomerulonephritis	• Associations: sickle cell disease, purpurea cutanea tarda, chronic bacterial infections (endocarditis), hepatitis B/C, cryoglobulinemia, SLE • Type II membranoproliferative glomerulonephritis (dense deposit disease): antibodies against C3 convertase lead to persistent activation of the complement system
	Focal segmental glomerulosclerosis	• Associations: sickle cell disease, human immunodeficiency virus, heroin use, Blacks, Hispanics
	Minimal change disease	• Most common cause of nephrotic syndrome in children • May be associated with Hodgkin lymphoma • Highly responsive to steroids; excellent prognosis
	Alport syndrome	• Defective type IV collagen • X-linked inheritance • Triad of progressive blindness (anterior lenticonus), sensorineural hearing loss, renal dysfunction
Nephritic syndrome	Poststreptococcal glomerulonephritis	• Preceded by streptococcal skin infection or strep throat 5–14 days prior to glomerulonephritis • Antistreptolysin (ASO), anti-DNAse antibodies; low complement levels • Antibiotics if streptococcal infection still present at the time of diagnosis
	Immunoglobulin A (IgA) nephropathy	• Most common cause of nephritic syndrome • Gross hematuria preceded by upper respiratory tract infection 1–2 days prior • Normal complement levels
	Cryoglobulinemia	• Associated with hepatitis C • Vasculitis presenting with arthralgias, palpable purpura, neuropathy, nephropathy, hepatosplenomegaly, lymphadenopathy • Elevated serum cryoglobulins; low complement levels
	Goodpasture disease	• Anti–basement membrane antibody (type IV collagen): glomerular and alveolar • Progressive pneumonitis (cough, hemoptysis) and renal dysfunction; similar to granulomatosis with polyangiitis; however, lacks upper respiratory tract symptoms • Biopsy: linear deposits on immunofluorescence microscopy • Management: corticosteroids +/– cyclophosphamide +/– plasmapheresis
	SLE	• Multiorgan systemic autoimmune disease • May be associated with nephrotic (membranous glomerulonephritis) or nephritic (rapidly progressive glomerulonephritis)
	Granulomatosis with polyangiitis (Wegener granulomatosis)	• Necrotizing granulomatous vasculitis • Triad of upper respiratory (rhinosinusitis, tracheal stenosis, saddle-nose deformity), lower respiratory (hemoptysis, lung nodules, cavitary lung lesions), progressive renal dysfunction • Other associated symptoms: constitutional (fatigue, weight loss), eyes (conjunctivitis, scleritis), musculoskeletal (arthralgias), painful oral ulcers, cardiac (pericarditis), neuropathy • c-ANCA antibody positive • Management: corticosteroids +/– cyclophosphamide

TABLE 7-13 Causes of Glomerulonephritis

GLOMERULONEPHRITIDES	KEY FEATURES
Polyarteritis nodosa (PAN)	• Medium vessel vasculitis without pulmonary involvement • Presents with abdominal pain (mesenteric vasculitis), polyneuropathy, mononeuritis multiplex, livedo reticularis • Diagnosis: p-ANCA, mesenteric angiography, biopsy • Associated with hepatitis B • Management: corticosteroids +/− cyclophosphamide
Churgg-Strauss	• Medium/small vessel vasculitis • Symptomatology similar to granulomatosis with polyangiitis and PAN: sinusitis, hemoptysis, mononeuritis multiplex, pulmonary infiltrates/nodules • p-ANCA, myeloperoxidase (MPO) antibody positive • Associated with refractory asthma and eosinophilia
Henoch-Schönlein purpura (leukocytoclastic vasculitis)	• Seen in children and adolescents • Small vessel vasculitis associated with systemic IgA deposition • Abdominal pain, intussusception, arthralgias, lower extremity palpable purpura
Rapidly progressive glomerulonephritis	• Also known as crescenteric glomerulonephritis; "crescents" on light microscopy • May be idiopathic or secondary to granulomatosis with polyangiitis, SLE, anti-GBM disease, microscopic polyangitis • Rapid progression to end stage renal disease
Amyloidosis	• Systemic deposition of abnormal proteins resulting in multiorgan dysfunction • May be primary or secondary to multiple myeloma, chronic infectious/inflammatory disease, rheumatoid arthritis, Alzheimer • Cardiac: restrictive cardiomyopathy, atrioventricular block • Neurologic: peripheral/autonomic neuropathy, cerebral amyloid angiopathy (parietal/occipital intracranial hemorrhage) • Dermatology: periorbital purpura, waxy skin, petechia • Gastrointestinal: macroglossia, hepatomegaly • Renal: nephrotic syndrome, nephrogenic diabetes insipidus, enlarged kidneys, type II renal tubular acidosis • Diagnostics: abdominal fat pad biopsy (apple-green birefringence on Congo red stain) • Management: treat underlying etiology. Various treatments available to decrease synthesis (patisiran, inotersen) and promote clearance (tafamidis, diflunisal) of amyloid proteins
Diabetes mellitus	• Complication of diabetic microvascular disease • Prevented with strict glycemic control; treated with ACE inhibitors or ARBs • Biopsy: nodular glomerulosclerosis (Kimmelstiel-Wilson nodules)
Fabry disease	• Lysosomal storage disease characterized by alpha galactosidase deficiency • X-linked recessive inheritance • Presents with angiokeratomas, peripheral neuropathy, visual disturbances (corneal opacities), cardiac (pericarditis, restrictive cardiomyopathy), cerebrovascular accident/transient ischemic attack and renal dysfunction • Treat with enzyme placement

ACE, Angiotensin-converting enzyme; *ARB*, angiotensin receptor blocker; *c-ANCA*, cytoplasmic-antineutrophil cytoplasmic antibodies; *p-ANCA*, perinuclear-anti-neutrophil cytoplasmic antibodies.

TABLE 7-14   Nephritic Versus Nephrotic Syndrome

	NEPHRITIC	NEPHROTIC
Pathophysiology	• Inflammation of the glomerular apparatus secondary to immune complex deposition	• Disruption of glomerular basement membrane → increased permeability and loss of proteins (albumin, antithrombin III, immunoglobulins, transferrin, cholecalciferol binding protein, thyroxine-binding globulin)
Degree of proteinuria	• <3.5 g/24 hr	• >3.5 g/24 hr
Associated features	• Hypertension • Hematuria • Oliguria • Red blood cell casts	• Hyperlipidemia • Bacterial infections (loss of immunoglobulins) • Hypercoagulability (loss of clotting factors, most commonly renal vein thrombosis) • Hypoalbuminemia, anasarca • Fatty casts
Treatment	• Treatment of underlying etiology • Management of associated complications and symptoms: +/− steroids, diuretics, antihypertensives, statins, anticoagulants, antibiotics	

TABLE 7-15   Types Of Proteinuria

	PATHOPHYSIOLOGY	MANAGEMENT
Transient	Benign minimal proteinuria without underlying etiology	Follow up with repeat urinalysis before further workup
Orthostatic	Proteinuria in the upright position	Measure urine protein in upright and supine position
Overflow	Overproduction of proteins secondary to underlying pathology (multiple myeloma, rhabdomyolysis, hemolysis)	Treat underlying etiology

NEPHROLITHIASIS
Nephrolithiasis:
- Types of stones include calcium phosphate, uric acid, ammonium magnesium phosphate (staghorn calculi), cystine (Table 7-17)
- All present similarly with colicky flank pain radiating to the groin, hematuria, dysuria
- May be complicated by pyelonephritis, ureteral obstruction, hydronephrosis

Special considerations
- Calcium oxalate: thiazide diuretics for idiopathic hypercalciuria (diagnosed with elevated 24-hour urine calcium)
- Uric acid stones: radiolucent and will not be visible on x-ray; treated with alkalization of the urine with potassium citrate
- Ammonia magnesium phosphate stones: typically form staghorn calculi requiring surgical intervention
- Cystine stones: positive urinary cyanide nitroprusside test and typical hexagonal crystals on urinalysis
- Medication-related causes of nephrolithiasis: indinavir, acyclovir

CYSTIC KIDNEY DISEASE
Renal cysts are extremely common findings discovered incidentally on CT and ultrasound performed for other reasons. The overwhelming majority are benign; however, there are key features to be aware of that increase the risk of cystic renal cell carcinoma (Table 7-18).

Autosomal Dominant Polycystic Kidney Disease (ADPKD)
- Signs and symptoms
  - Most commonly asymptomatic
  - Flank pain, abdominal pain/distention
  - Hematuria, dysuria
  - Hypertension
- Diagnostics
  - Ultrasound: multiple, large renal cysts
  - Genetic testing: PKD1, PKD2 mutation in patient and first-degree relatives
- Management
  - Blood pressure control: ACE inhibitors or ARBs
  - Extrarenal complications managed as they would for any other patient

TABLE 7-16   Differentiating Renal Tubular Acidosis

RENAL TUBULAR ACIDOSIS	PATHOPHYSIOLOGY	ASSOCIATIONS	MANAGEMENT
Type I (distal)	• Defective distal convoluted tubules resulting in inability to excrete acids and acidify urine • Acid infusion (ammonium chloride) should result in acidic urine; however, in distal renal tubular acidosis urine remains inappropriately alkaline	• Sjögren syndrome, systemic lupus erythematosus • Nephrolithiasis (secondary to alkaline urine) • Amphotericin B, lithium • Chronic hepatitis	• Bicarbonate replacement
Type II (proximal)	• Defective proximal tubular reabsorption of HCO_3^- • Bicarbonate infusion should result in reabsorption in the proximal tubules to correct the acidosis; however, due to proximal tubule defect bicarbonate cannot be reabsorbed and urine pH remains elevated (alkaline)	• Osteomalacia (acidosis resulting in bone resorption) • Fanconi syndrome • Carbonic anhydrase inhibitors (acetazolamide, topiramate) • Heavy metals • Multiple myeloma, amyloidosis	• High-dose bicarbonate • Thiazide diuretic (enhances proximal tubular bicarbonate reabsorption)
Type IV (hyporeninemic hypoaldosteronism)	• Dysfunctional cortical collecting tubule resulting in hyporeninemic hypoaldosteronism	• Uncontrolled diabetes • Hyperkalemia • NSAIDs, calcineurin inhibitors, ACE inhibitors • Heparin • Adrenal insufficiency	• Fludrocortisone

ACE, Angiotensin-converting enzyme; *NSAID,* nonsteroidal antiinflammatory drug.

TABLE 7-17   Differentiating, Diagnosing, and Managing Renal Stones

	RISK FACTORS	DIAGNOSTICS	MANAGEMENT
Calcium oxalate	• Hypercalcemia, primary hyperparathyroidism • Malabsorption syndromes, inflammatory bowel disease (fat malabsorption results in increased oxalate absorption and subsequent hyperoxaluria) • Ethylene glycol intoxication • Idiopathic hypercalciuria • Family history	• Urinalysis: blood, red blood cells • Noncontrast abdominal computed tomography • Stone analysis • Workup and treatment of underlying etiology	• Hydration, analgesia • Stones <7mm: ureteral dilation (tamsulosin, nifedipine), increase fluid intake • Stones >7mm: lithotripsy, ureteral stent • Decompression (nephrostomy, ureteral stent) if septic and obstructed
Uric acid	• Hyperuricemia, tumor lysis syndrome • Acidic urine		• Urinary alkalization: potassium citrate • Allopurinol
Ammonium magnesium phosphate	• Protease producing bacteria *(Proteus, Klebsiella, Pseudomonas, Staphylococcus, Ureaplasma)*		• Antibiotics
Cystine	• Dibasic amino acid transporter abnormality • Family history (autosomal recessive inheritance)		• Hydration, analgesia

– Complications
  • Chronic kidney disease, ESRD, renal cell carcinoma
  • Recurrent UTIs, nephrolithiasis
  • Diverticulosis, hepatic/pancreatic cysts
  • Ventral/inguinal hernias
  • Mitral valve prolapse, aortic stenosis
  • Cerebral aneurysm
Autosomal Recessive Polycystic Kidney Disease
– Similar to ADPKD with development of multiple renal cysts resulting in progressive renal failure

- Associated with Potter syndrome as renal dysfunction leads to decreased urine output → decreased amniotic fluid production → pulmonary hypoplasia and restricted growth in utero
- Management is similar to ADPKD

Medullary Sponge Kidney
- Definition: malformation of terminal collecting ducts in the pericalyceal region of the renal pyramids
- Signs and symptoms
  - Recurrent UTIs
  - Hematuria
  - Nephrolithiasis
- Diagnostics
  - Renal ultrasound
  - IV pyelogram: paintbrush pattern
- Management: supportive care

MALIGNANCY
Renal Cell Carcinoma
- Risk factors
  - Smoking
  - Hypertension, obesity
  - Phenacetin analgesics abuse
  - ADPKD, von Hippel-Lindau syndrome
  - Chronic dialysis
  - Heavy metals (mercury, cadmium)
- Signs and symptoms
  - Abdominal distention, flank pain, hematuria
  - Scrotal varices, testicular pressure (secondary to inferior vena cava or renal vein invasion)
  - Weight loss, night sweat, cachexia
- Paraneoplastic syndromes
  - SIADH
  - Ectopic erythropoietin, adrenocorticotropic hormone
  - Thrombocytosis
  - Hypercalcemia (PTH-like peptide)
- Diagnostics
  - CT abdomen/pelvis
  - Chest and brain imaging for staging
- Management
  - Partial/radical nephrectomy depending on the degree of invasion
  - Immunotherapy for advanced disease

Bladder Carcinoma
- Risk factors
  - Smoking
  - Schistosoma haematobium infection (chronic cystitis)
  - Pioglitazone, cyclophosphamide (acrolein metabolites)
  - Chemical exposures (painters, metal workers, aniline dyes)
  - Radiation
- Subtypes
  - Transitional cell carcinoma
  - Squamous cell carcinoma (associated with S. haematobium infection in North Africa)
- Symptoms
  - Hematuria, dysuria, frequency
  - Abdominal pain, oliguria (secondary to postobstructive uropathy)
  - Suprapubic mass
- Diagnostics
  - Urinalysis looking for hematuria and/or cytology
  - CT pelvis
  - Cystoscopy with biopsy
- Management: cystectomy +/− chemoradiation depending on degree of invasion and metastasis

Infections
Cystitis
- Risk factors
  - Female (shorter anus to urethra distance)
  - Indwelling catheter
  - Benign prostatic hyperplasia (BPH)

- Neurogenic bladder
- Genitourinary procedure
- Signs and symptoms
  - Burning, frequency, urgency with urination
  - Suprapubic pain
  - +/− Hematuria, fever
- Diagnostics
  - Urinalysis: positive nitrites, leukocyte esterase, numerous WBCs
  - Urine culture
- Management: empirically cover gram-negative rods (most commonly Escherichia coli)
  - Outpatient
    - Amoxicillin: simultaneously covers enterococcus, seen more commonly after genitourinary procedure; safe during pregnancy
    - Nitrofurantoin
    - TMP-SMX
    - Fosfomycin
  - Inpatient
    - Ceftriaxone
    - Ciprofloxacin
- Complications: pyelonephritis

Pyelonephritis
- Pathophysiology: ascending UTI often starting in the bladder, therefore caused by same organisms as cystitis (gram-negative rods, E. coli); less likely to spread hematogenous
- Signs and symptoms: similar to cystitis plus costovertebral angle tenderness
- Diagnostics: primarily clinical diagnosis, which may be supported by imaging
  - Urinalysis consistent with UTI plus symptoms
  - CT abdomen and pelvis: edematous renal parenchyma, perinephric stranding
- Management
  - Inpatient (ceftriaxone) or outpatient (ciprofloxacin) depending on severity and ability to take by mouth
  - Add extended-spectrum beta-lactmase (carbapenems) and/or methicillin-resistant Staphylococcus aureus coverage (vancomycin) if there is high suspicion for multidrug-resistant organism
- Complications: perinephric abscess, emphysematous pyelonephritis
  - Should be suspected if patient fails to respond to initial treatment (persistent hypertension, fevers)
  - Further evaluation with renal imaging (renal ultrasound, CT abdomen and pelvis) and urologic consultation

MISCELLANEOUS

Nephrogenic systemic fibrosis: acute on chronic renal failure secondary to administration of gadolinium-containing contrast; no cure, treatment is prevention.

Analgesic Nephropathy
- Acute or chronic renal failure secondary to analgesic abuse (NSAIDs)
- Presents with hematuria and/or renal colic (papillary necrosis, ischemia, sloughing)
- Associated with papillary necrosis, chronic tubulointerstitial nephritis, type I RTA
- Urinalysis: hematuria, sterile pyuria, proteinuria
- CT abdomen and pelvis: small kidneys with bilateral papillary calcification

TABLE 7-18   Benign Versus Malignant Cyst

	BENIGN	MALIGNANT
Size	• <3 cm diameter	• >3 cm diameter
Appearance	• Round, thin smooth walls • Cystic components	• Irregular, thick walled • Solid and cystic components
Enhancement	• Nonenhancing	• Enhancing with contrast indicating vascularity
Septations	• Few	• Multiple
Clinical presentation	• Asymptomatic, discovered incidentally, no follow-up required	• Flank pain, hematuria, hypertension • Will require urologic evaluation

CHAPTER 8 Endocrinology

Hypothalamic pituitary axis principles
- Negative feedback system whereby releasing hormones are secreted by the hypothalamus (Fig. 8-1)
- Releasing hormones from the hypothalamus are released directly into a primary plexus (hypophyseal portal system) to reach the anterior pituitary (Fig. 8-2)
- Nerve terminals from the hypothalamus connect directly to the posterior pituitary
- Hypothalamic-posterior pituitary axis (hypothalamic hypophyseal tract) hormones are produced in the hypothalamus and stored in the posterior pituitary
- From the pituitary, various stimulating hormones are released, which have an end-organ effect (Fig. 8-3)

> The melanocyte-stimulating hormone (MSH) secreted from the anterior pituitary stimulates melanocytes to make melanin. MSH is made from the same propeptide as adrenocorticotropic hormone (ACTH). Therefore, in disorders resulting in elevated ACTH, you will also have elevated MSH.

Posterior Pituitary Disorders
Syndrome of Inappropriate Antidiuretic Hormone (SIADH)
- Causes
  - Drugs
    - Carbamazepine, selective serotonin reuptake inhibitors
    - Cyclophosphamide
    - Nonsteroidal antiinflammatory drugs (NSAIDs)
    - Vincristine
    - Chlorpropamide
    - Oxytocin
  - Pulmonary
    - Lung cancer (small cell), pancreatic cancer
    - Pneumonia
    - Tuberculosis
  - Central nervous system (CNS; cerebral salt wasting)
    - Trauma
    - Meningitis
    - Stroke, hemorrhage
- Pathophysiology: autonomous secretion of ADH resulting in excess reabsorption free water
- Key manifestations: dependent upon rapidity of sodium change
  - Most commonly asymptomatic due to slow, gradual decrease in sodium
  - Headache, visual disturbances
  - Confusion, altered mental status, disorientation
  - Seizures, cerebral edema
- Diagnostics
  - Elevated urine sodium (>40 mEq): secondary to highly concentrated urine lacking free water
  - Urine osmolality > serum osmolality
  - Low serum uric acid level; low blood urea nitrogen
  - Elevated plasma and urine ADH levels
- Management: treat underlying etiology and correct sodium no more than 8 mEq/L over 24 hours
  - Fluid restriction +/– salt tablets +/– loop diuretics (for urine osmolality 2× greater than serum osmolality)

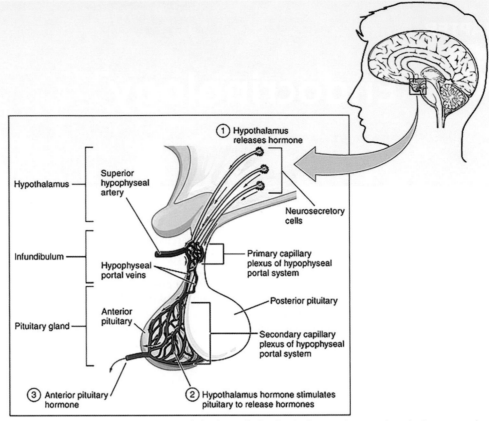

Figure 8-1: Diagrammatic representation of the hypothalamic pituitary axis, anterior pituitary complex. (Image courtesy of OpenStax College.)

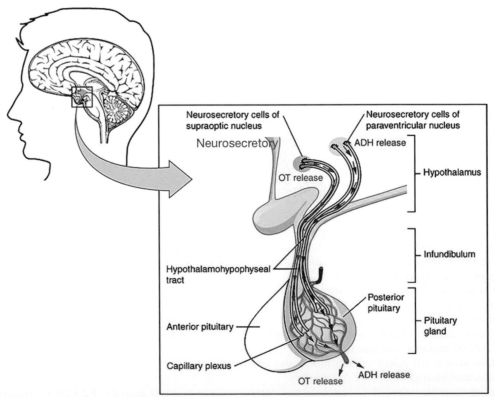

Figure 8-2: Diagrammatic representations of the hypothalamic pituitary axis, posterior pituitary complex. Nerve terminals of the hypothalamus directly connect to the posterior pituitary, which then stores and secretes oxytocin *(OT)* or antidiuretic hormone *(ADH)*. (Image courtesy of OpenStax College.)

Posterior Pituitary Hormones

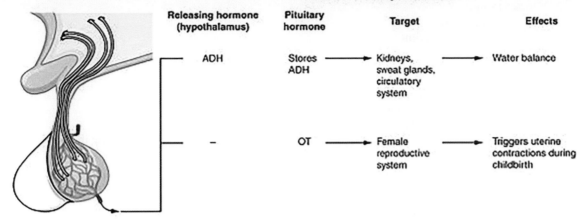

Releasing hormone (hypothalamus)	Pituitary hormone	Target	Effects
ADH	Stores ADH	Kidneys, sweat glands, circulatory system	Water balance
–	OT	Female reproductive system	Triggers uterine contractions during childbirth

Anterior Pituitary Hormones

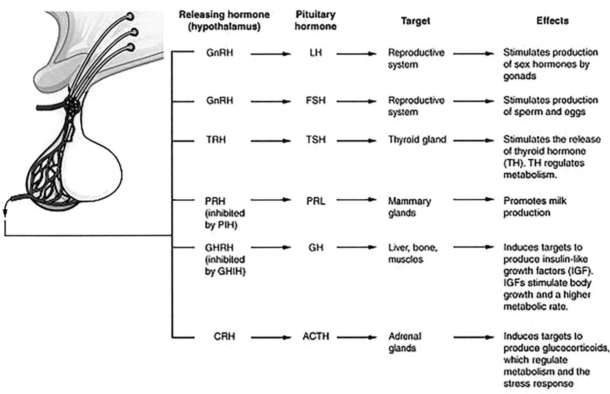

Releasing hormone (hypothalamus)	Pituitary hormone	Target	Effects
GnRH	LH	Reproductive system	Stimulates production of sex hormones by gonads
GnRH	FSH	Reproductive system	Stimulates production of sperm and eggs
TRH	TSH	Thyroid gland	Stimulates the release of thyroid hormone (TH). TH regulates metabolism.
PRH (inhibited by PIH)	PRL	Mammary glands	Promotes milk production
GHRH (inhibited by GHIH)	GH	Liver, bone, muscles	Induces targets to produce insulin-like growth factors (IGF). IGFs stimulate body growth and a higher metabolic rate.
CRH	ACTH	Adrenal glands	Induces targets to produce glucocorticoids, which regulate metabolism and the stress response

Figure 8-3: Diagrammatic representation of the hypothalamus pituitary and end-organ axis. Release of prolactin is inhibited by dopamine, prolactin inhibitory hormone. *GnRH*, gonadotropin-releasing hormone; *LH*, luteinizing hormone; *FSH*, follicle-stimulating hormone; *TRH*, thyrotropin-releasing hormone; *TSH*, thyroid-stimulating hormone; *PRH*, prolactin-releasing hormone; *GHRH*, growth hormone–releasing hormone; *CRH*, corticotrophin-releasing hormone; *ACTH*, adrenocorticotropic hormone. (Image courtesy of OpenStax College.)

- 3% hypertonic saline is severe cases (seizures, cerebral edema)
- ADH antagonist (tolvaptan, conivaptan): last line that does not respond to standard therapy
- Complications: central pontine myelinolysis (secondary to rapid overcorrection)

Diabetes Insipidus
- Causes
  - Central
    - Pituitary tumor
    - Trauma, resection of pituitary stalk
    - Infarction, infection
    - Infiltrative diseases
      - Hemochromatosis
      - Sarcoidosis
      - Langerhans histiocytosis X
      - Lymphocytic hypophysitis

- Nephrogenic
  - Drugs
    - Lithium
    - Demeclocycline
    - Foscarnet
    - Amphotericin B
    - Cidofovir
  - Hypokalemia, hypercalcemia
  - Tubulointerstitial renal disease
  - Mutation in ADH receptor or aquaporin gene
- Pathophysiology: deficiency (central) or resistance (nephrogenic) of ADH resulting in excess loss of free water
- Signs and symptoms
  - Polyuria (>5 L daily), polydipsia
  - CNS manifestations secondary to hyponatremia if unable to keep up with free water loss
    - Altered mental status, confusion
    - Headaches, cerebral edema
    - Seizures
- Diagnostics: water deprivation test: monitor urine osmolality to determine true diabetes insipidus vs psychogenic polydipsia (Table 8-1)
  - Psychogenic polydipsia: urine osmolality appropriately increases as free water is reabsorbed during water deprivation test
  - Diabetes insipidus: urine osmolality remains inappropriately dilute
    - To differentiate central (deficiency of ADH) vs nephrogenic (resistance to ADH) DDAVP is administered
      - Urine osmolality appropriately increases in central diabetes insipidus after DDAVP administration as you supplement the ADH deficiency
      - Urine osmolality remains inappropriately dilute in nephrogenic diabetes insipidus due to lack of response to ADH
- Management
  - Centrawl: ADH replacement (DDAVP)
  - Nephrogenic
    - Treat or stop offending agent
    - Hydrochlorothiazide: increased excretion of sodium resulting in increased reabsorption of sodium and water in the proximal tubules
    - Triamterene, amiloride
    - NSAIDs
- Complications: cerebral edema (secondary to rapid overcorrection)

Histiocytosis X: abnormal proliferation of histiocytes (Langerhans cells of the skin). High prevalence in cigarette smokers. Primarily interstitial lung disease associated with spontaneous pneumothorax, lytic bone lesions, cystic upper lung lesions, and diabetes insipidus. Two systemic variance: Hand-Schüller-Christian disease and Letterer-Siwe disease.

Anterior Pituitary Disorders
Prolactinoma
- Epidemiology: most common cause of hyperprolactinemia and pituitary adenoma
- Pathophysiology
  - Autonomous secretion of prolactin from a pituitary adenoma
  - Excessive prolactin inhibits gonadotropin-releasing hormone (GnRH) → decreased follicle-stimulating hormone (FSH) and luteinizing hormone (LH)
- Signs and symptoms

TABLE 8-1   Summary of urine deprivation test results

	URINE OSMOLARITY IN RESPONSE TO WATER DEPRIVATION	URINE OSMOLARITY IN RESPONSE TO DDAVP
Psychogenic polydipsia	Increased	Increased
Central diabetes insipidus	Dilute	Increased
Nephrogenic diabetes insipidus	Dilute	Dilute

- Headaches, decreased libido
- Females: present primarily due to hormonal symptoms
  - Amenorrhea, galactorrhea
  - Infertility
  - Decreased bone density
- Males: present primarily due to symptoms of mass effect
  - Erectile dysfunction, gynecomastia
  - Visual disturbances (bitemporal hemianopsia)
- Diagnostics
  - Rule out other causes of elevated prolactin: beta-human chorionic gonadotropin, thyroid-stimulating hormone (TSH)
  - Elevated serum prolactin (>200) level
  - Magnetic resonance imaging (MRI) pituitary
- Management
  - Dopamine agonists: cabergoline, bromocriptine
  - Transsphenoidal surgery for refractory cases

Acromegaly

> Other causes of hyperprolactinemia:
> - Idiopathic
> - Pituitary stalk transection
> - Medications: dopamine antagonists (methyldopa, typical antipsychotics, metoclopramide), verapamil, opioids, tricyclic antidepressants
> - Pregnancy
> - Chest wall stimulation
> - Hypothyroidism (increased thyrotropin-releasing hormone stimulates prolactin secretion)
> - Renal insufficiency (due to decreased clearance)

- Pathophysiology
  - Insidious, autonomous secretion of growth hormone → enlargement of soft tissue, cartilage, bones, and visceral organs
  - Growth of long bones will occur if growth hormone excess occurs during childhood prior to fusion of the epiphyseal plates
- Key manifestations
  - Headache, visual disturbances: due to mass effect
  - Macroglossia, protuberant jaw, widely spaced teeth
  - Coarse facial features
  - Increased hat size, ring size, shoe size
  - Carpal tunnel syndrome, early osteoarthritis
  - Obstructive sleep apnea
  - Goiter
  - Cardiomyopathy, hypertension
  - Colonic polyps/cancer, diverticula
  - Diabetes mellitus
- Diagnostics
  - Elevated insulin-like growth factor-1 (IGF-1)
  - Glucose suppression test: oral glucose load should normally suppress growth hormone; lack of growth hormone suppression indicates autonomous secretion of growth hormone
  - MRI pituitary
- Management
  - Surgical: transsphenoidal pituitary resection
  - Medical
    - Somatostatin analogues (octreotide, lanreotide)
    - Cabergoline
    - Pegvisomant (growth hormone receptor antagonist)

Other Hypothalamic Pituitary Disorders
Panhypopituitarism
- Causes: destruction of the pituitary secondary to infection, infiltration, infarction, or mass effect
- Signs and symptoms: related to deficiencies of anterior pituitary hormones (Table 8-2); timing of hormone symptom-related deficiencies is dependent on current body stores; initial presentation is most commonly related to hypocortisolism

TABLE 8-2   Differentiating primary versus secondary versus tertiary eendocrinologic disorders

TYPES	SITE OF ABNORMALITY
Primary	Target organ dysfunction (thyroid, adrenal gland, gonads)
Secondary	Anterior pituitary
Tertiary	Hypothalamus

- Hypocortisolism
  - Orthostatic hypotension, tachycardia
  - Hypoglycemia
  - Eosinophilia
- Hypothyroidism
  - Bradycardia, hypothermia
  - Lethargy
- Hyposomatotropism
  - Decreased muscle mass
  - Increased low-density lipoprotein
- Hypogonadotropism
  - Amenorrhea, decreased libido
  - Infertility
- Hypoprolactinemia: failure to lactate
- Diagnostics: TSH, ACTH, IGF-I, prolactin
- Management: hormone replacement

Pituitary Apoplexy
- Pathophysiology: untreated pituitary adenoma that undergoes growth, bleeding, and necrosis
- Signs and symptoms
  - Severe headache, altered mental status, confusion
  - Meningeal signs (neck pain/stiffness, photophobia)
  - Acute symptoms of hypocortisolism (hypoglycemia, altered mental status, refractory hypotension)
  - Symptoms of other hormone deficiencies (thyroid, gonadotropins, somatomedin) present days to weeks later
- Diagnostics
  - Neuroimaging (computed tomography [CT] head)
  - Lumbar puncture
  - Hormone levels: TSH, ACTH, IGF-I, prolactin
- Management
  - High-dose steroids to prevent vascular collapse and shock
  - Replacement of other anterior pituitary hormones

Empty Sella Syndrome
- Incidental finding on neuroimaging when working up other causes of intracranial pathology
- Associated with idiopathic intracranial hypertension as pressure compresses pituitary to the bottom of the sella as arachnoid mater herniates into the pituitary's suprasellar space
- No signs of hormone deficiencies

Sheehan Syndrome
- Pituitary gland prone to ischemia during pregnancy as it doubles in size to meet hormonal demands of pregnancy
- Acute ischemia and infarction of pituitary gland secondary to significant postpartum hemorrhage
- Presents with acute symptoms of anterior pituitary hormone deficiencies
- Treat with hormone replacement

Kallmann Syndrome
- Hypothalamic hypogonadism: GnRH deficiency → decreased FSH and LH
- Anosmia due to involvement of olfactory bulb
- Other defects include renal agenesis, congenital heart defects, adrenocortical insufficiency
- Lack of secondary sexual characteristics
  - Decreased testicular volume
  - Absent breast development
  - Lack of pubic and axillary hair
- Treat with GnRH replacement

Thyroid Disorders

Hyperthyroidism
Hyperthyroidism is the clinical presentation of elevated thyroid hormone, which may be due to a primary, secondary, or exogenous source (Table 8-3).

Thyroid Storm
- Causes: underlying or uncontrolled hyperthyroidism followed by precipitating event, which results in increased serum or sensitivity to thyroid hormone
- Triggers
  - Stress, surgery, infection, childbirth
  - Trauma
  - Acute iodine load (iodine contrast)
- Key manifestations: worsening of existing hyperthyroid symptoms
  - High fever
  - Delirium, confusion, seizures, coma

TABLE 8-3   Differentiating causes of hyperthyroidism

	PATHOPHYSIOLOGY	SIGNS AND SYMPTOMS	DIAGNOSTICS	TREATMENT
Graves disease	• Thyroid stimulating immunoglobulins (TSI) stimulate production and release of thyroid hormone • Type II hypersensitivity reaction	• Diffuse goiter • Exophthalmos, proptosis (Fig. 8-4) • Myxedema (nonpitting edema and induration over the shins) • Similar symptoms as other causes of hyperthyroidism; above are specific to Graves disease	• High T4, low TSH • Thyroid stimulating immunoglobulin (TSH receptor antibody) • Diffuse uptake on radioactive iodine uptake (RAIU) scan	• Hyperadrenergic symptoms: propranolol, atenolol • Thionamides (decrease thyroid hormone): methimazole, propylthiouracil • Radioactive iodine ablation after achievement of euthyroid state • Steroids for exophthalmos, proptosis
Toxic adenoma	• Single or multiple thyroid nodules autonomously secreting thyroid hormone	• Tachycardia, atrial fibrillation, palpitations • Tremors, anxiety, heat intolerance • Weight loss, increased appetite, diarrhea • Osteoporosis	• High T4, low TSH • Ultrasound • Solitary uptake on RAIU scan	• Thionamides • Radioactive iodine ablation
DeQuervain subacute thyroiditis	• Acute inflammation of thyroid gland secondary to viral infection resulting in release of preformed thyroid hormone and transient hyperthyroidism		• High T4, low TSH • Elevated ESR • Tender thyroid on physical exam	• NSAIDs
Surreptitious use of thyroid hormone	• Exogenous intake of thyroid hormone		• High T4, low TSH • Low thyroglobulin	• Cessation of exogenous thyroid hormone
Pituitary adenoma	• Autonomous secretion of TSH		• High TSH, high T4 • MRI pituitary	• Somatostatin analog (octreotide, lanreotide) to achieve euthyroidism • Transsphenoidal surgery for definitive treatment

Thyroglobulin is hormone that is produced concurrently with thyroid hormone allowing differentiation between endogenous and exogenous thyroid hormone. Similar to insulin and C-peptide.
ESR, Erythrocyte sedimentation rate; *MRI*, magnetic resonance imaging; *NSAID*, nonsteroidal antiinflammatory drug; *TSH*, thyroid-stimulating hormone.

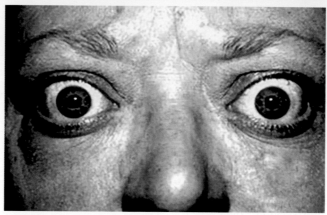

Figure 8-4: Proptosis, exophthalmos in a patient with Graves disease. (Image courtesy of Jonathan Trobe, M.D. - University of Michigan Kellogg Eye Center.)

- • High output congestive heart failure, tachyarrhythmias (atrial fibrillation), hypotension/hypertension
  • Tremor, lid lag, warm and moist skin
  • Nausea, vomiting, abdominal pain, hepatic dysfunction
- Diagnostics
  • Clinical
  • High T4, low TSH
- Management
  • Supportive care: IV fluids, cooling blankets
  • Beta blocker (propranolol): decreases adrenergic symptoms
  • Glucocorticoids: decreased conversion of T4 to T3; prevent vasomotor collapse
  • Thionamides: decreases thyroid hormone production
  • Iodine solution: prevents further release of thyroid hormone
  • Bile acid sequestrants: prevent enterohepatic recycling of thyroid hormone

Hypothyroidism
Hypothyroidism
- Causes
  • Hashimoto thyroiditis (chronic lymphocytic; autoimmune thyroiditis): most common cause of hypothyroidism
  • Medications: amiodarone, lithium
- Signs and symptoms (Fig. 8-5)
  • Myopathy, weakness
  • Fatigue, lethargy, depression
  • Bradycardia
  • Decreased deep tendon reflexes, carpal tunnel syndrome
  • Cold intolerance, weight gain
  • Dry skin, lateral eyebrow hair loss
  • Nonpitting edema
  • Constipation, decreased appetite
  • Menorrhagia
- Diagnostics
  • Primary hypothyroidism: high TSH, low T4
  • Secondary hypothyroidism: low TSH, low T4
  • Hashimoto thyroiditis (chronic lymphocytic; autoimmune thyroiditis): antithyroid peroxidase, antimicrosomal antibodies
  • Supporting labs
    ▪ Normocytic anemia
    ▪ Euvolemic hyponatremia
    ▪ Dyslipidemia
- Management: thyroid hormone replacement
- Complications: myxedema coma
- Caused by prolonged, untreated hypothyroidism
- Precipitated by infection, cold exposure, medication (narcotics), trauma

Hypothyroidism

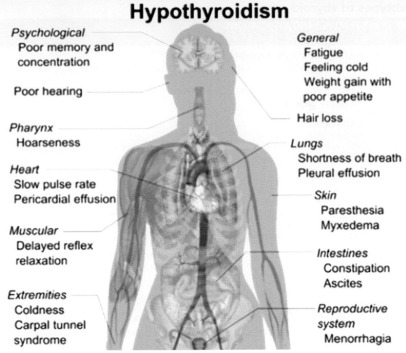

Psychological
Poor memory and
concentration

Poor hearing

Pharynx
Hoarseness

Heart
Slow pulse rate
Pericardial effusion

Muscular
Delayed reflex
relaxation

Extremities
Coldness
Carpal tunnel
syndrome

General
Fatigue
Feeling cold
Weight gain with
poor appetite

Hair loss

Lungs
Shortness of breath
Pleural effusion

Skin
Paresthesia
Myxedema

Intestines
Constipation
Ascites

*Reproductive
system*
Menorrhagia

Figure 8-5: Diagrammatic representation of the signs and symptoms of hypothyroidism. (Image courtesy of Mikael Häggström.)

TABLE 8-4   Other thyroid disease entities

Riedel thyroiditis	• Extensive fibrosis of the thyroid gland extending into the mediastinal structures (esophagus, trachea) • Treated with prednisone
Subclinical hypothyroidism	• Increased TSH, normal T4 levels • Treat with thyroid hormone replacement if symptomatic
Euthyroid sick syndrome	• Seen in critically ill patients; thyroid hormones should generally not be checked in this setting • Low T3/T4, low/low-normal TSH
Cretinism	• Inadequate thyroid hormone during fetal and neonatal development • Results in significant intellectual disability and growth delay

TSH, Thyroid-stimulating hormone.

- Signs and symptoms
  - Altered mental status, stupor, delirium, hypothermia
  - Hypoventilation, bradycardia, hypotension
  - Hypoglycemia, hyponatremia
  - Diffuse nonpitting edema
- Management
  - IV T3/T4 plus stress dose steroids (hydrocortisone)
  - Supportive care

Any cause of hypothyroidism can initially present with hyperthyroid symptoms due to release of preformed thyroid hormone, followed by a euthyroid state, and eventually hypothyroidism (Table 8-4).

Thyroid Nodule and Cancer

Principles and evaluation of thyroid nodule
- Vast majority of thyroid nodules are benign
- Workup of thyroid nodule should begin with TSH levels to differentiate functioning vs nonfunctioning nodule
- Functioning nodules are rarely malignant and should be managed as a toxic adenoma
- Nonfunctioning nodules should be examined with ultrasound to determine their size and composition; large nodules or those with suspicious features should undergo fine-needle aspiration (Table 8-5)

TABLE 8-5 Subtypes of thyroid cancer

TYPE OF THYROID CANCER	KEY FEATURES AND ASSOCIATIONS
Papillary	• Most common thyroid cancer (>70%) • Risk factors: childhood radiation exposure, positive family history • Best prognosis • Histopathology: psammoma bodies, ground glass cytoplasm, pale nuclei with inclusion bodies and central grooving
Follicular	• Spread hematogenously • Risk factors: similar to papillary thyroid cancer • Often require diagnostic lobectomy as fine-needle aspiration cannot distinguish follicular adenoma from malignancy (capsular invasion)
Medullary	• Tumor of the parafollicular C cells • Associated with MEN2A/2B syndromes • Secretes calcitonin, serotonin (flushing, diarrhea)
Anaplastic	• Locally and widely invasive • Aggressive, poorly differentiated, poor prognosis

Postthyroidectomy, higher doses of levothyroxine are needed to suppress thyroid-stimulating hormone and subsequent tumor growth.

Parathyroid Disorders

Function of parathyroid hormone (PTH) and calcium metabolism (Fig. 8-6; Table 8-6)
– PTH is a hormone secreted by the parathyroid glands located posterior to the thyroid glands
– PTH secreted in response to hypocalcemia and works at the kidneys and bone to maintain calcium homeostasis
– Functions at the distal convoluted tubules to increase calcium reabsorption and phosphate excretion
– Stimulates 1-alpha hydroxylase in the kidneys to convert 25-hydroxylase to 25-hydroxylase (active form of vitamin D)
– Functions at the bone by stimulating osteoclasts and bone resorption

Primary Hyperparathyroidism
– Causes
  • Parathyroid adenoma: most common cause
  • Parathyroid hyperplasia
  • Parathyroid malignancy
– Key manifestations: related to hypercalcemia
  • Neurologic
    ▪ Confusion, lethargy
    ▪ Seizures
  • Gastrointestinal
    ▪ Peptic ulcer disease
    ▪ Abdominal pain, constipation
  • Renal
    ▪ Nephrolithiasis
    ▪ Nephrogenic diabetes insipidus
  • Musculoskeletal
    ▪ Bone pain, osteoporosis
    ▪ Pseudogout
    ▪ Osteitis fibrosa cystica (brown tumors of the bone)
    ▪ Subperiosteal bone resorption (radial aspect of middle phalanges, distal clavicular tapering), "salt-and-pepper" skull
  • Cardiovascular
    ▪ Hypertension
    ▪ Short QT interval
    ▪ Vascular/valvular calcifications
– Diagnostics: biochemical testing followed by parathyroid localization (Fig. 8-7)
  • Biochemical pattern
    ▪ High PTH
    ▪ High calcium, low phosphate
    ▪ High alkaline phosphatase
  • Parathyroid localization: sestamibi scintigraphy, neck ultrasound

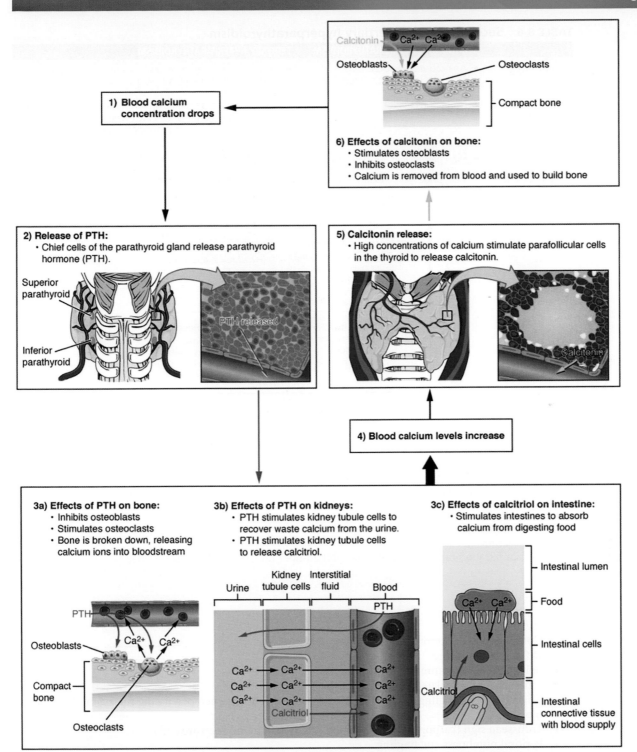

Figure 8-6: Diagrammatic representation of parathyroid hormone and calcium homeostasis. (Image courtesy of OpenStax College.)

– Management
  • Medical: for asymptomatic and/or poor surgical candidates; treatment targeted toward the resulting hypercalcemia
    ▪ IV fluids
    ▪ Bisphosphonates
    ▪ Cinacalcet
  • Surgical
    ▪ Parathyroid adenoma: parathyroidectomy of enlarged gland
    ▪ Parathyroid hyperplasia: removal of 3.5 glands and autotransplantation of 0.5 gland into the neck or forearm muscles

TABLE 8-6   Secondary versus tertiary hyperparathyroidism

	SECONDARY HYPERPARATHYROIDISM	TERTIARY HYPERPARATHYROIDISM
Causes	• Any cause of hypocalcemia (vitamin D deficiency, chronic kidney disease) except for hypoparathyroidism	• Persistent hyperparathyroidism despite correction of long-standing hyperparathyroidism (seen in end-stage renal disease) • Persistence of hyperparathyroidism likely secondary to parathyroid hyperplasia and increased parathyroid gland mass in response to long-standing hypocalcemia
Diagnostics	• Low calcium • High parathyroid hormone (PTH)	• High calcium • High PTH
Management	• Treat underlying etiology	• Same as parathyroid hyperplasia

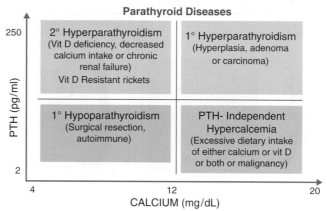

Figure 8-7: Summary of parathyroid diseases.
(Image courtesy of Dr.Vijaya Chandar, MBBS.)

Parathyroid hormone (PTH) related peptide: hormone secreted as part of paraneoplastic syndrome related to multiple malignancies (renal, head and neck, breast, ovarian), most commonly squamous cell carcinoma of the lung. Biochemical testing will show low PTH, high PTHrP, high calcium, low phosphate. Presents with symptomatic and significantly elevated calcium levels.
Surgical indications for parathyroidectomy:
- Serum calcium >1 mg/dL above the upper limit of normal
- Osteoporosis, vertebral fracture
- Nephrolithiasis, glomerular filtration rate <60 mL/min, elevated 24-hour urinary calcium >400 mg/day
- Age <50 years

Hypoparathyroidism
- Causes
  - Complication of thyroidectomy
  - DiGeorge syndrome
  - Polyglandular autoimmune syndrome type I
- Key manifestations: related to hypocalcemia
  - Chvostek sign (tingling along with facial nerve distribution when percussing the zygoid bone below the ear)
  - Trousseau sign (carpopedal spasms upon inflation of blood pressure cuff)
  - Perioral numbness and tingling
  - Anxiety, irritability, seizures
  - Prolonged QT
  - Early cataracts
- Diagnostics
  - Low PTH
  - Low calcium, high phosphate
  - Low 1, 25 vitamin D
- Management: calcium and vitamin D replacement

Pseudohypoparathyroidism
- Mutation of *GNAS-1* gene resulting in resistance of tissues to PTH
- Biochemical test: elevated PTH, elevated phosphate, low/normal calcium (see Fig. 8-7)

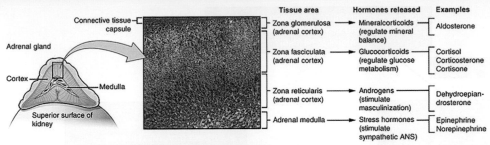

Figure 8-8: Normal anatomy and physiology of the adrenal gland. (Image courtesy of OpenStax College.)

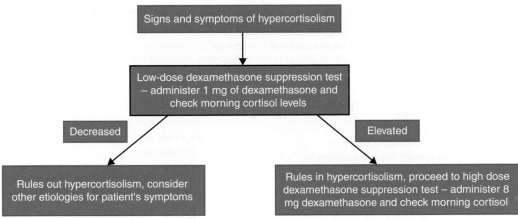

Figure 8-9: Approach to hypercortisolism. First determine whether patient has true hypercortisolism with low-dose dexamethasone depression test. If present, proceed to step two, high-dose dexamethasone suppression test to determine the exact etiology of hypercortisolism.

– Associated with Albright hereditary osteodystrophy (short stature, shortened fourth metacarpal, obesity, developmental delay)

Adrenal Disorders

The adrenal gland is divided into three layers, which secrete their own distinct hormones that play roles in blood pressure control, sodium management, stress hormones, and androgens (Fig. 8-8).

Cushing disease vs syndrome: Cushing disease refers to a pituitary adenoma secreting ACTH resulting in excess cortisol; Cushing syndrome is state of excess cortisol regardless of etiology (Figs. 8-9 and 8-10).

Hypercortisolism

– Causes
  • Cushing disease (pituitary adenoma)
  • Iatrogenic (excess glucocorticoids)
  • Adrenal adenoma
  • Ectopic ACTH-producing tumor (small cell lung cancer)
– Key manifestations (Fig. 8-11)
  • Truncal obesity, thin extremities, "buffalo hump"
  • Abdominal streaky, skin atrophy, easy bruising
  • Depression, mania, psychosis
  • Peptic ulcer disease
  • Hypertension, venous thromboembolism
  • Osteoporosis, avascular necrosis of the hip, myopathy
  • Amenorrhea, erectile dysfunction
  • Acne, hirsutism
  • Cataracts, glaucoma
  • Immunosuppression
  • Hyperglycemia, hypokalemia
– Diagnostics: step-by-step biochemical workup to determine the source of hypercortisolism
  • Low-dose dexamethasone suppression test: administer 1 mg dexamethasone, followed by checking morning cortisol levels

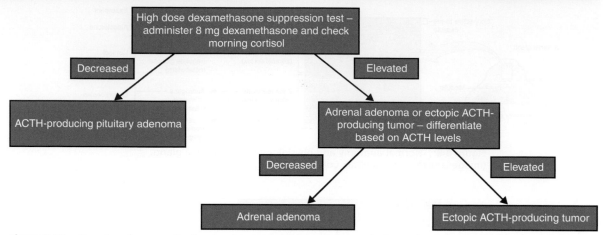

Figure 8-10:   Once true hypercortisolism has been established, the cause is determined via a high-dose dexamethasone suppression test and checking the morning cortisol and adrenocorticotropic hormone *(ACTH)* levels to differentiate the various causes.

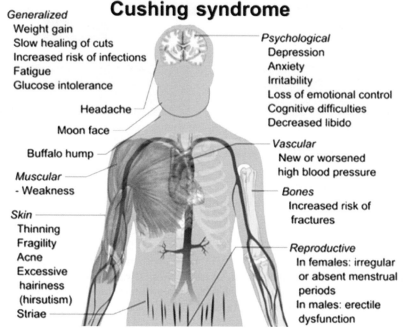

Figure 8-11:   Diagrammatic representation of the symptoms of excess cortisol, by organ system. (Image courtesy of Mikael Häggström.)

- - Low morning cortisol → rules out hypercortisolism
  - High morning cortisol → rules in hypercortisolism; will require further workup with high-dose dexamethasone suppression test
- High-dose dexamethasone suppression test: administered 8 mg dexamethasone, followed by checking morning cortisol levels
  - Low morning cortisol → ACTH-producing pituitary tumor
  - High morning cortisol → adrenal adenoma or ectopic ACTH-producing tumor; differentiate adrenal adenoma or ectopic ACTH-producing tumor by checking ACTH levels
    - Low ACTH → adrenal adenoma
    - High ACTH → ectopic ACTH-producing tumor
- Management: treat underlying etiology
  - Cushing disease: surgical resection
  - Iatrogenic: stop or decrease dose of glucocorticoids; use alternative steroid-sparing agents if possible
  - Adrenal adenoma: surgical resection
  - Ectopic ACTH-producing tumor: treat primary tumor

The cause of hypercortisolism can also be established using a 24-hour urine free cortisol level.

Cushing reflex: physiologic response to elevated intracranial pressures with hypertension, bradycardia, and irregular respirations.

Addison Disease (Adrenal Insufficiency)
– Causes
  • Autoimmune (most common cause in developing world)
  • Infectious
    ▪ Tuberculosis (most common cause in developing world)
    ▪ *Neisseria meningitides* (acute hemorrhagic adrenal crisis)
    ▪ Human immunodeficiency virus, *Mycobacterium avium* complex, cytomegalovirus
    ▪ Systemic mycoses
  • Metastatic cancer (small cell lung cancer)

Melanocyte-stimulating hormone and adrenocorticotropic hormone are produced simultaneously as they are both derived from the same propeptide (pro-opiomelanocortin).
Waterhouse-Friderichsen syndrome: *Neisseria meningitidis* infection resulting in hemorrhagic destruction of adrenal glands and adrenal crisis. Presents with characteristic purpuric rash. Treat as an adrenal crisis.

  • Adrenoleukodystrophy (accumulation of very long-chain fatty acids in the adrenal gland)
  • 21-hydroxylase deficiency
  • Sudden cessation or inappropriate tapering after chronic steroids
– Signs and symptoms
  • Orthostatic hypotension
  • Weakness, lethargy
  • Nausea, vomiting, weight loss
  • Hyperpigmentation of mucous membranes (secondary to melanocyte-stimulating hormone)
– Diagnostic
  • Low morning cortisol, high ACTH
  • ACTH stimulation test: elevated cortisol after administration of cosyntropin (synthetic ACTH)
  • Supporting labs
    ▪ Hyponatremia, hyperkalemia: due to lack of aldosterone
    ▪ Hypoglycemia (due to lack of cortisol)
    ▪ Eosinophilia
– Management: steroid +/− mineralocorticoid (fludrocortisone) replacement
– Complications: adrenal crisis
  • Typically occurs after rapid destruction of adrenal gland or acute stressor (surgery, trauma, hypotension, childbirth)
  • Presents with shock, vascular collapse, coma
  • Treat with aggressive IV fluids and high-dose stress steroids

Addison disease is typically associated with other autoimmune disease such as vitiligo, rheumatoid arthritis, type I diabetes, pernicious anemia, Hashimoto thyroiditis.

Hyperaldosteronism (Conn syndrome)
– Pathophysiology: autonomous secretion of aldosterone without feedback regulation (Fig. 8-12)
– Causes
  • Solitary adenoma: most common
  • Bilateral adrenal hyperplasia
– Key manifestations
  • Mild hypernatremia
  • Hypokalemia
  • Metabolic alkalosis
  • No peripheral edema due to aldosterone escape-induced diuresis
– Diagnostics
  • Elevated aldosterone after trial of high-salt diet
    ▪ Aldosterone-renin ratio >20
    ▪ Easily induced hypokalemia after use of loop/thiazide diuretics

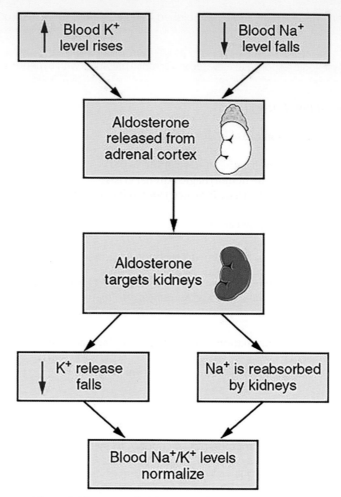

Figure 8-12: Normal aldosterone feedback mechanism. (Image courtesy of OpenStax College.)

– Management
  • Solitary adenoma: surgical resection
  • Bilateral hyperplasia: aldosterone antagonists (spironolactone, eplerenone)

Pheochromocytoma
– Pathophysiology: adrenal medullary tumor producing excessive catecholamines
– Signs and symptoms
  • Paroxysms of headache
  • Severe hypertension
  • Palpitations
  • Diaphoresis, tremors
  • Panic attack
– Diagnostics
  • Elevated urinary and serum metanephrine
  • CT/MRI or MIBG scan for localization
– Associations: rule of 10 s
  • 10% bilateral
  • 10% in children
  • 10% familial (associated with MEN 2 A/2B syndromes, von Hippel-Lindau disease)
  • 10% extraadrenal (organ of Zuckerkandl located at aortic bifurcation)
  • 10% recur
  • 10% malignant
– Management
  • Control blood pressure with nonselective alpha blockers (phenoxybenzamine, phentolamine) first
  • Avoid use of beta blockers if suspected due to potential unopposed alpha vasoconstriction and development of severe life-threatening hypertension
  • Surgical resection after optimizing blood pressure control

Diabetes Mellitus
Diabetes Mellitus
- Risk factors
  - Family history
  - Obesity
  - Gestational diabetes
  - Hereditary hemochromatosis
- Subtypes
  - Type I
  - Type II
- Pathophysiology (Fig. 8-13)
  - Type I: autoimmune destruction of insulin producing pancreatic beta cells
  - Type II: insulin resistance secondary to excess adipose resulting in burnout of pancreatic beta cells

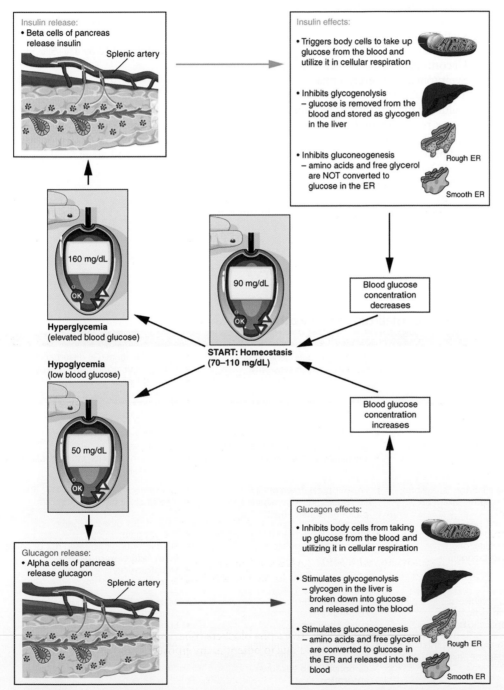

Figure 8-13: Glucose homeostasis via insulin and glucagon. (Image courtesy of OpenStax College.)

- Signs and symptoms
  - Asymptomatic (most common)
  - Polyuria, polydipsia, polyphagia
- Diagnostics
  - Any one of the three can be used to diagnose diabetes mellitus
    - Fasting blood sugar >125 on two separate occasions
    - Glucose >200 mg/dL plus symptoms of hyperglycemia
    - Hemoglobin A1c >6.5%
  - Supporting autoantibodies
    - Antiinsulin (IAA)
    - Antiislet cell cytoplasm (ICA)
    - Antiglutamic acid decarboxylase (GAD)
    - Antityrosine phosphatase (IA2)
- Management
  - Lifestyle changes: low carbohydrate diet, exercise, weight loss
  - Pharmacotherapy (Tables 8-7 and 8-8)
    - Oral antihyperglycemic: preferred for mild cases (hemoglobin A1c <9%) as these can only lower hemoglobin A1c by 2%
    - Insulin: indicated for the following cases as it can lower hemoglobin A1c by 4%–5%
      - Uncontrolled diabetes (hemoglobin A1c >9%)
      - Symptomatic hyperglycemia
      - Type I diabetics
      - Failure of oral antihyperglycemics
- Complications: related to long-term uncontrolled diabetes and can be managed/prevented with strict glycemic control (hemoglobin A1c <7%); require periodic reassessment (every 6–12 months) to monitor and prevent progression to end-stage complications (blindness, end-stage renal disease)

Complications of Diabetes
- Microvascular damage (microangiopathy)
  - Retinopathy
    - Epidemiology: most common cause of blindness in US adults
    - Types
      - Nonproliferative
      - Proliferative
    - Signs and symptoms: seen on fundoscopy
      - Exudates, hemorrhage

TABLE 8-7   Diabetes mellitus pharmacotherapy

DRUG	MECHANISM OF ACTION	SIDE EFFECTS
Metformin (first line)	• Inhibits gluconeogenesis • Increases insulin sensitivity	• Gastrointestinal (GI) disturbances • Rarely, lactic acidosis in renal dysfunction • B12 deficiency
Sulfonylureas (glyburide, glipizide)	• Stimulate release of insulin from the pancreas	• Hypoglycemia • Weight gain
GLP-1 analogues (exenatide, liraglutide)	• Increases insulin and decreases glucagon release from the pancreas • Decreases gastric motility	• Administered as an injection • Weight loss • Caution in patients with medullary thyroid cancer or MEN2 syndrome
DPP-4 inhibitors (sitagliptin, linagliptin, saxagliptin)	• Prevent breakdown of GLP-1 analogues (incretin mimetics) prolonging their effect	• GI disturbances • Nasopharyngitis
Thiazolidinediones (rosiglitazone, pioglitazone)	• Increases insulin sensitivity through transcription regulators	• Weight gain • Fluid retention (increased risk of congestive heart failure exacerbation) • Hepatotoxicity • Fractures, osteoporosis
SGLT2 inhibitors (canagliflozin, dapagliflozin)	• Blocks sodium-glucose cotransporter at the proximal convoluted tubule	• Mycotic urinary infections • Glucosuria • Euglycemic diabetic ketoacidosis
Alpha-glucosidase inhibitors (acarbose, miglitol)	• Blocks enzyme at intestinal brush border resulting in delayed carbohydrate breakdown absorption	• Abdominal cramping, flatulence

TABLE 8-8   Insulin subtypes

TYPES OF INSULIN	ONSET OF ACTION	DURATION OF ACTION
Short acting (aspart, lispro)	15–45 min	3–5 hr
Medium acting (NPH)	3 hr	18–26 hr
Long-acting (glargine, detemir)	2–3 hr	24 hr
70/30 mixture (70% NPH, 30% aspart)	30 min	14 hr

- ○ Macular edema, cotton-wools spots
- ○ Neovascularization
  - ▪ Management
    - ○ Nonproliferative: strict glycemic control
    - ○ Proliferative: laser photocoagulation
    - ○ Regular ophthalmologist follow-up
- Nephropathy (nephrotic syndrome, chronic kidney disease)
  - ▪ Pathophysiology: intercapillary glomerulosclerosis initially results in increased glomerular filtration rate (GFR) (later followed by decreased GFR after prolonged hyperfiltration injury), increased basement membrane thickening and permeability
  - ▪ Histopathology: diffuse glomerulosclerosis, nodular glomerulosclerosis (Kimmelstiel-Wilson nodules), mesangial expansion
  - ▪ Management: angiotensin-converting enzyme inhibitor or angiotensin receptor blocker initiation once microalbuminuria (30–300 mg protein per 24 hours) is detected to decrease intraglomerular and systemic hypertension (130/80)
- Neuropathy
  - ▪ Autonomic neuropathy
    - ○ Gastroparesis
- Pathophysiology: decreased gastric emptying time and contractility secondary to vagus nerve dysfunction
- Signs and symptoms
  - ▪ Nausea, vomiting
  - ▪ Abdominal pain, early satiety, bloating, constipation
  - ▪ Anorexia, hiccups, dyspepsia
  - ▪ Recurrent hypoglycemia
- Diagnostics: gastric emptying study
- Management
  - ▪ Lifestyle modifications: small frequent, high-fiber meals
  - ▪ Promotility agents
  - ▪ Acute: erythromycin (motilin receptor agonist; limited by tachyphylaxis)
  - ▪ Chronic: metoclopramide (D_2 receptor antagonist; prokinetic, antiemetic)
    - ○ Overflow incontinence
- Pathophysiology
  - ▪ Dysfunction of parasympathetic nerves supplying bladder smooth muscle (detrusor) resulting in decreased contractility and increased postvoidal urine
  - ▪ Passage of urine only when bladder pressure exceeds external urethral sphincter pressure; urine stream stops once pressures equilibrate
- Signs and symptoms
  - ▪ Lower abdominal fullness
  - ▪ Suprapubic tenderness
  - ▪ Recurrent urinary tract infection
- Diagnostics: voiding cystourethrogram
- Management: bethanechol or intermittent catheterization
    - ○ Postural hypotension
    - ○ Impotence
  - ▪ Peripheral neuropathy
    - ○ Signs and symptoms
- Stocking-glove distribution (distal sensorimotor neuropathy involving bilateral hands and feet) numbness and tingling
- Decreased vibratory sensation, proprioception
- Charcot arthropathy
- Initially painful, later becomes painless

- Chronic nonhealing lower extremity wounds
  - Diagnostics: monofilament testing
  - Management
- Neuropathic pain
  - Gabapentin, pregabalin
  - Duloxetine, TCAs
  - Carbamazepine
- Chronic lower extremity wounds: regular podiatrist follow-up, wound care, IV antibiotics if osteomyelitis +/− amputation
  - Cranial nerve neuropathy
    - Secondary to ischemia involving vasculature supplying nerves (most commonly cranial nerve III, IV, or VI)
    - Large nerves also affected (peroneal, radial)
- Diabetic ketoacidosis (DKA)
  - Epidemiology: most commonly in type I diabetics
  - Causes
    - Insulin noncompliance or inadequate amount
    - Acute illness (infection, acute coronary syndrome)
    - Trauma, surgery
  - Pathophysiology
    - Lack of insulin or insulin unresponsiveness results in starvation state as cells are deprived of glucose for adenosine triphosphate production
    - Cells switch to fatty acid metabolism for energy resulting in production of ketones as a byproduct
  - Signs and symptoms
    - Polyuria, polydipsia: secondary to hyperglycemia-induced osmotic diuresis
    - Anorexia, nausea, vomiting, abdominal pain
    - Kussmaul respirations (rapid deep breathing), "fruity" acetone breath
    - Hypotension, tachycardia, dry mucous membranes
    - Altered mental status, confusion, coma
  - Diagnostics
    - Elevated blood glucose >400
    - Elevated serum ketones, acetone, beta-hydroxybutyrate
    - Elevated anion gap metabolic acidosis
    - Supporting labs
      - Hyperkalemia (however, decreased total body potassium stores)
      - Pseudohyponatremia
  - Management: goal of therapy is to close the anion gap
    - Aggressive IV fluids
    - IV insulin infusion
    - Supplemental potassium and glucose: prevent insulin-induced hypokalemia and hypoglycemia
    - Replace electrolytes as needed
    - Correct precipitating cause
    - Bridge IV to subcutaneous insulin once anion gap is closed, glucose <200, or able to eat
- Hyperosmolar hyperglycemic nonketotic syndrome
  - Similar causes, signs and symptoms, and treatment as indicated
  - Occurs more commonly in type II diabetics
  - Blood glucose >800 without ketoacidosis
  - Low levels of insulin in type II diabetics prevent transition to fatty acid metabolism and ketoacidosis

Strict glycemic control resulting in prevention of macrovascular complications (stroke, myocardial infarction) has not been established.
Hyperkalemia in diabetic ketoacidosis occurs secondary to cellular hydrogen-potassium exchange pump (hydrogen in, potassium out) to correct acidosis.

Facts about insulin:
- Hormone produced by pancreatic islet beta cells; simultaneously secreted with C-peptide
- Released in response to hyperglycemia
- Functions by driving glucose into cells to be used for adenosine triphosphate (ATP) production
- Activate lipoprotein lipase in adipose to decrease triglyceride levels and treat significant hypertriglyceridemia (>1000)
- Stimulates sodium-potassium ATPase to cause intracellular shifts of potassium and temporarily treat hyperkalemia

TABLE 8-9   Labs differentiating causes of hypoglycemia

	C-PEPTIDE	SULFONYLUREA SCREEN
Insulinoma	Elevated	Negative
Sulfonylurea abuse	Elevated	Positive
Surreptitious insulin	Decreased	Negative

Hypoglycemia
- Causes
  - Excess insulin administration
  - Sulfonylurea abuse
  - Insulinoma
  - Decreased by mouth intake (alcoholism, malnutrition)
  - Sepsis
  - Cortisol deficiency
  - Glycogen storage diseases
- Signs and symptoms
  - Palpitations, tremulousness, diaphoresis
  - Confusion, altered mental status, seizure, coma
  - Whipple triad
    - Hypoglycemia when fasting
    - Hypoglycemic symptoms concurrent with low glucose
    - Hypoglycemic symptoms relieved by glucose administration
  - Diagnostics (Table 8-9)
  - Serum or fingerstick glucose <70 or symptoms of hypoglycemia
  - C-peptide levels: distinguishes surreptitious insulin use vs true hyperinsulinemia causing hypoglycemia
    - If elevated, indicates endogenous hyperinsulinemia (insulinoma, sulfonylurea abuse)
    - If decreased, indicates exogenous hyperinsulinemia (excessive insulin intake)
  - Sulfonylurea screen
- Management: glucose replacement
  - Vitamin B1 prior to administration of glucose to prevent Wernicke encephalopathy
  - High-sugar foods if patient able to take orally
  - IV D50
  - IM glucagon

Pancreatic Neuroendocrine Tumors

Pancreatic neuroendocrine tumors are a group of hormone-producing tumors resulting in symptomatology related to excess hormone production. All are associated with MEN1 syndrome (pituitary, parathyroid, and pancreatic endocrine tumors).

Gastrinoma
- Pathophysiology: autonomously secreting gastrin tumor resulting in hypersecretion of gastric acid and virulent peptic ulcer disease
- Signs and symptoms
  - Abdominal pain, nausea, dyspepsia
  - Anorexia, weight loss
  - Diarrhea, heartburn
- Diagnostics
  - Biochemical studies
    - Elevated serum gastrin (>1000)
    - Secretin stimulation test: normally, secretin should inhibit gastric; however, gastrin levels remain persistently elevated in gastrinoma
  - Localization studies
    - CT abdomen/pelvis to evaluate for metastatic disease
    - Somatostatin receptor scintigraphy
  - Upper endoscopy: multiple, large ulcers extending into jejunum
- Management
  - Localized disease: surgical resection
  - Metastatic disease: somatostatin analogues (octreotide)

- Complications
  - Perforated peptic ulcer
  - Gastrointestinal bleed
  - Gastric outlet obstruction

Insulinoma
- Pathophysiology: autonomously secreting insulin tumor
- Signs and symptoms: related to hypoglycemia
  - Palpitations, diaphoresis, tremors
  - Headache, visual disturbances
- Diagnostics
- Biochemical studies
  - Fasting hypoglycemia
  - Low serum glucose, elevated C-peptide
  - Localization studies: CT/MRI abdomen and pelvis to rule out metastatic disease
- Management
  - Acute management: supplemental glucose (IV dextrose, IM glucagon)
  - Localized disease: surgical resection
  - Metastatic disease: diazoxide, octreotide

Glucagonoma
- Pathophysiology: autonomously secreting glucagon tumor resulting in hyperglycemia
- Signs and symptoms
  - Refractory diabetes mellitus
  - Necrolytic migratory erythema
  - Glossitis, stomatitis
  - Abdominal pain, diarrhea, weight loss
  - Venous thrombosis
  - Depression, psychosis, ataxia
- Diagnostics
  - Elevated serum glucagon
  - CT abdomen and pelvis
  - Somatostatin receptor scintigraphy
- Management
  - Localized disease: surgical resection
  - Metastatic disease: octreotide, sunitinib, everolimus

VIPoma
- Pathophysiology: autonomously secreting vasoactive intestinal peptide (VIP) resulting in activation of intestinal chloride channels
- Signs and symptoms
  - Severe watery diarrhea: commonly referred to as pancreatic cholera
  - Nausea, vomiting
  - Abdominal pain
- Diagnostics
  - Elevated serum VIP
  - Stool osmolality suggestive of secretory etiology (stool osmolar gap <50)
  - Supporting labs
    - Hypokalemia
    - Nonanion gap metabolic acidosis, achlorhydria
    - Hyperglycemia, hypercalcemia
- Management
  - IV fluid resuscitation, electrolyte repletion
  - Localized disease: surgical resection
  - Metastatic disease: octreotide

Somatostatinoma: extremely rare; triad of cholelithiasis, steatorrhea, diabetes

BASICS OF HEMATOLOGY

Understanding the origins and functions of the different cell lines allows for better mastery of the various blood dyscrasias and their associated symptomatology (Figs. 9-1 and 9-2).

ANEMIA

General principles of anemia
- Definition: deficiency of red blood cells: <13 g/dL in men and <12 g/dL in women
- Pathophysiology: secondary to production abnormalities, destruction disorders, or bleeding (Fig. 9-3)
- Signs and symptoms
  - Palpitations, tachycardia, chest pain, dyspnea on exertion/rest
  - Lightheadedness, dizziness, orthostatic hypotension
  - Fatigue, lethargy
  - Pallor, pale conjunctiva
- Diagnostics
  - Mean corpuscular volume (MCV): average size of red blood cells (RBCs); normal range 80–100
  - Red cell distribution width (RDW): variation in size between RBCs; higher values indicate greater size difference between RBCs
  - Reticulocyte count: precursor of RBCs that will mature into erythrocytes within 24 hours; indicator of bone marrow response to anemia
  - Lactate dehydrogenase (LDH), haptoglobin, indirect bilirubin: indicators of hemolytic anemia; LDH and indirect bilirubin will be elevated, haptoglobin levels decreased
  - Bone marrow biopsy: evaluate production abnormalities of anemia
  - Peripheral smear
- Management
  - Treat underlying cause
  - Transfusion if necessary (Fig. 9-4; Table 9-1)
    - Hemoglobin <7
    - Hemoglobin <8 with preexisting coronary artery disease
    - Hemoglobin <10 with symptoms

Severe hypocalcemia can result following massive transfusion secondary to citrate in transfused blood binding ionized calcium.

Macrocytic Anemia
vitamin B12 Deficiency
- Causes
  - Dietary deficiency (strict vegan diet without vitamin B12 supplementation)
  - Pernicious anemia (antibodies against intrinsic factor), chronic atrophic gastritis
  - Gastric bypass, gastrectomy: loss of intrinsic factor producing parietal cells
  - Terminal ileitis (Crohn disease): inability to absorb B12-intrinsic factor complex
  - *Diphyllobothrium latum:* parasitic infection associated with undercooked fish
  - Pancreatic insufficiency (inability to separate vitamin B12 from R-binder)
  - Bacterial overgrowth
- Signs and symptoms: symptoms of anemia with neurologic abnormalities
  - Glossitis, stomatitis

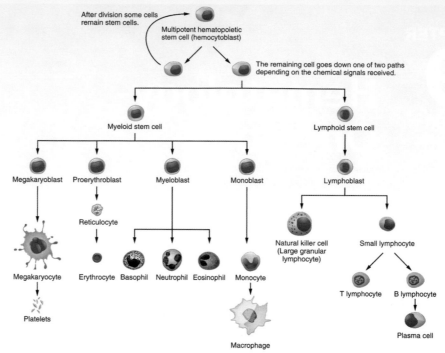

Figure 9-1: Hematopoeiosis of the cell lines from the bone marrow to the peripheral circulation. (Image courtesy of OpenStax College.)

- Reversible dementia, confusion, altered mental status
- Positive Romberg sign, peripheral neuropathy, ataxia: spinocerebellar degeneration
- Hyperactive reflex, spasticity: corticospinal tract generation
- Loss of vibratory and positional sensation: dorsal column degeneration
- Charcot joint (neurogenic arthropathy)
– Diagnostics
- MCV >100
- Peripheral smear: hypersegmented neutrophils, megaloblastic macrocytic RBCs (Fig. 9-5)
- Decreased vitamin B12 levels
- Methylmalonic acid (MMA) levels if vitamin B12 levels are equivocal; elevated MMA levels are diagnostic
- Antiintrinsic factor, antiparietal cell antibodies: pernicious anemia
- Elevated LDH, indirect hyperbilirubinemia, decreased reticulocyte: hemolysis
– Management: parenteral vitamin B12 replacement

Vitamin B12 metabolism and absorption: vitamin B12 is bound to R-binder from salivary glands as vitamin B12 is ingested. Intrinsic factor made in the stomach from parietal cells travels with B12 R-binder complex into duodenum. vitamin B12 is separated from R-binder by pancreatic enzymes allowing B12-intrinsic factor complex to form. Lastly, B12-intrinsic factor complex is absorbed at the terminal ileum. Therefore, pathology of the stomach, pancreas, or terminal ileum can potentially result in vitamin B12 deficiency. Vitamin B12 is stored in the liver with supplies lasting for years.

Folate Deficiency
– Causes
- Dietary deficiency, alcoholism, goat's milk
- Medications
    - Methotrexate
    - TMP-SMX
    - Phenytoin
- Pregnancy
- Chronic hemolysis
- Hemodialysis
– Signs and symptoms: anemia
– Diagnostics
- MCV >100
- Decreased RBC folate levels
- Peripheral smear: hypersegmented neutrophils, megaloblastic macrocytic RBCs
- Elevated LDH, indirect hyperbilirubinemia, decreased reticulocyte

Formed element	Major subtypes	Numbers present per microliter (µL) and mean (range)	Appearance in a standard blood smear	Summary of functions	Comments
Erythrocytes (red blood cells)		5.2 million (4.4–6.0 million)	Flattened biconcave disk; no nucleus; pale red color	Transport oxygen and some carbon dioxide between tissues and lungs	Lifespan of approximately 120 days
Leukocytes (white blood cells)		7000 (5000–10,000)	Obvious dark-staining nucleus	All function in body defenses	Exit capillaries and move into tissues; lifespan of usually a few hours or days
	Granulocytes including neutrophils, eosinophils, and basophils	4360 (1800–9950)	Abundant granules in cytoplasm; nucleus normally lobed	Nonspecific (innate) resistance to disease	Classified according to membrane-bound granules in cytoplasm
	Neutrophils	4150 (1800–7300)	Nuclear lobes increase with age; pale lilac granules	Phagocytic; particularly effective against bacteria. Release cytotoxic chemicals from granules	Most common leukocyte; lifespan of minutes to days
	Eosinophils	165 (0–700)	Nucleus generally two-lobed; bright red-orange granules	Phagocytic cells; particularly effective with antigen- antibody complexes. Release antihistamines. Increase in allergies and parasitic infections	Lifespan of minutes to days
	Basophils	44 (0–150)	Nucleus generally two-lobed but difficult to see due to presence of heavy, dense, dark purple granules	Promotes inflammation	Least common leukocyte; lifespan unknown
	Agranulocytes including lymphocytes and monocytes	2640 (1700–4950)	Lack abundant granules in cytoplasm; have a simple-shaped nucleus that may be indented	Body defenses	Group consists of two major cell types from different lineages
	Lymphocytes	2185 (1500–4000)	Spherical cells with a single often large nucleus occupying much of the cell's volume; stains purple; seen in large (natural killer cells) and small (B and T cells) variants	Primarily specific (adaptive) immunity: T cells directly attack other cells (cellular immunity); B cells release antibodies (humoral immunity); natural killer cells are similar to T cells but nonspecific	Initial cells originate in bone marrow, but secondary production occurs in lymphatic tissue; several distinct subtypes; memory cells form after exposure to a pathogen and rapidly increase responses to subsequent exposure; lifespan of many years
	Monocytes	455 (200–950)	Largest leukocyte with an indented or horseshoe-shaped nucleus	Very effective phagocytic cells engulfing pathogens or worn out cells; also serve as antigen-presenting cells (APCs) for other components of the immune system	Produced in red bone marrow; referred to as macrophages after leaving circulation
Platelets		350,000 (150,000–500,000)	Cellular fragments surrounded by a plasma membrane and containing granules; purple stain	Hemostasis plus release growth factors for repair and healing of tissue	Formed from megakaryocytes that remain in the red bone marrow and shed platelets into circulation

Figure 9-2: Number, appearance, and function of the hematologic cell types. (Image courtesy of OpenStax College.)

– Management: folate replacement

Folate deficiency is particularly catastrophic in pregnant women as deficiency can result in fetal neural tube defects. Both vitamin B12 and folate deficiency will have elevated homocysteine levels. Only vitamin B12 will have elevated methylmalonic acid levels.

Pharmacologic mechanisms of folic acid deficiency:
- Trimethoprim and methotrexate inhibit dihydrofolate reductase.
- ulfamethoxazole inhibits dihydropterate synthase.
- Phenytoin inhibits intestinal conjugate.

Orotic aciduria: congenital disorder of uridine monophosphate synthase deficiency (de novo pyrimidine synthesis pathway) resulting in macrocytic megaloblastic anemia and developmental delay; treat with replacement of uridine monophosphate

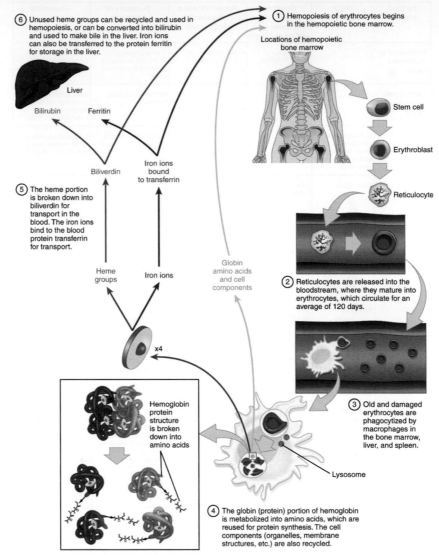

Figure 9-3: A normal red blood cell (RBC) life cycle. Anemia results in disruption of this process resulting in decreased RBC life span. (Image courtesy of OpenStax College.)

Other hematologic manifestations of alcoholism include thrombocytopenia and/or normocytic anemia of chronic disease secondary to bone marrow suppression, iron deficiency anemia secondary to gastritis-induced chronic blood loss.

Other causes of macrocytic nonmegaloblastic anemia:
- Alcoholism
- Myelodysplastic syndrome
- Diffuse reticulocytosis
- Hypothyroidism

Normocytic Anemia
Aplastic Anemia
- Pathophysiology: bone marrow suppression of all cell lines secondary to infectious, pharmacologic, or chemical insult
- Causes
  - Idiopathic
  - Medications
    - Thioamides: methimazole, propylthiouracil
    - Antiepileptics: phenytoin, carbamazepine, lamotrigine
    - Antibiotics: chloramphenicol, sulfonamides
    - Antipsychotics: clozapine

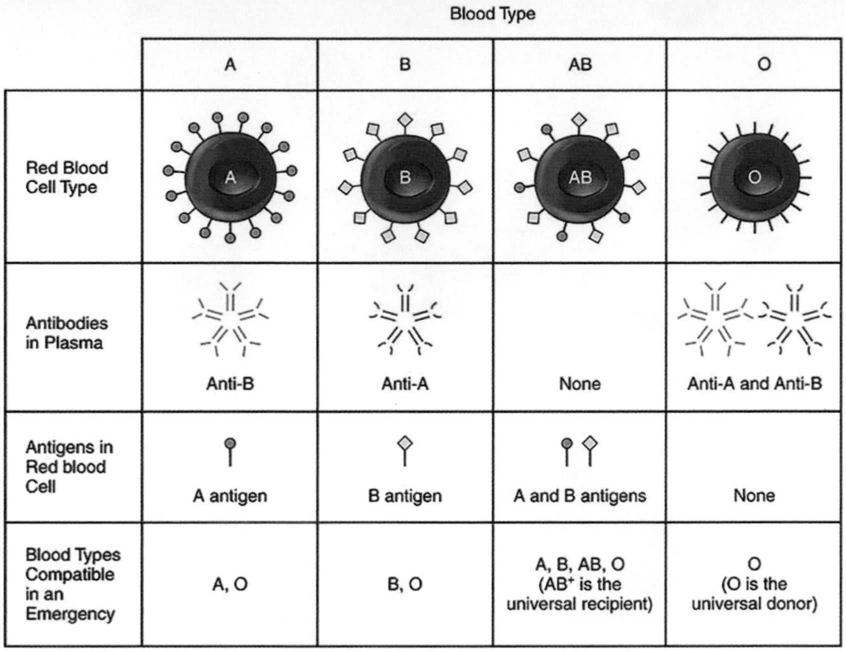

Blood Type

	A	B	AB	O
Red Blood Cell Type	A	B	AB	O
Antibodies in Plasma	Anti-B	Anti-A	None	Anti-A and Anti-B
Antigens in Red blood Cell	A antigen	B antigen	A and B antigens	None
Blood Types Compatible in an Emergency	A, O	B, O	A, B, AB, O (AB⁺ is the universal recipient)	O (O is the universal donor)

Figure 9-4: Comparison of blood types and blood compatibility. This is important for understanding what type of blood can be transfused based on a patient's blood type. (Image courtesy of OpenStax College.)

TABLE 9-1   Types of transfusion reactions

TYPE OF REACTION	PATHOPHYSIOLOGY	KEY FEATURES	TREATMENT/PREVENTION
Hemolytic transfusion reaction	• Type II hypersensitivity reaction • ABO incompatibility • Preformed antibodies bind host red blood cells resulting in hemolysis	• Onset within 1 hr • Fever, hypotension, flank pain • Dark urine (hemoglobinuria), jaundice • Renal failure, DIC, shock	• Most commonly due to clerical error
Febrile nonhemolytic transfusion reaction	• Prereleased cytokines from leukocytes during blood storage	• Onset within 1–6 hr • Fever, malaise	• Leukoreduced blood in the future • Premedication with antipyretics and antihistamines
Anaphylactic	• Blood with anti-IgA antibodies administered to patient with IgA deficiency	• Sudden onset, within seconds • Respiratory distress • Hives, urticaria, angioedema • Wheezing	• Intramuscular epinephrine • Antihistamines, glucocorticoids • IgA deficiency plasma and washed red cell products in future transfusions
Transfusion-related acute lung injury	• Donor antileukocyte antibodies	• Onset within 6 hr • Noncardiogenic pulmonary edema • Interstitial edema on chest x-ray	• Respiratory support • IV diuresis

Whenever a transfusion reaction is suspected, first step is always to stop the transfusion.
DIC, Disseminated intravascular coagulation; *Ig*, immunoglobulin.

- Infections
  - Viral hepatitis
  - Epstein-Barr virus (EBV)
  - Cytomegalovirus (CMV)
  - Human immunodeficiency virus (HIV)
  - Parvovirus B19
- Radiation exposure
- Congenital
- Benzene, insecticides

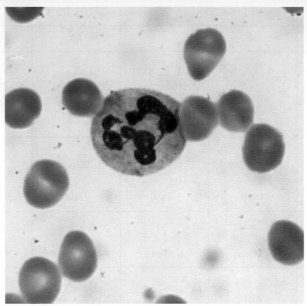

Figure 9-5: Hyperlobulated neutrophil in a patient with megaloblastic anemia. (Image courtesy of Ed Uthman from Houston, TX, USA.)

- Signs and symptoms
  - Fatigue, malaise, pallor: anemia
  - Easy bruising, petechiae, mucosal bleeding: thrombocytopenia
  - Recurrent bacterial infections: neutropenia
- Diagnostics
  - Complete blood count (CBC): pancytopenia
  - Reticulocytopenia
  - Bone marrow biopsy: hypoproliferative bone marrow
- Management
  - Treat underlying etiology
  - Packed RBCs (PRBCs) and platelet transfusion as needed

Chronic Kidney Disease
- Pathophysiology: decreased erythropoietin from the kidneys resulting in decreased erythropoiesis stimulation
- Causes
  - Hypertension, diabetes: most common causes
  - Polycystic kidney disease
  - Glomerulonephritis
  - Chronic ascending urinary tract infection (UTI)
- Signs and symptoms: anemia and electrolyte derangements
- Diagnostics: decreased renal function >3 months
- Management: erythropoietin stimulating agents

Hemolytic Anemia
Principles of hemolytic anemia: hemolytic anemias can be differentiated into intravascular versus extravascular hemolysis. Intravascular hemolysis as the name suggests results in hemolysis within the blood vessels resulting in indirect hyperbilirubinemia, elevated LDH, and low haptoglobin. Haptoglobin is a protein that binds to free hemoglobin in the blood so that hemoglobin can be removed by the reticuloendothelial system (spleen, liver). Therefore, haptoglobin levels will be low during intravascular hemolysis as it is utilized to bind free hemoglobin. In extravascular hemolysis, abnormal RBCs are phagocytosed by the reticuloendothelial system without release of intracellular RBC contents.

Sickle Cell Disease
- Pathophysiology: chronic hemolytic anemia due to beta-globin gene mutation at position 6 resulting in a valine for glutamic substitution and recurrent vasoocclusive crises
- Key manifestations
  - Neurologic: stroke, retinopathy
  - Cardiac
    - Hyperdynamic changes, high output heart failure
    - Systolic flow murmur

- Pulmonary
  - Acute chest syndrome (cough, shortness of breath)
  - Pulmonary embolism (PE), pulmonary hypertension
- Gastrointestinal (GI)
  - Bilirubin gallstones
  - Autosplenectomy (autoinfarction)
  - Acute abdomen
  - Splenic sequestration crisis: acute splenomegaly, drop in hemoglobin, diffuse reticulocytosis, hypovolemic shock; treat with exchange transfusion and splenectomy

Painful vasoocclusive crises are typically caused by hypoxia, infections, dehydration, acidosis.

- Rheumatologic
  - Osteomyelitis: increased incidence of Salmonella osteomyelitis; however, *Staphylococcus aureus* still the most common cause overall
  - Avascular necrosis of femoral head
  - Dactylitis
  - Growth delay
- Renal
  - Hematuria, recurrent UTIs, papillary necrosis
  - Diabetes insipidus (DI)
  - Distal renal tubular acidosis (RTA)
  - Membranoproliferative glomerulonephritis, focal segmental glomerulosclerosis
- Dermatologic: dermal occlusions, nonhealing skin ulcers

Diffuse reticulocytosis vs reticulocytopenia is a key differentiator between splenic sequestration crisis and aplastic crisis.

- Hematologic
  - Sepsis: secondary to encapsulated organisms (*Streptococcus pneumoniae, Neisseria, Haemophilus*) after splenic autoinfarction
  - Priapism
  - Howell-Jolly bodies (secondary to splenic infarct/dysfunction and inability to remove nuclear remnants inside RBCs)
  - Increased protection against malaria
  - Aplastic crisis: parvovirus B19 infection, reticulocytopenia
- Diagnostics
  - Hemoglobin electrophoresis: hemoglobin S >50%
  - Elevated LDH, indirect hyperbilirubinemia, reticulocytosis
  - Peripheral smear: sickle-shaped RBCs (Fig. 9-6)
- Management
  - Symptomatic management of pain crises: IV fluids, pain control (typically requires opioids), supplemental oxygen
  - Penicillin prophylaxis until 5 years of age
  - Low threshold to initiate antibiotics
  - Pneumococcal, Neisseria, and influenza vaccination
  - Folate supplementation
  - Hydroxyurea: prevents recurrent sickle cell crisis
  - Exchange transfusion indications
    - Stroke
    - Acute chest syndrome
    - Symptomatic anemia, reticulocytopenia,
    - Splenic sequestration crisis

Hereditary Spherocytosis

Hydroxyurea: inhibits ribonucleotide reductase and increases hemoglobin F levels to prevent recurrent pain crises. Also used in chronic myeloid leukemia. Common side effect is bone marrow suppression.

Sickle cell trait: ~50% hemoglobin S, 50% hemoglobin A on electrophoresis. Asymptomatic. May have painless hematuria, isosthenuria. No intervention required.
Hemoglobin SC: ~50% hemoglobin S, 50% hemoglobin C. Similar signs and symptoms as sickle cell disease; however, with less frequency and severity.

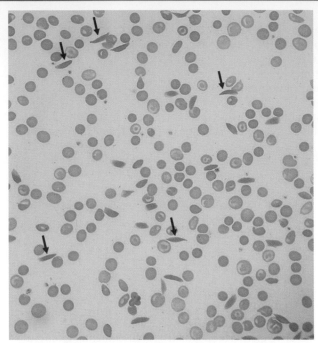

Figure 9-6: Sickled cells on peripheral smear.

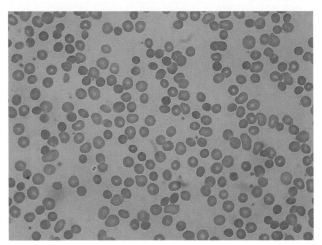

Figure 9-7: Peripheral blood smear in a patient with hereditary spherocytosis showing spherocytes. (Image courtesy of Paulo Henrique Orlandi Mourao.)

- Pathophysiology
  - Autosomal dominant extravascular hemolytic anemia characterized by ankyrin gene RBC membrane defect resulting in spectrin deficiency
  - Abnormal scaffolding proteins results in less deformable RBCs and increased splenic sequestration
- Key manifestations
  - Anemia, jaundice
  - Bilirubin gallstones, acute cholecystitis, splenomegaly
  - Parvovirus B19 aplastic anemia
- Diagnostics
  - Increased osmotic fragility on acidified glycerol lysis test
  - Eosin-5-maleimide binding test (flow cytometry)
  - Elevated mean corpuscular hemoglobin concentration: due to cellular dehydration and membrane loss
  - Peripheral smear: spherocytes (Fig. 9-7)
- Management: symptomatic
  - Transfusion as needed

- Folate supplementation
- Splenectomy as last resort

Paroxysmal Nocturnal Hemoglobinuria
- Pathophysiology
  - Acquired stem cell defect resulting in deficiency of cell membrane regulatory proteins (decay-accelerating factors, CD55/59) and increased susceptibility to complement mediated cell lysis
  - Phosphatidylinositol class A (PIG-A) gene mutation
- Signs and symptoms
  - Pancytopenia (fatigue, petechiae, recurrent infections)
  - Jaundice
  - Hematuria (typically nocturnal: mild respiratory acidosis during sleep results in increased complement activation and RBC lysis)
- Diagnostics
  - Flow cytometry: deficiency of CD55 and CD59
  - CBC: pancytopenia
  - Elevated LDH, indirect hyperbilirubinemia, reticulocytosis
- Management
  - Eculizumab (terminal complement C5 monoclonal antibody)
  - Allogeneic hemopoietic cell transplantation
  - PRBC transfusion, anticoagulation as needed
- Complications
  - Venous thrombosis (hepatic, mesenteric, cerebral)
  - Transformation to hematologic malignancy (myelodysplasia, acute leukemia)
  - Aplastic anemia

> Decay-accelerating factor functions to protect RBC membranes from complement-mediated lysis.

> Hereditary spherocytosis is a Coombs-negative hemolytic anemia. Autoimmune hemolytic anemia is Coombs positive. Previously used osmotic fragility test has poor sensitivity for diagnosing hereditary spherocytosis.

> Vaccinate against *Neisseria* prior to administering eculizumab.

Glucose-6-Phosphate Dehydrogenase (G6PD) Deficiency
- Epidemiology: Black, Mediterranean ancestry
- Definition: hemolytic anemia secondary to decrease G6PD after exposure to hemolytic triggers (infection, sulfa drugs, antimalarials, fava beans)
- Pathophysiology: deficiency of G6PD dehydrogenase → decrease RBC nicotinamide adenine dinucleotide phosphate → decrease glutathione production (antioxidant) → increased RBC radical damage
- Signs and symptoms
  - Abdominal pain
  - Nausea, vomiting
  - Jaundice
  - Fever
  - Dark urine (hemoglobinuria)
- Diagnostics
  - Elevated LDH, low haptoglobin
  - Peripheral smear: "bite" cells, Heinz bodies
  - Reticulocytosis
  - RBC G6PD levels after hemolytic crisis
- Management
  - Symptomatic management
  - Avoid hemolysis triggers

Thrombotic Thrombocytopenic Purpura (TTP)
- Epidemiology: hereditary form is more common in children, and acquired form more common in adults

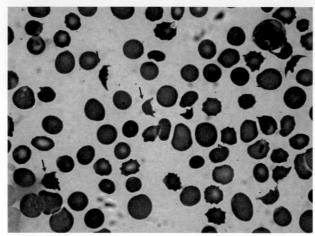

Figure 9-8: Schistocytes in a patient with hemolytic anemia. May be seen with any of the causes of hemolytic anemia discussed in this section.

- Pathophysiology
  - Decreased ADAMTS13 activity (plasma protease) secondary to autoantibody leading to inability to break down von Willebrand factor (vWF) multimers → development of diffuse small vessel thrombi, which consume platelets and shear RBCs
  - ADAMTS13 functions to cleave vW multimers from endothelial surface
- Signs and symptoms: classic pentad of symptoms (FAT RN)
  - Fever
  - Microangiopathic hemolytic anemia
  - Thrombocytopenia
  - Renal insufficiency
  - Neurologic symptoms (altered mental status, seizures)
- Diagnostics: do not need all five symptoms to make diagnosis, only requirement is evidence of hemolytic anemia and thrombocytopenia
  - Peripheral smear: schistocytes (Fig. 9-8)
  - Decreased ADAMTS13 levels
  - Elevated hemolysis markers (elevated LDH, indirect hyperbilirubinemia)
- Management: plasmapheresis +/− glucocorticoids

Thrombotic thrombocytopenic purpura is associated with ticlopidine, cyclosporine, clopidogrel, valproic acid, systemic lupus erythematosus, and acquired immunodeficiency syndrome.

Disseminated Intravascular Coagulation (DIC)
- Pathophysiology: coagulopathy characterized by overactivation of coagulation cascade resulting in consumption of platelets and coagulation factors seen in critically ill patients
- Causes
  - Gram-negative sepsis
  - Exertional heat stroke
  - Acute pancreatitis
  - Transfusion reaction (ABO incompatibility)
  - Major surgery, burn, trauma
  - Retained placental contents, abruptio placenta, amniotic fluid emboli
  - Malignancy (lung, colon, pancreas, acute promyelocytic leukemia)
- Key manifestations
  - Bleeding from orifices (venipuncture, oral, rectal)
  - Shock, end-organ dysfunction, thrombosis
- Diagnostics: clinical and laboratory
  - Elevated D-dimer, low fibrinogen
  - Elevated International Normalized Ratio (INR), prothrombin time (PT)/partial thromboplastin time (PTT)
  - Peripheral smear: schistocytes
  - Elevated hemolysis markers (elevated LDH, indirect hyperbilirubinemia)
  - CBC: anemia, thrombocytopenia

- Management
  - Treat underlying etiology
  - Cryoprecipitate, fresh frozen plasma

Autoimmune Hemolytic Anemia

- Pathophysiology: development of autoantibodies (immunoglobulin M [IgM] or IgG mediated) bind RBC membranes resulting in chronic extravascular (IgG) or intravascular (IgM cold agglutinin) hemolysis
- Causes
  - Infectious: EBV, Mycoplasma, herpes simplex virus
  - Systemic lupus erythematosus (SLE)
  - Chronic lymphocytic leukemia (CLL)
  - Penicillins, cephalosporins, methyldopa
  - Congenital immunodeficiencies
- Signs and symptoms: anemia, jaundice
- Diagnostics
  - Coombs positive: IgM cold agglutinin; IgG warm agglutinin
  - Peripheral smear: spherocytes
  - Elevated LDH, indirect hyperbilirubinemia, reticulocytosis
- Management
  - IgG warm agglutinin
    - Steroids: first line
    - +/− splenectomy or rituximab if unresponsive to steroids
  - IgM cold agglutinin
    - Cold avoidance
    - Rituximab

Partial immunity against malaria is seen in patients with hemoglobinopathies.

Malaria

- Microbiology
  - Intraerythrocytic infection caused by Plasmodium parasite
  - Transmitted by Anopheles mosquito; infects RBCs and hepatocytes depending on the species
- Species
  - *Plasmodium falciparum:* most lethal
  - *P. vivax, ovale:* remains dormant in the liver
  - *P. malaria:* most associated with nephrotic syndrome
- Signs and symptoms
  - Cyclic fevers, chills, pallor
  - Headaches, myalgias
  - Abdominal pain, splenomegaly, diarrhea, nausea, vomiting
- Diagnostics: clinical and laboratory
  - Peripheral smear
    - Banana-shaped gametocytes
    - Intraerythrocytic parasites on Giemsa stain (Fig. 9-9)
  - Elevated liver function test (LFTs; only in P. vivax and P. ovale infections)
  - Hemolysis markers (elevated LDH, low haptoglobin, reticulocytosis)
  - Anemia, thrombocytopenia
- Management
  - Intrahepatic *(P. vivax, P. ovale):* primaquine
  - Intraerythrocytic (all species): depends on region and resistance patterns
    - Chloroquine, hydroxychloroquine
    - Artemether
    - Mefloquine
    - Quinine
- Complications
  - Stroke, visual disturbances, seizures
  - Hematuria, renal failure
  - Pulmonary edema
- Prophylaxis
  - Lifestyle modifications: long-sleeve clothing, insect repellent
  - Pharmacologic: choice depends on side effect profile

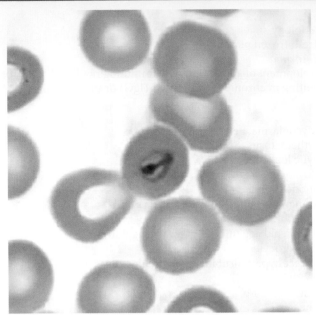

Figure 9-9: Intraerythrocytic parasite in a patient with malaria on Giemsa stain. (Image courtesy of the CDC.)

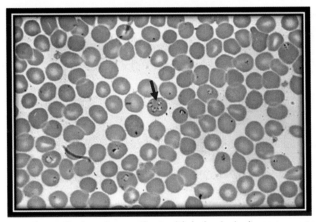

Figure 9-10: Intraerythrocytic rings in a patient with babesiosis. (Image courtesy of the CDC.)

- Mefloquine
- Chloroquine
- Doxycycline
- Atovaquone-proguanil

Malaria is endemic to South America, Africa, South Euthanasia. Most common cause of malaria in the United States is from travelers returning from endemic areas without appropriate prophylaxis.

Babesiosis
- Microbiology
  - Tickborne illness caused by *Babesia microti*
  - Associated with Exodes tick (also transmits Lyme disease, human granulocytic anaplasmosis)
- Signs and symptoms: similar to malaria
- Diagnostics
  - Peripheral smear: intraerythrocytic rings ("Maltese cross") (Fig. 9–10)
  - Anemia, thrombocytopenia
  - Hemolysis markers (LDH, haptoglobin, reticulocytosis)
- Elevated LFTs
- Management
  - Azithromycin + atovaquone: first line
  - Severe cases: quinine + clindamycin in severe cases

- Complications
  - Acute respiratory distress syndrome, congestive heart failure
  - DIC
  - Splenic rupture

Peripheral smear comparing malaria vs babesiosis

Microcytic Anemia

Iron metabolism/homeostasis

- Absorbed in the proximal intestine (duodenum) through divalent metal transporters
- Absorption is regulated by hepcidin, a protein produced by the liver that prevents excessive iron absorption; deficiency of hepcidin results in unopposed iron absorption and iron overload (hemochromatosis), and excess hepcidin is produced in inflammatory or infectious states preventing iron absorption and iron deficiency
- After absorption through divalent metal transporters, iron is transported through the blood by transferrin proteins and stored intracellularly as ferritin

Iron Deficiency Anemia

- Causes
  - Blood loss (GI, menorrhagia, antiplatelets, anticoagulants)
  - Insufficient dietary intake (lack of animal protein)
  - Increased requirements (pregnancy, infants, adolescents)
  - Malabsorption (celiac disease, small bowel resection, inflammatory bowel disease)
  - Plummer-Vinson syndrome: triad of iron deficiency anemia, esophageal webs, increased risk of esophageal carcinoma
- Signs and symptoms
  - Fatigue, malaise
  - Pallor
  - Palpitations, chest pain, dyspnea
  - Lightheadedness, dizziness
  - Pica, ice craving
  - Restless leg syndrome
- Diagnostics
  - Low MCV
  - Elevated RDW
  - Reactive thrombocytosis
  - Iron studies
- Peripheral smear: hypochromic, microcytic RBCs (Fig. 9–11)
- Management: oral or IV iron replacement

Additional notes regarding iron:
- Monitor for allergic reaction when administering IV iron transfusion.
- Iron replacement is sometimes given with vitamin C to increase absorption, as vitamin C is a reducing agent converting Fe^{3+} to Fe^{2+}.
- Side effects of oral iron replacement include nausea, constipation, dark stools.

Basics of hemoglobin: a peptide tetramer that requires two alpha-globin groups and two nonalpha blood globin groups (beta, gamma, or delta) to form hemoglobin (Table 9-2)
- Normal adult hemoglobin (HbA) = 2 alphas + 2 betas
- Fetal hemoglobin (HbF) = 2 alphas + 2 gammas
- Deficiency of either alpha- or beta-globin results in formation of abnormal tetramers; these abnormal hemoglobin result in decreased RBC life span

Lead Poisoning

- Causes
  - Ingestion from lead painted older houses: most commonly in children
  - Occupational exposure (batteries, plumbing, painting, construction): most commonly in adults
- Signs and symptoms
  - Neurologic
    - Headache, irritability
    - Encephalopathy
    - Peripheral neuropathy
  - GI

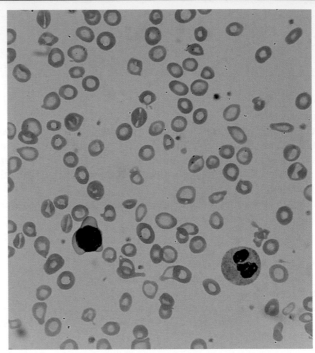

Figure 9-11: Peripheral smear in a patient with iron deficiency anemia showing microcytosis, hypochromasia, anisocytosis, and poikilocytosis.

- Nausea, vomiting
- Abdominal pain, constipation
  - Hematologic: microcytic sideroblastic anemia
  - "Lead line": pigmentation of gum-tooth line

> Lead inhibits ferrochelatase and ALA dehydratase resulting in defective heme synthesis. Basophilic stippling is also seen in sideroblastic anemia, thalassemia, sickle cell disease.

- Diagnostics
  - Elevated venous lead level
  - Elevated zinc protoporphyrin
  - X-ray fluorescence: detects lead levels in bone
  - Peripheral smear: basophilic stippling
- Management: depends on lead levels
  - <45 mcg/dL: no treatment, removal from work exposure
  - >45 mcg/dL: lead chelators
    - Ethylenediaminetetraacetic acid, dimercaprol
    - Succimer (most preferred in children)
    - Penicillamine

Sideroblastic anemia: genetic or acquired defect in heme synthesis; acquired causes include alcoholism, drugs (isoniazid, alcoholism, chloramphenicol), myelodysplastic syndrome; ringed sideroblasts on bone marrow

Anemia of Chronic Disease
- Pathophysiology
  - Inflammation and/or infection stimulates release of hepcidin from the liver resulting in decreased iron absorption from the GI tract
  - Inflammatory state increases production of acute phase reactant such as ferritin, which drives iron intracellularly and "hides" it from bacteria
- Causes
  - Autoimmune (SLE, rheumatoid arthritis), vasculitis
  - Infections: tuberculosis, endocarditis, lung abscess
  - Alcoholism
  - Malignancy
  - Chronic kidney disease
- Signs and symptoms: anemia and underlying chronic disease

TABLE 9-2 Alpha- versus beta-thalassemia. Hemoglobinopathies characterized by decreased synthesis or absence of alpha- or beta-globin

	ALPHA-THALASSEMIA	BETA-THALASSEMIA
Pathophysiology	• Defect in alpha-globin production due to deletion in up to four alpha-globin genes resulting in formation of beta-globin tetramers	• Defect in beta-globin production due to mutation in up to two beta-globin genes
Signs and symptoms	Depends on number of alpha genes deleted: • One-gene deletion: normal phenotype, no symptoms • Two-gene deletion: mild anemia under stress, mostly asymptomatic • Three-gene deletion: moderate anemia requiring occasional transfusion • Four-gene deletion: fatal in newborns, hydrops fetalis	Depends on number of beta genes mutated: • One-gene mutation: normal phenotype, no symptoms • Two-gene mutation: moderate anemia requiring transfusions, growth retardation, extramedullary hematopoiesis (hepatosplenomegaly, chipmunks facies, "crew-cut" appearance on head x-ray), jaundice
Diagnostics	Hemoglobin (Hb) electrophoresis: • One- or two-gene deletion: normal • Three-gene deletion: HbH • Four-gene deletion: Hb Barts • Peripheral smear: hypochromic microcytic red blood cells • Hemolysis markers (elevated lactate dehydrogenase, decreased haptoglobin, reticulocytosis)	Hemoglobin electrophoresis: • One-gene mutation: increased HbF, HbA$_2$ • Two-gene mutation: no HbA, increased HbF • Similar peripheral smear and hemolysis markers as alpha-thalassemia
Management	• One- or two-gene deletion: no treatment necessary • Three-gene deletion: transfusions as needed, folate replacement, iron chelators (deferoxamine, deferasirox) to prevent iron overload. Consider splenectomy in severe cases. Allogeneic hematopoietic cell transplantation is potentially curative • Four-gene deletion: no treatment, death in utero	• One-gene mutation: no treatment necessary • Two-gene mutation: similar to three alpha gene deletion

- Diagnostics: iron studies (Table 9-3)
- Management
  • Treat underlying disease
  • Erythropoietin-stimulating agents for chronic kidney disease

Pregnancy-associated anemia: overall increase in red blood cell mass; however, even greater increase in intravascular volume results in hemodilution and relative anemia

Bleeding Disorders
Primary hemostasis (Fig. 9–12): formation of platelet plugs via platelet adhesion and aggregation
  1. Endothelial injury exposes subendothelial collagen
  2. vWF binds subendothelial collagen
  3. Platelet glycoprotein 1B binds to vWF (platelet adhesion)
  4. Platelets release adenosine diphosphate resulting in expression of glycoprotein IIb/IIIa
  5. Fibrinogen binds to glycoprotein IIB/IIIa and links platelets (platelet aggregation)
Secondary hemostasis (see Fig. 9–12): activation of clotting factors to convert fibrinogen into fibrin and formation of fibrin clot
  1. Tissue factor activates extrinsic pathway (factor VII) and clotting cascade
  2. Activation of intrinsic pathway begins with factor XII
  3. Extrinsic and intrinsic clotting pathways function to activate combined pathway (factor X)
  4. Combined pathway converts fibrinogen into fibrin resulting in formation of fibrin clot

Platelet Quantity Disorders
Thrombocytopenia
- Causes
  • Destruction

TABLE 9-3   Iron studies

	SERUM IRON	IRON SATURATION	FERRITIN	TOTAL IRON BINDING CAPACITY (TIBC)
Iron deficiency anemia	Decreased	Decreased	Decreased	Increased
Anemia of chronic disease	Decreased	Decreased	Increased	Normal/low
Thalassemia	Normal	Normal	Normal	Normal
Lead poisoning; sideroblastic anemia	Normal	Increased	Increased	Decreased
Hemochromatosis	Increased	Increased	Increased	Decreased

Interpreting iron deficiency iron studies: low serum iron → low iron saturation → increased number of circulating transferrin not bound to iron (increased TIBC) → low intracellular iron stores

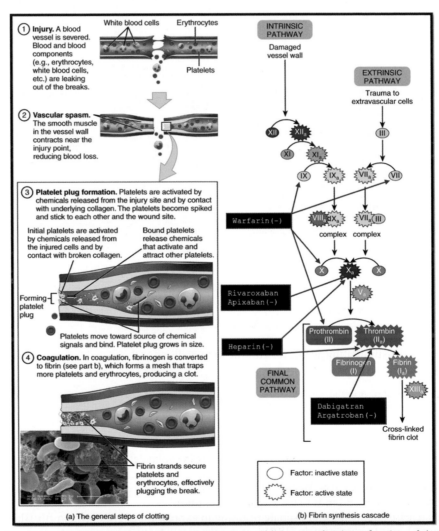

Figure 9-12: Summary of primary and secondary hemostasis. In addition, mechanism of action of drugs commonly used to manipulate the coagulation cascade. *(-)*, Inhibits. (Image courtesy of OpenStax College.)

- Heparin-induced thrombocytopenia (HIT)
- SLE (antibodies against platelets; type II hypersensitivity reaction)
- TTP/hemolytic uremic syndrome
- DIC
- Production/suppression
  - Alcohol, chemotherapy, valproate, quinine, interferon, linezolid
  - Bone marrow dysfunction, leukemia
  - Sepsis

- Viral infections (EBV, CMV, HIV, hepatitis)
- Babesia, malaria, Rocky Mountain spotted fever, dengue
- Nutritional deficiencies (B12, folate, copper)
- Consumption: splenic sequestration
- Other causes
  - Wiskott-Aldrich syndrome (immunodeficiency associated with eczema and thrombocytopenia)
  - Pseudothrombocytopenia (platelet clumping)
  - Immune thrombocytopenic purpura (ITP): diagnosis of exclusion
- Signs and symptoms
  - Petechiae, ecchymosis, easy bruising
  - Gingival bleeding
- Diagnostics
  - CBC: platelets <150,000
  - Peripheral smear: elevated megakaryocytes
- Management
  - Treat underlying disorder
  - ITP
    - Prednisone, IV immunoglobulin
    - Splenectomy last resort
  - Platelet stimulators if severe bleeding is present and platelets <30,000
    - Synthetic thrombopoietin: romiplostim, eltrombopag
    - Oprelvekin (interleukin-11)
  - Platelet transfusion if needed under the following circumstances
    - Asymptomatic: <10,000
    - Severe bleeding: <30,000
    - Intracranial bleeding or prior to central nervous system (CNS) surgery: <100,000
    - Prior to major surgery: <50,000

Platelet Function Disorders
vWF Deficiency
- Epidemiology
  - Most common inherited bleeding disorder
  - Autosomal dominant inheritance
- Subtypes
  - Type I: decreased vWF
  - Type II: defective vWF
  - Type III (most severe): complete deficiency of vWF multimers
- Signs and symptoms
  - Epistaxis, gingival bleeding
  - Petechiae, ecchymosis
  - Easy bruising/bleeding
  - Mucosal bleeding (GI, genitourinary [GU])
  - Significant bleeding after initiation of aspirin or antiplatelets
- Diagnostics
  - Decreased serum vWF antigen
  - Ristocetin cofactor assay (measures ability vWF binds to glycoprotein IB)
  - Decreased factor VIII activity
  - Slightly elevated PTT (vWF stabilizes factor VIII)
- Management
  - DDAVP: stimulates release of vWF and factor VIII from Weibel-Palade bodies located in endothelial cells
  - vWF replacement
Bernard-Soulier Syndrome
- Defective glycoprotein 1B resulting in inadequate platelet adhesion
- Mild thrombocytopenia
- Giant platelets
- Bleeding out of proportion to the degree of thrombocytopenia
Glanzmann Thrombasthenia
- Defective glycoprotein IIB/IIIa resulting in inadequate platelet aggregation
- Mucocutaneous bleeding
- Associated with defects in leukocyte function (leukocyte adhesion deficiency)

Aspirin and clopidogrel increase risk of bleeding by causing platelet dysfunction through enzymatic inhibition.

Inherited Coagulopathies

Hemophilia A/B
– Pathophysiology: X-linked inherited disorder (affects only males) resulting in deficiency of factor VIII (hemophilia A) or IX (hemophilia B)
– Signs and symptoms
  • Muscle hematomas
  • Retroperitoneal bleeds
  • Hemarthroses
  • Early osteoarthritis
– Diagnostics: decreased serum factor VIII or IX
– Management
  • Factor replacement
  • Desmopressin for mild hemophilia A

Acquired Coagulopathies

Vitamin K Deficiency
– Causes
  • Prolonged antibiotic use (destroys vitamin K–producing bacterial flora)
  • Newborns (lack of colonization by vitamin K–producing flora)
  • Malnutrition
  • Fat malabsorption syndromes (cystic fibrosis, celiac disease, inflammatory bowel disease, obstructive biliary disease)
  • Liver disease
  • Warfarin
– Signs and symptoms: bleeding
– Diagnostics
  • Elevated PT/PTT (PT increases first)
  • Decreased plasma levels of factor II, VII, IX, X, protein C/S
– Management
  • Fresh frozen plasma for severe bleeding
  • Vitamin K replacement for mild to asymptomatic cases

Coagulopathy of Liver Disease
– Decreased synthetic liver function results in inability to produce vitamin K–dependent clotting factors (factor II, VII, IX, X, protein C and S).
– Severe bleeding, most commonly GI
– Elevated PT/PTT; however, PT increases first due to short half-life of factor VII
– Coagulopathy does not improve with vitamin K administration

CLOTTING DISORDERS

Venous Thromboembolism (VTE)
– Risk factors
  • Venous stasis
    ▪ Prolonged immobility
  • Hypercoagulable state
    ▪ Factor V Leiden mutation
    ▪ Antiphospholipid (APL) syndrome
    ▪ Malignancy
    ▪ Oral contraceptive pills
    ▪ Pregnancy
  • Endothelial injury
    ▪ Surgery
    ▪ Trauma
– Signs and symptoms
  • Deep venous thrombosis (DVT)
    ▪ Unilateral lower extremity erythema/edema
    ▪ Pain on forceful dorsiflexion (Homans sign)
    ▪ Calf circumference asymmetry

- PE
  - Acute onset of dyspnea
  - Tachycardia, hypoxemia
  - Pleuritic chest pain, cough, hemoptysis
- Diagnostics
  - DVT: noncompressible vein on lower extremity Doppler ultrasound
  - PE
    - CT pulmonary angiogram
      - Test of choice, assuming normal renal function
      - Presence of "filling defect" confirms diagnosis of PE
    - V/Q scan
      - Requires normal chest x-ray
      - Utilized when there is a contraindication to contrast administration (renal dysfunction) or radiation (pregnancy)
      - Interpreted as low, moderate, or high probability for PE
    - Echocardiogram: evaluates for signs of right ventricular dilation, right heart strain, pulmonary hypertension
    - Arterial blood gas: hypoxia, respiratory alkalosis
    - Electrocardiogram: sinus tachycardia (most common finding); S1Q3T3 (less common)
    - Chest x-ray: usually normal; however, some characteristic findings may be present
      - Hapten hump: pleural-based abnormalities suggesting wedge-shaped infarct
      - Westermark sign: lung lobe oligemia, lack of vascular markings distal to the PE
      - Atelectasis
    - D-dimer
      - High sensitivity, low specificity test used when there is low to moderate suspicion of PE
      - Used to guide management to determine if additional testing (CT pulmonary angiogram) is needed
  - Wells criteria for DVT/PE: risk stratification tool to determine next step in management (Tables 9-4, 9-5, 9-6, and 9-7)

TABLE 9-4   Wells criteria for deep vein thrombosis (DVT)

CRITERIA	SCORING
• Alternative diagnosis is more likely than DVT	−2 point
• Lower extremity paralysis/paresthesias • Recent surgery or immobilization • Lower extremity tenderness • Swelling of entire leg • Calf circumference discrepancy >3 cm • Pitting edema in the symptomatic light • Collateral nonvaricose superficial veins • Active or recent cancer within the last 6 mo	1 point each for any of these

TABLE 9-5   Wells criteria deep vein thrombosis score interpretation

PROBABILITY	SCORE	MANAGEMENT
High	3–8 points	Immediate anticoagulation +lower extremity Doppler ultrasound
Moderate	1–2 points	Lower extremity Doppler ultrasound
Low	−2–0 points	D-dimer

TABLE 9-6   Wells criteria for pulmonary embolism

CRITERIA	SCORING
• DVT or PE is most likely diagnosis	3 points
• Heart rate >100 • >3 days immobilization • Surgery within the last 4 wk • Previous PE or DVT	1.5 points each
• Hemoptysis • Malignancy	1 point each

DVT, Deep vein thrombosis; *PE*, pulmonary embolism.

TABLE 9-7 Wells criteria pulmonary embolism (PE) score interpretation

PROBABILITY	SCORE	MANAGEMENT
PE likely	<4	D-dimer
PE unlikely	>5	CT pulmonary angiogram

Three-tier model is also used, which divides patients into low risk (<2 points), moderate risk (2–6 points), high risk (>6 points). CT, Computed tomography.

TABLE 9-8 Anticoagulation pharmacology

MEDICATION	INDICATIONS	MECHANISM OF ACTION	SIDE EFFECTS	REVERSAL AGENTS
Heparin	• Acute anticoagulation due to rapid onset of action and short half-life • Also used in NSTEMI	• Increases antithrombin III activity	• Bleeding • Heparin-induced thrombocytopenia	• Protamine sulfate
Low-molecular-weight heparin (enoxaparin)	• Anticoagulant of choice in cancer patients	• Indirectly inhibits factor Xa	• Bleeding	• Protamine sulfate (less effective reversal compared to heparin)
Warfarin	• Anticoagulant of choice in patients with valvular atrial fibrillation • Requires initial bridging therapy with heparin until goal INR is achieved	• Epoxide reductase inhibitor resulting in inactivation of vitamin K–dependent clotting factors (factor II, VII, IX, X, protein C/S)	• Bleeding • Warfarin-induced skin necrosis (initial transient hypercoagulable state with depletion of anticoagulants protein C/S) • Teratogenic	• Immediate: fresh frozen plasma, cryoprecipitate • Chronic: vitamin K
Xa inhibitors (rivaroxaban, apixaban, betrixaban, edoxaban)	• Venous thromboembolism, nonvalvular atrial fibrillation	• Inhibits factor Xa (common pathway) activity	• Bleeding	• Andexanet alfa • Four-factor prothrombin complex concentrate
Direct thrombin inhibitors (dabigatran, argatroban)	• Anticoagulant of choice in patients with heparin-induced thrombocytopenia	• Inhibits thrombin (factor IIa) activity	• Bleeding	• Idarucizumab (dabigatran)
Thrombolytics (alteplase; tPA)	• Anticoagulant of choice in patients with pulmonary embolism and hemodynamic instability • Also used in nonhemorrhagic ischemic strokes, STEMI (if PCI is unavailable)	• Stimulates conversion of plasminogen to plasmin resulting in cleavage of thrombin and fibrin clots	• Bleeding	• Aminocaproic acid • Tranexamic acid

Avoid low-molecular-weight heparin, fondaparinux, Xa inhibitors in patients with renal dysfunction.
INR, International Normalized Ratio; NSTEMI, non-ST-segment myocardial infarction; PCI, percutaneous coronary intervention; STEMI, ST-segment myocardial infarction; tPA, tissue plasminogen activator.

- Management
  - Anticoagulation for 3–6 months (3 months for provoked, 6 months for unprovoked DVT); choice depends on patient preference for continuous monitoring, bleeding reversibility, and side effect profile (Table 9-8)
    - Heparin
    - Warfarin
    - Xa inhibitors
    - Direct thrombin inhibitors
  - Thrombolytics: if hemodynamically unstable
  - Inferior vena cava filter: indicated if developed VTE while on therapeutic anticoagulation or contraindication to anticoagulation (bleeding, high fall risk)
- Prevention: sequential compression devices, early mobilization, prophylactic subcutaneous anticoagulation

Acquired and Inherited Thrombophilia

Superficial Vein Thrombosis
- Pain, erythema, induration along the venous course; palpable tender cord may be present
- Migratory thrombophlebitis (Trousseau syndrome) associated with underlying malignancy, especially pancreatic cancer
- Diagnosed with venous duplex ultrasound
- Extensive superficial thrombophlebitis (>5 cm) or those near deep vein system are treated as DVT with systemic anticoagulation
- All other superficial vein thromboses are treated symptomatically with NSAIDs and warm compresses
- Suppurative thrombophlebitis will have fevers in addition to the abovementioned features and is treated with systemic antibiotics

Type II HIT
- Pathophysiology
  - Development of platelet factor 4 antibodies (IgG autoantibody) approximately 5–10 days after initiation of heparin therapy resulting in >50% decrease in platelets from baseline and increased risk of thrombosis
  - Platelet factor 4 antibody results in platelet aggregation and release of procoagulant factors
- Signs and symptoms
  - Venous/arterial thrombosis
  - Pain
  - Swelling, erythema
  - Limb ischemia, necrotic skin lesions at heparin injection sites
  - Petechiae, easy bruising
  - Bleeding uncommon
- Diagnostic
  - Four Ts of HIT: used to estimate the pretest probability of HIT prior to obtaining laboratory data; if determined to be moderate or high probability, further laboratory testing can be obtained
    - Thrombocytopenia
    - Timing
    - Thrombosis
    - Other causes of thrombocytopenia
  - Laboratory data
    - Enzyme-linked immunosorbent assay for platelet factor 4 antibody
    - Serotonin-release assay: measures platelet activation in the presence of heparin
- Management: initiate treatment prior to obtaining final laboratory data
  - Discontinue all heparin products
  - Anticoagulate with nonheparin analogues (direct thrombin inhibitors, Xa inhibitors, fondaparinux)

Antiphospholipid (APL) syndrome caused by IgM or IgG antibodies against membrane phospholipids. APL syndrome is one of the causes of false-positive Venereal Disease Research Laboratory rapid plasma reagin.

Type I heparin-induced thrombocytopenia: nonimmune-mediated platelet aggregation resulting in mild thrombocytopenia. Occurs within 2 days upon initiation of heparin injection. No treatment or testing necessary.

Development of autoantibodies may occur earlier in patients previously exposed to heparin.

APL Syndrome
- Associations
  - Idiopathic (most common)
  - SLE and other autoimmune disease
- Key manifestations
  - Arterial or venous thrombosis
    - VTE
    - Stroke
  - Pregnancy complications
    - Multiple early spontaneous abortions
    - Preeclampsia
    - Placental insufficiency

- Thrombocytopenia, microangiopathic hemolytic anemia
- Livedo reticularis
– Diagnostics: requires both clinical and laboratory findings
  - Serology
    - Anticardiolipin antibody
    - Lupus anticoagulant
    - Anti-beta-2 glycoprotein antibody
  - Elevated PTT
  - Mixing study: patient's plasma is mixed with normal plasma; normally, if PTT is elevated from clotting factor deficiency then it should normalize with mixing study. In patients with APL, PTT remains elevated due to presence of antibody.
  - Russell viper venom test (most specific)
– Management
  - No treatment if asymptomatic
  - Thrombosis treated with warfarin; no indication for direct oral anticoagulants
  - Recurrent spontaneous abortion: heparin and aspirin

Other examples of thrombophilia are less common but have unique DNA mutations and allow for testing of the clotting cascade (Table 9-9).

Medication-induced thrombophilia:
- Oral contraceptive pills
- Hormone replacement therapy
- Tamoxifen
- Glucocorticoids

WHITE BLOOD CELL (WBC) DYSCRASIAS

Myelodysplastic Syndrome
– Definition: heterogenous group of hematopoietic stem cell disorders resulting in abnormal blood cell production and increased risk of transformation to hematologic malignancy
– Causes
  - Idiopathic
  - Radiation
  - Toxins (benzene)
  - Chemotherapy
  - Immunosuppressive agents
  - Paroxysmal nocturnal hemoglobinuria
– Key manifestations
  - Fatigue, shortness of breath: anemia
  - Easy bruising, bleeding: normocytic anemia
  - Recurrent infections: neutropenia
  - Autoimmune phenomenon

TABLE 9-9 Other inherited thrombophilia

TYPE OF THROMBOPHILIA	KEY FEATURES
Factor V Leiden	• Most common inherited thrombophilia in whites • Mutation in factor V causes resistance to activated protein C activity and uninhibited activation of coagulation cascade • Routine testing of patients or relatives is not indicated
Prothrombin G20210A mutation	• Second most common inherited thrombophilia • Elevated prothrombin levels
Protein C/S deficiency	• Inability to inactivate factor Va and VIIIa • Increased risk of warfarin-induced skin necrosis (protein C deficiency)
Antithrombin III deficiency	• Resistance to activation by heparin, therefore anticoagulate with nonheparin products • Autosomal dominant inheritance • Most commonly acquired in the setting of cirrhosis, nephrotic syndrome, or disseminated intravascular coagulopathy
Paroxysmal nocturnal hemoglobinuria	• Deficiency of cell membrane regulatory proteins (decay-accelerating factors, CD55/59) and increased susceptibility to complement mediated cell lysis • Phosphatidylinositol class A (PIG-A) gene mutation • Transformation to hematologic malignancy

All inherited thrombophilia is diagnosed with DNA mutation testing.

- - - Rheumatic heart disease
    - Rheumatoid arthritis
    - Pernicious anemia
  - Acquired hemoglobin H disease
  - Dermatologic: sweet syndrome (acute febrile neutrophilic dermatosis)
- Diagnostics
  - CBC: macrocytic anemia, neutropenia, thrombocytopenia/thrombocytosis
  - Peripheral smear: dysplastic RBCs and WBCs (<20% blast forms), Howell-Jolly bodies, basophilic stippling, hypolobulated neutrophilic nuclei (pseudo-Pelger-Huet anomaly), ringed sideroblasts
  - Bone marrow aspirate/biopsy: <20% myeloblasts
  - Flow cytometry, genetic testing
- Management
  - Asymptomatic: serial laboratory studies
  - Symptomatic
    - PRBCs and platelet transfusion as needed
    - Chemotherapy (azacitidine), antiangiogenesis agents
    - Lenalidomide in RBC transfusion-dependent patients with 5q deletion
    - Bone marrow transplantation is potentially curative
- Complications: conversion to hematologic malignancy (acute myeloid leukemia [AML], acute lymphoid leukemia [ALL])

AML

- Definition: hematologic malignancy characterized by excessive production of immature granulocyte (>20% myeloblasts)
- Associations
  - Trisomy 21
  - Klinefelter syndrome
  - Radiation/toxin exposure
  - Chemotherapy
  - Myelodysplastic syndrome, polycythemia vera
- Subtypes: seven total subtypes
  - AML M3 (acute promyelocytic leukemia)
    - Auer rods on peripheral smear; DIC
    - 15:17 translocation
    - Treated with all-trans-retinoic acid
  - AML M4/M5 (myelocytic leukemia)
    - Mimics meningitis due to CNS involvement
    - Skin and soft tissue nodules
    - Gingival hyperplasia
  - AML M6: periodic acid-Schiff–positive blasts
- Signs and symptoms
  - Fatigue, shortness of breath: anemia
  - Easy bruising, bleeding: thrombocytopenia
  - Recurrent infections: malfunctioning granulocytes
  - Hepatosplenomegaly: extramedullary hematopoiesis
  - Lymphadenopathy
  - Bone and joint pain
- Diagnostics
  - CBC: anemia, thrombocytopenia, leukocytosis
  - Peripheral smear: Auer rods (Fig. 9–13), >20% blasts
  - Chromosomal studies, cytogenetics
  - Flow cytometry
  - Myeloperoxidase positive
- Management: induction chemotherapy (cytarabine + daunorubicin) followed by allogeneic hematopoietic cell transplantation

Chronic Myeloid Leukemia (CML)

- Definition: myeloproliferative disorder characterized by abnormal gene fusion (BCR-ABL) resulting in constitutively active tyrosine kinase
- Signs and symptoms
  - Anemia, thrombocytopenia, neutropenia
  - Hepatosplenomegaly
  - Lymphadenopathy

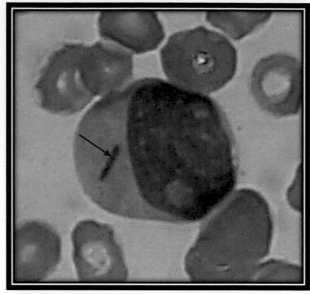

Figure 9-13: Peripheral smear showing myeloblast Auer rod *(red arrow)*. The Auer rod is what makes acute my-elogenous leukemia highly thrombogenic. (Image courtesy of Paulo Henrique Orlandi Mourao.)

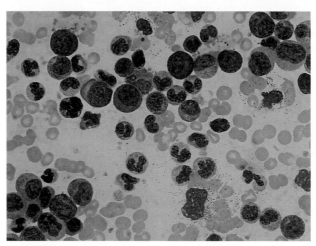

Figure 9-14: Peripheral blood smear of a patient with chronic myelogenous leukemia showing myeloid cell types in various stages of development. (Image courtesy of Paulo Henrique Orlandi Mourao.)

- Diagnostics
  - CBC: leukocytosis, basophilia, increased neutrophil precursors
  - Peripheral smear: myeloid cells in various stages of development (promyelocytes, metamyelocytes, myelocytes, bands, neutrophils) (Fig. 9–14)
  - Chromosomal studies: BCR-ABL fusion gene (9:22 translocation; Philadelphia chromosome)
  - Leukocyte alkaine phosphatase score: differentiates CML from leukemoid reaction
    - Low score: CML
    - High score: leukemoid reaction
- Management
  - Tyrosine kinase inhibitors (imatinib, dasatinib, nilotinib): first line
  - Allogeneic hematopoietic cell transplantation
- Complications: transformation to acute leukemic blast crisis (AML, ALL)

Chronic Lymphoid Leukemia
- Epidemiology: most common leukemia after age 50; typically presents between age 60 and 80 years
- Definition: lymphocytic proliferative disorder characterized by mature lymphocyte
- Signs and symptoms
  - Asymptomatic (most common presentation)
  - Fever, night sweats, weight loss

- Fatigue, easy bruising/bleeding, recurrent depression
- Generalized lymphadenopathy
- Hepatosplenomegaly
– Diagnostics
- CBC: lymphocytosis
- Peripheral smear: mature lymphocytes, smudge cells (fragile leukemic cells)
- Flow cytometry: CD markers positive for both B and T cells
- Bone marrow biopsy
– Management
- Asymptomatic, early disease: observation
- Symptomatic, advanced disease: chemotherapy
– Complications
- Richter phenomenon: transformation to high-grade lymphoma
- Autoimmune hemolytic anemia/thrombocytopenia: treated with glucocorticoids

> When treating patients with hematologic malignancies, prophylaxis with allopurinol and/or rasburicase is needed prior to initiation of chemotherapy due to rapid cell destruction and risk of tumor lysis syndrome.

Hairy Cell Leukemia
– Signs and symptoms
- Pancytopenia
- Massive splenomegaly, early satiety
- Increased risk of atypical mycobacteria infection
– Diagnostics
- Flow cytometry: CD11c, CD25
- Peripheral smear: hairy cells
- Tartrate-resistant acid phosphatase stain positive
- Bone marrow biopsy: "dry" tap, hypercellular bone marrow (increased reticulin fibrosis)
– Management
- Asymptomatic, early stage: observation
- Symptomatic, advanced disease: purine-based analog (cladribine, pentostatin)

> Other causes of agranulocytosis:
> - Bone marrow suppressive chemotherapy
> - Clozapine
> - Methimazole
> - Propyltiouracil

RBC DYSCRASIAS
Polycythemia Vera
– Pathophysiology: JAK2 tyrosine kinase mutation resulting in recruitment of STAT (signal transducer activators of transcription) and proliferation of erythrocytes
– Signs and symptoms
- Hyperviscosity
  - Headache, visual disturbances, neuropathy
  - Erythromelalgia (burning cyanosis in extremities)
  - Facial plethora, ruddy cyanosis
- Aquagenic pruritus (secondary to mast cell degranulation, histamine release)
- Thrombosis
- Gout
- Hepatosplenomegaly
– Diagnostics
- JAK2 V617F mutation
- CBC: polycythemia, thrombocytosis, leukocytosis
- Low erythropoietin levels
– Management
- Phlebotomy with goal hematocrit <45
- Low-dose aspirin
- Hydroxyurea: decreases the risk of thrombosis
- Alternative agents: pegylated interferon, ruxolitinib (JAK inhibitor)
– Complications: transformation to AML or myelodyplastic syndrome

Other causes of polycythemia:
- Erythropoietin-producing tumor (renal cell carcinoma, hepatocellular carcinoma, hemangioblastoma, leiomyoma)
- Chronic hypoxemia (obstructive sleep apnea, chronic obstructive pulmonary disease)
- Hemoconcentration

Thrombocytosis

Essential Thrombocytosis
- Pathophysiology: JAK2 tyrosine kinase mutation resulting in recruitment of STAT and proliferation of platelets
- Key manifestations
  - Bleeding, arterial/venous thrombosis
  - Headaches, dizziness, visual disturbances
  - Erythromelalgia
  - Spurious hypocalcemia (pseudohyperkalemia)
- Diagnostics
  - CBC: thrombocytosis >1 million
  - JAK2 tyrosine kinase mutation
- Management
  - Low-dose aspirin
  - Hydroxyurea
  - Systemic anticoagulation for venous thrombosis
  - Anagrelide

Other causes of thrombocytosis:
- Sepsis
- Iron deficiency anemia
- Malignancy
- Postsplenectomy
- Chronic inflammatory disease (malignancy, inflammatory bowel disease, collagen vascular disease)

Plasma Cell Dyscrasias

Multiple Myeloma
- Pathophysiology: proliferation of plasma cells resulting in excess production of abnormal immunoglobulins (IgG or IgA)
- Key manifestations
  - Hypercalcemia
    - Lethargy, confusion
    - Malaise
    - Constipation
  - Renal dysfunction: oliguria, nephrolithiasis
  - Normocytic anemia: fatigue, dyspnea on exertion
  - Bony lesions: bone pain, pathologic fractures
  - Recurrent infections
- Diagnostics: symptomatology plus bone marrow biopsy
  - CRAB symptoms:
    - Hypercalcemia (release of osteoclast-activating factor; direct bony destruction)
    - Renal dysfunction
      - Myeloma nephropathy secondary to deposition of Bence-Jones proteins into renal tubules
      - Nephrogenic DI
      - Overflow proteinuria
      - RTA type I/II
    - Normocytic anemia
      - Anemia of chronic disease
      - Renal dysfunction
      - Plasma cell bone marrow infiltration
    - Punched-out lytic bony lesions (release of osteoclast-activating factor) on x-ray/CT; cord compression if lytic lesions involve the spine resulting in pathologic fractures
  - Bone marrow biopsy: >10% plasma cells
  - Serum/urine protein electrophoresis: elevated monoclonal proteins (M-spike)

- Other supportive findings
  - Gamma gap: elevated protein with normal albumin
  - Peripheral smear: RBC rouleaux formation
  - Hyperuricemia: increased cell turnover
  - Amyloidosis: light chain deposition
- Management
  - Younger, asymptomatic: autologous hematopoietic cell transplantation
  - Older, asymptomatic, not transplant candidates: chemotherapy (bortezomib, lenalidomide, dexamethasone)

Waldenström Macroglobulinemia
- Pathophysiology: proliferation of IgM resulting in hyperviscosity symptoms due to IgM being a large pentameric protein
- Key manifestations
  - Fever, night sweats, weight loss
  - Headache, visual disturbances (retinal vasodilation, hemorrhage, blindness)
  - Neuropathy, Raynaud phenomenon
  - Bleeding, facial plethora
  - Lymphadenopathy, organomegaly
- Diagnostics
  - Serum protein electrophoresis: IgM spike
  - Bone marrow biopsy: >10% infiltration by small lymphocytes with plasmacytoid or plasma cell differentiation
- Management
  - Asymptomatic: observation
  - Symptomatic
    - Plasmapheresis: removes IgM proteins and decreases blood viscosity
    - Chemotherapy: rituximab + bendamustine

Monoclonal gammopathy of unknown significance: asymptomatic M-spike on protein electrophoresis; 1% per year transform into multiple myeloma; no treatment unless transformation into myeloma occurs

Smoldering multiple myeloma: M-spike, >10% plasma cells in bone marrow biopsy, without CRAB symptoms

LYMPHOMA

Basic principles of lymphoma
- Cancer of the lymphatic system
- Has the potential to spread into the blood causing leukemia
- Presents with painless lymphadenopathy plus A symptoms (asymptomatic) or B symptoms (fever, weight loss, night sweats); presence of B symptoms indicates a worse prognosis
- Location of lymphadenopathy results in local compressive symptoms: mediastinal (cough, shortness of breath, superior vena cava syndrome), mesenteric (abdominal pain), retroperitoneal (back pain)
- May invade other organs such as spleen (splenomegaly), liver (hepatomegaly), and bone marrow (bone pain)
- Divided into Hodgkin and non-Hodgkin lymphoma
- Hodgkin lymphoma staging (Ann Arbor system) is determined based on number of lymph nodes involved, location of lymph nodes (above or below the diaphragm), and extralymphatic spread

> Lymph nodes may become tender when drinking alcohol.

- Some lymphoma subtypes are characterized by chromosomal translocation

> Hodgkin lymphoma most commonly presents during localized early-stage disease treated with radiation.

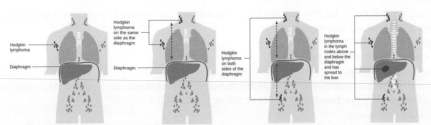

Figure 9-15: Ann Arbor staging of Hodgkin lymphoma, stages 1 to 4 from left to right. (Images courtesy of Cancer Research UK; CC BY-SA 4.0 [https://creativecommons.org/licenses/by-sa/4.0])

Hodgkin Lymphoma
- Epidemiology: bimodal distribution, 15–30 years old and >50 years old
- Subtypes
  • Nodular sclerosing: most common
  • Mixed cellularity
  • Lymphocytic rich: best prognosis
  • Lymphocyte depleted: worse prognosis
- Signs and symptoms: painless lymphadenopathy plus A or B symptoms
- Diagnostics
  • Excisional lymph node biopsy: Reed-Sternberg cells (owl's-eye nucleus; CD15, CD30 positive)
  • Elevated LDH
  • Ann Arbor staging (Fig. 9–15)
    ▪ CT chest abdomen and pelvis
    ▪ Bone marrow biopsy
- Management
  • Localized disease: radiation +/− chemotherapy
  • Advanced disease: chemotherapy
- Complications: related to radiation therapy
  • Increased risk of future solid organ malignancy (lung, breast, thyroid, GI, bone)
  • Non-Hodgkin lymphoma
  • Leukemia from chemoradiation

Associated with minimal change disease (nephrotic syndrome), hypervitaminosis D (increased production of 1, 25-dihydroxyvitamin D), Lambert-Eaton syndrome (antibodies against presynaptic voltage-gated calcium channels), Guillain-Barré syndrome

Non-Hodgkin Lymphoma
- Risk factors
  • Autoimmune disease
  • Genetic syndromes
    ▪ Klinefelter
    ▪ Down syndrome
    ▪ Wiskott-Aldrich
  • Environmental exposures: benzene, pesticides, herbicide
  • Infections/associations
    ▪ HIV: diffuse large B-cell lymphoma, Burkitt lymphoma, CNS lymphoma
    ▪ EBV: Burkitt lymphoma
    ▪ Human T-cell leukemia virus: T-cell lymphoma
    ▪ *Helicobacter pylori*: gastric lymphoma, MALToma
- Subtypes: most commonly B-cell lymphomas
  • Low grade
    ▪ Follicular: a 14:18 translocation
    ▪ Small lymphocytic lymphoma: CLL of the lymph nodes
  • Intermediate/high grade
    ▪ Diffuse large B-cell lymphoma: most common subtype
    ▪ Burkitt lymphoma: a 8:14 translocation; abdominal/mandibular mass, "starry sky" appearance on histology
    ▪ Lymphoblastic lymphoma
  • Other subtypes
    ▪ Marginal zone, MALToma: a 11:18 translocation
    ▪ Mantle cell: a 11:14 translocation
- Signs and symptoms: painless lymphadenopathy plus A or B symptoms
- Diagnostics
  • Excisional lymph node biopsy: allows for evaluation of the entire lymph node architecture
  • Elevated LDH, beta-2 microglobulin
  • Staging
    ▪ CT chest abdomen and pelvis
    ▪ Bone marrow biopsy
- Management: R-CHOP chemotherapy (rituximab, cyclophosphamide, hydroxydaunorubicin, vincristine [oncovin], prednisone)

Cutaneous T-cell Lymphoma
- Signs and symptoms

- • Pruritus, eczematous skin lesions
- • Fungoid-like rash
- • Generalized erythroderma
- – Diagnostics
  - • Skin biopsy
  - • Peripheral smear: T cells with cerebriform-shaped nucleus (referred to as Sezary syndrome; leukemic version of T-cell lymphoma)
- – Management: topical/systemic chemotherapy

MISCELLANEOUS ONCOLOGY

Certain chemotherapy agents have unique side effects that may warrant cessation and switching to a new regimen (Table 9–10). Additonlly, there characteristic syndromes that result in increased frequency of certain malignancies, often related to their DNA mutations (Table 9–11).

Paraneoplastic syndromes are clinical presentations associated with typical cancers that may be the first clue that a patient has a cancer. These symptoms often occur due to autonomous secretion of a hormone or new onset physicial manifestation (Table 9–12). Efforts to combat malignancy and provide patients with the best chance of cure is often through screening programs. Several studies have been performed to screen for a myriad of cancer; however, only a few screening programs have been shown to reduce overall mortality (Table 9–13).

TABLE 9–10   Chemotherapeutics and associated side effects

CHEMOTHERAPY AGENT	SIDE EFFECTS
Bleomycin Busulfan	Pulmonary fibrosis
Cisplatin	Nephrotoxicity (prevented with amifostine) Neurotoxicity (ototoxicity)
Cyclophosphamide	Hemorrhagic cystitis (prevented with mesna) Bladder cancer
Doxorubicin Daunorubicin Trastuzumab	Cardiotoxicity Trastuzumab cardiotoxicity is reversible upon cessation
Methotrexate	Hepatotoxicity Pulmonary fibrosis
Nitrosoureas	Central nervous system toxicity (ataxia, seizures)
Prednisone	Weight gain Hyperglycemia Osteoporosis
Vincristine	Peripheral neuropathy

Most chemotherapy agents target rapidly dividing cells resulting in bone marrow suppression (pancytopenia), diarrhea, dermatitis, mucositis, and hair loss.

TABLE 9–11   Oncology-related syndromes

DISEASE	KEY FEATURES
Lynch syndrome (hereditary nonpolyposis colorectal cancer)	• Colon cancer arises spontaneously without development of polyps • DNA mismatch repair gene mutation • Increased risk of endometrial and ovarian cancer • Suspected when colorectal cancer occurs in three family members, two generations, one prematurely
Familial adenomatous polyposis (FAP)	• APC gene mutation • Development of 1000 colon polyps • 100% of patients will develop colorectal cancer • Treat with prophylactic colectomy
Turcot syndrome	• Colorectal cancer plus soft tissue tumors (osteomas, desmoid tumors, lipomas)
Gardner syndrome	• Colorectal cancer plus central nervous system malignancy (glioma, medulloblastoma)

TABLE 9–11   Oncology-related syndromes

DISEASE	KEY FEATURES
Peutz-Jeghers syndrome	• Multiple hamartomatous polyps • Hyperpigmented lips and skin lesions • Increased risk of gonadal, pancreatic, breast cancer
BRCA gene mutation	• Increased risk of breast, ovarian, and prostate cancer
Li-Fraumeni	• *P53* gene mutation • Increased risk of several cancers, particularly sarcomas
Neurofibromatosis	• Neurofibromatosis type I: optic glioma, meningiomas, café au lait spots, iris hamartomas (Lisch nodules) • Neurofibromatosis type II: bilateral vestibular schwannomas
Polycystic kidney disease	• *PKD1/PKD2* gene mutation • Enlarged bilateral palpable kidneys with multiple renal cysts • Hypertension, recurrent urinary tract infection, proteinuria • Multiple prolapsing organs: cerebral aneurysms, mitral valve prolapse, diverticulosis, inguinal hernias • Increased risk of renal cell carcinoma
Wiskott-Aldrich syndrome (WAS)	• WAS gene mutation • Triad of immunodeficiency, thrombocytopenia, eczema • B-cell lymphoma (associated with Epstein-Barr virus) and leukemia
Von Hippel-Lindau	• Associated with development of hemangioblastoma, renal cell carcinoma, pheochromocytoma
Multiple endocrine neoplasia (MEN)	• MEN1: pancreatic neuroendocrine tumors, parathyroid adenoma, pituitary adenoma • MEN2A: medullary thyroid cancer, pheochromocytoma, parathyroid hyperplasia • MEN2B: medullary thyroid cancer, pheochromocytoma, mucosal neuromas • MEN2A/2B associated with RET protooncogene mutation

TABLE 9–12   Paraneoplastic syndromes

PARANEOPLASTIC SYNDROME	ASSOCIATED MALIGNANCIES	CLINICAL MANIFESTATIONS
Syndrome of inappropriate antidiuretic hormone	Small cell lung cancer	• Asymptomatic hyponatremia (most common) • Headache, visual disturbances, seizures
Cushing syndrome	Small cell lung cancer	• Hypertension, hyperglycemia • Weight gain, buffalo hump, central adiposity
Lambert-Eaton syndrome	Small cell lung cancer	• Muscle weakness improved by use
Myasthenia gravis (acetylcholine receptor antibodies)	Thymoma	• Ptosis, diplopia worsened by use and at the end of the day • Dysphagia, dysarthria
Parathyroid hormone–related peptide	Squamous cell carcinoma the long	• Hypercalcemia-related symptoms
Erythropoietin	Renal cell carcinoma, hepatocellular carcinoma, hemangioblastoma, leiomyoma, pheochromocytoma	• Hyperviscosity syndrome: headache, visual disturbances, peripheral neuropathy • Facial plethora
Dermatomyositis/polymyositis	Gastrointestinal (GI) adenocarcinoma, ovarian cancer, visceral malignancy	• Proximal muscle weakness • Gottron papules, heliotrope rash
Acanthosis nigricans	GI adenocarcinoma, visceral malignancy	• Hyperpigmented, velvety skin involving posterior neck and axilla
Leser-Trélat sign	GI adenocarcinoma, visceral malignancy	• Sudden onset appearance of multiple seborrheic keratosis
Trousseau syndrome	Pancreatic adenocarcinoma	• Superficial migratory thrombophlebitis
Anti-NMDA receptor encephalitis	Ovarian teratoma	• Confusion, neurocognitive deficits, seizures

NMDA, N-methyl-D-aspartate.

TABLE 9–13 Cancer screening guidelines

TYPE OF CANCER	SCREENING MODALITY	SCREENING RECOMMENDATIONS
Breast cancer	Mammogram (preferred)Breast MRI (high-risk patients)	• Start at age 50, every 2 yr until 74 yr old • Screening for women >75 only if life expectancy is at least 10 yr
Cervical cancer	Pap smear +/− HPV DNA testing	• Start at age 21, regardless of age of first sexual encounter • Age 21–30, Pap smear only every 3 yr • Age 30–65, Pap smear plus HPV DNA testing every 5 yr
Colon cancer	Colonoscopy (most preferred), alternatives include sigmoidoscopy, FOBT, virtual colonoscopy, FIT	• Start at age 50, every 10 yr until 75 yr old • Screening for patients >75 only if life expectancy is at least 10 yr
Lung cancer	Low-dose contrast CT chest	Age 55–80, every 1 yr who meet all the following criteria: • 30-pack-year smoking history • Previous smokers who quit within the last 15 yr • Otherwise good health without comorbidities limiting life expectancy

CT, Computed tomography; *FIT*, fecal immunochemical test; *FOBT*, fecal occult blood test; *HPV*, human papillomavirus; *MRI*, magnetic resonance imaging.

Radiation side effects
– Radiation-induced organ dysfunction
  • Musculoskeletal: joint immobility, lymphedema, muscle atrophy
  • Pulmonary: pulmonary fibrosis
  • Cardiac: constrictive pericarditis, coronary artery disease
  • GI/GU: strictures/fistulas, urethral stenosis, cystitis
– Miscellaneous: secondary malignancies years later

Other additional notes regarding cancer screening:
  • Screening for other cancers such as prostate cancer remains controversial.
  • Screening guidelines given in Table 9-13 are per US Preventive Services Taskforce recommendations. Other societies may have different screening recommendations and/or modalities.
  • For all types of cancer screening, if abnormal results are noted screening interval becomes more frequent. See specific sections regarding further details.

COLLAGEN VASCULAR DISEASES

Systemic Lupus Erythematosus (SLE)
- Epidemiology: primarily affects middle-aged women with personal or family history of other autoimmune disease (rheumatoid arthritis [RA], Sjögren, scleroderma)
- Definition: systemic, multiorgan autoimmune disorder
- Key manifestations (Fig. 10-1)
  - Cutaneous
    - Photosensitive malar rash (Fig. 10-2)
    - Painless oral ulcers
    - Discoid rash
    - Raynaud phenomenon
  - Musculoskeletal
    - Avascular necrosis of the hip
    - Migratory, symmetric arthritis/arthralgias
  - Hematologic/immunologic
    - Autoimmune thrombocytopenia, hemolytic anemia, leukopenia: type II hypersensitivity reaction
    - Anemia of chronic disease
    - Diffuse lymphadenopathy
    - Antiphospholipid syndrome (anticardiolipin, lupus anticoagulant, anti-beta-2 glycoprotein antibody)
  - Serology
    - Antinuclear antibody (highly sensitive)
    - Anti-dsDNA (highly specific), anti-Smith (highly specific)
    - Hypocomplementemia (low C3/C4)
    - Elevated inflammatory markers (erythrocyte sedimentation rate [ESR], C-reactive protein [CRP])
  - Renal
    - Rapidly progressive glomerulonephritis (crescenteric glomerulonephritis)
    - Membranous nephropathy
  - Neurologic
    - Cerebritis
    - Stroke (secondary to vasculitis)
    - Seizures
    - Cognitive deficits
  - Pulmonary
    - Pleuritis
    - Pleurisy
    - Interstitial lung disease
    - Pleural effusion
  - Cardiac
    - Libman-Sacks endocarditis
    - Pericarditis, pericardial effusion
    - Early atherosclerosis/coronary arter disease (CAD)
    - Myocarditis
- Diagnostics: 4 of 11 diagnostic criteria (SOAP BRAIN MD [see text box])
- Management
  - Acute flare: glucocorticoids

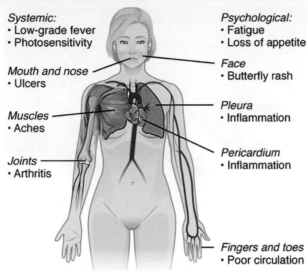

Systemic:
• Low-grade fever
• Photosensitivity

Psychological:
• Fatigue
• Loss of appetite

Mouth and nose
• Ulcers

Face
• Butterfly rash

Muscles
• Aches

Pleura
• Inflammation

Joints
• Arthritis

Pericardium
• Inflammation

Fingers and toes
• Poor circulation

Figure 10-1: Diagrammatic representation of the symptoms of systemic lupus erythematosus, system by system. (Image courtesy of OpenStax College.)

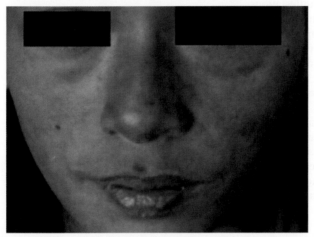

Figure 10-2: Malar rash in a patient with systemic lupus erythematosus. (Image courtesy of CNX OpenStax.)

Drug-induced systemic lupus erythematosus (SHIPPE): sulfasalazine, hydralazine, isoniazid, procainamide, phenytoin, etanercept

Drug-induced lupus does not have central nervous system or renal manifestations. Associated with antihistone antibodies, which are highly specific.

Anti-Ro and anti-La associated with neonatal lupus. These babies present with complete heart block requiring pacing at birth.

• Chronic disease
  ▪ Mild disease: hydroxychloroquine, nonsteroidal antiinflammatory drugs (NSAIDs)
  ▪ Moderate disease: methotrexate, azathioprine
  ▪ Severe disease (life-threatening renal or central nervous system [CNS] disease): steroid-sparing agents (cyclophosphamide, mycophenolate)
• Steroids also used for lupus with renal, CNS, and hematologic manifestations

Rheumatoid Arthritis
– Definition: polyarticular symmetric inflammatory arthritis resulting in damage to bone and cartilage
– Epidemiology: young to middle-aged women
– Signs and symptoms
  • Arthritis involving wrist, metacarpophalangeal (MCP), proximal interphalangeal (PIP) joints

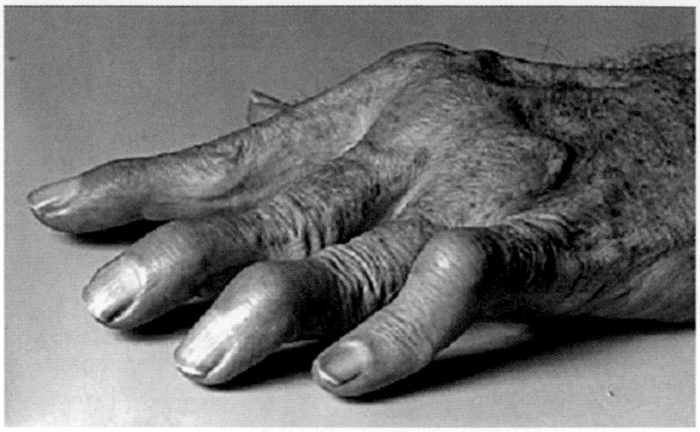

Figure 10-3: Swan neck deformity in a patient with rheumatoid arthritis. (Image courtesy of Abdulaziz Alkanderi.)

- Morning joint stiffness lasting >1 hour
- Ulnar deviation of MCP joint
- Boutonniere deformity (PIP flexed, distal interphalangeal [DIP] hyperextended)
- Swan neck deformity (MCP flexed, PIP hyperextended, DIP flexed) (Fig. 10-3)
- Extraarticular manifestations
  - Musculoskeletal
    - Carpal tunnel syndrome
    - C1/C2 joint instability
    - Rheumatoid nodules
  - Pulmonary
    - Pleural effusions (exudative, very low glucose)
    - Pulmonary nodules
    - Bronchiectasis
  - Cardiac: pericarditis, CAD
  - Hematologic: anemia of chronic disease
  - Ocular: episcleritis, scleritis
  - Neurologic: mononeuritis multiplex
  - Systemic: vasculitis, amyloidosis

Felty syndrome: triad of long-standing rheumatoid arthritis, splenomegaly, and neutropenia

Kaplan syndrome: triad of long-standing rheumatoid arthritis, pneumoconiosis, and lung nodules

- Diagnostics: symptomatology involving small/large joints lasting >6 weeks plus serology
  - Rheumatoid factor positive
  - Anti-CCP antibodies
  - Elevated inflammatory markers (ESR, CRP)
  - Imaging: x-ray or computed tomography (CT)
    - Periarticular osteopenia
    - Joint erosions
    - Joint space narrowing
- Management
  - Acute flares: glucocorticoids
  - Early disease: NSAIDs, glucocorticoids; used as bridging agent to disease-modifying antirheumatic drugs (DMARDs)
  - Advanced disease (erosive joint disease): DMARDs
    - Methotrexate
    - Hydroxychloroquine
    - Leflunomide
    - Sulfasalazine
    - Tumor necrosis factor (TNF) inhibitors

CREST syndrome has similar features as scleroderma (diffuse) with less cutaneous and visceral organ involvement (lack of renal, pulmonary, or cardiac dysfunction).

Sjögren Syndrome
- Pathophysiology: autoimmune disorder characterized by salivary and lacrimal gland destruction
- Signs and symptoms
  - Glandular manifestations
    - Xerostomia (dry mouth)
    - Keratoconjunctivitis sicca (dry eyes)
    - Dental caries
  - Extraglandular manifestations
    - Interstitial lung disease
    - Arthralgias
    - Renal tubular acidosis type 1, acute interstitial nephritis
    - Vasculitis
    - Non-Hodgkin B-cell lymphoma
    - Cytopenias, cryoglobulinemia
    - Manifestations of other autoimmune diseases (RA, inflammatory bowel disease [IBD], SLE, primary biliary cirrhosis, Hashimoto)
- Diagnostics
  - Serology: anti-SSA/SSB
  - Biopsy: lymphoid infiltration of the salivary gland
  - Positive Schirmer test: decreased tears on filter paper placed against the eye
- Management: symptomatic
  - Frequent sips of water; chewing gum
  - Artificial tears
  - Saliva stimulants: cevimeline, pilocarpine

Scleroderma
- Pathophysiology: autoimmune disorder characterized by diffuse fibrotic deposition and organ dysfunction
- Subtypes
  - Diffuse
  - Limited (CREST syndrome)
- Key manifestations
  - Cutaneous
    - Thick, waxy skin
    - Loss of wrinkles
    - Pruritus
  - Musculoskeletal: arthritis, arthralgias
  - Pulmonary
    - Interstitial lung disease
    - Pulmonary hypertension
  - Cardiac
    - Dilated/restrictive cardiomyopathy
    - Pericarditis
  - Renal
    - Scleroderma renal crisis (sudden-onset hypertensive emergency)
    - Nephrolithiasis
  - Gastrointestinal (GI)
    - Gastroesophageal reflux disease (GERD): secondary to relaxation of the lower esophageal sphincter from fibrotic deposition
    - Bowel dysmotility, small intestinal bacterial overgrowth (SIBO)
  - Limited scleroderma (CREST syndrome)
    - Calcinosis (calcium deposition into skin and other tissues)
    - Raynaud syndrome (vasospasm of digital vessels)
    - Esophageal dysmotility
    - Sclerodactyly (loss of skin folds, ulcerations)
    - Telangiectasia
- Diagnostics: clinical features plus serology
  - Serology
    - Anti-Scl 70 (anti-DNA topoisomerase I): diffuse type
    - Anticentromere antibody: limited type, CREST syndrome
- Management: symptomatic
  - Diffuse skin sclerosis: methotrexate, mycophenolate
  - Arthralgias: NSAIDs, acetaminophen

TABLE 10-1 Ehlers-danlos versus Marfan syndrome

	EHLERS-DANLOS SYNDROME	MARFAN SYNDROME
Pathophysiology	• Collagen synthesis gene mutation (specific collagen type characterizes clinical manifestations and Ehlers-Danlos syndrome subtype)	• Fibrillin-1 gene mutation
Key manifestations	• Rheumatologic: hypermobile joints, kyphoscoliosis • Cardiac: mitral valve prolapse (MVP), valvular regurgitation, aortic aneurysm/dissection • Neurologic: cerebral aneurysm, subarachnoid hemorrhage	• Musculoskeletal: decreased upper limbs to lower limb length ratio, arachnodactyly, pectus deformity • Cardiac: MVP, aortic aneurysm/dissection (cystic medial necrosis) • Ocular: ectopia lentis (downward displaced lens) • Pulmonary: emphysematous bullae, spontaneous pneumothorax • Neurologic: dural ectasia
Diagnostics	• Clinical +/– genetic testing	
Management	• No treatment • Screening and management of complications as they occur	

- Scleroderma renal crisis: angiotensin-converting enzyme inhibitor
- GERD: PPI
- SIBO: antibiotics
- Raynaud phenomenon: calcium channel blockers
- Pulmonary hypertension
  - Phosphodiesterase inhibitors: sildenafil, tadalafil
  - Endothelin antagonist: bosentan, ambrisentan, macitentan
  - Another connective tissue disorder that results in abnormal collagen production is Ehlers-Danlos (Table 10-1).
  - Prostaglandin analogues: epoprostenol, treprostinil

Another connective tissue disorder that results in abnormal collagen production is Ehlers-Danlos (Table 10-1).

Mixed Connective Tissue Disease
- Overlap disease characterized by features of SLE, RA, systemic sclerosis, and polymyositis
- Does not meet criteria for one specific collagen vascular disease
- Anti-U1-RNP (ribonucleoprotein) antibodies

Many disease-modifying agents are used in autoimmune disorders as antiinflammatories and immuno-suppressives (Table 10-2). The downside of this is that patients are at increased risk of opportunistic infections. Other disease-modifying agents have unique side effects making them highly testable.

Other drugs besides hydroxychloroquine that affect the eyes:
- Ethosuximide: red-green discoloration
- Thioridazine: retinal deposits
- Chlorpromazine: corneal deposits
- Latanoprost: browning of the iris

Autoimmune serology is important as these markers are highly sensitive and/or specific for their associated autoimmune disease, and often necessary for diagnosis (Table 10-3).

SERONEGATIVE SPONDYLOARTHROPATHIES
General principles
- Spondyloarthropathies present primarily with axial skeletal symptoms with characteristic extraaxial manifestations
- Commonly affect young to middle-aged males
- Highly associated with HLA-B27

Psoriatic Arthritis
- Signs and symptoms
  - Cutaneous: plaque psoriasis
    - Silver, scaly lesions involving extensor surfaces
    - Nail pitting, onychomycosis, onycholysis

TABLE 10-2   Pharmacotherapy of disease-modifying agents used in autoimmune disorders

MEDICATION	MECHANISM OF ACTION	SIDE EFFECTS
Cyclophosphamide	DNA alkylating agent	• Hemorrhagic cystitis, bladder cancer
Hydroxychloroquine	Antimalarial/antiinflammatory	• Retinal toxicity • Myopathy • Hemolysis in G6PD
Sulfasalazine	Antibacterial/ antiinflammatory metabolites	• Hemolysis in G6PD • Azoospermia
Methotrexate	Folate antagonist	• Bone marrow suppression • Pulmonary fibrosis • Hepatotoxicity
Anti-TNF (infliximab, etanercept, adalimumab)	TNF receptor decoy; monoclonal antibody	• Increased risk of tuberculosis, opportunistic infections
Azathioprine	Antimetabolite	• Myelosuppression • Increased toxicity when used with xanthine oxidase inhibitors (allopurinol, febuxostat)
Leflunomide	Inhibits pyrimidine synthesis	• Hypertension, hepatotoxicity
Rituximab	CD20 monoclonal antibody	• Hepatitis B reactivation • Increased risk of progressive multifocal leukoencephalopathy

TNF, Tumor necrosis factor.

TABLE 10-3   Summary of autoimmune serologies

AUTOIMMUNE DISEASE	SEROLOGY
Systemic lupus erythematosus	ANA (sensitive) Anti-Smith, anti-dsDNA
Antiphospholipid syndrome	Anticardiolipin, lupus anticoagulant, Anti-beta-2 glycoprotein
Rheumatoid arthritis	Rheumatoid factor, anti-CCP
Type I diabetes	Antiglutamic acid decarboxylase, islet autoantibodies, insulin autoantibodies
Graves disease	Thyroid-stimulating immunoglobulin
Hashimoto thyroiditis	Antithyroid peroxidase, antimicrosomal
Primary biliary cirrhosis	Antimitochondrial
Sjögren syndrome	Anti-SSA/SSB (anti-Ro/anti-La)
Scleroderma	Anti-Scl-70 (anti-DNA topoisomerase)
CREST syndrome	Anticentromere
Goodpasture syndrome	Antiglomerular basement membrane
Pemphigus vulgaris	Antidesmosome
Bullous pemphigoid	Antihemidesmosome
Polymyositis/dermatomyositis	Anti-Jo-1, anti-Mi-2
Pernicious anemia	Antiparietal, antiintrinsic factor
Drug-induced lupus	Antihistone
Celiac disease	Antiendomysial, antitissue transglutaminase
Granulomatosis with polyangitis	c-ANCA
Mixed connective tissue disease	Anti-U1 RNP (ribonucleoprotein)
Autoimmune hepatitis	ANA, anti-smooth muscle, anti-liver-kidney-microsomal (LKM)
Myasthenia gravis	Anti-acetylcholine receptor
Pulmonary alveolar proteinosis	Anti-GM-CSF

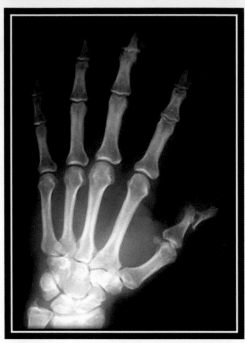

Figure 10-4: "Pencil in cup" deformities in a patient with psoriatic arthritis. Note *(red arrows)* subluxation of the first distal phalangeal joint.

- Musculoskeletal
  - DIP joint involvement: dactylitis ("sausage" digits)
  - Arthritis mutilans (bony joint destruction)
  - Enthesopathy (tendon inflammation)
  - Lower back and hip pain/stiffness
- Ocular: uveitis, conjunctivitis
- Diagnostics
  - Clinical diagnosis
  - Imaging: x-ray/CT
    - "Pencil in cup" deformity (Fig. 10-4)
    - Bony erosions
    - Sacroiliitis, spondylitis
- Management
  - NSAIDs
  - ± disease-modifying agents, similar to RA

Ankylosing Spondylitis
- Signs and symptoms
  - Musculoskeletal
    - Lower back and hip pain/stiffness, improved with exercise
    - Enthesitis
    - Dactylitis
    - Osteoporosis, increased risk of spinal fracture
    - Cauda equina syndrome
  - Extraarthritic
    - Cardiac: aortitis, aortic regurgitation, atrioventricular block
    - Pulmonary: restrictive lung disease, apical lung fibrosis
    - Ocular: anterior uveitis
- Diagnostic: clinical plus imaging
- Imaging: x-ray/CT
  - Sacroiliitis
  - "Bamboo" spine (fusion of vertebral bodies by bridging syndesmophytes) (Fig. 10-5)
- Management
  - Exercise, physical therapy/occupational therapy
  - NSAIDs: initial treatment
  - Disease-modifying agents, similar to RA

Triad of uveitis ("can't see"), urethritis ("can't pee"), and arthritis ("can't climb a tree") is classic for reactive arthritis.

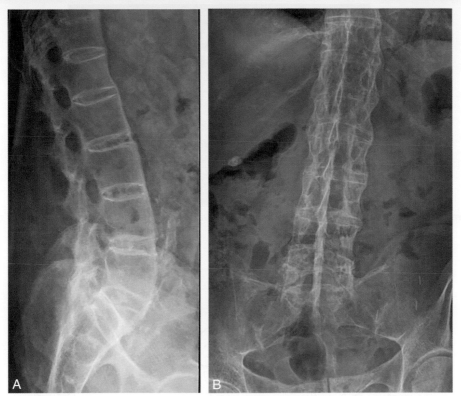

Figure 10-5: Characteristic bamboo spine in a patient with ankylosing spondylitis on lateral (A) and anterior-posterior (B) views.

Reactive Arthritis (previously known as Reiter syndrome)
– Signs and symptoms
  • Preceding GI (Salmonella, Shigella, Campylobacter, Yersinia) or genitourianary (GU) infection (chlamydia, ureaplasma) 1–4 weeks prior to other symptomatology
    ▪ Diarrhea, abdominal pain
    ▪ Dysuria, urgency
    ▪ Purulent vaginal/penile discharge (urethritis)
  • Ocular: conjunctivitis, uveitis
  • Musculoskeletal
    ▪ Spondylitis, sacroiliitis
    ▪ Peripheral arthritis, dactylitis
    ▪ Enthesitis
    ▪ Bursitis
  • Cutaneous
    ▪ Keratoderma blennorrhagica (hyperkeratotic lesions on palms and soles, similar to pustular psoriasis) (Fig. 10-6)
    ▪ Balanitis circinata
  • Cardiac: aortic regurgitation
– Diagnostics: clinical
– Management
  • No antibiotics for preceding GI/GU infection
  • Arthritis
    ▪ NSAIDs: initial treatment
    ▪ Intraarticular steroid injections (Fig. 10-7)
    ▪ ± disease-modifying agents, similar to RA

Enteropathic Arthritis
– Inflammatory arthritis associated with IBD; less commonly associated with celiac disease and Whipple disease
– Arthritic symptoms wax and wane with bowel disease
– Arthritis is considered an extraintestinal manifestation of the bowel disease
– Treatment is directed toward both arthritic (NSAIDs, sulfasalazine, anti-TNF) and GI symptoms

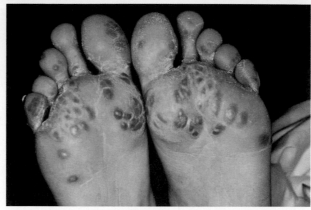

Figure 10-6: Keratoderma blennorrhagica in a patient with reactive arthritis. (Image courtesy of the CDC.)

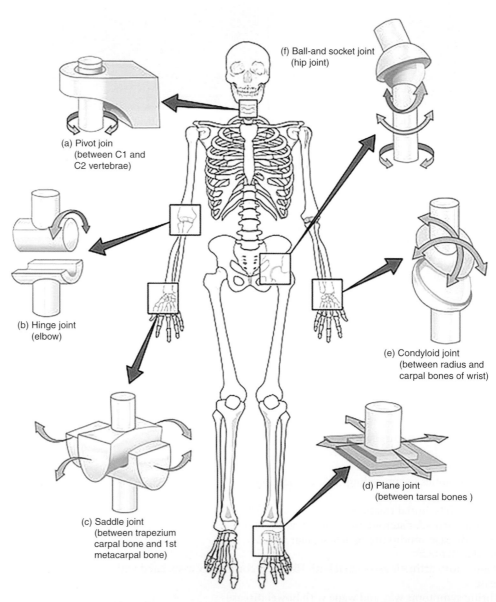

Figure 10-7: Autoimmune, inflammatory, and degenerative arthritis primarily affects the synovial joints *(arrow)*. Various types of arthritides have a propensity to affect a select few joints. (Image courtesy of OpenStax College.)

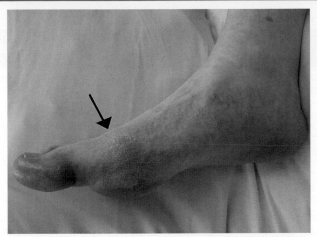

Figure 10-8: Acute gouty arthritis of the first metatarsophalangeal joint (arrow). (Image courtesy of James Heilman, MD.)

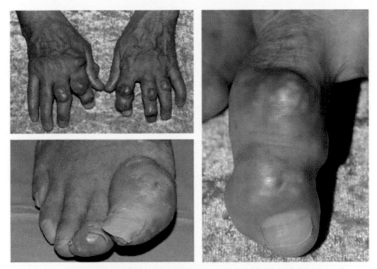

Figure 10-9: Multiple images depicting gouty tophi. (Image courtesy of Arthritis Research UK Primary Care Centre, Primary Care Sciences, Keele University, Keele, UK.)

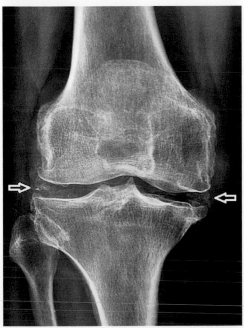

Figure 10-10: Chondrocalcinosis involving the knee in a patient with pseudogout. This is the most common location for chondrocalcinosis. Arrows pointing to areas of chondrocalcinosis. (Images courtesy of OpenStax College.)

TABLE 10-4   Comparison of gout versus pseudogout

	GOUT	PSEUDOGOUT (CALCIUM PYROPHOSPHATE DEPOSITION DISEASE)
Causes/ associations	• Idiopathic (most common) • Hyperuricemia • Drugs: thiazide/loop diuretics, niacin, pyrazinamide, cyclosporine, alcohol • Foods (high purine): red meat, seafood • Metabolic: Lesch-Nyhan syndrome, glycogen storage disease • Increased cell turnover (release of intracellular uric acid): tumor lysis syndrome (treatment of lymphoma, leukemia, myeloproliferative disorder), psoriasis • Renal insufficiency (decreased excretion)	• Hemochromatosis • Wilson disease • Diabetes mellitus • Hyperparathyroidism, hypothyroidism
Signs and symptoms	• Acute: sudden-onset, unilateral severe joint tenderness (most commonly first MTP joint), erythema overlying affected joint (Fig. 10-8) • Chronic: tophi (deposition of urate crystals into soft tissues such as knees, achilles, extensor surfaces of forearms, pinna of the ear), uric acid nephropathy (Fig. 10-9)	• Acute: similar to gout with monoarticular inflammatory joint (more commonly affects large joints such as knees and wrists)
Diagnostics	• Arthrocentesis: • Intraneutrophilic urate crystals • <50, 000 WBCs • Negative Gram stain and culture • Negatively birefringent crystals under polarized microscopy • Imaging: bony erosions with overhanging rim of cortical bone ("rat bite" lesion)	• Arthrocentesis: similar to gout except for rhomboid-shaped positively birefringent crystals under polarized microscopy • Imaging: chondrocalcinosis (calcification) of cartilage (Fig. 10-10), "squared off" bones and hooked osteophytes

Management	• Acute: NSAIDs, colchicine, intraarticular glucocorticoid
	• Chronic:
	  • Avoid offending agent
	  • Xanthine oxidase inhibitors: allopurinol, febuxostat
	  • Uricosuric agents: probenecid, sulfinpyrazone, rasburicase, pegloticase
		• Acute: similar to gout
		• Chronic: prophylactic colchicine, hydroxychloroquine, or methotrexate

MTP, Metatarsophalangeal; *NSAID*, nonsteroidal antiinflammatory drug; *WBC*, white blood cell.

CRYSTALLINE ARTHROPATHY

Crystalline arthropathy refers to the deposition of crystals within the joint secondary to gout or pseudogout. These are differentiated with an arthrocentesis in examining the crystals under polarized microscopy (Table 10-4).

Presence of urate crystals within synovial fluid is common in patients with gout; however, acute gout flares will have presence of urate crystals within neutrophils. Neutrophils phagocytose urate crystals resulting in degranulation of inflammatory enzymes.

Lesch-Nyhan syndrome is characterized by deficiency of hypoxanthine guanine phosphoribosyltransferase.
Colchicine side effects: leukopenia, diarrhea
Allopurinol side effects: hypersensitivity reaction, Stevens-Johnson syndrome
Losartan and calcium channel blockers are the best antihypertensives for patients with gout due to their uric acid–lowering effect.

Synovial fluid analysis involves sampling the joint via an arthrocentesis in examining the fluid using various parameters such as appearance, white blood cells, polymorphonuclear leukocytes (PMNs), and Gram stain to determine the etiology of the joint effusion (Table 10-5).

VASCULITIS
Large-Vessel Vasculitis
General principles
- Inflammation involving large, medium, or small vessels
- Often present with constitutional symptoms (fever, weight loss, fatigue)
- All will have elevated inflammatory markers (ESR, CRP) and anemia of chronic disease
- Inflammation of involved vessels can result in stenosis and ischemia
- Many vasculitides have associations with other diseases that occur concurrently or must be ruled out prior to treating underlying vasculitis
- Differentiated based on serology, angiography, and biopsy findings
- Typically treated initially with corticosteroids and maintained with steroid-sparing immunosuppressants

TABLE 10-5 Synovial fluid analysis

	NORMAL	NONINFLAMMATORY	INFLAMMATORY	SEPTIC
Appearance	Clear	Clear	Translucent	Opaque
WBCs	<200	200–2000	2000–20, 000	>20, 000, more often >100, 000
PMNs percentage	<25%	<25%	>50%	>75%
Gram stain and culture	Negative	Negative	Negative	Positive

PMNs, Polymorphonuclear leukocytes; *WBCs,* white blood cells.

Giant Cell Arteritis (GCA)
– Pathophysiology: granulomatous inflammation of the branches of the external carotid artery
– Signs and symptoms
  • Headache, fever, weight loss
  • Jaw claudication
  • Visual disturbances, transient ischemic attack (TIA)/stroke
  • Hearing disturbances, vertigo
  • Scalp tenderness
  • Carotid/axillary bruits, decreased pulses, arm claudication
  • 50% associated with polymyalgia rheumatica
– Diagnostics
  • Elevated ESR, CRP
  • Temporal artery biopsy: granulomatous inflammation with multinuclear giant cells
– Management: high-dose prednisone; initiated prior to obtaining biopsy results if clinically suspicious for GCA
– Complications
  • Blindness (anterior ischemic optic neuropathy)
  • Aortic aneurysm/dissection

Takayasu Arteritis
– Epidemiology: young, Asian females
– Pathophysiology: granulomatous inflammation involving the aorta and its branches
– Signs and symptoms
  • Coarctation of the aorta, aortic aneurysm
  • Arthralgias, myalgias
  • Carotidynia (tenderness of the carotid artery)
  • Diminished pulses in upper extremities (radial, ulnar, axillary), arm claudication
  • Subclavian steal syndrome, posterior circulation ischemia (vertigo, dizziness, syncope)
  • Visual disturbances
  • Discrepant blood pressure between upper extremities
  • Secondary hypertension due to coarctation of the aorta and/or renal artery stenosis
– Diagnostics
  • Elevated inflammatory markers (ESR, CRP)
  • Imaging
    ▪ Chest x-ray: widened mediastinum, aortic dilation
    ▪ CT/magnetic resonance imaging (MRI) chest: thickening of arterial walls, luminal narrowing
    ▪ Arteriogram: narrowing of involved vessels (Fig. 10–11)
  • Biopsy: last resort, rarely needed
– Management
  • High-dose steroids
  • Refractory cases: immunosuppressants
    ▪ Azathioprine
    ▪ Methotrexate
    ▪ Mycophenolate
    ▪ Leflunomide
      ○ Angioplasty to recanalize stenosed vessels

Medium-Vessel Vasculitis
Polyarteritis Nodosa
– Signs and symptoms
  • Neurologic

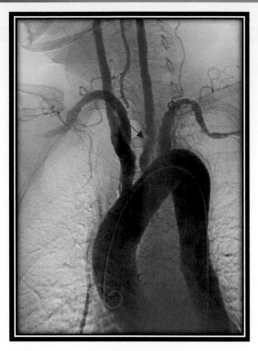

Figure 10-11: Angiography in a patient with Takayasu arteritis showing irregularity and narrowing of the left common carotid artery *(red arrow)*.

- - Polyneuropathy
    - Mononeuritis multiplex
    - TIA/stroke
  - Musculoskeletal: arthralgias, myalgias
  - Cardiac: pericarditis, CAD
  - Renal
    - Hematuria, proteinuria
    - Chronic kidney disease
    - Renal artery stenosis (secondary hypertension)
  - GI: abdominal pain worsened by eating (mesenteric vasculitis)
  - Cutaneous
    - Livedo reticularis
    - Ulcers, digital gangrene
    - Subcutaneous nodules
  - No pulmonary involvement
- Diagnostic
  - Check hepatitis panel: associated with chronic hepatitis B/C
  - Mesentery/renal/hepatic angiography ("beads on a string")
  - Biopsy of involved site
  - P-ANCA positive in 20% of cases
- Management
  - Treat underlying hepatitis B/C
  - Initial management: glucocorticoids
  - Mild disease: azathioprine, methotrexate
  - Severe disease: cyclophosphamide

Granulomatosis With Polyangiitis (Wegener)
- Key manifestations: vasculitis associated with pulmonary-renal syndrome
  - Upper respiratory tract
    - Chronic, recurrent sinusitis
    - Perforated nasal septum, saddlenose deformity
    - Epistaxis
    - Otitis media
    - Oral/auditory canal ulcers
    - Mastoiditis
    - Tracheitis, tracheal ulceration, tracheomalacia
  - Lower respiratory tract
    - Hemoptysis, alveolar hemorrhage

- Lung cavity
- Interstitial lung disease
  - Renal: rapidly progressive glomerulonephritis (hematuria, proteinuria)
  - Cutaneous: recurrent ulcers, livedo reticularis
  - Ocular: conjunctivitis, scleritis
  - Cardiac: pericarditis
- Diagnostics
  - c-ANCA, antiproteinase-3 antibody
  - Biopsy
- Management
  - High-dose glucocorticoids
  - Immunosuppressants: cyclophosphamide, rituximab

Microscopic Polyangiitis
- Similar presentation as granulomatosis with polyangiitis (weakness)
- No involvement of nasal septum
- p-ANCA positive, myeloperoxidase (MPO) antibody
- Differentiated from Wegner based on biopsy findings (negative granulomatous inflammation)
- Similar treatment and complications as granulomatosis with polyangitis

Churg Strauss (Eosinophilic Granulomatosis With Polyangiitis)
- Overlap syndrome with features of polyarteritis nodosa, microscopic polyangiitis, and granulomatosis with polyangiitis
- P-ANCA positive, MPO antibody
- Characteristic features include severe refractory asthma and eosinophilia
- Chest imaging with transient patchy and nodular infiltrates
- Treated similarly as other ANCA-positive vasculitides

Kawasaki disease: further details in pediatric cardiology
- Pediatric vasculitis characterized by frequent cardiac involvement
- Commonly affects children (<5 years old) of Asian descent
- Other key features
  - Prolonged fever
  - Bilateral nonexudative conjunctivitis
  - Strawberry tongue
  - Desquamation of palms and soles
  - Rash
  - Cervical adenopathy
- Treated with aspirin and IV immunoglobulin

Small-Vessel Vasculitis

Henoch-Schönlein Purpura
- Pathophysiology: immune-mediated vasculitis secondary to deposition of IgA immune complexes
- Signs and symptoms
  - GI: abdominal pain, bloody diarrhea, intussusception
  - Musculoskeletal: arthralgias, myalgias
  - Renal: hematuria, proteinuria
  - Cutaneous: lower extremity palpable purpura (Fig. 10–12)

> Hepatitis C is also associated with porphyria cutanea tarda, lichen planus, polyarteritis nodosa, and membranoproliferative glomerulonephritis.

- Diagnostics
  - Clinical
  - Biopsy: leukocytoclastic vasculitis
  - Normal complement levels
- Management
  - Supportive care, most cases resolve spontaneously
  - Steroids for severe refractory cases

Behcet Disease
- Affects individuals of Asian or Middle Eastern descent
- Variable vessel vasculitis, commonly affects small vessels; however, may also affect medium and large vessels
- Characterized by features
  - Painful oral/genital ulcers
  - Pathergy (development of >2 mm-papule after needle prick)

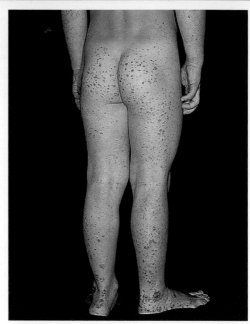

Figure 10-12: Lower extremity palpable purpura of an Henoch-Schönlein purpura.

- • Ocular (uveitis, iritis, conjunctivitis)
- • CNS involvement (optic neuritis, meningoencephalitis)
- • Less common features: erythema nodosum and aortic disease
- – Treated with steroids +/– immunosuppressants

Other Vasculitides
Buerger Disease (thromboangiitis obliterans)
- – Affects men and heavy smokers
- – Characterized by
  - • Superficial thrombophlebitis
  - • Raynaud phenomenon
  - • Ischemia, gangrene, paresthesias, and autoamputation of the distal extremities
- – Treatment is smoking cessation to decrease disease progression

Cryoglobulinemia
- – Pathophysiology: immune-mediated vasculitis resulting in deposition of IgM immune complexes into small and medium sized vessels
- – Signs and symptoms
  - • Musculoskeletal: arthralgias, myalgias, collagen vascular disease
  - • Neurologic: peripheral neuropathy
  - • Renal: membranoproliferative glomerulonephritis
  - • Cutaneous: palpable purpura
- – Associations
  - • Chronic hepatitis C
  - • Endocarditis
  - • Collagen vascular disease
- – Diagnostics
  - • Elevated cryoglobulin levels
  - • Decreased C4 complement levels
  - • Positive rheumatoid factor
  - • Check hepatitis C serologies
- – Management
  - • Treat underlying cause
  - • Severe disease: steroids +/– rituximab +/– plasmapheresis

INFECTIONS
Osteomyelitis
- – Definition: infection of the bone involving any part from the periosteum to the bone marrow

- Pathophysiology: hematogenous spread (children) or direct invasion from overlying skin/soft tissue infection (adults)
- Microbiologic associations
  - *Staphylococcus aureus:* most common cause overall
  - Salmonella: sickle cell disease
  - Pseudomonas: nail puncture wounds, malignant necrotizing otitis externa, IV drug abuse
  - Polymicrobial: diabetics
  - Coagulase negative Staphylococcus: prosthetic joint
  - Eikenella: human bite
  - *Pasteurella multicoda:* cat bite
  - Capnocytophaga: dog bite
  - Fungus: central catheter (total parenteral nutrition), neutropenia
  - *Mycobacterium tuberculosis* (Pott disease): active pulmonary tuberculosis with dissemination
- Signs and symptoms
  - Fevers, chills
  - Bone pain, muscle aches
  - Decreased range of motion
  - Overlying erythema, edema, and tenderness
  - Purulent sinus tract +/− probe to bone
  - Diagnostics
    - Imaging
      - X-ray: initial test; however, usually negative
      - MRI: bone marrow edema, periosteal elevation
      - CT or bone scan are alternative imaging modalities for patients who cannot tolerate MRI
    - Bone biopsy: gold standard
    - Blood cultures
    - Elevated inflammatory markers (ESR, CRP)
- Management
  - Long-term (6 weeks) IV antibiotics pending culture results
  - Empiric treatment with vancomycin (gram-positive coverage) and third- or fourth-generation cephalosporin (gram-negative coverage)
  - +/− amputation/debridement

Infectious/Septic Arthritis
- Definition: infection involving joint space (synovial membrane)
- Pathophysiology: same as osteomyelitis
- Microbiology
  - *S. aureus:* most common cause
  - *Neisseria gonorrhea:* young, sexually active
  - *Streptococcus pneumoniae:* splenic dysfunction
  - Gram negative: GI infection, immunocompromised, IV drug abuse
  - Eikenella: human bites
  - *Borrelia burgdorferi* (Lyme disease): "bulls-eye" rash, hiking, tick bite
- Signs and symptoms
  - Acute, painful, erythematous monoarticular arthritis
  - Palpable effusion
  - Decreased range of motion
  - Fevers, chills
- Diagnostics
  - Arthrocentesis: always initial step in patient with painful, erythematous joint
  - Opaque, purulent fluid
  - >50,000 RBCs, >75% PMNs, positive Gram stain and culture
  - Polymerase chain reaction if gonococcal arthritis is suspected
  - Imaging (x-ray or ultrasound): joint effusion
- Management
  - Joint washout
  - Empiric treatment with vancomycin (gram-positive coverage) and third- or fourth-generation cephalosporin (gram-negative coverage)
  - Antibiotics tailored to Gram stain and culture results

Neisseria gonorrhea septic arthritis is associated with tenosynovitis (wrists, ankles, knees), dermatitis (vesicular pustules, bullae), and terminal complement deficiency. Be sure to check STD panel (HIV, syphilis, hepatitis B, chlamydia).

TABLE 10-6 **Pharmacotherapy for treatment of infectious rheumatologic disease**

MICROBIOLOGY	TREATMENT OPTIONS
MRSA	• Vancomycin • Daptomycin • Linezolid
MSSA	• Oxacillin • Nafcillin • Dicloxacillin • Cefazolin
Gram negatives	• Third-generation cephalosporin (ceftriaxone, cefotaxime) • Fluroquinolones • Piperacillin-tazobactam • Aztreonam • Aminoglycosides

MRSA, Methicillin-resistant *Staphylococcus aureus; MSSA*, methicillin-susceptible *S. aureus.*

Epidural Abscess
– Pathophysiology: hematogenous spread resulting in seeding of the vertebral body or direct invasion from overlying vertebral osteomyelitis
– Risk factors
  • IV drug abuse
  • Recent neurologic procedure (laminectomy)
  • Epidural anesthesia
  • Spinal steroid injection
– Microbiology: *S. aureus* (most common cause)
– Signs and symptoms
  • Exquisite tenderness over vertebral body
  • Muscle spasms
  • Decreased range of motion
  • Fever, chills
  • +/− neurologic deficits
– Diagnostics
  • MRI spine
  • Elevated inflammatory markers (ESR, CRP)
– Management
  • Surgical decompression/drainage
  • Steroids if acute neurologic deficits are present
  • Empiric treatment with vancomycin (gram-positive coverage) and third- or fourth-generation cephalosporin (gram-negative coverage); specific antibiotics pending culture and sensitivities (Table 10-6)

INFLAMMATORY MYOPATHIES
Polymyositis/Dermatomyositis
– Definition: autoimmune inflammatory myopathy resulting in muscle damage and characteristic cutaneous manifestations

Lumbosacral strain is the most common cause of lower back pain with lifetime risk of approximately 80%.

– Signs and symptoms
  • Fever, malaise, lethargy
  • Muscle aches, weakness
  • Symmetric, proximal myopathy (difficulty getting up from seated position, raising arms above shoulder level)
  • No neurologic deficits
  • Cutaneous (associated with dermatomyositis)
    ▪ Gottron papules (patchy, erythematous rash involving dorsum of hand) (Fig. 10–13)
    ▪ Heliotrope rash (purplish discoloration around periorbital region) (Fig. 10–14)
    ▪ Shawl sign (rash involving upper neck, back, chest, and shoulders)
    ▪ Mechanics hand (dark, dirty-appearing hands with cracks and fissures)
    ▪ Malar rash

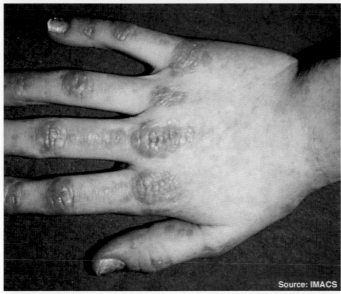

Figure 10-13: Gottron papules in a patient with dermatomyositis.

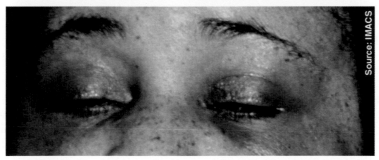

Figure 10-14: Heliotrope rash in a patient with dermatomyositis.

- Other associated findings
  - Dysphasia
  - Interstitial lung disease
  - Myocarditis
  - Raynaud disease
  - Malignancy (ovarian, GI, longer, lymphoma): polymyositis/dermatomyositis may be paraneoplastic syndrome of underlying visceral malignancy
- Diagnostics
  - Elevated creatinine phosphokinase (CPK), aldolase
  - Anti-Jo-1, anti-SRP, anti-Mi-2, antisynthetase
  - Muscle biopsy: mononuclear infiltrate and necrosis
  - CT chest/abdomen/pelvis searching for underlying malignancy and age-appropriate cancer screening
- Management
  - Glucocorticoids: initial treatment
  - Steroid-sparing agents for steroid unresponsive
    - Methotrexate
    - Azathioprine

Polymyalgia Rheumatica
- Epidemiology: primarily affects patients >50 years old
- Definition: bilateral proximal inflammatory myopathy without signs of muscle damage or neurologic deficits
- Signs and symptoms
  - Fatigue, malaise, fevers, weight loss
  - Proximal muscle aches and pains
  - Decreased range of motion
  - Synovitis, tenosynovitis
  - Profound morning stiffness involving proximal muscles (hips, neck, knees, and torso) lasting >1 month

TABLE 10-7 Other Causes of myopathy

Endocrine	• Thyroid • Hypercortisolism
Electrolyte derangements	• Potassium • Phosphorus
Medications	• Statins • Daptomycin • Corticosteroids • Antiretrovirals
Genetics	• Myotonic dystrophy (CTG trinucleotide repeat) • Becker muscular dystrophy (defective dystrophin gene) • Duchenne muscular dystrophy (defective dystrophin gene) • Mitochondrial myopathies (children of affected mothers will have the phenotype)
Infectious	• Trichinella (uncooked pork, periorbital edema) • Viral syndrome (influenza, adenovirus)
Miscellaneous	• Inclusion body myositis (distal and proximal, asymmetric muscle weakness unresponsive to steroids)

– Associations: GCA
– Diagnostics
  • Elevated ESR
  • Normal CPK, aldolase
– Management: low-dose steroids with rapid improvement in symptoms

In a patient presenting with myopathy it should be performed as several other etiologies aside from auto-immune causes can be the source of myopathy (Table 10-7).

LOWER BACK PAIN

Lower back pain is extremely common and increases in incidence with age. Most patients with lower back pain do not require imaging. When presented with the patient with lower back pain, it is important to rule out any acute pathology that may involve the spinal cord, in which case an urgent MRI should be performed (Table 10-8).

One of the most common reasons for lower back pain and radiculopathy is due to herniation of the intervertebral disc into the neural foramina resulting in compression of the exiting nerve roots (Figs. 10–15 and 10–16).

OSTEOARTHRITIS

Osteoarthritis
– Risk factors
  • Age
  • Trauma
  • Inflammatory arthritis
  • Obesity
  • Hemophilia (hemarthroses)
  • Metabolic
    ▪ Hemochromatosis
    ▪ Wilson disease
    ▪ Gaucher disease
    ▪ Alkaptonuria
– Pathophysiology: noninflammatory arthritis resulting in joint degeneration and loss of articular cartilage from chronic wear and tear
– Signs and symptoms
  • Joint pain involving large weight-bearing joints (knees, hips)
  • Hip osteoarthritis may present with groin pain
  • DIP enlargement (Heberden nodes)
  • PIP enlargement (Bouchard nodes)
  • Joint crepitation
  • Morning stiffness <30 minutes
  • Decreased range of motion secondary to pain
– Diagnostics
  • Clinical

TABLE 10-8 Differentiating causes of lower back pain

	SIGNS AND SYMPTOMS	DIAGNOSTICS	MANAGEMENT
Lumbar strain	• Lumbar pain after increased physical activity • Paraspinal muscle spasm • +/- radiation to the buttocks or thighs	Clinical	• Nonopioid analgesics • Continue physical activity
Lumbar spinal stenosis	• Commonly seen in elderly (>60) • Associated with degenerative arthritis, thickened ligamentum flavum, spondylolisthesis, and bulging intervertebral discs • Pain worsened by lumbar extension (i.e., walking downhill) • Pain relieved with lumbar flexion ("shopping cart sign") • Radiation to the buttocks and thighs • No neurologic deficits	MRI: narrowing of spinal canal with compression of nerve roots	• Nonopioid analgesics • Surgery for persistent/disabling symptoms
Lumbar disk herniation (radiculopathy)	• Herniation of nucleus pulposus through the annulus fibrosis resulting in nerve root compression and radicular symptoms • Acute back pain with unilateral radiation of pain involving a specific dermatome • Positive straight leg test • No vertebral tenderness	Clinical	Nonopioid analgesics Surgery for persistent/disabling symptoms
Vertebral fracture	Associated with osteoporosis, inflammatory arthritis, Paget disease, bony metastasis, hyperparathyroidism Acute back pain, may be asymptomatic in chronic cases • Point tenderness • Pain worsened with standing, coughing, lying down • Progressive kyphosis • Loss of stature	X-ray	• Nonopioid analgesic • +/- nasal calcitonin • +/- vertebral augmentation (kyphoplasty/vertebroplasty) • Bisphosphonates for osteoporosis
Cord compression (cauda equina syndrome)	• Acute onset lower back pain with neurologic deficits • Lower extremity paralysis • Bladder/bowel incontinence	MRI	• Surgical decompression • +/- high-dose steroids
Malignancy	• Fever, weight loss, anorexia • Pain worse at night • History of cancer	MRI, CT, or bone scan	• Treat underlying malignancy
Infection (epidural abscess, osteomyelitis, discitis)	• Fever, chills • Recent bacteremia • Exquisite point tenderness	MRI	• Antibiotics +/- surgical debridement

CT, Computed tomography; *MRI*, magnetic resonance imaging.

- Radiographic
  - Asymmetric joint space narrowing
  - Osteophytes (new bone formation secondary to bone-on-bone friction)
  - Subchondral cysts/sclerosis
- Arthrocentesis only if effusion is present and suspicious for inflammatory arthritis
  - Clear/yellow color
  - <2000 WBCs
  - <25% PMNs
- Normal labs
- Management
  - Lifestyle modifications: weight loss, moderate exercise
  - Oral analgesics: acetaminophen, NSAIDs
  - +/− intraarticular steroids
  - Joint replacement if severe and limiting quality of life

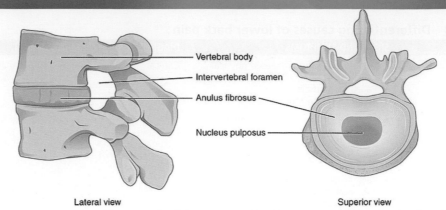

Figure 10-15: Normal intervertebral disc anatomy. (Images courtesy of OpenStax College.)

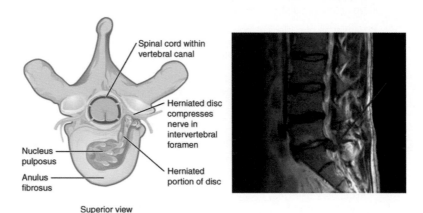

Figure 10-16: Tear of the annulus fibrosis resulting herniation of nucleus pulposus with compression of the exiting nerve root *(red arrow)*. (Images courtesy of OpenStax College.)

JOINTS, LIGAMENTS, AND TENDONS

Carpal Tunnel Syndrome
- Risk factors
  - Excessive typing
  - RA
  - Acromegaly
  - Pregnancy
  - Hypothyroidism
  - Diabetes mellitus
  - Amyloidosis
- Pathophysiology: compression of the median nerve as it traverses underneath the flexor retinaculum (Fig. 10–17)
- Signs and symptoms
  - Numbness and tingling following median nerve distribution (lateral 3.5 fingers, including nail beds)
  - Pain worse at night
  - Atrophy of thenar eminence
  - Positive Phelan sign (palmar flexion resulting in paresthesias in the median nerve distribution)
  - Positive Tinel sign (tapping over median nerve results in paresthesias in the median nerve distribution)
- Diagnostic
  - Clinical
  - Electromyography, nerve conduction studies
- Management
  - Wrist splint promoting wrist extension
  - Nonanalgesic pain medication
  - Corticosteroid injections
  - Surgery (excision of flexor retinaculum) for persistent symptoms

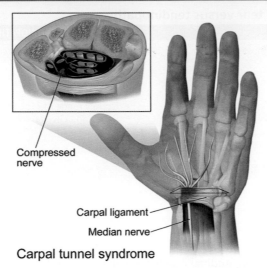

Compressed
nerve

Carpal ligament
Median nerve

Carpal tunnel syndrome

Figure 10-17: Pathophysiology of carpal tunnel syndrome demonstrating compression of the median nerve as it traverses underneath the flexor retinaculum. (Image courtesy of Blausen Medical.)

Rotator cuff tear and tendinopathy can be seen as to pathologies on a spectrum with tendinopathy eventually progressing to a rotator cuff tear. Differentiation of these is important as rotator cuff tear is made beneficial to surgical repair (Table 10-9).

Dupuytren Contracture
- Fibroproliferative disorder with hyperplasia of the palmar fascia resulting in nodule formation and chronically contracted fourth/fifth fingers
- Associated with Norwegian descent, alcoholism
- Treated with intralesional glucocorticoid injections or fasciotomy in refractory cases

Plantar Fasciitis
- Signs and symptoms
  - Pain on the plantar surface of the foot worse with the first few steps in the morning, improved throughout the day with increased activity, then worsens at the end of the day after prolonged weight bearing
  - Pain worsened by dorsiflexion of the foot
  - +/− areas of local point tenderness
- Commonly seen in runners secondary to repeated microtrauma
- Treat with conservative therapy: stretching, proper-fitting shoes, NSAIDs

Bursitis
- Inflammation of the bursa (fluid-filled structure between muscle and bone allowing for smooth joint mobility)
- Occurs secondary to trauma, injections, infection, chronic direct pressure
- Pain worsened by palpation and usage of affected joint
- Commonly affects the greater trochanter, olecranon, pes anserine, subacromial, and ischia
- Treat with joint protection, analgesics, +/− glucocorticoid injections

DeQuervain Disease
- Commonly affects new mothers who hold their infants with their thumb abducted and extended
- Pain on radial side of the hand worsened by movement
- Results in inflammation of the extensor pollicis brevis and abductor pollicis longus tendons
- Positive Finkelstein test: pain worsened when flexed thumb is placed into the fingers
- Treat with splinting and NSAIDs; glucocorticoid injections or surgery for refractory cases

Epicondylitis
- Inflammation of the medial or lateral epicondyle tendons as they insert into their respective bony prominences
- Worsened by repeated wrist extension and supination (lateral epicondylitis; "tennis elbow") or wrist extension and pronation (medial epicondylitis; "golfer's elbow")
- Pain upon palpation epicondyles
- Conservative management with activity modification and biomechanics, bracing, splinting

TABLE 10-9   Rotator cuff tear versus tendinopathy

ROTATOR CUFF TEAR	ROTATOR CUFF TENDINOPATHY
• Tear of rotator cuff tendons (most commonly supraspinatus)	• Impingement of rotator cuff tendons
• Pain worse at night, when lying on affected shoulder • Positive empty can test • Positive Neer test • Weakness with external rotation	• Positive empty can test • Positive Neer test • Normal range of motion • Pain with active range of motion • Subacromial tenderness
• MRI diagnostic	• Clinical diagnosis
• Treat with analgesics, physical therapy, surgery	• Treat with analgesics, physical therapy

MRI, Magnetic resonance imaging.

Diffuse Idiopathic Skeletal Hyperostosis
– Ossification of the anterior longitudinal ligament involving multiple consecutive vertebrae
– Presents with morning stiffness, dorsal lumbar pain, decreased range of motion
– Most commonly affects the thoracic spine

Fibromyalgia
– Epidemiology: young to middle-aged women associated with other medical-psychiatric conditions (migraines, irritable bowel syndrome, chronic pain syndrome)
– Signs and symptoms
  • Chronic musculoskeletal pain involving tenderness of the trigger points (11 of 18 involved: trapezius, medial knee, lateral epicondyle) (Fig. 10–18)
  • Numbness, stiffness
  • Generalized fatigue, weakness
  • Nonrestorative sleep
– Diagnostics
  • Clinical
  • Diagnosis of exclusion
– Management
  • Lifestyle modifications
    ▪ Relaxation, yoga
    ▪ Regular exercise
    ▪ Good sleep hygiene
  • Pharmacotherapy
    ▪ Tricyclic antidepressants (amitriptyline)
    ▪ Gamma-aminobutyric acid agonists (pregabalin, gabapentin)
    ▪ Serotonin-norepinephrine reuptake inhibitors (milnacipran, duloxetine)
  • Cognitive behavioral therapy

MINERAL BONE DISEASE
Osteoporosis
– Epidemiology: chronic bone degeneration commonly affecting elderly woman (Fig. 10–19)
– Pathophysiology: increased osteoclastic and decreased osteoblastic activity resulting in decreased bone density, mineralization, and architectural distortion
– Risk factors
  • Nonmodifiable
    ▪ Age (postmenopausal)
    ▪ Low body mass index, slim build
    ▪ White, Asian
    ▪ Family history
    ▪ Decreased peak bone mass
  • Modifiable
    ▪ Medications
      ◦ Glucocorticoids
      ◦ Phenytoin
      ◦ Tenofovir
      ◦ Aromatase/estrogen inhibitors
      ◦ Heparin

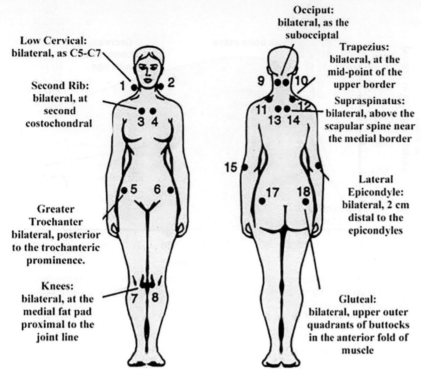

Figure 10-18: Eighteen tender points of fibromyalgia. (Image courtesy of Hang Pham; CC BY-SA 4.0 [https://creativecommons.org/licenses/by-sa/4.0])

- Endocrine
  - Hypercortisolism
  - Hyperparathyroidism
  - Hyperthyroidism
  - Hypogonadism
- Malabsorption syndromes: result in calcium/vitamin D deficiency
  - Celiac disease
  - Cystic fibrosis
  - Primary biliary cholangitis
- Alcoholism, smoking
- Inflammatory arthritis
- Chronic liver or kidney disease
- Signs and symptoms
  - Asymptomatic
  - Pathologic fractures (vertebral compression fractures, hip fractures)
  - Loss of stature
  - Kyphosis
  - Localized tenderness to palpation at fracture sites
- Diagnostics
  - Plain film for suspected fractures
  - DEXA scan
    - T-score <2.5 standard deviations → osteoporosis
    - T-score <1–2.5 standard deviations → osteopenia
  - Normal serum calcium, phosphorus, and parathyroid
- Management
  - Bisphosphonates (alendronate, residronate, zoledronate)
    - Indications
      - T-score <2.5 standard deviations
      - Fragility fractures
      - Increased risk of hip or combined major osteoporotic fractures
    - Side effects: flulike symptoms, arthralgias, osteonecrosis of the jaw, esophagitis
  - Calcium, vitamin D supplementation
  - Weight-bearing exercise

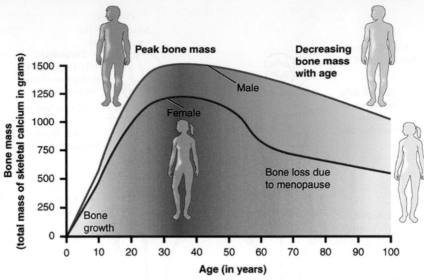

Figure 10-19: Relationship between bone mass and age. Bone density and mass increase until age 30, afterwards bone density decreases with age. Higher peak bone density will result in less risk of developing osteoporosis. Men on average have higher peak bone masses.

- Smoking/alcohol cessation
- Alternatives
  - Raloxifene
  - Denosumab (RANK-L monoclonal antibody)
  - Teriparatide (parathyroid hormone analogue that stimulates new bone formation through increased osteoblastic activity)

Paget Disease of the Bone (Osteitis Deformans)
- Epidemiology: age >40
- Pathophysiology: abnormal bone remodeling secondary to increased osteoclastic activity followed by a period of increased osteoblastic activity and disorganized new bone formation
- Signs and symptoms
  - Most commonly asymptomatic
  - Bone pain, deformity, arthritis
  - Increased skull size (increased hat size)
  - Frontal bossing, chronic headaches
  - Hearing loss (cranial nerve VIII entrapment)
  - Bowing of the long bones, pathologic fractures
  - Radiculopathies
- Diagnostics
  - Elevated alkaline phosphatase
  - Elevated urine hydroxyproline, procollagen type I N-terminal propeptide
  - Normal calcium, phosphorus
- Imaging
  - X-ray: mixed osteolytic and sclerotic lesions (hip, pelvis, skull, long bones)
  - Bone scan: increased focal uptake
  - Histopathology: disorganized "mosaic" lamellar bone
- Management
  - Asymptomatic: no treatment
  - Symptomatic: bisphosphonates +/− calcitonin
- Complications
  - High-output cardiac failure
  - Osteosarcoma
  - Giant cell tumor of the bone

BONE NEOPLASMS
Bone neoplasms have a propensity to arise from typical locations in long bones allowing the radiologist to provide better specificity when presented with bone neoplasm imaging (Fig. 10–20). Additionally, the

age of the patient is extremely important as certain neoplasms are found almost exclusively in adult or pediatric populations.

Osteosarcoma
- Epidemiology: most common primary bone tumor in young adults and adolescents most commonly affecting the distal femur (metaphysis of long bones)
- Risk factors
  - Paget disease of the bone
  - Prolonged use of teriparatide
  - Chemoradiation
  - Retinoblastoma gene mutation
- Signs and symptoms
  - Bone pain, muscle aches
  - Tender soft tissue mass
  - Pathologic fractures
- Diagnostics

> Metastasis is the most common cause of bone tumors. Common sources include lung, breast, and prostate.

  - Imaging (MRI/CT):
    - Periosteal elevation (Codman triangle)
    - Spiculated "sunburst" pattern
  - Staging: CT chest (lung is common site of metastasis)
  - Biopsy
  - Elevated lactate dehydrogenase, alkaline phosphatase
- Management
  - Surgical resection
  - Chemotherapy

Osteochondroma
- Most common benign bone tumor
- Bony exostosis with cartilaginous cap
- Affects adolescents and young adults

Chondrosarcoma
- Bone tumor affecting patients >50 years old
- Most commonly affects pelvis and femur

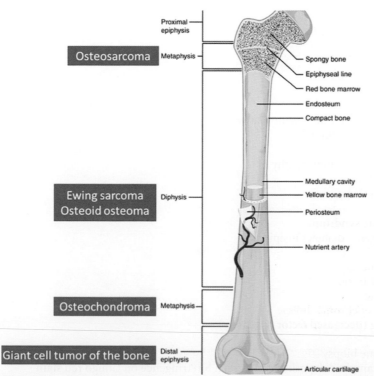

Figure 10-20: Normal long bone anatomy with associated bone tumors arising from different locations of the bone.

– May arise from osteochondroma

Ewing Sarcoma
– Commonly affects young boys and adolescents
– Malignant anaplastic small blue cell tumor arising from diaphysis of long bones
– "Onion skin" pattern on x-ray due to the tumor pushing out the periosteum and the body responding by laying down additional layers of bone
– 11:22 translocation

Giant Cell Tumor of the Bone
– Benign, locally aggressive bone tumor commonly affecting young adults arising from the epiphyses of long bones
– "Soap-bubble" appearance on x-ray (expensive, eccentric lytic lesion)
– MRI shows both cystic and hemorrhagic components
– May arise from Paget disease of the bone
– Biopsy shows large osteoclast giant cells
– Treat with surgical resection

Osteoid Osteoma
– Benign bone tumor that presents with severe localized pain, worse at night, swelling and tenderness (most commonly involving diaphysis of long bones) relieved by NSAIDs
– Radiographically appears as small lucency with reactive sclerosis
– May regress spontaneously; however, symptoms relieved via surgical excision or radiofrequency ablation

AMYLOIDOSIS
Amyloidosis
– Risk factors
  • RA, SLE
  • Multiple myeloma
  • Alzheimer disease
– Subtypes
  • AL amyloidosis (deposition of immunoglobulin light chain)
  • AA amyloidosis (chronic inflammatory disease)
  • Hereditary
  • Dialysis related (beta-2 microglobulin deposition)
– Pathophysiology: abnormal protein production that deposits systemically resulting in organ dysfunction
– Signs and symptoms
  • HEENT
    ▪ Periorbital purpura
    ▪ Macroglossia
  • Cutaneous
    ▪ Waxy thickened skin
    ▪ Easy bruising
  • Neurologic
    ▪ Peripheral/autonomic neuropathy
    ▪ Intracerebral hemorrhage
  • Cardiac
    ▪ Restrictive cardiomyopathy
    ▪ Myocarditis
    ▪ Arrhythmias
  • Renal
    ▪ Nephrotic syndrome
    ▪ Nephrogenic diabetes insipidus
  • GI
    ▪ Hepatomegaly
    ▪ Malabsorption
  • Hematologic
    ▪ Anemia of chronic disease
    ▪ Bleeding (decreased factor X activity)
– Diagnostics
  • Fat pad tissue biopsy
  • Pathology: amyloid deposits, apple-green birefringence on Congo red stain
  • Cardiac MRI for cardiac amyloidosis

- Management: symptomatic, no cure
  - Treat underlying cause
  - Colchicine: AA amyloidosis, familial Mediterranean fever
  - Melphalan, steroids: AL amyloidosis

MISCELLANEOUS

Morton Neuroma
- Inflammation of the digital nerve at the third metatarsal space
- Palpable tender nodule
- Occur secondary to ill-fitting shoes
- Diagnosis is clinical
- Treatment is symptomatic with proper fitting shoes; surgical removal for refractory cases

Adhesive Capsulitis
- Inflammation, fibrosis, and contractures of the glenohumeral joint capsule secondary to chronic rotator cuff tendinopathy; may be idiopathic
- Presents with shoulder pain, stiffness, and decreased range of motion
- Diagnosis is clinical
- Treatment is conservative management with NSAIDs, physical therapy, and glucocorticoid injections

CHAPTER 11 Dermatology

BASICS OF DERMATOLOGY

Dermatology has a specific lexicon that is used to describe the size, appearance, and texture of skin lesions (Table 11-1). Understanding this lexicon is important as it allows for easier communication of skin lesions to other providers and are specific for certain pathologies. Additionally, understanding the anatomy of the skin can make it easier to localize pathologies when a particular area of the skin becomes overactive or underactive (Fig. 11-1).

AUTOIMMUNE DERMATOLOGIC DISORDERS

Pemphigus Vulgaris
– Causes
  • Most commonly idiopathic
  • May be associated with angiotensin-converting enzyme inhibitors, penicillamine
  • Associated with malignancies (non-Hodgkin lymphoma, chronic lymphocytic leukemia, Castleman disease)

TABLE 11-1 Dermatologic Descriptions

SKIN LESION	DESCRIPTION
Macule	Flat, <1 cm
Patch	Flat, >1 cm
Papule	Solid, elevated, <1 cm
Plaque	Solid, elevated, >1 cm, flat topped
Nodule	Palpable, >1 cm, not flat topped
Vesicle	Elevated, <5 mm, filled with clear fluid
Bulla	Elevated, >5 mm, filled with clear fluid

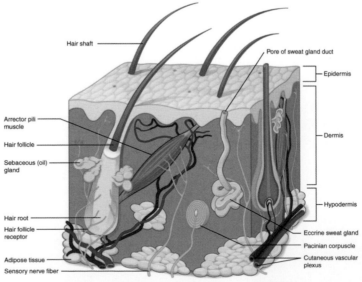

Figure 11-1: Anatomy of the skin. (Image courtesy of OpenStax College.)

- Pathophysiology: type II hypersensitivity reaction with antidesmosomal antibodies (antidesmoglein)
- Signs and symptoms
  - Fragile, painful, blistering skin lesions
  - Positive Nikolsky sign: sloughing of skin when applying minimal pressure
  - Mucosal involvement
- Diagnostics: skin biopsy with immunofluorescence (antibodies present between epidermal cells resulting in acantholysis)
- Management
  - Steroids
  - Steroid-sparing agents
    - Mycophenolate
    - Azathioprine
    - Cyclophosphamide
    - Rituximab

> Nikolsky sign is also present in staphylococcal scalded skin syndrome and toxic epidermal necrolysis.

Bullous Pemphigoid
- Pathophysiology: antihemidesmosome antibodies
- Signs and symptoms
  - Thick-walled, tense intact bulla
  - Prodromal pruritus, urticaria
  - Few, open skin lesions
  - No mucosal involvement
- Diagnostics
  - Skin biopsy with immunofluorescence (antibodies present at the dermal-epidermal junction)
- Management
  - Topical/systemic steroids
  - Steroid-sparing agents
  - Tetracyclines + nicotinamide
  - Dapsone

Psoriasis
- Key manifestations
- Silvery, scaly, erythematous plaque lesions (Fig. 11-2)
- Extensor surfaces involvement
- Auspitz sign: pinpoint bleeding when plaque is removed

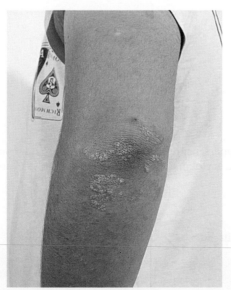

Figure 11-2: Silvery, scaly plaquelike lesion involving the extensor surfaces in a patient with psoriasis.

- Nail pitting, onycholysis
- Koebner phenomenon: development of lesion at the site of epidermal injury (scratching)
- Associated with arthritis, gout (thickened skin has high cell turnover and increases uric acid burden)
- Diagnostics
  - Clinical
  - Biopsy
    - Hyperkeratosis and parakeratosis (nucleus in stratum corneum)
    - Elongated rete ridges
    - Neutrophils in stratum corneum (Monroe microabscesses)
- Management
  - Topical: emollients, steroids, vitamin A/D derivatives
  - Methotrexate
  - Tumor necrosis factor inhibitors (infliximab, adalimumab, etanercept)
  - Immunosuppressants (cyclosporine)

Dermatitis Herpetiformis
- Pathophysiology: autoimmune dermal reaction to gluten
- Signs and symptoms: erythematous, pruritic vesicular papular lesions on the extensor surfaces
- Associations
  - Celiac sprue (diarrhea, weight loss, vitamin deficiencies)
  - Autoimmune disorders (hypothyroidism, type I diabetes, pernicious anemia)
  - Non-Hodgkin lymphoma
- Diagnosis
  - Clinical
  - Biopsy: subepidermal microabscesses at the dermal papillae
  - Immunofluorescence: immunoglobulin A (IgA) transglutaminase deposition in the dermis
- Management
  - Dapsone for symptomatic relief
  - Gluten-free diet for definitive treatment

Systemic Lupus Erythematosus (SLE)
- Signs and symptoms
  - Photosensitivity malar rash, sparing of the nasolabial fold
  - Discoid rash
  - Oral/nasopharyngeal ulcers
  - Other signs and symptoms of SLE: joints, pleuritic, cardiac, central nervous system (CNS), renal involvement
- Diagnostics: 4 of 11 diagnostic criteria must be met
- Management: treat underlying SLE

SOAP BRAIN MD lupus diagnostic criteria:
- Serositis
- Oral ulcers
- Arthralgias, arthritis
- Photosensitivity rash
- Blood dyscrasias (anemia, thrombocytopenia, leukopenia)
- Renal
- Antinuclear antibodies+
- Immunologic (anti-dsDNA, anti-Smith)
- Neurologic
- Malar rash
- Discoid rash

Erythema Nodosum
- Pathophysiology: type IV hypersensitivity reaction toward subcutaneous tissues
- Signs and symptoms: tender, erythematous, subcutaneous nodules (panniculitis) located over the anterior tibia (Fig. 11-3)
- Associations
  - Autoimmune
    - Sarcoidosis
    - Inflammatory bowel disease
    - Behcet
  - Infectious
    - Tuberculosis
    - Streptococcus
    - Fungal (Coccidioides)

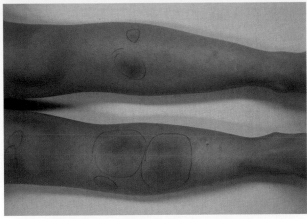

Figuer 11-3: Patient with erythema nodosum. (Image courtesy of James Heilman, MD.)

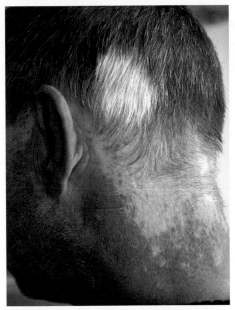

Figure 11-4: Patient with vitiligo involving the posterior neck. (Image courtesy of OpenStax College.)

- Syphilis
- Hepatitis
  - Medications
    - Oral contraceptive pills (OCPs)
    - Amiodarone
    - Sulfa drugs
  - Pregnancy
  - Lymphoma
  - Sweet syndrome (dermal neutrophilic infiltrate)
- Diagnostics: workup for underlying etiology based on related signs and symptoms
- Management
  - Pain control with nonsteroidal antiinflammatory drugs (NSAIDs); treat underlying etiology
  - Nodules are eventually self-limiting

Vitiligo
- Pathophysiology: autoimmune destruction of melanocytes
- Signs and symptoms
  - Patchy, well-demarcated, gradually progressive areas of hypopigmentation (milky, chalky white) (Fig. 11-4)
  - Nonpruritic, nonerythematous
  - Most commonly involves the face
- Associations: other autoimmune disorders (hypothyroidism, pernicious anemia, Addison disease)

- Diagnostics: clinical
- Management
  - Localized disease: topical steroids or calcineurin inhibitors depending on location
  - Extensive disease: oral corticosteroids +/− ultraviolet B (UVB) phototherapy

Pyoderma Gangrenosum
- Signs and symptoms
  - Inflammatory papule, vesicle, nodule
  - Progresses to expanding purulent ulcer
  - Pathergy: skin lesions triggered by minimal trauma
  - Primarily involves the lower extremities or trunk
  - Associated with inflammatory bowel disease (diarrhea, abdominal pain), hematologic malignancy, other systemic inflammatory disorders (rheumatoid arthritis)
- Diagnosis
  - Clinical
  - Biopsy: neutrophilic infiltration
- Management
  - Directed toward underlying inflammatory bowel disease
  - Systemic/topical steroids

Henoch-Schönlein Purpura
- Pathophysiology: immune-mediated IgA deposition into multiple organs (skin, kidneys, gastrointestinal, joints)
- Signs and symptoms
  - Palpable purpura primarily involving the lower extremity and buttocks
  - Arthralgias
  - Abdominal pain, diarrhea, intussusception
  - Renal dysfunction (glomerulonephritis), hematuria, hypertension
- Diagnostics
  - Clinical
  - Biopsy: leukocytoclastic vasculitis
- Management
  - Typically, not indicated as most cases resolve spontaneously with supportive care
  - Steroids for severe cases

DRUG-RELATED SKIN DISORDERS
Erythema Multiforme
- Pathophysiology: type IV hypersensitivity reaction
- Causes
  - Infectious: herpes simplex virus (HSV), Mycoplasma, Coccidioides
  - Drugs
    - Penicillin
    - Anticonvulsants
    - Sulfa drugs
    - NSAIDs
    - Barbiturates
  - Postvaccination
- Signs and symptoms
  - Erythematous, iris-shaped macules, targetoid-like lesions involving the palms and soles (Fig. 11-5)
  - Painful or pruritic lesions
  - Occasional bullae and desquamation
  - No mucous membrane involvement
- Diagnostic
  - Clinical
  - Biopsy: perivascular lymphocytic infiltrate, epidermal necrosis
- Management: treat underlying infection, stop offending agent

Stevens-Johnson Syndrome (SJS)/Toxic Epidermal Necrolysis (TEN)
- Causes
  - Drug related (Table 11-2)
    - Anticonvulsants (lamotrigine)
    - Sulfa drugs
    - NSAIDs
    - Penicillins

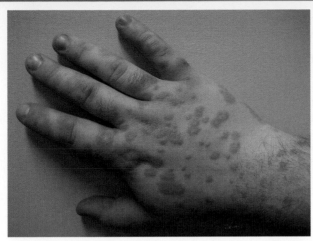

Figure 11-5: : Erythema multiforme of the hand. (Image courtesy of James Heilman, MD.)

TABLE 11-2 Drugs and Their Associated Skin Conditions

DRUG	REACTION
Tetracyclines	Photosensitivity
Glucocorticoids	Skin atrophy, striae, acne
Warfarin	Skin-induced necrosis
Penicillins	Morbilliform rash
Phenytoin, cyclosporine, calcium channel blockers	Gingival hyperplasia
Contrast dye, opiates	Urticaria

- Antiretrovirals (abacavir)
- Allopurinol
  - Nondrug related
    - Mycoplasma
    - Postvaccination
    - Graft-versus-host disease
- Signs and symptoms
  - Prodromal fever, myalgias, nausea followed by rapid onset of skin lesions
    - Blistering, desquamating
    - Sloughing, necrotic
    - Bullous lesions involving the skin and mucous membranes (oral cavity, conjunctiva)
  - Differentiated based on percent of body surface area involved:
    - <10% for SJS
    - >30% for TEN
  - Positive Nikolsky sign
  - Systemic signs such as tachycardia, hypotension, altered mental status, seizures, and coma more commonly seen in TEN
- Diagnostics: clinical
- Management
  - Stop offending agent
  - Management in burn unit: IV fluids, analgesics, wound care

DRESS (Drug Rash, Eosinophilia, Systemic Symptoms)
- Causes
  - Anticonvulsants
  - Antibiotics (TMP-SMX)
  - Allopurinol
- Key manifestations
  - Skin lesions similar to erythema multiforme (targetoid-like lesions involving the palms and soles), morbilliform rash
  - Lymphadenopathy

- Eosinophilia, leukocytosis
- May have hepatic, renal, or pulmonary involvement
  - Diagnostics: clinical
  - Management: stop offending agent

INHERITED SKIN DISORDERS
Porphyria Cutanea Tarda
- Pathophysiology: deficiency of uroporphyrinogen decarboxylase (porphobilinogen deaminase) resulting in accumulation of phototoxic porphyrins
- Signs and symptoms
  - Photosensitive vesicles and erosions
  - Increased skin fragility
  - Hypotrichosis of the face
  - Skin hyperpigmentation
  - Pseudoscleroderma (thickening, scarring, and calcification of the skin)
- Associations
  - Hepatitis C
  - Liver disease
  - OCPs
  - Diabetes mellitus
  - Iron overload
- Diagnostics: elevated serum/urinary uroporphyrins
- Management
  - Treat and avoid associations
  - Phlebotomy, hydroxychloroquine

Albinism
- Pathophysiology: deficiency/decreased function of tyrosinase enzyme preventing conversion of DOPA to melanin
- Signs and symptoms
  - Hypopigmented, chalky, white skin and hair
  - Rough, thickened skin in sun-exposed areas
  - Increased actinic keratoses and freckles
  - Blue/green irises, ocular sensitivity
  - Nystagmus, delayed/decreased visual acuity for age
- Associations
  - Chédiak-Higashi
  - Wardenburg syndrome
- Diagnostics: clinical
- Management
  - Sun protection
  - Periodic comprehensive eye exams with treatment of refractive errors
- Complications: increased risk of skin cancer (most commonly squamous cell carcinoma; increased risk of amelanotic melanoma)

Chédiak-Higashi: immunodeficiency secondary to microtubule dysfunction in phagosome-lysosomal fusion. Microtubular dysfunction results in inability to transfer melanin from basal cell melanocytes to epidermal cells resulting in albinism.

ITCHY DERMATITIDES
Atopic Dermatitis
- Risk factors
  - Family history
  - Change in weather immunity
  - Irritant clothing
  - Environmental exposure
  - Immunodeficiency
- Pathophysiology: mutation of filaggrin gene, which is responsible for strengthening of epidermal cell layers and acts as a natural moisturizing factor

- Signs and symptoms
  - Erythema, pruritus
  - Lichenification (thickening of the epidermis secondary to chronic scratching)
  - Involving the flexor surfaces in adults and extensor surfaces in children
- Associations
  - Atopy, asthma, allergies (AAA)
  - Wiskott-Aldrich syndrome
- Diagnostics
  - Clinical
  - Elevated IgE levels
- Management
  - Emollients, moisturizing agents
  - Avoidance of triggers
  - Topical steroids, antihistamines
  - Topical calcineurin inhibitors (tacrolimus, cyclosporine)
  - Severe cases: systemic immunosuppressants, phototherapy
- Complications: secondary to chronic scratching and skin breakdown
  - Superimposed cellulitis: treat with topical mupirocin; oral antistaphylococcal/streptococcal for extensive disease
  - Eczema herpeticum: treat with oral HSV antivirals (acyclovir, valacyclovir)

Contact Dermatitis
- Pathophysiology
  - Irritant-type contact dermatitis requires no previous exposure
  - Allergic-type contact dermatitis often requires previous exposure and sensitization; type IV hypersensitivity reaction
- Causes: prolonged and repetitive contact with irritant
  - Latex
  - Detergents, soaps
  - Poison ivy
  - Nickel, copper
  - Medications (neomycin, benzoyl peroxide)
- Signs and symptoms
  - Scaly, erythematous, pruritic
  - Well-demarcated rash involving area of contact (Fig. 11-6)
  - Vesicles, bullae
  - Chronically develop excoriations, hyperkeratosis, fissures, and lichenification
- Diagnostics
  - Clinical
  - Patch testing if etiology is unclear

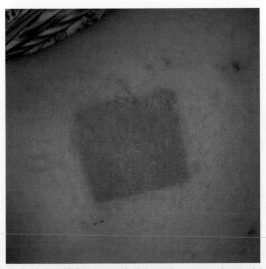

Figure 11-6: Well-demarcated rash in a patient who developed contact dermatitis from a buprenorphine drug patch.

– Management
  • Avoid offending agent
  • Emollients and others skin hydrating agents
  • Topical steroids, antihistamines

Urticaria

– Pathophysiology: type I hypersensitivity IgE-mediated reaction resulting in mast cell degranulation of histamine and localized anaphylaxis
– Causes
  • Drugs
    ▪ Penicillins
    ▪ Sulfa drugs
    ▪ NSAIDs
    ▪ Anticonvulsants
    ▪ Narcotics, radiocontrast dye: both result in direct mast cell degranulation
  • Foods
    ▪ Peanuts
    ▪ Shellfish
  • Infections
    ▪ Acute hepatitis B
    ▪ Strongyloides
  • Insect bites/sting
  • Chronic urticaria triggered by pressure (dermatographism), cold, vibration
  • Systemic disorders (vasculitis, autoimmune, malignancy)
  • Systemic mastocytosis
  • Idiopathic
– Signs and symptoms
  • Prodromal/localized anaphylaxis
  • Sudden onset wheal and flare reaction: well-circumscribed erythematous plaques with central pallor
  • Severe pruritus
– Diagnostics: clinical
– Management
  • Epinephrine if there are signs of anaphylaxis (respiratory compromise, hypotension)
  • Antihistamines
  • Oral glucocorticoids for severe unresponsive cases
  • Desensitization for unavoidable triggers

Systemic mastocytosis: infiltration of mast cells in various tissues resulting in release vasoactive mediators such as histamine, prostaglandins, leukotrienes; presents with chronic urticaria, pruritus, facial flushing, abdominal pain, diarrhea, hepatomegaly, and peptic ulcer disease

Seborrheic Dermatitis

– Signs and symptoms
  • Erythematous, pruritic, greasy, yellowish scaly plaques involving the areas with multiple sebaceous glands (face, scalp, chest, trunk)
  • Dandruff occurring on the face, eyebrows, and nasolabial folds
  • Severe cases seen in Parkinson disease and human immunodeficiency virus (HIV)
  • Chronic cases seen in Langerhans cell histiocytosis
  • Cradle cap in infants
– Diagnostics: clinical
– Management
  • Antifungal shampoo (ketoconazole, ciclopirox, zinc pyrithione, selenium sulfide)
  • Topical corticosteroids for severe cases

Purulent cellulitis: think Staphylococcus
Nonpurulent cellulitis: think Streptococcus
Be sure to differentiate cellulitis from deep venous thrombosis with lower extremity Doppler.

Infection by Malassezia species is considered to play a role in seborrheic dermatitis.

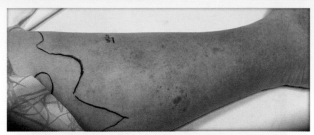

Figure 11-7: Cellulitis of the lower extremity with marker outlining the extent of the erythema. (Image courtesy of Stephen Ewen.)

INFECTIONS

Cellulitis
- Definition: infection of the deep dermis and subcutaneous fat
- Risk factors
  - Trauma, insect bite
  - Chronic irritation (scratching)
  - Previous cellulitis secondary to damaged and impaired local lymphatic vessels (lymphedema)
  - Immunosuppressed (diabetes mellitus, HIV)
- Microbiology
  - Staphylococcus
  - Streptococcus
- Signs and symptoms
  - Localized erythematous, tender, indolent, expanding edematous patch (Fig. 11-7)
  - Poorly demarcated
  - Systemic signs (fever, tachycardia) may be present
  - Regional lymphadenitis/lymphadenopathy
  - +/− fluctuance, drainage, purulence: suspicious for underlying abscess secondary to methicillin-resistant Staphylococcus aureus (MRSA)
- Diagnostics: clinical
- Management
  - Antibiotics covering gram-positive Staphylococcus/Streptococcus
    - First-generation cephalosporin (cephalexin, cefadroxil)
    - Dicloxacillin

> Fournier gangrene: necrotizing fasciitis of the perineum

  - Presence of fluctuance, drainage, purulence raises suspicion for MRSA
    - Vancomycin
    - Clindamycin
    - Doxycycline
    - TMP-SMX
  - Topical mupirocin for localized infection

Cellulitis in particular clinical settings should raise suspicions for atypical organisms, and these patients should be treated empirically, including coverage for these organisms (Table 11-3).

TABLE 11-3 Other Cellulitis-Related Organisms and Their Associations

ORGANISM	ASSOCIATIONS
Pseudomonas aeruginosa	Puncture wounds Tennis shoes Folliculitis Hot tub
Vibrio vulnificus	Hemochromatosis Liver disease Marine environment Raw oysters
Pasteurella	Dog/cat bites
Streptococcus pneumonia *Haemophilus influenza* *Moraxella catarrhalis*	Orbital/periorbital cellulitis
Aeromonas hydrophila	Fresh-water exposure

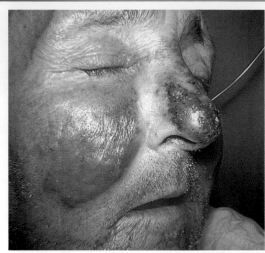

Figure 11-8: Well-demarcated, facial erysipelas. (Image courtesy of CDC/Dr. Thomas F. Sellers/Emory University.)

Erysipelas
- Definition: infection of the superficial dermis and lymphatics
- Risk factors: similar to cellulitis
  - Lymphatic obstruction (postradical mastectomy)
  - Local trauma
  - Diabetes mellitus
- Microbiology
  - Group A Streptococcus (*S. pyogenes*)
  - Less commonly *S. aureus*
- Signs and symptoms
  - Well-demarcated, erythematous, tender lesion (Fig. 11-8)
  - Systemic symptoms may be present
- Diagnostics: clinical
- Management: antibiotics covering gram-positive cocci; similar to cellulitis with less concern for MRSA coverage

Ludwig angina: bilateral cellulitis of the submandibular and sublingual spaces

Necrotizing Fasciitis
- Definition: life-threatening soft tissue infection that dissects through the fascial planes associated with destruction of muscle fascia and subcutaneous tissue resulting in production of air and necrosis within the tissues
- Causes
  - Group A Streptococcus
  - Clostridium
- Signs and symptoms
  - Preexisting cellulitis, bullae
  - Pain out of proportion extending beyond area of erythema
  - Palpable crepitus
  - High fevers, hemodynamic instability
- Diagnostics
  - X-ray/computed tomography (CT): air in the tissues
  - Surgical debridement
- Management
  - Surgical debridement
  - Broad-spectrum antibiotics covering gram positives, gram negatives, and anaerobes
    - Carbapenem (meropenem) or beta-lactam/beta-lactamase inhibitor (ampicillin-sulbactam, piperacillin-tazobactam)
    - PLUS

- Vancomycin or daptomycin for MRSA
- PLUS
- Clindamycin for antitoxin effects

Syphilis
- Microbiology: *Treponema pallidum*
- Signs and symptoms: dermatologic involvement typically occurs during secondary syphilis
  - Diffuse symmetric maculopapular rash involving the palms and soles
  - Alopecia areata
  - Condylomata lata: flat-topped, wartlike lesion
- Diagnostics
  - Serology: rapid plasma reagin, fluorescent treponemal antibody absorption
  - Biopsy: spirochetes on dark-field microscopy
- Management
  - Penicillin

> Primary syphilis: self-resolving painless genital chancre with associated adenopathy
> Tertiary syphilis: tabes dorsalis, Argyll Robertson pupils, meningitis, vasculitis, endarteritis obliterans (aortitis, aortic regurgitation, aortic aneurysm), and gummas

  - Doxycycline for penicillin allergic

Lyme Disease
- Microbiology: *Borrelia burgdorferi* infection secondary to Ixodes tick bite
- Signs and symptoms
  - Localized disease: erythema migrans presenting as circular area of erythema surrounded by central clearing (target shaped, bull's-eye) (Fig. 11-9)
  - Disseminated/late disease
    - Migratory arthralgias
    - Atrioventricular block, myocarditis
    - Cranial nerve palsies
- Diagnostics
  - Early/primary Lyme disease diagnosed clinically based on appearance of skin lesion
  - Secondary/tertiary
    - Enzyme-linked immunosorbent assay (screening) followed by Western blot (confirmatory)
    - Synovial/cerebrospinal fluid polymerase chain reaction (PCR)
- Management
  - Doxycycline for most cases except CNS Lyme
  - Alternatives if doxycycline is contraindicated (children, pregnancy): cefuroxime, amoxicillin
  - Early disseminated, carditis: IV ceftriaxone or cefotaxime

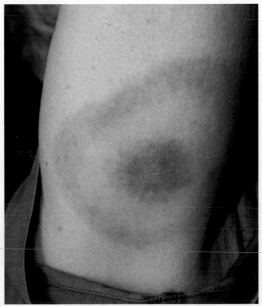

Figure 11-9: Bull's-eye rash in a patient with Lyme disease. (Image courtesy of the CDC.)

Toxic Shock Syndrome
- Causes: chronic indwelling packing
  - Tampon
  - Surgical wound infections
  - Rhinoplasty
- Pathophysiology: *S. aureus* exotoxin (toxic shock syndrome toxin-1), which acts as superantigen resulting in overactivation of T cells and release of excessive cytokines
- Signs and symptoms
  - High fever, hypotension, tachycardia
  - Desquamating rash involving the palms and soles
  - More than three dysfunctional organs, including but not limited to gastrointestinal, renal, hepatic, CNS, musculoskeletal, and mucous membranes
- Diagnostics: clinical
- Management
  - Removal of foreign body
  - IV fluid resuscitation
  - Antistaphylococcal antibiotics

Sporotrichosis (Sporothrix schenckii)
- Risk factors
  - Gardening
  - Landscaping
- Signs and symptoms: ascending lymphangitis/lymphadenopathy from the site of skin prick
- Diagnostics
  - Microscopy: cigar-shaped budding yeast
  - Culture
- Management: itraconazole

Acne
- Causes
  - *Propionibacterium acnes*
  - Glucocorticoids
  - Hyperandrogenism
- Pathophysiology (Fig. 11-10)
  - Follicular hyperkeratinization
  - Excessive sebum production
  - Inflammation
  - *P. acnes* proliferation
- Signs and symptoms: dependent on the type of acne
  - Inflammatory
    - Erythematous papules, pustules, and cysts
    - Involves the face, upper chest/arms, and back
  - Comedonal
    - Follicular occlusion secondary to hyperkeratosis
    - Blackheads and whiteheads
  - Nodulocystic
    - Large nodules
    - Cystic appearing with sinus tract formation and scarring

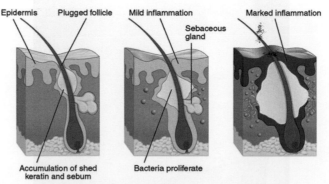

Figure 11-10: Diagrammatic representation of the pathophysiology of acne. (Image courtesy of OpenStax College.)

– Diagnostics: clinical
– Management: dependent on the type of acne and severity
  • Mild: benzoyl peroxide
    ▪ +/− topical retinoids
    ▪ +/− topical antibiotic (erythromycin, clindamycin)
    ▪ +/− topical salicylates
  • Moderate: benzoyl peroxide + topical retinoids + oral antibiotics (tetracyclines)
  • Severe, unresponsive: oral isotretinoin
  • Alternatives: OCPs, spironolactone

> Ensure patient is not pregnant and on appropriate contraception before starting oral isotretinoin due to deleterious fetal side effects.

Dermatophytosis
– Causes
  • Microsporidium, Trichophyton, Epidermophyton
  • Malassezia species (furfur, globosa)
– Signs and symptoms
  • Papulosquamous, annular erythematous, scaly lesions with central area of clearing
  • Located in body skinfolds (groin, armpits, inframammary, interdigital) (Fig. 11-11)
  • Hypopigmentation and/or hyperpigmentation
  • Satellite lesions (small erythematous lesions adjacent to the main area of infection)
– Diagnostics
  • Clinical
  • Wood lamp positive (bluish green tinge indicates presence of fungi)
  • Potassium hydroxide skin test
  • Fungal culture for resistant cases or if long-term treatment is required (onychomycosis, tinea capitis)
– Management
  • Topical antifungals
    ▪ Clotrimazole, miconazole
    ▪ Terbinafine
  • Topical selenium sulfide shampoo
  • Oral antifungals (only for onychomycosis, tinea capitis) for 6–12 weeks
    ▪ Terbinafine
    ▪ Ketoconazole, itraconazole
    ▪ Griseofulvin

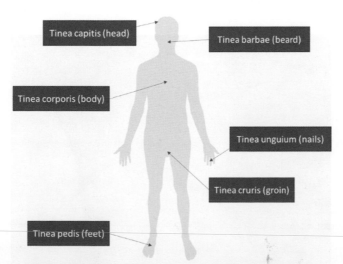

Figure 11-11: Dermatophytosis and their names by location.

Herpes Simplex Virus
- Causes: HSV1, HSV2
- Signs and symptoms
  - Prodromal tingling, itching, and burning
  - Painful, erythematous, grouped weeping vesicles
  - Located in the genitalia (sexually transmitted disease), mouth (cold sores)
- Diagnostics
  - Clinical
  - Viral PCR
- Management
  - Acyclovir or valacyclovir
  - Foscarnet for acyclovir-resistant cases

Herpes Zoster Virus
- Signs and symptoms
  - Grouped vesicles on an erythematous base
  - Prodromal tingling, numbness, burning
  - Often reactivation (elderly, immunosuppression, stress), which follows a dermatomal distribution without crossing midline (Fig. 11-12)
- Diagnostics
  - Clinical
  - Viral PCR
- Management: same as HSV (see earlier)
- Prevention: herpes zoster vaccine for adults >50 years old
- Complications: postherpetic neuralgia (persistent hypersensitivity of afferent pain fibers)
  - Early treatment decreases risk and duration of postherpetic neuralgia
  - Treat with tricyclic antidepressants (amitriptyline, nortriptyline), gabapentin, pregabalin

Other manifestations of herpes zoster:
- Ramsey Hunt syndrome (vesicles in the auditory canal)
- Herpes zoster ophthalmicus (herpes of V1 may present as orbital/periorbital cellulitis, blindness, or corneal anesthesia)

Molluscum Contagiosum
- Microbiology: poxvirus
- Signs and symptoms
  - Waxy, skin-colored papules with central umbilication (Fig. 11-13)
  - Tend to be grouped due to autoinoculation
  - Widespread, large, hundreds of lesions indicative of impaired cellular immunity (HIV)
- Diagnostics: clinical
- Management: cryotherapy, curettage, cantharidin

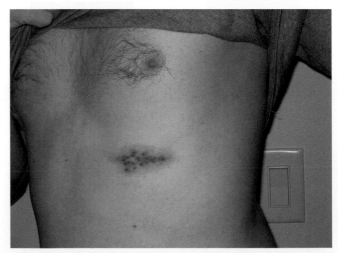

Figure 11-12: Herpes zoster infection affecting a thoracic dermatome and does not cross the midline. (Image courtesy of Preston Hunt.)

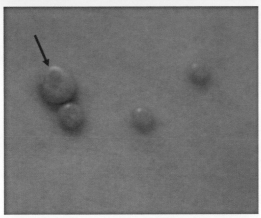

Figure 11-13: Skin lesion of molluscum contagiosum with characteristic central umbilication. (Image courtesy of Dave Bray, MD, Walter Reed Army Medical Center.)

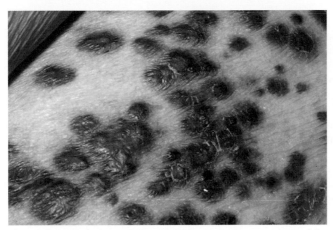

Figure 11-14: Bright, violaceous lesions of Kaposi sarcoma. (Image courtesy of OpenStax College.)

Kaposi Sarcoma
– Definition: microvascular endothelial cell tumor; spindle cell proliferation
– Causes
  • Human herpesvirus 8
  • Associated with immunosuppression (transplant, HIV)
– Signs and symptoms
  • Papules, plaques, nodules that may be brown, pink, or violaceous color (Fig. 11-14)
  • Located on the trunk, face, extremity, genitals
  • In severe cases located in the mucous membranes and visceral organs
– Diagnostics
  • Clinical
  • Biopsy for atypical cases (may present similarly to bacillary angiomatosis)
  • Check HIV antigen/antibody; CD4 count: acquired immunodeficiency syndrome–defining illness
– Management
  • Interferon-alfa
  • Highly active antiretroviral therapy
  • Chemotherapy (anthracycline) for advanced cases

Scabies
– Microbiology: Sarcoptes scabiei mite
– Transmission: direct person-to-person contact
– Signs and symptoms
  • Erythematous, pruritic (type IV hypersensitivity reaction to the scabies), burrows involving the web spaces between the fingers, toes, elbows, genitalia, breasts
  • Excoriations, small pruritic vesicles
  • Highly contagious; likely other household contacts with similar symptoms
– Diagnostics: burrow scrapings (visualization of mites, ova, feces under light microscopy)

- Management
  - Topical permethrin OR oral ivermectin: first-line treatment
  - Lindane (however, typically avoided due to neurotoxicity)
  - Wash all clothing and linen used in the last 48–72 hours (mites can only live 2–3 days without a human host)
  - Treat the whole family

Norwegian (crusted) scabies: severe case scabies involving the entire body associated with immunocompromise; treat with ivermectin

PREMALIGNANT SKIN DISORDERS

Acanthosis Nigricans
- Pathophysiology: abnormalities in tyrosine kinase, epithelial growth factor, and fibroblast growth factor receptors
- Causes
  - Obesity, insulin resistance, diabetes mellitus
  - Polycystic ovarian syndrome
  - Visceral malignancy (gastric, genitourinary malignancy)
  - Medications
    - Glucocorticoids
    - OCPs, human growth hormone
    - Niacin
  - Hypothyroidism/hyperthyroidism
- Signs and symptoms
  - Thickened, velvety, hyperpigmented skin (Fig. 11-15)
  - Typically involves the posterior neck, axilla, groin
  - Lesions in atypical locations (mucous membranes, palms, and soles), rapid onset, and elderly should raise suspicion for malignant etiology
  - Associated with skin tags (acrochordons): pedunculated outgrowths of normal skin
- Diagnostics
  - Clinical diagnosis
  - Diabetes screening: hemoglobin A1c, fasting blood sugar
  - Age-appropriate cancer screening
- Management
  - Stop or treat underlying etiology
  - Topical retinoids or vitamin D analogs for cosmetic benefits if underlying etiology is not identified

Polymyositis/Dermatomyositis
- Definition: autoimmune inflammatory myopathy resulting in muscle damage and characteristic cutaneous manifestations
- Key manifestations

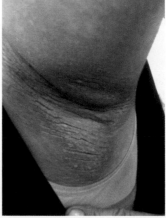

Figure 11-15: Hyperpigmented, velvety, thickened skin in a patient with acanthosis nigricans.

- Fever, malaise, lethargy
- Muscle aches, weakness
- Symmetric, proximal myopathy (difficulty getting up from seated position, raising arms above shoulder level)
- No neurologic deficits
- Cutaneous (associated with dermatomyositis)
  - Heliotrope rash (purplish discoloration around periorbital region)
  - Gottron papules (patchy, erythematous rash involving dorsum of hand)
  - Shawl sign (rash involving upper neck, back, chest, and shoulders)
  - Mechanics hand (dark, dirty-appearing hands with cracks and fissures)
  - Malar rash
- Malignancy (ovarian, gastrointestinal, longer, lymphoma): may be paraneoplastic syndrome of underlying visceral malignancy
– Diagnostics
  - Elevated creatine phosphokinase, aldolase
  - Anti-Jo-1, anti-SRP, anti-Mi-2, antisynthetase
  - Muscle biopsy: mononuclear infiltrate and necrosis
  - CT chest/abdomen/pelvis searching for underlying malignancy and age-appropriate cancer screening
– Management
  - Glucocorticoids: initial treatment
  - Steroid-sparing agents for steroid unresponsive (methotrexate, azathioprine)

Actinic Keratosis (also known as solar keratosis)

Leser-Trélat sign: sudden onset of multiple seborrheic keratoses associated with occult internal malignancy (gastrointestinal adenocarcinoma).
Acanthosis nigricans, dermatomyositis, and Leser-Trélat sign are all cutaneous manifestations of visceral malignancies.

– Definition: premalignant lesion associated with squamous cell carcinoma
– Signs and symptoms
  - Rough, scaly papules on chronically sun-exposed areas (face, neck, scalp, dorsal, hands)
  - Sandpaper-like texture
  - Most common in fair-skinned individuals
– Diagnostics
  - Clinical
  - Biopsy to exclude squamous cell carcinoma for lesions >1 cm, indurated, ulcerated, or rapidly growing
  - Histopathology
    - Parakeratosis (retention of nuclei in the stratum corneum)
    - Acanthosis (epidermal thickening)
    - Thickened stratum corneum, basal atypical keratinocytes
    - Solar elastosis
– Management
  - Medical: topical medications used for multiple lesions
5-fluorouracil
Imiquimod
- Surgical: cryotherapy, curettage

MALIGNANT SKIN LESIONS
There are three main cell types that make up the epidermis, each of which haa potential to undergo malignant degeneration (Fig. 11-16).
Basal Cell Carcinoma
– Epidemiology: most common skin cancer; accounts for up to 75% of all skin cancers
– Risk factors
  - Chronic UV exposure
  - Fair-skinned individuals
  - Chronic arsenic exposure
  - Ionizing radiation

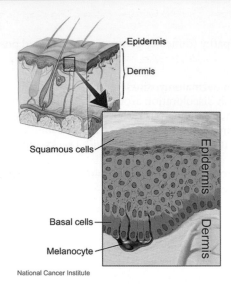

Figure 11-16: Layers of the skin showing the origin of malignant skin lesions. (Image courtesy of Don Bliss via the National Cancer Institute.)

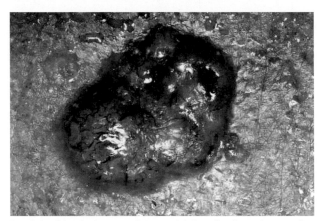

Figure 11-17: Telangiectatic, pink, shiny lesion consistent with basal cell carcinoma. (Image courtesy of OpenStax College.)

– Signs and symptoms
  • Pearly, pink, shiny papule or plaque (Fig. 11-17)
  • Central depression, telangiectasias
  • Itchy, ulcerating, oozing, crusting, chronically open sores
  • Tends to favor upper lips, nose
  • Locally invasive, metastasis extremely rare
– Diagnostics: biopsy
  • Invasive clusters of spindle cells surrounded by palisaded basal cells
  • Differentiates superficial, nodular, and sclerosing subtypes
– Management
  • Surgical resection (Mohs microsurgery for cosmetically sensitive areas), electrodessication, and curettage
  • Topical 5-fluorouracil for superficial basal cell carcinoma
Squamous Cell Carcinoma
– Epidemiology: second most common skin cancer
– Risk factors
  • Chronic UV exposure
  • Fair-skinned individuals
  • Actinic keratosis
  • Smoking/chewing tobacco, alcohol
  • Chronic inflammation/immunosuppression

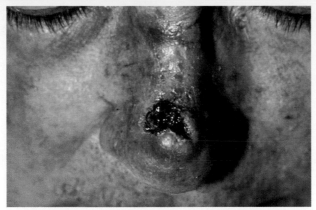

Figure 11-18: Scaly, ulcerating lesions involving the tip of the nose secondary to squamous cell carcinoma. (Image courtesy of OpenStax College.)

> Marjolin ulcer: squamous cell carcinoma that occurs after a severe burn or chronic wound resulting in chronic inflammation, dysplasia, and invasive cancer.
> Bowen disease: squamous cell carcinoma in situ

- Previous severe burns
- Chronic arsenic exposure
- HPV infection
- Cyclosporine
– Signs and symptoms
  - Chronic, ulcerating, irregular lesion (Fig. 11-18)
  - Easily bleeds
  - Scaly, hyperkeratotic, nodular appearance
  - Favors the lower lips
  - Numbness, paresthesia secondary to local perineural invasion
– Diagnostic: biopsy (cords of invasive squamous cell with keratin pearls)
– Management: surgical resection

Melanoma
– Risk factors
  - White, fair-skinned individuals
  - Chronic UV exposure, tanning booths
  - Family history
  - Severe, blistering sunburn
  - Dysplastic nevus syndrome
  - Xeroderma pigmentosum (autosomal recessive disease impairing DNA repair caused by UV light)
  - Chronic inflammatory disease (inflammatory bowel disease, autoimmune)
– Signs and symptoms: ABCDE (Fig. 11-19)
  - A: asymmetry
  - B: irregular borders
  - C: color variegation
  - D: diameter >6 mm
  - E: evolving, evolution
    - "Ugly duckling" sign: in a patient with multiple nevi, one or more nevi will look significantly different than the others
– Subtypes
  - Lentigo maligna: more superficial; good prognosis
  - Superficial spreading: most common type; radial spread
  - Acral lentiginous: most common in dark-skinned individuals; involves palms, soles, and subungual regions; positive Hutchinson sign (darkening of the nail bed and plate extending out to the skin)
  - Nodular: vertical growth pattern; worst prognosis
  - Amelanotic melanoma
– Diagnostics
  - Excisional biopsy with 1- to 3-mm margins

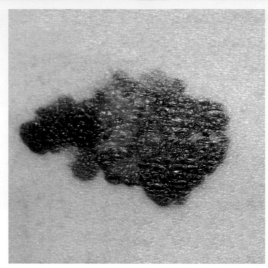

Figure11-19: Melanoma showing several of the ABCDE features. (Image courtesy of OpenStax College.)

- • Breslow staging for depth of invasion: determines prognosis
- • Lymphatic mapping, sentinel lymph node biopsy
- – Management
  - • Localized disease: surgical resection
  - • Metastatic disease
    - ▪ Metastectomy for limited metastatic disease (oligometastatic)
    - ▪ Immunotherapy: pembrolizumab, nivolumab, ipilimumab
    - ▪ Vemurafenib (BRAF-positive mutation)
    - ▪ Alternatives: interferon-alfa, interleukin 2

Mycosis Fungoides (Cutaneous T-Cell Lymphoma)

Xeroderma pigmentosum: autosomal recessive disease resulting in defective DNA repair mechanisms (nucleotide excision repair); increased risk of all skin cancers.

- – Definition: cutaneous T-cell lymphoma, monoclonal proliferation of CD4+ cells
- – Key manifestations
  - • Erythematous, pruritic, scaly rash; often confused for fungal infection, psoriasis, or eczema
  - • Generalized erythroderma
  - • Lymphadenopathy, hepatosplenomegaly
  - • Sezary syndrome (T-cell leukemia): hematologic variant with atypical lymphocytes (cerebriform nuclei)
- – Diagnostics: biopsy
  - • Mononuclear cells with cerebriform nuclei involving the upper dermis
  - • Intraepidermal aggregates (Pautrier microabscesses)
- – Management: topical (localized disease) or systemic chemotherapy (advanced disease)

MISCELLANEOUS DISORDERS
Pityriasis Rosea
- – Signs and symptoms
  - • Diffuse, symmetric erythematous pruritic, scaly eruption
  - • Preceded by herald patch: oval, rose-colored plaque located on the trunk that resolves followed by multiple smaller lesions; resembles ringworm with central area of clearing
  - • Christmas tree distribution on the back: follows cleavage lines on the trunk (Fig. 11-20)
- – Diagnostics
  - • Clinical
  - • Venereal Disease Research Laboratory to rule out secondary syphilis
- – Management: self-resolving

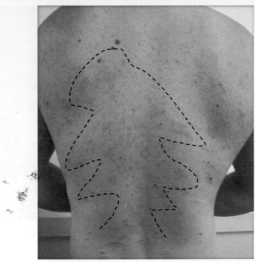

Figure 11-20: Pityriasis rosea involving the trunk, in a classical Christmas tree distribution. (Image courtesy of James Heilman, MD.)

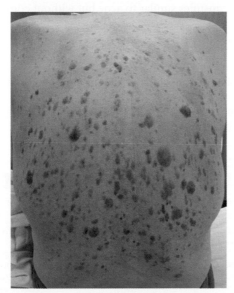

Figure 11-21: Multiple seborrheic keratoses, indicative of Leser-Trélat sign and underlying visceral malignancy. However, when seen in isolation or scattered this is completely benign. (Image courtesy of James Heilman, MD.)

Seborrheic Keratosis
- Definition: benign pigmented epidermal (keratinocyte) tumor
- Signs and symptoms
  - Waxy, velvety, well-demarcated, scaly, raised papular lesions with stuck-on appearance (Fig. 11-21)
  - Located on the trunk
  - Increased number in the elderly
  - Leser-Trélat sign: sudden onset of multiple seborrheic keratosis; cutaneous manifestation of a visceral malignancy
- Diagnostics: clinical
- Management: none; resection for cosmetic purposes

Keratoacanthoma: benign cutaneous tumor presenting as dome-shaped (volcano-like) nodules with central keratotic plug; regresses spontaneously

Rosacea
- Subtypes
  - Erythematotelangiectatic
  - Papulopustular
- Signs and symptoms

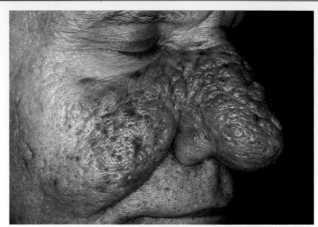

Figure 11-22: Rosacea involving the nose and cheeks showing facial erythema and telangiectasias. (Image courtesy of M. Sand, and others.)

- • Facial erythema, telangiectasias involving nose and cheeks (Fig. 11-22)
- • Recurrent facial flushing worsened by alcohol, emotional stress, temperature changes
- • Inflammatory papules and pustules similar to acne but without comedones
- • Ocular blepharitis
- – Diagnostics: clinical
- – Management
  - • Behavioral modification and avoidance of triggers
  - • Facial erythema: topical brimonidine, laser or intense pulsed light therapy
  - • Papules, pustules: topical metronidazole; oral tetracyclines

Venous stasis and arterial insufficiency ulcers result in abnormal discoloration of the lower extremities secondary to issues with venous return and lower extremity perfusion, respectively (Table 11-4).

TABLE 11-4   Venous Stasis Dermatitis Versus Arterial Insufficiency

	VENOUS STASIS ULCER	ARTERIAL INSUFFICIENCY ULCER
Pathophysiology	• Venous valve incompetence; venous hypertension	• Atherosclerosis
Location	• Medial malleolus • Pretibial area	• Distal toes
Signs and symptoms	• Lower extremity pitting edema worse after prolonged standing • Stasis dermatitis: thickened, brawny, indurated, darkening skin discoloration • Venous varicosities, telangiectasias • Lipodermatosclerosis	• Lower extremity claudication • Skin atrophy • Lower extremity hair loss • Leg elevation worsens symptoms • Symptoms worsen at night • Pain improved by standing and hanging legs over the side of the bed
Treatment	• Lower extremity elevation • Compression stockings	• Antiplatelets • Smoking cessation • Exercise • Reperfusion (stenting, bypass)

Calciphylaxis (Calcific Uremic Arteriolopathy)
- – Causes
  - • End-stage renal disease
  - • Hyperparathyroidism
  - • Hyperphosphatemia
- – Pathophysiology: precipitation of calcium and phosphate resulting in a vascular calcifications and necrotic skin lesions
- – Signs and symptoms
  - • Painful, violaceous nodules
  - • Ulcerations in areas of high adiposity (buttocks, abdomen, thighs)
- – Diagnostics
  - • Clinical
  - • Biopsy: arteriolar occlusion, calcification

- Management
  - Strict wound care
  - Sodium thiosulfate
  - Lower calcium-phosphate product
    - Dialysis
    - Phosphate binders (sevelamer, lanthanum)
    - Parathyroid hormone downregulator (cinacalcet)

Hidradenitis Suppurativa
- Pathophysiology: folliculopilosebaceous occlusion, rupture, and inflammation preventing shedding of keratinocytes
- Signs and symptoms
  - Inflammatory nodules and abscesses located in the intertriginous areas (axilla, groin, inframammary)
  - Sinus tracts: results in chronic relapsing nodule formation
  - Comedones
  - Scarring
- Diagnostics: clinical
- Management
  - Avoid skin trauma
  - Gentle cleansing

Lichen Planus
- Signs and symptoms
  - Purple, pruritic, polygonal, papular plaques involving the flexor surfaces, genitals (Fig. 11-23)
  - Wickham striae: white lacy pattern along the surface of the plaques and papules; may also involve mucous membranes
- Diagnostics: clinical
- Associations: hepatitis C, HIV
- Management: medium- to high-potency topical corticosteroids

---

Estrogen-related skin changes:
- Melasma
- Palmar erythema
- Spider angiomas

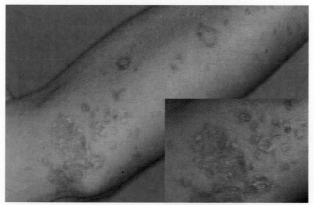

Figure 11-23: Purple, polygonal papules in a patient with lichen planus. (Image courtesy of Tag-El -Din Anbar MD and others.)

TABLE 11-5 Ulcer Staging

Stage I	Intact skin, mild erythema at the site of pressure
Stage II	Superficial, skin break without visualization of subcutaneous tissues
Stage III	Full thickness, visualization of subcutaneous tissues
Stage IV	Destruction and visualization of the muscle and bone necrosis

Ulcers most commonly occur at pressure points in debilitated patients as they are unable to reposition themselves. This results in prolonged pressure at bony protrusions resulting in worsening skin defects that can eventually progress to the bone (Table 11-5; Figs. 11-24 and 11-25).

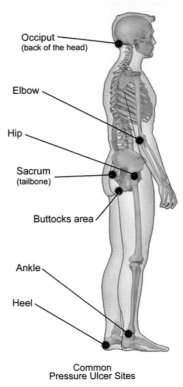

Figure 11-24: Diagram depicting the common locations for pressure ulcers. Locations involve bony protrusions in a supine patient.

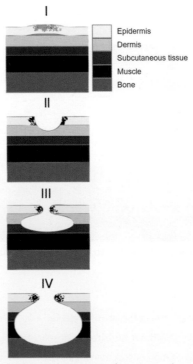

Figure 11-25: Illustration depicting the stages of pressure ulcers from stage I to stage IV.

CHAPTER 12 Emergency Medicine

TOXICOLOGY

Most patients presenting to the emergency room found to have drug toxicity are often too ill to provide a good history, placing greater emphasis on the use of physical examination and laboratory studies; however, if present some key history, physical, and laboratory findings are specific for certain drug toxicities (Table 12-1).

- Acetaminophen
  - Right upper quadrant pain
  - Aspartate transaminase/alanine transaminase >1000
  - Suicide attempt
- Benzodiazepines
  - History of insomnia
  - May be combined with alcohol

TABLE 12-1 Drug Toxicities, Mechanisms, and Treatment

DRUG	MECHANISM OF TOXICITY	MANAGEMENT
Acetaminophen	• Production of toxic metabolite and depletion glutathione	• N-acetylcysteine (replenishes glutathione stores)
Beta blockers	• Negative chronotropic effect	• Glucagon (increases cAMP)
Benzodiazepines	• Respiratory depression	• Respiratory support +/− flumazenil (may induce withdrawal seizures)
Carbon monoxide	• Binds to hemoglobin with higher affinity than oxygen	• 100% oxygen (decreases carbon monoxide half-life)
Cyanide	• Inhibits electron transport chain reactions	• Nitrite (converts iron in hemoglobin from normal Fe^{2+} to Fe^{3+}, which binds to cyanide with higher affinity) • Thiosulfate • Hydroxocobalamin
Ethylene glycol	• Metabolized into toxic metabolites	• Fomepizole (inhibits alcohol dehydrogenase)
Iron	• Production of free radicals	• Deferoxamine, deferasirox
Lead	• Systemic organ deposition and disruption of hematopoiesis	• Dimercaprol, succimer, EDTA
Methemoglobin	• Converse iron in hemoglobin from Fe^{2+} to Fe^{3+}	• Methylene blue
Opioids	• Respiratory depression	• Naloxone, naltrexone
Organophosphates	• Inhibition of acetylcholinesterase	• Atropine, pralidoxime
Salicylates	• Stimulates ventilatory centers of the brain • Mitochondrial toxin	• Sodium bicarbonate
SSRIs	• Excess serotonergic activity	• Cyproheptadine
TCAs	• Anticholinergic toxicity (cardiotoxicity, convulsions, coma) • Disruption of myocardial sodium channels	• Sodium bicarbonate

cAMP, Cyclic adenosine monophosphate; *EDTA*, ethylenediaminetetraacetic acid; *SSRI*, selective serotonin reuptake inhibitor; *TCA*, tricyclic antidepressants.

- Carbon monoxide
  - Elevated anion gap metabolic acidosis (lactic acidosis)
  - Kerosene lamps, heaters, or stoves
- Cyanide
  - Nitroprusside for treatment of hypertensive emergency
  - Elevated anion gap metabolic acidosis (lactic acidosis)
  - Flushing (cherry-red skin color)
- Ethylene glycol
  - Antifreeze
  - Sweet tasting
  - Elevated anion gap metabolic acidosis (lactic acidosis)
- Iron
  - Accidental ingestion by infant
  - Abdominal pain, necrotizing gastroenteritis
  - Radiopaque tablets seen on x-ray
- Lead
  - Accidental ingestion by infant living in an old house with paint chips
  - Neuropathy
  - Lead lines on x-ray (dense metaphyseal bands)
- Methemoglobin
  - Chocolate-colored blood
  - Recent use of anesthetic agent (i.e., benzocaine)
- Opioids
  - Respiratory depression
  - Pinpoint pupils
- Organophosphates
  - Farmer using pesticides
  - Cholinergic overdrive: diarrhea, urination, bronchoconstriction, lacrimation, diaphoresis
- Salicylates
  - Overdose attempt with aspirin
  - Tinnitus
  - Metabolic acidosis, hyperventilation
- Selective serotonin reuptake inhibitor
  - Myoclonus, hypertension, rigidity
  - Accidental combination with another serotonin-containing drug (St. John wort, tramadol, linezolid, meperidine): thoroughly review medication list

13 Infectious Disease

Human Immunodeficiency Virus (HIV)
- Risk factors
  - Unprotected sex
  - Men who have sex with men
  - IV drug user
  - History of other sexually transmitted diseases (STDs) (syphilis, chlamydia/gonorrhea, hepatitis B)
- Pathophysiology: retroviruses primarily infect CD4 cells incorporating its viral genome into the host cell DNA
- Signs and symptoms
  - Acute: mononucleosis-like syndrome
    - Fever, malaise, night sweats
    - Generalized lymphadenopathy
    - Maculopapular rash
    - Mucocutaneous ulcerations
  - Chronic
    - Most commonly asymptomatic
    - Opportunistic infections (Tables 13-1, 13-2)
- Diagnostics: HIV polymerase chain reaction (PCR)/antibodies
- Management
  - Initiate treatment in all patients regardless of CD4 count (Fig. 13-1)
  - Antiretroviral therapy targeted based on patient-specific virus resistance patterns (Table 13-3)
- Screening
  - One-time screening for patients aged 15–65
  - Screening for high-risk individuals
    - IV drug abusers
    - Men who have sex with men
    - Homeless
    - HIV-positive partner
    - Incarceration
    - Presence of other STDs

HIV During Pregnancy

HIV postexposure prophylaxis: initiated in patients with significant exposures from patients with known HIV or unknown HIV status while waiting for HIV tests. Treat for 4 weeks with antiretrovirals followed by periodic testing for seroconversion.

- Mother
  - If mother is already on antiretroviral at the time of pregnancy, continue same regimen; only efavirenz is teratogenic and will need to switch to an alternative
  - If mother is found to be HIV positive during pregnancy, initiate antiretroviral in a similar manner as a nonpregnant patient
  - Intrapartum zidovudine in addition to antiretrovirals further decreases the risk of transmission to the baby
- Fetus
  - Best method of preventing perinatal transmission is to treat the mother with antiretrovirals
  - Should be delivered by cesarean section if viral load >1000 copies/mL
  - Additional 2–6 weeks of HIV prophylaxis depending on mother's viral load, use of antiretrovirals, and whether she received intrapartum prophylaxis

TABLE 13-1   HIV Opportunistic Infections (appear after CD4 count <200)

CD4 COUNT	INFECTION	KEY MANIFESTATIONS	DIAGNOSTICS	TREATMENT/PROPHYLAXIS

<200	Pneumocystis pneumonia	• Dyspnea
		• Bilateral interstitial markings
		• +/− hypoxia
			• Sputum culture
			• Bronchoalveolar lavage
				• Prophylaxis: TMP-SMX
				• Management:
				  • TMP-SMX: first line
				  • Atovaquone
				  • Dapsone
				  • Pentamidine
				• Add steroids if patient has A-a gradient >35 mm Hg or P_aO_2 <55

<150	Histoplasma capsulatum	• Cough, dyspnea • Lymphadenopathy • Hepatosplenomegaly • Mucocutaneous papules/nodules • Diffuse interstitial and reticulonodular infiltrates	• Urine or serum histoplasma antigen • Pancytopenia • Elevated LFTs, LDH	• Initial treatment: amphotericin B • Itraconazole maintenance therapy • Consider itraconazole prophylaxis in endemic areas
<100	Cryptococcus	• Headache, visual disturbances, neck stiffness • Elevated opening pressure on LP	• CSF cryptococcal antigen • India ink stain	• Initial treatment: amphotericin B • Fluconazole secondary prophylaxis
	Toxoplasma gondii	• Encephalitis • Focal neurologic deficits	• CT head +/− brain biopsy • Multiple ring-enhancing lesions on CT	• Prophylaxis: TMP-SMX • Treatment: pyrimethamine + sulfadiazine
<50	Mycobacterium avium complex (MAC)	• Fever, weight loss • Lymphadenopathy • Diarrhea	• Blood cultures • Bone marrow or lymph node biopsy • Elevated alkaline phosphatase	• Prophylaxis: macrolides • Treatment: macrolide + ethambutol

TMP-SMX, Trimethoprim-sulfamethoxazole; *A-a gradient*, alveolar–arterial gradient; P_aO_2, partial pressure of oxygen; *LFT*, liver function tests; *LDH*, lactate dehydrogenase; *CSF*, cerebrospinal fluid; *LP*, lumbar puncture.

HIV immune reconstitution syndrome: paradoxic worsening of infectious symptoms upon initiation of antiretroviral therapy due to recovery of immune system and enhanced ability to combat underlying infection.

Syphilis
- Risk factors
  • Unprotected sex
  • Men who have sex with men
  • Multiple sexual partners
- Signs and symptoms
  • Primary: painless chancre
  • Secondary
    ▪ Maculopapular rash involving the palms and soles
    ▪ Alopecia areata
    ▪ Condyloma lata
  • Tertiary: central nervous system (CNS) and vascular involvement
    ▪ Argyll Robertson pupil
    ▪ Tabes dorsalis (posterior column demyelination: loss of vibratory and position sensation)
    ▪ Meningitis
    ▪ Vasculitis, aortitis
    ▪ Gummas
- Diagnostics
  • Screening: rapid plasma reagin, Venereal Disease Research Laboratory (VDRL)
  • Confirmatory: fluorescent treponemal antibody (FTA)
  • Tertiary syphilis: cerebrospinal fluid (CSF)–VDRL/FTA
- Management
  • Penicillin: first line
  • Doxycycline: alternative to penicillin allergy for primary and secondary

TABLE 13-2   Other HIV-Related Manifestations

NEUROLOGIC	KEY MANIFESTATIONS

Dermatologic	• Kaposi sarcoma
	  • Purplish. brown nonpruritic violaceous rash
	  • May involve oral mucosa or visceral organs
	  • Highly vascular tumor with spindle cells on histology
	  • Associated with HHV-8
	
	• Bacillary angiomatosis
	  • Bright red, firm papules/plaque
	  • Treat with macrolides or tetracycline
	
	• Seborrheic dermatitis
	  • Diffuse widespread erythematous plaques, greasy yellowish scales
	  • Severe intractable cases seen in HIV and Parkinson disease
	  • Treated with topical steroids, shampoo, antifungals
	
	• Molluscum contagiosum
	  • Widespread papules with central umbilication
	  • Similar to seborrheic dermatitis, severe cases with multiple papules seen in HIV

Pulmonary	• Systemic mycoses • Tuberculosis

Gastrointestinal	• Esophagitis
	  • HSV: ovoid, punched-out lesions; treat with valacyclovir
	  • CMV: large, linear lesion; treat with ganciclovir
	  • Candida: oral thrush; treat with fluconazole
	
	• Cryptosporidium
	  • Chronic nonremitting watery diarrhea
	  • Self-limiting in nonimmunocompromised pulse
	  • Treat with nitazoxanide
	
	• CMV colitis

Renal	• Focal segmental glomerulosclerosis • BK virus

Neurologic	• HIV dementia
	
	• Progressive multifocal leukoencephalopathy
	  • JC virus reactivation
	  • Patchy areas of demyelination on MRI
	
	• CNS lymphoma
	  • Associated with EBV
	  • Solid, ring-enhancing solitary lesion on neuroimaging

Ophthalmologic	• CMV retinitis
	  • Commonly seen in patients with CD4 count <50
	  • Treat with ganciclovir

HHV, Human herpesviruses; *HSV*, herpes simplex virus; *CMV*, cytomegalovirus; *JC*, John cunningham

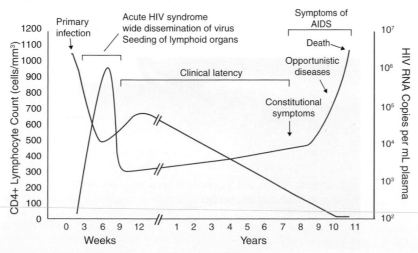

Figure 13-1: Time course of untreated human immunodeficiency virus *(HIV)* infection until death caused by opportunistic infection. *AIDS*, Acquired immunodeficiency syndrome.

TABLE 13-3   Antiretrovirals Pharmacotherapy

CLASS OF MEDICATION	EXAMPLE	SIDE EFFECTS
Nucleoside reverse transcriptase inhibitors	Tenofovir Emtricitabine Abacavir Didanosine Stavudine Zidovudine	• Didanosine, stavudine: pancreatitis, peripheral neuropathy • Abacavir: hypersensitivity reaction and human leukocyte antigen B5701 • Zidovudine: bone marrow suppression, macrocytic anemia • Tenofovir: renal insufficiency, osteopenia/osteoporosis
Nonnucleoside reverse transcriptase inhibitors	Efavirenz Nevirapine Etravirine	• Rash, hepatotoxicity • Efavirenz: vivid dreams, teratogenic
Protease inhibitors	Atazanavir Indinavir Ritonavir	• Hyperglycemia, hyperlipidemia, lipodystrophy • Indinavir: hematuria
Integrase inhibitor	Raltegravir	• Rhabdomyolysis
Fusion inhibitors	Enfuvirtide	• Injection site reaction
CCR5 antagonists	Maraviroc	• Hepatotoxicity • Arthralgias • Upper respiratory infections

CCR5, CC chemokine receptor 5.

Chloramphenicol typically avoided due to side effect profile: blood dyscrasias, gray baby syndrome (in premature infants) Chloramphenicol is also used to treat Ehrlichiosis.

Jarisch-Herxheimer reaction: fever, rash, lymphadenopathy, arthralgias after treatment of syphilis; occurs secondary to release of immunogenic antigens from dying spirochetes

Pregnant women with tertiary syphilis will need to be desensitized as doxycycline is an inappropriate option due to side effect of fetal bone growth abnormalities and teeth deformities.

Rocky Mountain Spotted Fever (RMSF)
- Microbiology
    • Rickettsia rickettsi (gram negative, obligate intracellular)
    • Tickborne illness
    • Predilection for vascular endothelial cells
- Signs and symptoms
    • High fever, myalgias
    • Headache, photophobia, meningismus
    • Blanching erythematous macular/petechial rash that spreads centripetally, initially involving extremities, including palms and soles (Fig. 13-2)

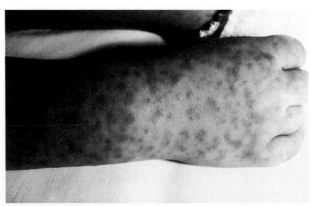

Figure 13-2: Spotted rash typical of Rocky Mountain spotted fever. (Image courtesy of Public Health Image Library [PHIL], Centers for disease control and prevention [CDC].)

- Diagnostics
  - Clinical
  - Confirmatory: immunoglobulin M (IgM)/IgG antibodies, immunofluorescent staining
  - Supporting findings
    - Transaminitis
    - Thrombocytopenia
    - Interstitial pneumonitis
- Management
  - Doxycycline: first line, even in pregnant women and children
  - Chloramphenicol: alternative agents in rare cases

Chlamydia
- Microbiology: chlamydia trachomatis
- Signs and symptoms
  - Typically, asymptomatic in both men and women
  - Men: painful, purulent penile discharge
  - Women
    - Purulent cervical discharge
    - Cervical erythema, vaginitis
    - Painful intercourse
    - Dysuria, urinary frequency
- Diagnostics: nucleic acid amplification test (NAAT)
- Management
  - Empiric (cover both chlamydia and gonorrhea): ceftriaxone + azithromycin
  - Confirmed: azithromycin or doxycycline

Gonorrhea
- Microbiology: *Neisseria gonorrhoeae* (intracellular gram-negative diplococci)
- Signs and symptoms

Urethritis is caused by chlamydia, gonorrhea, mycoplasma, ureaplasma.
Both chlamydia and gonorrhea are associated with high-risk sexual behaviors and commonly coinfected with other sexually transmitted diseases such as HIV, syphilis, and hepatitis B.

  - Typically, asymptomatic, especially in women
  - Mucopurulent discharge
  - Cervical erythema, vaginitis
  - Dysuria, urinary frequency
  - Disseminated disease: triad of purulent dermatitis, tenosynovitis, septic arthritis
- Diagnostics
  - NAAT
  - Obtain swab from cervix, rectum, oropharynx based on sexual practices
- Management: ceftriaxone + azithromycin

Genital ulcers are often sexually transmitted, each with their own unique appearance. The presence or absence of pain is a useful differential (Table 13-4).

Noninfectious genital ulcers are caused by Behcet syndrome.

Epididymitis

Complications of chlamydia/gonorrhea infection include Fitz-Hugh-Curtis syndrome (perihepatitis), pelvic inflammatory disease, epididymitis, urethritis, prostatitis, proctitis, conjunctivitis, reactive arthritis (chlamydia only).

- Microbiology
  - Young men, <35 years old: STDs (chlamydia, gonorrhea)
  - Older men, >35 years old: non-STDs (*Escherichia coli*, Pseudomonas)
- Signs and symptoms
  - Tender, enlarged testicles
  - Fever, chills
  - Dysuria, increased frequency
  - Scrotal tenderness +/− hydrocele

TABLE 13-4   Comparison of Genital Ulcers

PAIN	CAUSE	CLINICAL FEATURES	DIAGNOSTICS	TREATMENT
Painful	Herpes simplex virus	• Vesicular, erythematous base	• Vesicular fluid PCR	Acyclovir or valacyclovir or famciclovir
	Haemophilus ducreyi	• Coalescing ragged edges • Small, tender papules that erode	• "School of fish" on Gram stain • NAAT	Ceftriaxone or azithromycin
Painless	Syphilis	• Chancre	• Dark-field microscopy • VDRL, FTA-ABS	Penicillin
	Lymphogranuloma venereum	• Transient, painless ulcerating lesion • Painful, suppurative lymph nodes	• NAAT	Doxycycline or erythromycin
	Klebsiella granulomatis	• Red, erythematous ulcerative lesion • Pungent, beefy red	• Wright/Giemsa stain: Donssovan bodies	Azithromycin

PCR, Polymerase chain reaction; *NAAT*, nucleic-acid amplification test; *VDRL*, venereal disease research laboratory; *FTA-ABS*, fluorescent treponemal antibody test absorption test.

- Diagnostics
  - Clinical
  - Urinalysis + culture
  - NAAT for chlamydia/gonorrhea
  - Scrotal ultrasound: will see an enlarged hyperemic epididymis; also performed to rule out testicular torsion
- Management: dependent upon suspicion for STDs vs non-STD etiology
  - Young, STDs: ceftriaxone + azithromycin
  - Older men, non-STD: fluoroquinolone or TMP-SMX

Prostatitis
- Microbiology: *E. coli* (gram-negative rod)
- Signs and symptoms
  - Fever, chills, malaise
  - Tender, bulging prostate on digital rectal examination
  - Pelvic or perineal pain
  - Dysuria, urinary frequency, incontinence, cloudy urine
- Diagnostics
  - Clinical
  - Urinalysis after prostate massage: increases culture yield
- Management
  - 4–6 weeks of antibiotics covering causative organism
  - Fluoroquinolone or TMP-SMX
- Complications: prostatic abscess

CHAPTER
14 Aging

As we get older there are various changes that occur throughout our organ systems as part of normal aging (Table 14-1). It is important to differentiate this decreased functionality from organic pathology to prevent overdiagnosis and unnecessary workup.

TABLE 14-1   Changes as We Get Older, System by System

ORGAN SYSTEM	CHANGES
Neurologic	• Occasional forgetfulness • Decreased rapid eye movement sleep, increased sleep latency, and early awakening • Decreased brain volume
Eyes, ears, nose, and throat	• Presbyopia • Presbycusis • Dental caries
Pulmonary	• Decreased functional reserve • Diaphragmatic flattening • Decreased surface area for gas exchange
Cardiovascular	• Hypertension • Coronary artery disease
Gastrointestinal	• Diverticulosis • Decreased hepatic metabolism
Musculoskeletal	• Osteoarthritis • Increased adipose • Decreased muscle • Decreased bone density
Nephrology	• Decreased renal mass • Decreased creatinine clearance
Genitourinary	• Urinary incontinence • Erectile dysfunction • Dyspareunia
Hematology	• Decreased immune response
Dermatology	• Wrinkles • Dermal thinning • Decreased vascularity, delayed wound healing

CHAPTER
15 Early Pregnancy

Early pregnancy occurs when the sperm meets the egg resulting in the formation of a zygote, which eventually implants into the uterine endometrium. This results in hormonal changes that produce recognizable signs and symptoms of pregnancy.

Fertilization and implantation

1. Sperm travels down the fallopian tube and penetrates the egg releasing enzymes that degrade the zona pellucida permitting fusion of gametes
2. Simultaneously, oocyte release enzymes causing zona pellucida to become impenetrable to additional sperm (Fig. 15-1)
3. Zygote replicates and travels toward the uterine endometrium with implantation occurring between days 6 and 10 (Fig. 15-2)
4. Implanted blastocyst secretes beta-human chorionic gonadotropin (beta-hCG), which prevents degeneration of the corpus luteum, which in turn secretes progesterone to maintain the fetus during first trimester of pregnancy (Table 15-1; Figs. 15-3 and 15-4)

Gestational age is counted from last menstrual period.

Additional notes regarding pregnancy hormones:
- Extremely high levels of beta-hCG indicative of molar pregnancy, choriocarcinoma, multiple gestation, or Down syndrome
- Low levels of beta-hCG indicative of ectopic pregnancy, impending miscarriage, trisomy 13/18
- Beta-hCG has a similar alpha subunit as luteinizing hormone, follicle-stimulating hormone, and thyroid-stimulating hormone
- Ectopic pregnancy occurs when implantation occurs outside the uterine endometrium
- Extremely high levels of human placental lactogen indicative of placental trophoblastic tumor

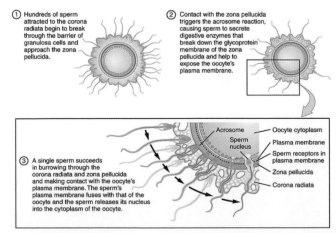

Figure 15-1: Diagrammatic representation of the physiology of fertilization. (Image courtesy of OpenStax College.)

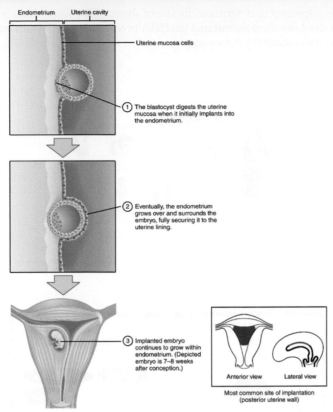

Figure 15-2: Diagrammatic representation of the physiology of implantation. (Image courtesy of OpenStax College.)

TABLE 15-1 Pregnancy Hormones, Sources, and Function

HORMONE	SOURCE	FUNCTION
beta-hCG	Placenta	• Main hormone of pregnancy • Used to determine pregnancy in pregnancy tests • Maintains corpus luteum during the first trimester
Progesterone	Corpus luteum in first trimester; placenta after first trimester	• Maintenance of pregnancy • Prevents premature urine contractions • Decrease in progesterone after delivery disinhibits prolactin and promotes lactation
Prolactin	Posterior pituitary	• Maintains lactation • Assists in preventing pregnancy during breastfeeding as it inhibits GnRH, and in effect FSH/LH
Human placental lactogen	Placenta	• Increases mother's insulin resistance allowing glucose and energy to reach the placenta for fetal metabolism • Potentially implicated in gestational diabetes

hCG, Human chorionic gonadotropin; *GnRH*, gonadotropin-releasing hormone; *FSH*, follicle-stimulating hormone; *LH*, luteinizing hormone.

Genetic embryology is important to determine the site of abnormality when there is abnormal internal or external genitalia in a newborn. Female internal genitalia predictably arises from paramesonephric ducts while male internal genitalia arises from mesonephric ducts (Table 15-2; Fig. 15-5).

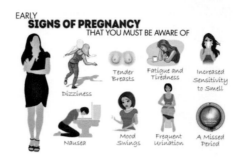

Figure 15-3: Diagrammatic representations of the earliest physical signs of pregnancy.

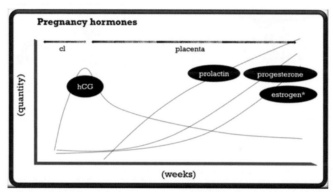

Figure 15-4: Relative quantity of pregnancy hormones by week of gestation. Early pregnancy hormones are supplied by the corpus luteum, and later source of hormones is taken over by the placenta.

TABLE 15-2   Genetic Embryology—Embryonic Structures and Their Adult Equivalents

EMBRYOLOGIC STRUCTURES	ADULT STRUCTURES EQUIVALENT
Paramesonephric (mullerian) ducts	Female internal structures (upper portion of vagina, uterus, fallopian tubes)
Mesonephric (wolffian) duct	Male internal structures (seminal vesicles, epididymis, ejaculatory ducts, ductus deferens)
Formation of male external structures (penis, prostate, scrotum) occurs via stimulation by dihydrotestosterone (DHT); 5-alpha-reductase enzyme converts testosterone to DHT	

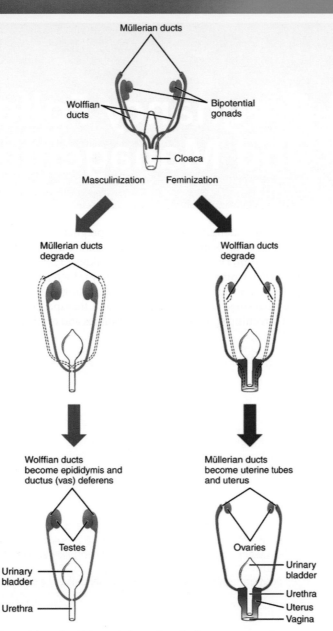

Figure 15-5: Normal male and female differentiation of mullerian structures. (Image courtesy of OpenStax College; CC BY 3.0 [https://creativecommons.org/licenses/by-sa/3.0])

16 Pregnancy Follow-Up and Management

There are several normal physiologic changes that occur during pregnancy to accommodate the developing fetus (Table 16-1). Pregnancy follow-up is important as it allows for early detection of fetal abnormalities providing the opportunity for early intervention and decision making (Tables 16-2 and 16-3). Additionally, it allows for risk stratification to determine whether the pregnancy is high or low risk, which will determine the frequency of follow-up. If an abnormality is detected on screening examination, additional interventions and procedures can be performed for both diagnostic and therapeutic purposes (Table 16-4). The more serious pathologies that screening studies detect are trisomies and erythroblastosis fetalis (Fig. 16-1).

Chorionic villus sampling and amniocentesis are being performed less and less as cell-free DNA testing improves and becomes both a screening and a diagnostic test.

Indications to give intrapartum antibiotics for group B streptococci (GBS):
- Positive GBS from urine or rectovaginal swab culture
- Previous baby with GBS neonatal infection
- Unknown screening results plus one of the following: intrapartum fever, preterm/premature rupture of membranes, preterm labor

Leopold maneuvers: physical maneuver often combined with ultrasound to determine fetal presentation. Beneficial to decrease need for cesarean section. Typically done after 32–34 weeks. Followed up by external cephalic version at 37 weeks of gestation whereby the fetus is maneuvered into a vertex position to enable vaginal delivery.
In most cases the fetus self-converts to the vertex position despite being in an abnormal delivery earlier in pregnancy.

TABLE 16-1 Normal Maternal Changes Associated With Pregnancy

Dermatologic	• Melasma • Palmar erythema • Telangiectasia • Linea nigra (dark line from umbilicus to pubis)
Pulmonary	• Increased tidal volume • Decreased total lung capacity: elevation of diaphragm secondary to gravid uterus
Cardiac	• Increased cardiac output (increased intravascular volume, stroke volume, and heart rate) • Decreased systemic vascular resistance: progesterone vasodilatory effects
Gastrointestinal	• GERD secondary to pressure from enlarging uterus • Morning sickness (nausea, vomiting)
Genitourinary	• Ureteral vasodilation: progesterone vasodilatory effects, increased risk of pyelonephritis • Urinary incontinence: gravid uterus compressing bladder
Hematologic	• Dilutional anemia • Increased RBC mass • Iron or folate deficiency: secondary to increased requirements of pregnancy • Hypercoagulable state, increased risk of thromboembolic events
Renal	• Decreased creatinine: secondary to increase GFR

GERD, Gastroesophageal reflux disease; *RBC,* red blood cell; *GFR,* glomerular filtration rate

TABLE 16-2 Trimester by Trimester Testing During Pregnancy

TRIMESTER	LAB TESTING	PURPOSE OF TESTING	INTERVENTION
First trimester	• Type and screen • Coombs testing	• Rh incompatibility in Rh-negative mothers to prevent erythroblastosis fetalis and subsequent pregnancies	• Rh immunoglobulin at 28 wk and anytime there is potential for maternal fetal blood mixing such as postprocedure (amniocentesis, chorionic villus sampling), miscarriage or abortion, and postdelivery
	• CBC	• Anemia	• Iron and/or folate supplementation to keep up with pregnancy demands
	• HIV • Syphilis • Hepatitis B • Chlamydia/gonorrhea	• Prevent vertical transmission and premature delivery	• HIV: antiretroviral therapy • Syphilis: penicillin; desensitize if penicillin allergic • Hepatitis B: antiviral therapy • Chlamydia/gonorrhea: ceftriaxone + azithromycin
	• Urinalysis and culture	• Prevent premature delivery and pyelonephritis	• Treat based on sensitivities (amoxicillin, nitrofurantoin, cephalosporins)
	• Pap smear	• Detect cervical dysplasia/malignancy	• Management based on stage of dysplasia or malignancy (see gynecology section for detailed management)
	• Rubella antibody	• Determine risk for primary rubella infection in mother and congenital rubella in fetus	• Immunize after delivery • Avoid sick contacts and settings with potential for contracting rubella
Optional first trimester testing	• PPD skin test	• Risk of TB in high-risk mother	• Treat based on active vs latent disease • Avoid streptomycin due to risk of ototoxicity in fetus
	• Fetal nuchal translucency, pregnancy-associated plasma protein A (PAPP-A), beta-hCG	• Early aneuploidy screening in high-risk mothers	• Confirmatory with chorionic villus sampling
Second trimester	• Quad screen: aFP, beta-hCG, estriol, inhibin-A • Increasingly common alternative to quad screen is maternal testing of cell-free DNA	• Differentiate between trisomy 13/18/21 • Evaluate for neural tube defects	• Confirm correct dating by ultrasound as most common cause of elevated aFP is incorrect dating • Amniocentesis for further evaluation and confirmation via karyotyping and acetylcholinesterase activity • Offer all options to mother including early termination • Mentally and physically prepare mother for potentially ill newborn
Third trimester	• Screening: 1-hr oral glucose tolerance test (OGTT) • Confirmatory: 3-hr OGTT	• Gestational diabetes	• Oral antihyperglycemics (metformin) +/− insulin
	• CBC	• Anemia	• Iron and/or folate supplementation
	• Rectal and vaginal culture at 35–37 wk	• Screen for group B streptococci if negative from urinalysis and culture from first semester • Group B streptococci associated with high risk of neonatal sepsis, pneumonia, and meningitis	• Intrapartum antibiotics (penicillin, ampicillin)

Rh, Rhesus; *PPD*, purified protein derivative; *hCG*, human chorionic gonadotropin; *AFP*, alpha-fetoprotein; *CBC*, complete blood count; *HIV*, human immunodeficiency virus

TABLE 16-3   Interpretation of Second Trimester Fetal Testing

	AFP	BETA-HCG	ESTRIOL	INHIBIN-A
Down syndrome	Increased	Increased	Decreased	Increased
Edwards	Decreased	Decreased	Decreased	Normal
Patau	-	-	-	-
Neural tube defects, ventricle wall defects, twins, renal disease	Increased	Normal	Normal	Normal

HCG, Human chorionic gonadotropin; *AFP,* alpha-fetoprotein

TABLE 16-4   Interventions During Pregnancy

PROCEDURE	PURPOSES
Chorionic villus sampling	• Invasive obstetric procedure where fluid is sampled from chorionic villi • Performed in the first trimester • Used to sample fetal cells for diagnostic purposes (karyotyping, FISH) of congenital disorder when screening tests (quad screen, cell-free DNA) are positive • Risk of fetal loss
Amniocentesis	• Invasive obstetric procedure where fluid is sampled from amniotic fluid • Performed in the second trimester • Used to sample fetal cells for diagnostic purposes (karyotyping, FISH, alpha-fetoprotein, acetylcholinesterase activity) of congenital disorder when screening tests (quad screen, cell-free DNA) are positive • Risk of fetal loss, injury, rupture of membranes
Ultrasound	• Safe, noninvasive procedure • Determining gestational age; earlier ultrasound allows for greater accuracy • Fetal dimensions
Transcranial Doppler	• Highly sensitive test to determine presence of fetal anemia • Increased intracranial blood flow is indicative of low hemoglobin and thus fetal anemia
Percutaneous umbilical blood sampling	• Ultrasound-guided sampling of umbilical vein • Directly samples fetal blood allowing for both diagnostic (karyotyping, antibody testing) and therapeutic interventions (transfusion for fetal anemia)

FISH, Fluorescence in situ hybridization

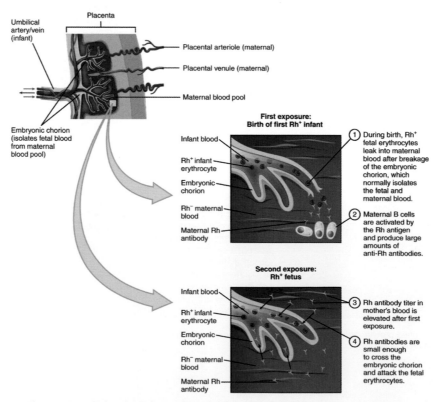

Figure 16-1: Pathophysiology of erythroblastosis fetalis from Rh sensitization.
(Image courtesy of OpenStax College.)

CHAPTER 17 Abnormal Fertilization and Implantation

TWINNING

Twin pregnancy principles

- Dizygotic twins occur when two different sperm fertilize two different eggs (Table 17-1)
- Dizygotic twins will always have two separate amniotic sacs and two placentas (chorion)
- Monozygotic twins occur when one sperm fertilizes one egg, which then splits into two zygotes during early pregnancy
- The number of amniotic sacs and placentas in monozygotic twins depends on when the fertilized egg splits into two cycles; as a principal, earlier splitting results in more placenta and more amnion, and later splitting results in a fewer number of placenta and amnion (Fig. 17-1)
- Splitting after implantation of the zygote will always only have one placenta
- Will present with uterus larger than dates, significantly elevated beta-human chorionic gonadotropin (beta-hCG)

ABNORMAL FERTILIZATION

Klinefelter Syndrome

- XXY karyotype, male phenotype
- Associated conditions
  - Neuropsychiatric
    - Learning disabilities
    - Behavioral disorders
    - Depression
  - Musculoskeletal
    - Slipped capital femoral epiphysis
    - Slim physique with long limbs
  - Gynecologic
    - Breast cancer
    - Gynecomastia
    - Gynecoid appearance
  - Reproductive
    - Infertility
    - Hypogonadism
  - Cardiac: mitral valve prolapse

Turner Syndrome

- XO karyotype, female phenotype
- Associated conditions
  - Cardiac
    - Bicuspid aortic valve
    - Coarctation of the aorta
  - Reproductive
    - Streak ovaries
    - Lack of secondary female sex characteristics
  - Musculoskeletal
    - Short stature
    - Webbed neck
    - Broad chest with widely spaced nipples
    - Cubitus valgus
  - Endocrine: hypothyroidism
  - Renal

TABLE 17-1   Differentiating Types of Twinning

DAY OF ZYGOTE SPLITTING	NUMBER OF CHORIONS AND AMNIONS	COMPLICATIONS	TREATMENT/ PREVENTION
Day 0–4	Dichorionic, diamniotic	None	-
Day 4–8 (after implantation)	Monochorionic, diamniotic	Twin-twin transfusion reaction: donor twin risk receives less blood supply and is delivered anemic and growth restricted However, has overall better outcome Recipient twin receives more blood resulting in excessive growth and polycythemia, however, results in poor outcome	Laser ablation of placental anastomoses in severe cases
Day 8–12	Monochorionic, monoamniotic	Umbilical cord entanglement	Close monitoring of fetal heart tracings for presence of variable decelerations
After day 13	Monochorionic, monoamniotic	Conjoined twins, no twinning	Separation surgery once able to tolerate depending on the conjoined body part

- Horseshoe kidney
- Double renal pelvis

Molar Pregnancy
- Definition: gestational trophoblastic disease resulting in abnormal proliferation of trophoblastic tissue and nonviable fetus
- Subtypes
  - Complete (46,XX)
  - Incomplete (69,XXY)
- Signs and symptoms

Preeclampsia is typically a disease of the third trimester, therefore its presence prior to that is concerning for hydatidiform mole.

- Vaginal bleeding
- Passage of grapelike vesicles from the vagina
- Uterus larger than dates
- Related to elevated beta-hCG (hyperemesis gravidarum, hyperthyroidism)
- Preeclampsia <20 weeks of gestation
- Diagnostics
  - Ultrasound: snowstorm appearance, theca-lutein cysts
  - Absence of fetal heart tones
- Management: suction curettage
- Complications: choriocarcinoma (higher risk with complete hydatidiform mole)
- Follow up: 1 year of contraception with serial monitoring of beta-hCG to evaluate for development of choriocarcinoma

Choriocarcinoma
- Risk factors

Contraception is important during the first year after treatment of hydatidiform mole as pregnancy during the first year will prevent detection of choriocarcinoma as both will cause rise in beta-hCG.

Consequences of significantly elevated beta-hCG: hyperemesis gravidarum, preeclampsia, hyperthyroidism, theca lutein cysts

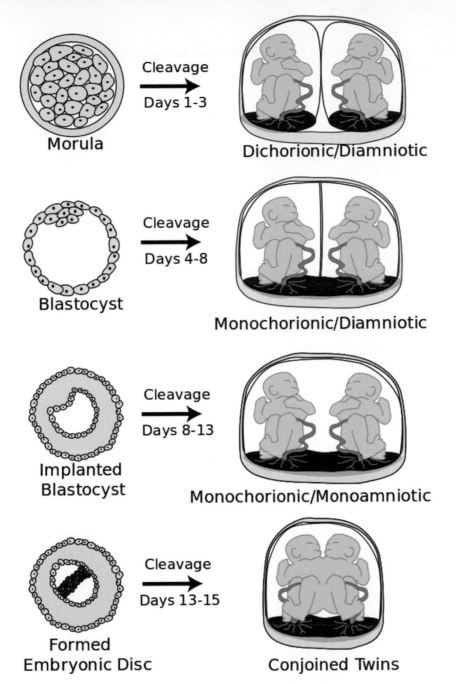

Figure 17-1: Summary of placentation in the formation of twins and the effect of cleavage on the number of placentas and amniotic sacs. (Image courtesy of Dufendach, K. [Artist].)

- Prior molar pregnancy
- Normal pregnancy
- Post miscarriage, abortion, ectopic pregnancy
- Advanced maternal age
- Signs and symptoms: similar to hydatidiform mole plus signs of metastases
  - Cough, hemoptysis, chest pain: lung metastases (most common site of spread)
  - Headache, dizziness, visual disturbances: central nervous system metastases
  - Right upper quadrant abdominal pain: liver metastasis
- Diagnostics
  - Plateau or rising beta-hCG after treatment of molar pregnancy
  - Pelvic ultrasound: necrotic, hemorrhagic uterine mass +/− parametrial invasion
  - Computed tomography chest, abdomen, and pelvis for staging

- Management: chemotherapy

Ectopic Pregnancy

- Risk factors
  - History of pelvic inflammatory disease (Neisseria/chlamydia infection)
  - Prior tubal surgery
  - Anatomic uterine deformities
  - Previous ectopic pregnancy
  - Intrauterine device
  - In vitro fertilization
  - Signs and symptoms
  - Lower-quadrant abdominal pain
  - Nausea, vomiting
  - Amenorrhea
  - Vaginal bleeding
  - +/– adnexal mass
- Diagnostics
  - Transvaginal ultrasound: absent intrauterine gestational sac, adnexal mass
  - Slow rising beta-hCG
- Management: depends on acuity and beta-hCG levels
  - Unruptured ectopic pregnancy
    - Methotrexate
      - Beta-hCG <5000
      - <5-cm pregnancy
      - Absence of fetal heart tones
    - Laparoscopic salpingostomy/salpingectomy: if parameters for methotrexate use not met
  - Ruptured ectopic pregnancy (hypotension, tachycardia, peritoneal signs): emergent laparotomy with salpingectomy

---

Most common location of ectopic pregnancy is the ampulla of the fallopian tubes.

18 Fetal Monitoring

Fetal heart tracings are used to determine presence of fetal distress so that they may be addressed by treating the underlying issue or delivering the baby.

Nonstress Test
- Principles
  - Transducer measures both maternal contractions and fetal heart rate
  - Appropriate rise and timing of fetal heart rate is termed a reactive nonstress test; inappropriate rise and timing of fetal heart rate (accelerations) is termed a nonreactive nonstress test (Table 18-1; Fig. 18-1)
  - Accelerations in fetal heart rate are indicative of fetal movement
- Indications: high-risk pregnancy due to fetal or maternal comorbidities
  - Fetal
    - Hypoxia
    - Acidemia
    - Decreased fetal movements
  - Maternal
    - Chronic medical conditions (hyper/hypothyroidism, diabetes, hypertension)
    - Previous fetal demise
    - Fetal growth restriction
- Interpretation
  - Reactive
    - Baseline heart rate 100–160 beats per minute
    - Moderate variability in fetal heart rate (6–25 beats per minute)
    - More than two accelerations in 20 minutes with rise in heart rate >15 beats per minute above baseline lasting >15 seconds
  - Nonreactive: criteria for reactive not met; should be followed up with biophysical profile

Most common cause of lack of accelerations during nonstress test is fetal sleep, therefore testing should be extended to ensure fetal activity is monitored outside the sleep cycle. The fetus can be awoken using vibroacoustic stimulation.

Biophysical Profile
- Principles: extensive testing performed in high-risk pregnancies to evaluate for fetal complications before they occur and in cases of nonreactive nonstress test
- Specific indications
  - Previous unexplained fetal demise
  - Diabetic mothers
  - Chronic hypertension
- Five components of biophysical profile
  - Nonstress test
  - Amniotic fluid volume
  - Fetal breathing
  - Fetal movement
  - Fetal tone (flexion/extension)
- Interpretation: each component of the biophysical profile is given a score of 0 or 2 (maximum score of 10, minimal score 0), depending if it is normal or abnormal
  - 8–10: normal
  - 6: equivocal, closer fetal monitoring
  - <4: immediate delivery

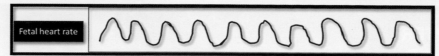

Figure 18-1: Various patterns of fetal heart rate tracings in response to maternal contractions (contraction stress test).

TABLE 18-1   Fetal Heart Tracing Categories

CATEGORIES	FEATURES
Category I	• Normal fetal heart tracing • Normal baseline heart rate • Moderate variability, no variable or late decelerations
Category II	• Unequivocal fetal heart tracing • +/− variable or late deceleration • +/− fetal bradycardia or tachycardia • +/− minimal variability
Category III	• Abnormal fetal heart tracing • Multiple and recurrent late or variable decelerations • Persistent fetal tachycardia or bradycardia • Sinusoidal (fetal anemia) (Fig. 18-2)

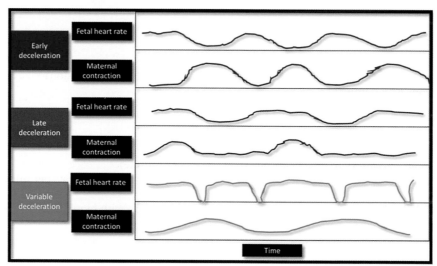

Figure 18-2: Sinusoidal pattern of fetal heart rate tracing seen in fetal anemia.

Contraction Stress Test
– Principles
  • Transducer is placed on mother and fetus visualizing the fetal heart rate in response to maternal contractions
  • Fetal heart rate is evaluated in response to maternal contractions, therefore contraction stress test is typically only performed during labor
  • Contraction stress test may be simulated with IV oxytocin; however, not routinely done
  • Fetal heart rate should decrease and then return to baseline in conjunction with maternal contractions and relaxations
– Interpretation
  • Early decelerations
    ▪ Gradual decrease in heart rate occurs simultaneously with maternal uterine contractions
    ▪ Overall reassuring
    ▪ Secondary to fetal head compression and vagal stimulation
  • Variable decelerations
    ▪ Rapid decrease in fetal heart rate occurring irrespective of maternal contractions
    ▪ Secondary to umbilical cord compression
    ▪ Multiple variable decelerations indicative of fetal distress and acidosis

- Late decelerations
  - Gradual decrease in heart rate occurring after uterine contractions
  - Secondary to uteroplacental insufficiency
  - Indicative of fetal distress and acidosis

Causes of fetal bradycardia:
- Beta blockers
- Local anesthetics
- Neonatal heart block (maternal lupus)

Abruptio Placentae
– Definition: separation of placenta from uterine wall (Fig. 19-1)
– Risk factors
  • Trauma
  • Maternal drug use (cocaine, tobacco)
  • Hypertension/preeclampsia/eclampsia
  • Previous abruptio placentae
  • Submucosal fibroids
– Key manifestations
  • Maternal
    • Severe lower abdominal/back pain
    • Hypertonic, high-frequency, low-intensity uterine contractions
    • Painful third trimester bleeding (hemorrhage may be concealed)
  • Fetus
    • Oligohydramnios
    • Tachycardia
    • Hypoxia
– Diagnostics
  • Clinical
  • Ultrasound: retroplacental hematoma; rules out placenta previa
– Management: delivery
– Complications: disseminated intravascular coagulation

Placenta Previa
– Definition: abnormal implantation of placenta at or near the cervical os (Fig. 19-2)
– Risk factors
  • Previous cesarean section
  • Multiparity
  • Prior placenta previa
  • Uterine fibroids
  • Smoking
  • Advanced maternal age

Painful third trimester bleeding: think abruptio placentae, uterine rupture
Painless third trimester bleeding: think placenta previa, vasa previa

– Subtypes
  • Complete: cervical os completely covered
  • Incomplete: cervical os partially covered
  • Marginal: placenta near cervical os
– Signs and symptoms: painless third trimester bleeding
– Diagnostics
  • If suspected, transabdominal ultrasound followed by transvaginal ultrasound
  • No intercourse or speculum examination
– Management
  • Commonly resolves prior to labor; however, if present at term will necessitate elective cesarean section
  • Pelvic rest, no intercourse

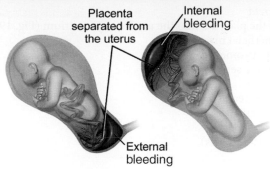

Placenta
separated from
the uterus

Internal
bleeding

External
bleeding

Figure 19-1: Diagrammatic representation of abruptio placentae and its two types of presentations. (Image courtesy of Blausen Medical.)

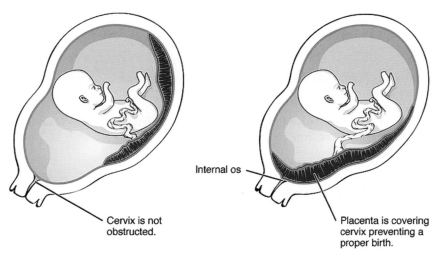

Internal os

Cervix is not
obstructed.

Placenta is covering
cervix preventing a
proper birth.

Normal location of placenta   **Placenta previa**

Figure 19-2: Diagrammatic representation of placenta previa versus normal placentation.

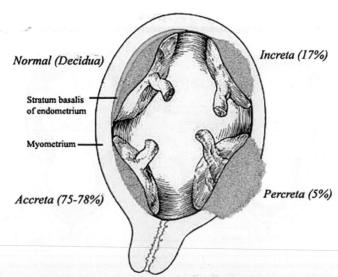

Normal (Decidua)

Stratum basalis
of endometrium

Myometrium

Increta (17%)

Accreta (75-78%)

Percreta (5%)

Figure 19-3: Diagrammatic representation of the three subtypes of abnormal placental penetration into the uterine myometrium and the frequency at which they occur by percentage.

Placenta Accreta/Increta/Percreta
- Definition: penetration of the placenta into the uterine myometrium (Fig. 19-3)
  - Accreta: attaches to superficial myometrium
  - Increta: penetrates deep myometrium
  - Percreta: penetrates uterine serosa
- Risk factors
  - Previous uterine scar (cesarean section)
  - Previous dilation and curettage
  - Placenta previa
  - Advanced maternal age (>35 years)
- Signs and symptoms
  - Retained placenta
  - Prolonged delivery of placenta
  - Postpartum hemorrhage
- Diagnostics: antenatal ultrasound (irregularity/absence of placental myometrial interface; intraplacental villous lakes)
- Management
  - Monitoring, transfusion as needed, maternal stabilization
  - Uterine massage, IV oxytocin
  - Cesarean hysterectomy for uncontrollable bleeding

Vasa Previa
- Definition: crossing of umbilical vessels over the cervical os resulting in rupture of umbilical vessels upon rupture of membranes (Fig. 19-4)
- Risk factors
  - Velamentous cord insertion (umbilical cord inserts into the fetal membranes and travels to the placenta unprotected by Wharton jelly)
  - Multiple gestations
  - Accessory placental lobe

Avoid amniotomy if vasa previa is suspected as it may result in injury to traversing fetal vessels.

- Signs and symptoms
  - Painless vaginal bleeding
  - Membrane rupture
  - Fetal bradycardia +/− exsanguination
  - Sinusoidal fetal heart tracing
- Diagnostic: antenatal ultrasound
- Management
  - Premembrane rupture: close monitoring, elective cesarean section
  - Postmembrane rupture: emergency cesarean section plus packed red blood cell transfusion

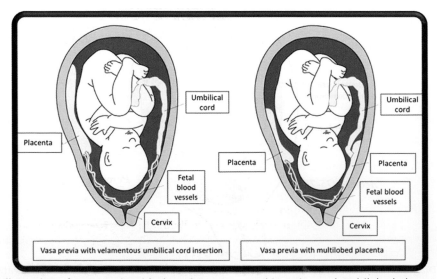

Figure 19-4: Illustration of vasa previa with the velamentous cord insertion and multilobed placenta. (Modified Image courtesy of www.vasaprevia.nl, Sigrid de Rooij.)

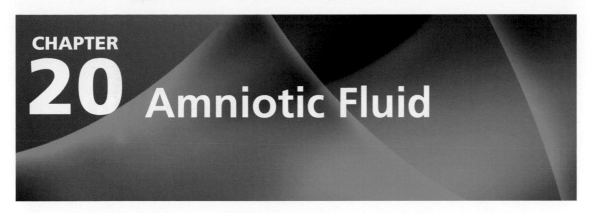

CHAPTER 20 Amniotic Fluid

The evaluation of amniotic fluid is important as it is used to assess for the presence of polyhydramnios or oligohydramnios (Table 20-1). Each of these findings is associated with underlying fetal anomalies, most commonly gastrointestinal abnormalities in oligohydramnios and renal abnormalities in oligohydramnios. Furthermore, oligohydramnios may be associated with both fetal and maternal complications.

Potter syndrome
- Renal agenesis results in decreased production of amniotic fluid.
- Amniotic fluid is inspired by the growing fetus to promote lung development, therefore lack of amniotic fluid results in pulmonary hypoplasia.
- Amniotic fluid protects growing fetus from compression against uterine wall, therefore lack of amniotic fluid results in restricted fetal movement and physical deformities known as Potter facies (hypertelorism, epicanthal folds, low-set ears, compressed flat nose).

TABLE 20-1   Polyhydramnios Versus Oligohydramnios

	POLYHYDRAMNIOS	OLIGOHYDRAMNIOS
Definition	• Excess amniotic fluid	• Insufficient amniotic fluid
Causes	• Idiopathic: most common cause • Gastrointestinal abnormalities (T-E fistula, duodenal/jejunal atresia, annular pancreas) • Forebrain anomalies (anencephaly) • Congenital diaphragmatic hernia (external esophageal compression) • Neural tube defects • Maternal hyperglycemia (fetal osmotic diuresis) • Fetal anemia • Multiple gestations • Twin-twin transfusion syndrome	• Renal abnormalities (renal agenesis, posterior urethral valves, autosomal recessive polycystic kidney disease) • Uteroplacental insufficiency • Preeclampsia • Postterm pregnancy • Premature rupture of membranes
Signs and symptoms	• Uterus larger than dates	• Uterus smaller than dates
Diagnostics	• Amniotic fluid index* >25 cm	• Amniotic fluid index* <5 cm
Complications	• Premature birth • Premature rupture of membranes • Uterine atony (secondary to overdistention) • Stillbirth • Preeclampsia • Cord prolapse	• Potter syndrome • Developmental dysplasia of the hip • Congenital muscular torticollis

*The amniotic fluid index divides the maternal abdomen into four quadrants and measures depth of amniotic fluid in each quadrant via ultrasound.

CHAPTER 21 Perinatal Infections

All congenital infections present with nonspecific symptoms such as jaundice, lymphadenopathy, hepatosplenomegaly, intrauterine growth restriction, and blueberry muffin spots.

TORCHS infections:

- Toxoplasma
- Other (varicella-zoster virus [VZV], parvovirus, listeria)
- Rubella
- Cytomegalovirus (CMV)
- Herpes/human immunodeficiency virus (HIV)/hepatitis
- Syphilis

Toxoplasmosis

- Microbiology: *Toxoplasma gondi*
- Risk factors
  - Cat feces
  - Uncooked meat
- Signs and symptoms
  - Chorioretinitis
  - Intracranial calcifications
  - Seizures
  - Microcephaly
- Diagnostics
  - Mother: toxoplasma immunoglobulin M (IgM)/IgG
  - Fetus: amniocentesis for toxoplasma DNA polymerase chain reaction (PCR)
- Management
  - Spiramycin: treats maternal disease, without evidence of fetal disease
  - Pyrimethamine/sulfadiazine + leucovorin: treats fetal disease

VZV

- Microbiology: human herpesvirus 3 (HHV-3) (DNA virus)
- Risk factors: primary maternal varicella infection
- Signs and symptoms
  - Mother
    - Erythematous, vesicular rash
    - Pneumonia
    - Encephalitis
  - Neonate
    - Limb hypoplasia
    - Cicatricial (scarring, zigzag) skin lesions
    - Microcephaly, microphthalmia
    - Seizures, chorioretinitis
- Diagnostics
  - Clinical
  - DNA PCR from vesicular lesions
- Management
  - Maternal
    - Pre/postpregnancy: live attenuated VZV vaccine
    - Postexposure prophylaxis: VZV immunoglobulin
    - Uncomplicated infection: oral acyclovir

- Isolation from fetus if active lesions are present
- Neonates: IV acyclovir +/− VZV immunoglobulin (if disease occurs between 5 days prior to delivery and 2 days postpartum)

Reactivation of varicella-zoster virus resulting in congenital varicella syndrome typically occurs anywhere from 5 days prior to delivery to 2 days postpartum.

Parvovirus
- Microbiology: parvovirus B19 (DNA virus)
- Risk factors: primary maternal infection
- Signs and symptoms
  - Mother: self-limiting arthritis
  - Neonatal
    - Hydrops fetalis
    - High-output cardiac failure
    - Anemia (cytotoxic to erythroid progenitor cells), thrombocytopenia
- Diagnostics
  - Maternal parvovirus IgM antibodies
  - Transcranial Doppler: monitor for fetal anemia
- Management: symptomatic
  - Transfuse as needed via percutaneous umbilical blood sampling
  - Drain pleural effusions and ascites

Listeriosis
- Microbiology: Listeria monocytogenes (gram-positive rod, tumbling motility)
- Risk factors
  - Deli meats
  - Goat cheese
  - Dairy products
- Signs and symptoms
  - Maternal: mild gastroenteritis
  - Neonate
    - Diffuse granulomas with microabscesses
    - Meningitis
    - Sepsis
    - Chorioamnionitis, spontaneous abortion, placental lesions
- Diagnostics: neonatal cerebrospinal fluid/blood cultures
- Management
  - Mother: supportive care
  - Neonate: IV ampicillin + gentamicin for the neonate

Rubella
- Microbiology: togaviridae (single-stranded RNA virus)
- Risk factors: primary maternal rubella infection
- Signs and symptoms
  - Maternal
    - Rash
    - Arthritis
  - Neonates
    - Patent ductus arteriosus
    - Cataracts
    - Congenital deafness
    - Intellectual disability
- Diagnostics: maternal rubella IgM antibodies
- Management
  - Mother: measles-mumps-rubella live attenuated vaccine before or after pregnancy
  - Neonates: supportive care

CMV
- Epidemiology: most common congenital viral infection
- Microbiology: CMV (HHV-5, DNA virus)

- Signs and symptoms
  - Mother: asymptomatic +/– mononucleosis-like syndrome
  - Fetus
    - Periventricular calcifications
    - Hearing loss: most common cause of congenital deafness
    - Chorioretinitis
    - Interstitial pneumonitis
    - Fetal hydrops
- Diagnostics
  - Maternal CMV IgG/IgM antibodies
  - Antenatal ultrasound determines severity of infection
- Management: ganciclovir (reduces neurologic sequelae)

Herpes
- Microbiology: herpes simplex virus (HSV) (DNA virus)
- Signs and symptoms
  - Mother
    - Vesicular, erythematous rash
    - Prodromal numbness/tingling
  - Neonate
    - Skin/mucous membranes: vesicular lesions, conjunctivitis
    - Central nervous system
      - Meningoencephalitis
      - Hydrocephalus
      - Lethargy, irritability
    - Pneumonia
    - Hepatitis
- Diagnostics
  - Clinical
  - HSV PCR
- Management: prevent genital herpes at the time of delivery to allow for vaginal delivery and prevent vertical transmission
  - Mother
    - Acyclovir: indicated for the following scenarios
      - Suppressive therapy starting at 36 weeks until time to deliver
      - Primary infection prior to delivery
    - Cesarean section: if active lesions present at time of delivery
  - Neonate
    - Asymptomatic: monitoring +/– prophylactic acyclovir depending on maternal history of HSV and presence of active lesions
    - Symptomatic: IV acyclovir

HIV
- Microbiology: HIV (retrovirus)
- Risk factors
  - IV drug abuse
  - Promiscuous sexual activity (multiple partners, unprotected sex)
- Signs and symptoms: asymptomatic
- Diagnostics
  - Mother: HIV antibody +/– RNA PCR
  - Fetus: HIV RNA PCR
    - Do not test for HIV antibodies immediately after birth in the fetus born to mother who is HIV positive as results will be positive due to transplacental transmission
    - Repeat testing with PCR should be done at 3 weeks, 6 weeks, 6 months
- Management: prevent vertical transmission
  - Mother
    - Known HIV prior to pregnancy: continue highly active antiretroviral therapy (HAART) (only efavirenz is teratogenic)
    - Diagnosed during antenatal testing: initiate HAART
    - Cesarean section if viral load is >1000 copies/mL and low CD4 count
    - Avoid breastfeeding
  - Fetus: intrapartum zidovudine (if high risk) plus 6 weeks after delivery

90% of vertical transmission rate of hepatitis B in actively infected mothers

Hepatitis B
- Microbiology: hepatitis B (DNA virus)
- Risk factors
  - Unprotected sex
  - Needlestick
- Signs and symptoms: asymptomatic
- Diagnostics: antenatal testing in mother
  - Hepatitis B surface antigen
  - If hepatitis B surface antigen positive, check the following
    - Hepatitis B core antibody
    - Hepatitis B e-antigen
    - Hepatitis B surface antibody
- Management: immunoprophylaxis in fetus
  - Hepatitis B immunoglobulin within 12 hours of birth
  - Hepatitis B vaccination at birth, 1 month, and 6 months

Syphilis
- Microbiology: Treponema pallidum (gram-negative spirochete)
- Risk factors: multiple sexual partners
- Signs and symptoms
  - Neonate to 2 years old
    - Desquamation of palms and soles
    - Snuffles (copious mucopurulent rhinorrhea)
    - Periostitis, osteochondritis
    - Interstitial keratitis, photophobia
    - Nonimmune hydrops fetalis
  - >2 years old
    - Hutchinson teeth
    - Cranial nerve VIII palsy
    - Saber shins
    - Frontal bossing, saddlenose
    - Rhagades (fissures at the corners of the mouth)
    - Mulberry molar (rounded enamel cusps)
- Diagnostics: antenatal or neonatal testing
  - Venereal Disease Research Laboratory/rapid plasma reagin
  - Antitreponemal antibodies
- Management: penicillin

If syphilis is diagnosed during antenatal testing in mother, treatment is with penicillin regardless of allergies. If mother is allergic to penicillin, treatment is to desensitize mother as alternative treatments (doxycycline) are contraindicated in pregnancy.

CHAPTER 22 Teratogens

The use of teratogenic medications is often a risk-benefit assessment for the mother and health care provider who must determine whether the benefit of the teratogenic medication outweighs the potential fetal harm it may cause. These medications are categorized from category A (safest) to category X (most harmful, absolute contraindication), with categories B, C, and D drugs considered to have unknown fetal effects or relative contraindications (Table 22-1).

Differentiating between symmetric and asymmetric intrauterine growth restriction is important as it allows the health care provider to narrow the differential as to the etiology of the growth restriction (Table 22-2).

TABLE 22-1 Teratogenic Medications

MEDICATIONS	ASSOCIATIONS
ACE inhibitors, ARBs	• Renal agenesis
Carbamazepine	• Neural tube defects • Genitourinary abnormality • Facial dysmorphism
Chloramphenicol	• Gray baby syndrome
Diethylstilbestrol	• Vaginal adenosis • Vaginal clear cell carcinoma • T-shaped uterus
Fluoroquinolone	• Cartilaginous defects
Isotretinoin	• Microtia (small ears) • Congenital deafness • Cardiac defects (heart and great vessels)
Lithium	• Ebstein anomaly (downward displacement of tricuspid valve)
NSAIDs	• Premature closure of PDA
Phenytoin	• Craniofacial abnormalities (cleft lip/palate, depressed nasal bridge, epicanthal folds, microcephaly) • Nail hypoplasia • Intellectual disability
Streptomycin	• Cranial nerve VIII palsy
Tetracyclines	• Bone abnormalities • Teeth discoloration
Thalidomide	• Phocomelia, limb reduction defects
Valproic acid	• Neural tube defects • Cleft lip • Cardiac defects
Warfarin	• Chondrodysplasia • Lamp/nail hypoplasia • Optic atrophy
Substance Abuse	
Alcohol	• Intellectual disability: most common cause of preventable intellectual disability • Microphthalmia • Short palpebral fissures • Long philtrum • Midfacial hypoplasia

Continued

TABLE 22-1   Teratogenic Medications—Cont'd

MEDICATIONS	ASSOCIATIONS
Cocaine	• Placental abruption • IUGR • Preterm delivery • Intraventricular hemorrhage
Marijuana	• Small for gestational age • Neurobehavioral abnormalities
Opioids	• Neonatal abstinence syndrome (seizures, high-pitched cry, irritability, feeding difficulties)

ACE, Angiotensin-converting enzyme; *ARB*, angiotensin receptor blocker; *PDA*, patent ductus arteriosus; *NSAIDs*, non-steroidal anti-inflammatory drugs; *IUGR*, intrauterine growth restriction.

TABLE 22-2   Intrauterine Growth Restriction: Symmetric Versus Asymmetric

SYMMETRIC	ASYMMETRIC
All fetal measurements are decreased	Some fetal measurements are decreased, others remain normal (head-sparing)
Caused by intrinsic fetal abnormalities	Caused by maternal or placental abnormalities resulting in decreased placental perfusion
Examples: aneuploidy, congenital defects, TORCH infections	Examples: uncontrolled maternal medical conditions, substance abuse, twin-twin transfusion, placental abruption

TORCH, Toxoplasmosis, other agents, rubella, cytomegalovirus, and herpes simplex.

Differentiating the type and subtypes of abortion using both physical exam and ultrasound allows the health care provider to predict the likely eventual outcome and thus guide management (Table 23-1).

Recurrent Pregnancy Loss
- Definition: three consecutive pregnancy losses

Abortion vs fetal demise: abortion is loss of fetus before <20 weeks vs >20 weeks in fetal demise.
Overview of abortion management:
- Expectant management for spontaneous abortion if <14 weeks of gestation
- Medical abortion if <70 days gestation
- Dilation and evacuation (D&E) or medical induction for second trimester fetal loss

---

- Causes
  - Antiphospholipid syndrome
  - Parental chromosomal abnormalities (i.e., Robertsonian translocation)
  - Luteal phase defect (inadequate progesterone levels)
  - Anatomic uterine abnormalities (congenital, fibroids, endometrial polyps)
  - Cervical insufficiency: most commonly associated with recurrent second trimester pregnancy loss
  - Thrombophilia
  - Diabetes, hypothyroidism, hyperprolactinemia
- Diagnostics
  - Karyotype
  - Antinuclear antibody, anticardiolipin antibody, lupus anticoagulant
  - Factor V Leiden mutation, antithrombin III, protein C/S, prothrombin G20210A mutation
  - Hysterosalpingogram +/− hysteroscopy
  - Transvaginal ultrasound (evaluate cervical insufficiency)
  - Thyroid-stimulating hormone, hemoglobin A1c, prolactin levels
- Management: correct underlying etiology; however, in most cases no underlying etiology is identified
  - Antiphospholipid syndrome: heparin + warfarin
  - Parental chromosomal abnormalities: genetic counseling +/− in vitro fertilization
  - Cervical insufficiency: cerclage + progesterone
  - Uterine abnormalities: surgical correction
  - Thrombophilia: anticoagulation
  - Optimize management of underlying medical condition (hypothyroidism, diabetes, hyperprolactinemia)

TABLE 23-1   Types of Abortion Differentiated Based on Presence/Absence of Parts of Conception and Dilation/Closure of Cervix

TYPE	SUBTYPES	FEATURES	MANAGEMENT
Induced abortion		• Vaginal bleeding • Passage of clots • Uterine contractions	Surgical evacuation, pain control (nonsteroidal antiinflammatory drug, local anesthetic, paracervical block +/− sedation), and prophylactic doxycycline (prevents perioperative endometritis) OR Medical abortion (misoprostol plus mifepristone) if <70 days gestation
Spontaneous abortion	Complete	• Most commonly occurs in first trimester secondary to fetal chromosomal abnormalities • Cervix closed • Products of conception absent	No management
	Threatened	• Cervix closed • Products of conception present • Intrauterine bleeding	Observation
	Incomplete	• Cervix dilated • Products of conception present (some products would have already been passed)	Expectant management or surgical aspiration or medical abortion
	Inevitable	• Cervix dilated • Products of conception present	
	Missed	• Nonviable intrauterine pregnancy	
	Septic	• Fever, chills, uterine tenderness after abortion	Surgical evacuation PLUS antibiotics (second-generation cephalosporin plus doxycycline)

Spontaneous abortions can be viewed as a spectrum with increasing likelihood of fetal loss: threatened → inevitable → incomplete → complete/missed.

Recognizing and treating maternal medical disorders (Table 24-1) prior to pregnancy is important as it allows the health provider time to optimize medical management to ensure a successful pregnancy. Additionally, certain medications used for the treatment of adult medical disorders may be teratogenic, and, therefore, this allows the opportunity to find a nonteratogenic alternative or to weigh the risks and benefits of continuing with the current teratogenic medication.

TABLE 24-1 Chronic Maternal Medical Disorders by Organ System

MEDICAL CONDITION		PREGNANCY ISSUES	MANAGEMENT
Cardiac	Hypertension	• Progesterone-induced vasodilation decreases blood pressure • Common medications used in nonpregnancy (ACE inhibitors, ARBs, diuretics) are contraindicated in pregnancy	• Hydralazine • Alpha-methyldopa • Labetalol • Nifedipine
	Valvular/septal defects	• Increased intravascular volume results in increased flow across septal and valvular defects	• Women with right-to-left shunts develop increased hypoxia and have high mortality rates, and therefore are encouraged to avoid pregnancy • Valvular defects such as mitral or pulmonary stenosis may require valvuloplasty to keep up with increased demands of pregnancy and prevent CHF (mitral stenosis)
Endocrine	Diabetes mellitus	• Human placental lactogen results in relative insulin resistance • Limited oral antihyperglycemic options • Uncontrolled diabetes associated with fetal malformations	• Metformin, glyburide • Insulin
	Hyperthyroidism	• Radioactive iodine ablation contraindicated • Uncontrolled hyperthyroidism associated with fetal loss	• PTU in first trimester • Methimazole in second/third trimester • Both PTU and methimazole cross the placenta and can cause fetal goiter
	Hypothyroidism	• Increased thyroid-binding globulin results in decreased free thyroxine levels • Uncontrolled hypothyroidism associated with intellectual disability and growth retardation	• Increase levothyroxine dose by 25%

TABLE 24-1 Chronic Maternal Medical Disorders by Organ System

MEDICAL CONDITION		PREGNANCY ISSUES	MANAGEMENT
Neurologic	Seizures	• Most antiepileptics are contraindicated in pregnancy	• Consider discontinuing or tapering depending on severity of seizures • Transition to less teratogenic alternative (lamotrigine, levetiracetam) or monotherapy
Psychiatric	Schizophrenia Bipolar Depression	• Lithium results in Ebstein anomaly	• SSRIs, first-generation antipsychotics, second-generation antipsychotics remain safe in pregnancy
Hematologic	Thromboembolism	• Warfarin contraindicated	• Low-molecular-weight heparin • Switch to unfractionated heparin prior to delivery as its shorter half-life decreases risk of epidural hematoma
Rheumatologic	SLE	• Anti-Ro and anti-La antibodies associated with neonatal heart block • Recurrent pregnancy loss concerning for antiphospholipid syndrome	• Pacemaker for neonatal heart block • Cyclophosphamide and methotrexate contraindicated
Renal	Chronic kidney disease	• Increased GFR increases creatinine clearance	• Normalization of creatinine may be sign of preeclampsia

PTU, Propylthiouracil; *SLE*, systemic lupus erythematosus; *SSRI*, selective serotonin reuptake inhibitors

Both hydatidiform mole and multiple gestations result in hyperemesis gravidarum due to causing significantly elevated beta-human chorionic gonadotropin.

Hyperemesis Gravidarum
- Definition: severe form of morning sickness unresponsive to antiemetics lasting past the first trimester
- Risk factors
  - Hydatidiform mole: related to significantly elevated beta-human chorionic gonadotropin
  - Multiple gestations
  - Gastroesophageal reflux disease
- Signs and symptoms
  - Severe nausea, vomiting
  - >5% prepregnancy weight loss
  - Severe dehydration (hypotension, tachycardia, dry mucous membranes)
  - Wernicke encephalopathy
- Diagnostics
  - Clinical
  - Supporting labs
    - Ketonuria, hypoglycemia, hypokalemia
    - Transaminitis
    - Hypochloremic, metabolic alkalosis
- Management
  - IV rehydration
  - IV thiamine followed by glucose
  - Nausea control
    - Vitamin B6, doxylamine
    - Diphenhydramine, meclizine
    - Promethazine, metoclopramide
  - Frequent small meals and oral hydration

HELLP Syndrome
- Definition: third trimester pregnancy complication along a similar spectrum of severe preeclampsia
- Risk factors
  - Preeclampsia
  - Advanced maternal age
  - Multigravida
- Clinical features
  - Fatigue, jaundice: hemolysis
  - Right upper quadrant abdominal pain (distention of [Glisson] hepatic capsule, subcapsular hematoma): elevated liver enzymes
  - Easy bruising/bleeding, petechiae: low platelets
  - Hypertension
- Diagnostics
  - Complete blood count: anemia, thrombocytopenia
  - Complete metabolic panel: transaminitis
  - Elevated lactate dehydrogenase, low haptoglobin, indirect hyperbilirubinemia: hemolysis
  - D-dimer, fibrinogen: disseminated intravascular coagulation (DIC)
  - Schistocytes on peripheral smear

- Management
  - Blood pressure control
  - IV magnesium for seizure prophylaxis
  - Delivery after maternal stabilization
- Complications
  - DIC
  - Acute respiratory distress syndrome
  - Hepatic rupture
  - Fetal demise
  - Abruptio placentae

Preeclampsia
- Definition: new-onset hypertension associated with proteinuria or end-organ damage >20 weeks of gestation
- Pathophysiology: abnormal placental artery spiralization resulting in vasospasm and uteroplacental insufficiency
- Risk factors
  - Chronic hypertension
  - History of preeclampsia
  - Chronic kidney disease
  - Primiparas, multiple gestation
  - Autoimmune disease
  - Extremes of maternal age (<18 or >40 years)
  - Substance abuse
- Signs and symptoms
  - New-onset hypertension (>140/90 or >160/110 if severe preeclampsia) PLUS
    - Proteinuria
         OR
    - End-organ damage
      - Acute kidney injury
      - Pulmonary edema
      - Right upper-quadrant pain, transaminitis
      - Visual disturbances
      - Thrombocytopenia, DIC
- Diagnostics: clinical
  - Complete blood count
  - Complete metabolic found
  - Chest x-ray
  - 24-hour urine protein collection >300 mg or urine protein/creatinine ratio >0.3
- Management (Fig. 25-1)
  - Antihypertensives (hydralazine, labetalol, nifedipine)
  - IV magnesium for seizure prophylaxis
  - Delivery
- Prevention: low-dose aspirin +/− calcium supplementation
- Complications
  - Eclampsia (severe preeclampsia plus generalized tonic-clonic seizures): treat with IV magnesium
  - Intrauterine growth restriction
  - Abruptio placentae

Signs of magnesium toxicity: decreased deep tendon reflexes, respiratory depression, cardiac arrest

Intrahepatic Cholestasis of Pregnancy
- Risk factors: white race, multiple gestation, increased estrogen
- Pathophysiology: impaired bile acid flow resulting in elevated serum bile acids and severe pruritus
- Management: ursodeoxycholic acid (decreases pruritus)

Acute Fatty Liver of Pregnancy
- Definition
  - Acute liver failure in third trimester or early postpartum
  - Associated with defective fatty acid metabolism (long chain 3-hydroxy acyl-CoA dehydrogenase deficiency)

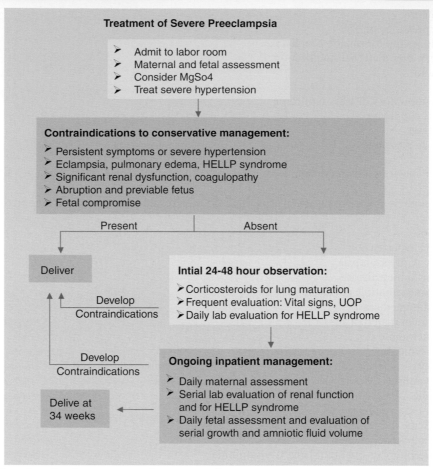

Figure 25-1: Flow chart for the treatment of severe preeclampsia. *MgSO₄*, magnesium sulfate; *UOP*, urine output. (Image courtesy of Dr. Vijaya Chandar.)

- Key features
  - Nausea, vomiting, jaundice
  - Hypertension, preeclampsia
  - Coagulopathy (elevated prothrombin time/partial thromboplastin time), hypoglycemia, hyperammonemia, encephalopathy
  - Acute kidney injury

Pruritic urticarial papules and plaques of pregnancy: red papules within striae and sparing around the umbilicus occurring during the third trimester of pregnancy

- Management: immediate delivery

Peripartum Cardiomyopathy
- Definition: congestive heart failure that develops between late pregnancy and early postpartum
- Risk factors
  - Preexisting cardiomyopathy
  - Preeclampsia
  - Multiple gestations
- Signs and symptoms
  - Orthopnea
  - Paroxysmal nocturnal dyspnea
  - Lower extremity edema
- Diagnostics: echocardiogram

- Management
  - During pregnancy
    - Beta blockers (carvedilol, metoprolol): improves mortality
    - Hydralazine/nitrate: improves mortality
    - Loop diuretics: no mortality benefit, treats symptomatic pulmonary edema
  - Postpartum: similar to nonpregnant cardiomyopathy
    - Angiotensin-converting enzyme inhibitors: avoid in pregnancy due to teratogenicity
    - Beta blockers (metoprolol, carvedilol)
    - Mineralocorticoid antagonist (spironolactone, eplerenone)
    - Loop diuretics
- Prognosis: most women return to normal heart function within months

CHAPTER 26 Preterm Complications

TERMINOLOGY

- Preterm delivery: delivery prior to 37 weeks of gestation associated with poor fetal and neonatal outcomes (Table 26-1)
- Preterm rupture of membranes: rupture of membranes prior to 37 weeks of gestation
- Premature rupture of membranes: rupture of membranes prior to maternal uterine contractions
- Prolonged rupture of membranes: rupture of membranes lasting >18 hours
  Chorioamnionitis
  - Definition: infection of the amniotic fluid, membranes, placenta, and/or umbilical cord
  - Risk factors
    - Prolonged rupture of membranes
    - Prolonged labor
    - Cervical insufficiency
    - Intrauterine monitoring devices
  - Signs and symptoms
    - Maternal/fetal tachycardia
    - Maternal fever
    - Uterine tenderness
    - Purulent, malodorous vaginal discharge
  - Diagnostics
    - Clinical plus positive amniotic fluid cultures
    - Leukocytosis

TABLE 26-1 Conditions Associated With Prematurity

DISEASE	KEY FEATURES	MANAGEMENT
Cerebral palsy	• Spastic diplegia • Intellectual disability, seizures • Strabismus	• Intrapartum IV magnesium provides neuroprotection and decreases risk
Neonatal respiratory distress syndrome	• Respiratory distress • Tachypnea • Nasal grunting	• Antenatal corticosteroids • Exogenous surfactant • CPAP
Patent ductus arteriosus (PDA)	• Continuous flow murmur • Wide pulse pressure • Bounding pulses	• Indomethacin: closes PDA • Prostaglandin: keeps it open in ductus-dependent heart defects
Intraventricular hemorrhage	• Increasing head circumference • Obstructive hydrocephalus • Lethargy, irritability, vomiting	• Prevent premature delivery • Avoid hyperoxia • +/− cerebrospinal fluid removal
Necrotizing enterocolitis	• Bloody diarrhea • Abdominal distention • Pneumatosis intestinalis	• Bowel rest • Broad-spectrum antibiotics • IV fluids plus nutrition • Surgery if necrosis or perforation
Retinopathy of prematurity	• Fundoscopy: abnormal retinal vascularization	• Avoid hyperoxia • Laser photocoagulation • VEGF inhibitors (bevacizumab)

CPAP, Continuous positive airway pressure; VEGF, vascular endothelial growth factor.

- Management
- Delivery
- IV antibiotics: ampicillin + gentamicin +/− clindamycin
- Complications
  - Maternal
    - Endometritis
    - Postpartum hemorrhage
    - Uterine atony
  - Neonate
    - Sepsis
    - Premature birth
    - Cerebral palsy

Interventions for premature neonates:
- Steroids between 23 and 34 weeks for fetal lung maturity
- Magnesium sulfate prior to 32 weeks for neuroprotection

CHAPTER 27
Post-Term Complications

Postterm Delivery
– Definition: delivery >42 weeks of gestation
– Risk factors
  • Inaccurate dating
  • Previous postterm pregnancy
  • Maternal obesity
  • Nulliparity
– Complications (Table 27.1)
  • Fetal
    ▪ Meconium aspiration
    ▪ Macrosomia (increased time for growth)
    ▪ Oligohydramnios (decreased placental perfusion to aging placenta → decreased urine output → oligohydramnios)
    ▪ Stillbirth
  • Maternal
    ▪ Postpartum hemorrhage
    ▪ Perineal laceration
    ▪ Chorioamnionitis
– Management: delivery
  • Labor induction
  • Cesarean section if emergent

TABLE 27.1 Postterm Pregnancy Complications, Features, and Management

CONDITION*	KEY FEATURES	MANAGEMENT
Meconium aspiration	• Respiratory distress • Hypoxemia • Chest x-ray: patchy infiltrates, flattened diaphragm	• Airway suctioning • Respiratory support
Oligohydramnios	• Amniotic fluid index <5 cm	• Cesarean section
Perenial laceration	• Perineal bleeding	• Surgical repair • Consider episiotomy prior to delivery if there is high risk
Chorioamnionitis	• Maternal fever • Uterine tenderness • Purulent uterine discharge	• IV antibiotics • Delivery

*Postpartum hemorrhage and macrosomia to be discussed in later sections.

28 Normal and Abnormal Labor

There is specific labor terminology that must be understood to determine the positioning of the fetus as it enters the birth canal. Furthermore, understanding the stages of labor, their length, and the causes for prolonged labor allows for better differentiation between normal and abnormal labor, and guides the decision as to the appropriate intervention (Tables 28.1 and 28.2; Fig. 28.1).

Interpretation of the Bishop score (Table 28.3):
- Score >8: cervix favorable for labor
- Score <5: cervix unfavorable for labor

TABLE 28.1 Labor Terminology

LABOR	UTERINE CONTRACTIONS THAT CAUSE CERVICAL CHANGES TO PREPARE MOTHER FOR FETAL DELIVERY; CAN BE INDUCED, AUGMENTED, OR DELAYED
Lie	Orientation of the long axis of the fetus to the long axis of the uterus; most common is longitudinal lie
Station	Degree of descent of the presenting part through the birth canal; expressed in centimeters above or below the maternal ischial spine. Positive numbers indicate fetus is closer to the birth canal
Presentation	Portion of the fetus overlying the pelvic inlet; most common is cephalic (head down)
Position	Relationship of a definitive fetal part to the maternal bony pelvis; most common is left occipital transverse

TABLE 28.2 Normal and Abnormal Labor

STAGES OF LABOR	FEATURES	NORMAL	ABNORMALITIES	MANAGEMENT
Stage I: latent phase	• Cervical effacement: softening of the cervix due to breakage of disulfide bonds • Cervical dilation up to 6 cm	• Primipara: <20 hr • Multipara: <12 hr	• Prolonged latent phase, most commonly due to analgesia	• Decrease analgesic dose and sedation
Stage I: active phase	• Accelerated cervical dilation from 6–10 cm	• Primipara: >1.0 cm/hr • Multipara: >1.2 cm/hr	• Power (inadequate uterine contractions) • Passenger (fetus too large) • Pelvis (maternal pelvis too small) • Active phase arrest: no change in cervical dilation or station for 2–4 hr despite adequate uterine contractions (>200 Montevideo units)	• Inadequate power: oxytocin • Passenger: cesarean section • Pelvis: birthing assist assess maneuvers, if this fail, proceed to cesarean section • Active phase arrest: cesarean section

TABLE 28.2   Normal and Abnormal Labor

STAGES OF LABOR	FEATURES	NORMAL	ABNORMALITIES	MANAGEMENT
Stage II	• Fetal descent and delivery	• Primipara: <3 hr • Multipara: <2 hr • Allow additional 1 hr if patient received epidural	• Power • Passage • Pelvis	• If fetus is close to delivery (positive station): continued management, oxytocin, operative vaginal delivery (forceps, vacuum), episiotomy
Stage III	• Delivery of placenta	• <30 min • Cord lengthening • Gush of blood • Uterine fundal rebound	• Retained placenta	• Manual extraction +/− curettage

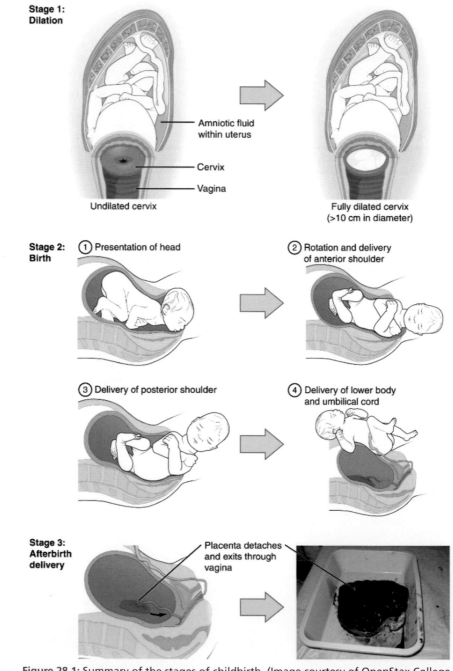

Figure 28.1: Summary of the stages of childbirth. (Image courtesy of OpenStax College.)

TABLE 28-3   Bishop Score—Scoring System Used to Determine Cervix Favorability for Labor

SCORE	0	1	2	3
Cervical consistency	Firm	Malleable	Soft	
Cervical dilation	Closed	1–2 cm	3–4 cm	>5 cm
% cervical effacement	0–30%	40–50%	60–70%	>80%
Cervical position	Posterior	Middle	Anterior	
Fetal station	−3	−2	−1, 0	>1

CHAPTER 29
Birthing Assistance and Complications

Macrosomia
- Risk factors
  - Maternal hyperglycemia
  - Maternal obesity
  - Advanced maternal age
  - Male fetus
  - Postterm pregnancy
  - Twin-twin transfusion
  - Beckwith-Wiedemann syndrome
- Diagnostics
  - Estimated fetal weight >90th percentile
  - Estimated fetal weight >4000 g
- Management
  - Expectant management +/− operative or nonoperative birthing assistance
  - Scheduled cesarean section
    - Estimated fetal weight >5000 g or 4500 g in diabetic mothers
    - Prior shoulder dystocia
- Complications
  - Maternal
    - Pelvic/vaginal injury
    - Postpartum hemorrhage (secondary to overdistended uterus)
  - Neonatal
    - Shoulder dystocia: turtle sign retraction of the fetal head into the perineum
    - Clavicular/humeral fracture: clavicular/humeral irregularity
    - Erb palsy
      - C5–C7 brachial plexopathy secondary to traction on the anterior shoulder due to being trapped behind the pubic symphasis
      - Elbow extended; forearm pronated
    - Klumpke palsy
      - C8–T1 brachial plexopathy secondary to traction when pulling arm from the birth canal
      - Claw hand: hyperextended metacarpophalangeal joint, extended wrist +/− Horner syndrome (ptosis, miosis)
    - Asphyxia
    - Hypoglycemia
    - Polycythemia
    - Respiratory distress (neonatal respiratory distress syndrome, transit tachypnea of the newborn, meconium aspiration)

When faced with a macrosomic baby, birthing assistance maneuvers can be utilized to increase the diameter of the birth canal and aid in delivery (Table. 29-1; Fig. 29-1). Additionally, other nonoperative devices can be used to move the baby out of the birthing canal.

Other measures to ensure safe delivery are the use of tocolytics, which function to decrease uterine contractions to delay delivery (Table 29-2). This is often used in cases of premature infants to provide sufficient time to deliver the necessary medications such as steroids and magnesium. Uterotonics function to increase maternal uterine contractions to aid in delivery (Table 29-3).

Pain management is also an important aspect of labor and delivery with a variety of methods, each with their own set of pros and cons (Table 29-4).

TABLE 29-1 Birthing Assistance Maneuvers and Interventions, Nonoperative Versus Operative

	TYPES OF INTERVENTIONS	PURPOSE	COMPLICATIONS
Nonoperative	McRoberts maneuver +/− suprapubic pressure	• Flex maternal thighs to rotate pubic symphysis cephalad and flatten sacral promontory	• Minimal
	Rubin maneuver	• Adduction of the fetal shoulder	
	Woods screw maneuver	• Rotation of the fetus by exerting pressure on the anterior clavicle	
	Gaskin maneuver	• Mother placed on all fours (hands and knees), which increases space in the sacrum, takes advantage of gravity	
	Zavenelli maneuver	• Replacement of fetal head into maternal birth canal followed by cesarean section	
	External cephalic version	• Manual reorientation of fetus by clinician from noncephalic presentation to cephalic to allow for vaginal delivery	
Operative	Forceps	• Aid fetal extraction during prolonged second stage of labor; forceps are slightly better if a difficult extraction is anticipated	• Facial nerve palsies • Lacerations • Maternal genital trauma
	Vacuum assisted		• Intracranial hemorrhage • Cephalohematoma
	Episiotomy (controlled perineal laceration)	• Generally avoided • Delivery with high risk of perineal laceration	• Bladder/bowel incontinence • Rectovaginal fistula

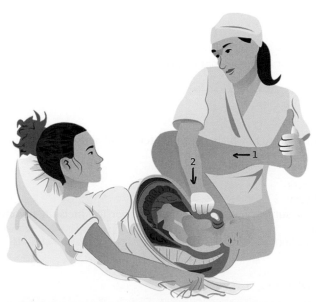

Figure 29-1: Illustration of McRoberts birthing assistance maneuver where the maternal thighs are flexed, and suprapubic pressure is applied to assist in widening the birth canal and relieve shoulder dystocia.

TABLE 29-2   Types of Tocolytics

MEDICATIONS	ADVERSE EFFECTS
Prostaglandin inhibitors (indomethacin)	Premature patent ductus arteriosus closure
Calcium channel blockers (nifedipine)	Hypotension
Beta-2 agonist (terbutaline)	Tachycardia
Magnesium	Decreased deep tendon reflexes, respiratory depression, cardiac arrest

These are used to decreased maternal uterine contractions in cases of tachysystole or hypertonic contractions.

TABLE 29-3   Types of Uterotonics

MEDICATIONS	ADVERSE EFFECTS
Oxytocin	Tachysystole Hyponatremia (secondary to water retention)
Methylergonovine	Hypertension Migraines Raynaud phenomenon
Carboprost	Bronchoconstriction (avoid in asthmatics)
Misoprostol	FeverShivering

These increase the frequency and power of uterine contractions.

TABLE 29-4   Pain Management

INTERVENTION	ADVERSE EFFECTS
Paracervical block	Hematoma
Neuraxial analgesia (epidural, spinal)	Epidural hematoma/abscess Hypotension Urinary retention
Pudendal nerve block	Transient fetal bradycardia
Systemic opioids	Respiratory depression

Trial of labor after cesarean section: may only be attempted if mother had previous horizontal uterine incision as there is less risk of uterine rupture.

Cesarean Section
- Definition: surgical procedure in which maternal uterus and abdomen is incised to help in delivery of fetus
- Indications
  - Maternal/fetal distress
  - Failed vaginal delivery
  - Previous intrauterine surgery (cesarean section with vertical incision, myomectomy)
  - Maternal preference
  - Fetal macrosomia (>5000 g)
  - Placenta previa
- Complications
  - Postpartum hemorrhage
  - Cosmetics
  - Inability for trial of labor after cesarean after vertical uterine incision

Uterine Rupture

Lower segment uterine transverse incision vs classical vertical incision: Lower segment transverse incision preserves the mother's cosmetic appearance and allows for trial of labor after cesarean section. Classic vertical incision is performed in emergencies and any fetal lie. Lower segment transverse incision is more commonly performed; however, it is only compatible with fetus in longitudinal lie.

- Risk factors
  - Previous uterine procedure (myomectomy)
  - Previous cesarean section with vertical incision
  - High-dose oxytocin
  - Fetal macrosomia
  - Congenital anatomic uterine anomalies
- Signs and symptoms
  - Sudden-onset abdominal pain
  - Sudden loss of fetal station (i.e., from 0 to −3)
  - Nonreassuring fetal heart tracing
  - Fetal parts palpated on abdominal examination
  - Vaginal bleeding
- Diagnostics: clinical
- Management: immediate laparotomy, delivery, and uterine repair

CHAPTER 30 Post-Partum Hemorrhage

Postpartum hemorrhage: >500 mL blood loss during vaginal delivery and >1000 mL during cesarean section

Postpartum hemorrhage differential diagnosis:

- Uterine atony
- Uterine inversion
- Retained placenta
- Obstetric laceration
- Disseminated intravascular coagulation (DIC)

Uterine Atony
- Epidemiology: most common cause of postpartum hemorrhage
- Pathophysiology: failure of postpartum uterine contraction secondary to uterine overdistention → inability to compress placental blood vessels after placental delivery
- Risk factors
  - Macrosomia
  - Multiple gestations
  - Precipitous delivery
  - Polyhydramnios
  - Grand multipara
  - Tocolytics
- Signs and symptoms
  - Soft, boggy uterus
  - Enlarged uterus palpated above the umbilicus
- Diagnostics: clinical
- Management
  - Uterine massage
  - Uterotonics (oxytocin, misoprostol, methylergonovine)

Uterine Inversion
- Pathophysiology: expulsion of uterus during delivery secondary to excessive traction
- Risk factors
  - Excessive placental cord traction while attempting to extract placenta
  - Excessive fundal pressure
  - Previous uterine inversion
  - Placenta accreta
  - Precipitous delivery
- Signs and symptoms
  - Profuse vaginal bleeding
  - Protrusion of uterine mass
  - Inability to palpate uterine fundus
  - Lower abdominal pain
  - +/− hemorrhagic shock
- Diagnosis: clinical
- Management: manual uterine replacement followed by IV oxytocin

Retained Placenta
- Definition: placenta not delivered within 30 minutes of fetal delivery
- Risk factors
  - Placenta accreta
  - Preterm delivery
  - Accessory placenta lobe

336

- Diagnostics: blood vessels running off the edge of the placenta (indicates possibility of accessory lobe or infiltration of placental villi)
- Management
  - Initial management: manual removal +/− uterotonics
  - Uncontrolled bleeding: curettage +/− hysterectomy
- Complications
  - Postpartum hemorrhage
  - Postpartum endometritis

Obstetric Laceration
- Epidemiology: second most common cause of postpartum hemorrhage
- Risk factors
  - Precipitous delivery
  - Macrosomia
  - Vacuum/forceps-assisted delivery
  - Iatrogenic (episiotomy)
- Signs and symptoms
  - Vaginal/cervical laceration
  - Urinary incontinence
  - Rectovaginal fistula (fourth-degree perineal laceration; malodorous brown vaginal discharge)
- Diagnostics: clinical
- Management: suture repair

Rectovaginal fistula: develop within weeks postpartum after third- or fourth-degree laceration. Presents with malodorous, brown vaginal discharge. Diagnosed on visual inspection of dark red, velvety rectal mucosa along the posterior vaginal wall. Treat via surgical repair.

DIC

> Rectovaginal fistula: develop within weeks postpartum after third- or fourth-degree laceration. Presents with malodorous, brown vaginal discharge. Diagnosed on visual inspection of dark red, velvety rectal mucosa along the posterior vaginal wall. Treat via surgical repair.

- Rare cause of postpartum hemorrhage
- Associated with abruptio placentae, amniotic fluid embolism, prolonged retention of dead fetus, severe preeclampsia
- Generalized bleeding/bruising from orifices and venipuncture sites

> Lochia: reddish-brown vaginal discharge secondary to shedding of the superficial layer of the uterus after delivery; may persist for weeks with discharge becoming clearer over time.

CHAPTER 31
Other Post-Partum Complications

Sheehan Syndrome
  – Pathophysiology: ischemia and necrosis of a physiologically enlarged pituitary gland secondary to hypotension from significant postpartum hemorrhage
  – Signs and symptoms: hypopituitarism
    • Weakness, lethargy
    • Orthostatic hypotension
    • Lactation failure
    • Prolonged postpartum amenorrhea
  – Diagnostics: thyroid-stimulating hormone, adrenocorticotropic hormone, prolactin, follicle-stimulating hormone/luteinizing hormone levels
  – Management: hormone replacement
Mastitis
  – Microbiology: Staphylococcus aureus
  – Signs and symptoms
    • Unilateral breast erythema/tenderness
    • Fevers, chills
    • +/− fluctuance (indicative of breast abscess)
  – Diagnostics: clinical
  – Management
    • Antistaphylococcal (dicloxacillin, nafcillin)
    • Continued breastfeeding from affected breast to aid in drainage
Postpartum Endometritis
  – Epidemiology: most common cause of postpartum fever
  – Risk factors
    • Prolonged rupture of membranes
    • Multiple vaginal exams
    • Internal fetal monitoring
    • Manual removal of placenta
    • Chorioamnionitis
    • Cesarean section
  – Signs and symptoms
    • Postpartum fever
    • Uterine tenderness
    • Purulent, foul-smelling lochia
  – Diagnostics: clinical
  – Management: clindamycin + gentamicin
Thromboembolic Disease
  – Most common cause of postpartum maternal mortality
  – Highest risk up to 6 weeks postpartum
  – Present similarly to nonpregnant with chest pain, shortness of breath, tachycardia, and hypoxia
  – Treat with low-molecular-weight heparin during pregnancy; may transition to warfarin postpartum
Septic Thrombophlebitis
  – Risk factors
    • Prolonged labor
    • Cesarean section
    • Endometritis/chorioamnionitis

- Signs and symptoms
  - Spiking fevers despite broad-spectrum antibiotics (usually for presumed endometritis)
  - Palpable, cordlike mass
- Diagnostics: clinical
- Management: systemic anticoagulation (2 days–6 weeks depending on severity)

Postpartum blues are quite common particularly in firsttime mothers. The key is differentiating this from postpartum depression or psychosis, both of which require additional management (Table 31.1).

Chronic endometritis is treated with doxycycline.

TABLE 31.1   Differentiating Postpartum Blues, Depression, and Psychosis

	KEY FEATURES	MANAGEMENT
Postpartum blues	• Emotional lability following childbirth • 2–3 days postpartum	• Emotional support, resolves within 2 wk
Postpartum depression	• Sleep disturbances • Depressed mood, anhedonia • Sensation of guilt/worthlessness • Lack of energy • Difficulty concentrating • Appetite changes • Psychomotor agitation/retardation • Suicidal ideation	• Antidepressants (SSRIs) • Ensure mother has no thoughts of infanticide
Postpartum psychosis	• Thoughts of infanticide • Hallucinations, delusions • Within 2 wk postpartum • Commonly seen in patients with history of bipolar	• Hospitalize mother • Avoid leaving mother and baby alone, may allow for supervised visits • Second-generation antipsychotics (quetiapine, risperidone, olanzapine) +/− mood stabilizer (lithium, valproate)

The breastfeeding feedback loop is a positive feedback loop that starts with stimulation of the maternal nipple from suckling by the baby (Fig. 32.1). This ultimately results in milk letdown. Breastfeeding is the preferred feeding method as it has both health and psychological benefits for the mother and baby (Table 32.1).

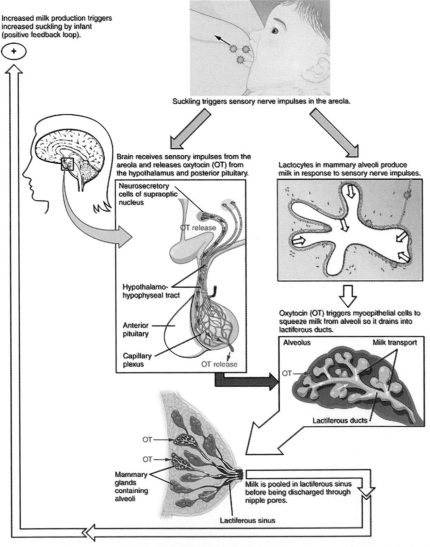

Fig. 32.1: Illustration demonstrating milk letdown positive feedback loop. (Image courtesy of OpenStax College; CC BY 3.0 [https://creativecommons.org/licenses/by-sa/3.0])

TABLE 32.1   Breastfeeding Benefits and Contraindications for Mother and Baby

	MOTHER	BABY
Benefits	• Maternal infant bonding • Weight loss • Uterine contraction • Temporary contraception for up to 3 mo (suppresses ovulation)	• Increased immunity (colostrum enriched with immunoglobulins, particularly IgA) • Decreased allergies, gastroenteritis, respiratory tract infections • Increased absorption of vitamins and Minerals • Decreased colic and reflux
Contraindications	• Human immunodeficiency virus • Herpes simplex virus lesion on the breast • Active varicella infection • Active untreated tuberculosis • Active substance abuse • Chemoradiation	• Galactosemia

Breastfeeding babies require supplementation with vitamin D. Exclusive breastfeeding is recommended until 6 mo of age.

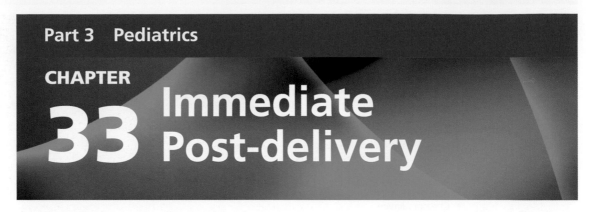

CHAPTER 33 Immediate Post-delivery

EARLY MANAGEMENT

Newborn management after delivery
- Check vitals and assess fetal well-being with Apgar scores (Tables 33.1 and 33.2)
- Suction oral and nasal airways
- Cleanse skin and umbilical cord with warm, soft soap solution
- Disinfect umbilical cord with bacitracin ointment
- Evaluate umbilical cord for the presence of two arteries and one vein (umbilical cord abnormalities may be indicative of fetal anomalies)
- Administration of erythromycin ophthalmic ointment: prevents gonococcal ophthalmia
- Administration of intramuscular vitamin K: prevents hemorrhagic disease of the newborn
- Administration of hepatitis B vaccine
- Hearing testing
- Routine neonatal screening (sickle cell, cystic fibrosis, human immunodeficiency virus, phenylketonuria, galactosemia, hypothyroidism)
- Bloody vaginal discharge in a female newborn after birth is normal due to progesterone withdrawal

TABLE 33.1   Normal Fetal Vital Signs

HEART RATE	120–160 BEATS/MIN
Respiratory rate	30–60 breaths/min
Blood pressure	50–70 systolic mm Hg
Temperature	97.3–100°C

TABLE 33.2   Apgar Scoring System

	SCORING		
	0	1	2
Appearance	Blue	Pink with blue extremities	Pink
Pulse	Absent	<100 bpm	>100 bpm
Grimace	No cry despite stimulation	Weak cry	Strong, vigorous cry
Activity	No movement	Moderate tone in arms and legs	Actively moving all extremities
Respiration	Absent	Slow, shallow, irregular	Regular

Apgar scoring system is used to determine early fetal well-being immediately after birth and need for early resuscitation. Performed at 1 min (to determine the need for resuscitation) and 5 min (to evaluate response to interventions).
Normal: 7–10 points
Abnormal: <6 points (indicative baby may need additional support and resuscitation)

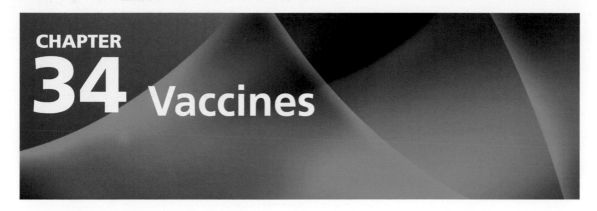

CHAPTER
34 Vaccines

Reactions After Vaccination (Table 34-1)
- Fever
- Redness, swelling, induration at injection site
- Mild illness
- Febrile seizure
- Arthralgias
- Inconsolable, persistent crying
  Contraindications to vaccines
- Anaphylaxis: all vaccines
- History of intussusception: rotavirus
- Immunocompromised: avoid live attenuated vaccines
- Progressive neurologic disorder, encephalopathy within 1 week from previous dose: pertussis

Herd immunity: immunization of >90% of the population against a certain disease will provide protection against those who are unimmunized due to extremely low disease prevalence and transmission.

Postexposure prophylaxis
  – Hepatitis B: immunoglobulin plus vaccine after birth if mother is hepatitis B surface antigen positive
  – Rabies: immunoglobulin plus vaccine if offending animal has signs of rabies
  – Tetanus
    • <3 doses or unknown
      • Give Td vaccine if wound is clean or minor
      • Give Td vaccine plus immunoglobulin for all other wounds
    • >3 doses
      • Give Td vaccine if last dose was >10 years for clean/minor wounds
      • Give Td vaccine if last dose was >5 years for all other wounds
  – Varicella
    • VZIG to newborns whose mother had varicella infection within 5 days of delivery to 48 hours after delivery
    • Varicella vaccine within 3–5 days of exposure for susceptible individuals (i.e., adults, children, household contacts who have not received the full two-dose series)
  Special consideration vaccines
- Traveler vaccines: yellow fever, meningococcal, typhoid, hepatitis A, hepatitis B, rabies, Japanese encephalitis, cholera
- Pneumococcal polysaccharide (PPSV23): high-risk individuals (asplenia, immunocompromised, chronic lung disease)
- Tdap: administered in pregnant woman between 27 and 36 weeks of gestation

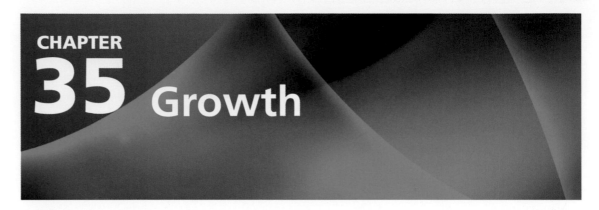

Normal growth principles
- Newborn loses ~10% of birthweight in the first week, and regains birthweight by the second week
- Birthweight doubles within 6 months, triples within 12 months, quadruples within 2 years
- Height percentile at 2 years old correlates with adult height percentile

Causes of abnormal growth: evaluated based on abnormal height and/or weight
- Lack of weight gain
  - Inadequate nutritional intake
  - Malabsorption syndromes
  - Psychosocial deprivation
- Lack of height gain
  - Endocrinologic abnormality (hypothyroidism, growth hormone deficiency
  - Skeletal dysplasia
- Lack of weight/height gain
  - Chronic infection/disease
  - Constitutional growth delay
- Excess weight gain
  - Obesity (excess caloric intake)
  - Endocrine abnormalities (hypercortisolism, hypothyroidism)
- Excess height gain
  - Familial tall stature
  - Excess growth hormone

Growth velocity: compares bone age to chronologic age to determine etiology of abnormal growth velocity
- Bone age = chronologic age
  - Normal: familial short stature (normal onset of puberty)
  - Abnormal: chromosomal, genetic abnormalities
- Bone age > chronologic age
  - Normal: familial tall stature
  - Abnormal: hyperthyroidism, precocious puberty, congenital adrenal hyperplasia
- Bone age < chronologic age
  - Normal: constitutional delay (late onset of puberty)
  - Abnormal: chronic disease, endocrinologic abnormality

Bone age reference standards are used to evaluate a child's bone age vs chronologic age. X-ray of the left wrist is taken, and ossification centers are compared with known standards.
Growth curves plot child's growth percentiles based on height, weight, length, and head circumference.

Failure to Thrive
- Definition: weight <2nd percentile with decreased velocity of weight gain
- Causes
  - Inadequate caloric intake
    - Inadequate food security
    - Oropharyngeal dysfunction
    - Lack of parental knowledge
    - Neglect

- Increased caloric requirement
  - Chronic medical disease
  - Chronic infection
  - Inadequate nutritional absorption
  - Celiac disease
  - Cystic fibrosis
- Signs and symptoms
  - Thin extremities, narrow face
  - Prominent ribs
  - Wasted buttocks
  - Flattened occiput
  - Avoidance of eye contact
  - Feeding aversion
- Management
  - Treat underlying medical etiology
  - Lack of parental knowledge: feed under supervision, may need hospitalization depending on severity of malnutrition
  - Neglect: contact Child Protective Services

NEUROCUTANEOUS SYNDROMES

Tuberous Sclerosis
- Inheritance: autosomal dominant
- Pathophysiology: abnormal TSC1/TSC2 genes
- Key features
  - Shagreen patches (thickened, rough, skin lesions)
  - Ash-leaf spots (hypopigmented macules)
  - Sebaceous adenomas (acnelike skin lesion) (Fig. 36-1)
  - Refractory seizures (calcified central nervous system [CNS] tubers), intellectual disability
  - Arrhythmias (cardiac rhabdomyomas)
  - Renal angiomyolipoma
- Diagnostics: clinical
- Associations
  - Infantile spasms
  - Pheochromocytoma
- Complications
  - Seizures
  - Brain tumor
  - Cardiac tumors

Sturge-Weber Disease
- Signs and symptoms
  - Port-wine stain involving trigeminal nerve distribution (**unilateral cavernous hemangioma**)
  - Intellectual disability
  - Seizures
  - Hemiparesis
  - Glaucoma
- Diagnostics
  - Clinical
  - Magnetic resonance imaging (MRI) brain: leptomeningeal capillary venous malformation, intracranial calcifications
- Associations: pheochromocytoma
- Management
  - Seizures: antiepileptics
  - Port-wine stain: argon laser therapy
  - Glaucoma: prostaglandin, beta blocker eyedrops

Neurofibromatosis are genetic disorders identified by development of multiple nerve tumors; however, there are specific features that allow you to differentiate type 1 and type 2 (Table 36-1; Figs. 36-2 and 36-3).

INFECTIONS

Meningitis in infants presents with fever and irritability, rather than the typical triad of headache, fever, and neck stiffness seen in older children and adults (Table 36-2).

Encephalitis
- Signs and symptoms: similar to meningitis with addition of confusion, focal neurologic deficits, personality changes
- Microbiology: herpes simplex virus
- Diagnostics
  - Computed tomography (CT) scan first due to symptoms

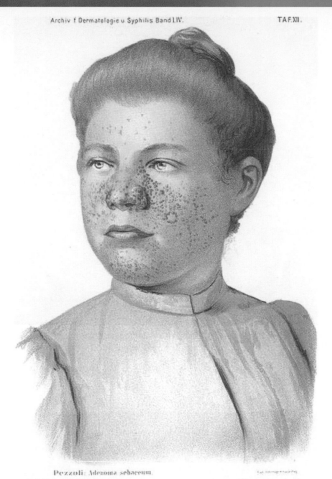

Archiv f Dermatologie u Syphilis Band LIV.   TAF.XII.

Pezzoli: Adenoma sebaceum.

Figure 36-1: Illustration of patient with tuberous sclerosis suffering with facial adenoma sebaceum. (From a journal article by Dr C. Pezzoli, but the artist isn't known for sure.)

TABLE 36-1   **Differentiating Neurofibromatosis Type 1 Versus Type 2**

NEUROFIBROMATOSIS TYPE 1	NEUROFIBROMATOSIS TYPE 2
• Café au lait spots	• Bilateral vestibular neuromas
• Macrocephaly	• Intracranial meningioma
• Intellectual disability	• Peripheral neuropathy
• Neurofibromas (benign peripheral nerve sheath tumors)	• Cataract
• Axillary/inguinal freckling	• Retinal hamartomas
• Optic nerve glioma, Lisch nodules (iris hamartomas)	• Plaquelike skin lesions
• Epilepsy, lymphoma	• Subcutaneous nodules

- • Lumbar puncture followed by cerebrospinal fluid (CSF) viral polymerase chain reaction (Table 36-3)
- – Management: acyclovir

SEIZURES
Seizures
- – Definition: neuronal excitotoxicity resulting in abnormal movements and altered consciousness
- – Subtypes
  - • Simple: no postictal state
  - • Complex: postictal state present
  - • Partial: tonic-clonic movements involving the face or single extremity; no postictal state
  - • Generalized: tonic-clonic movements involving the face, eyes, and all extremities; postictal state present

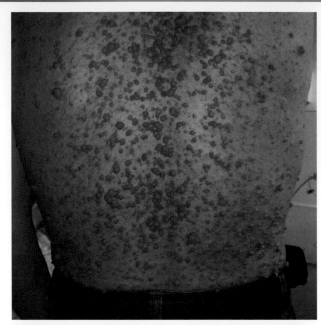

Figure 36-2: Extensive neurofibromas in a patient with neurofibromatosis type 1. (Klaus D. Peter, Gummersbach, Germany; CC BY 3.0 DE [https://creativecommons.org/licenses/by/3.0/de/deed.en])

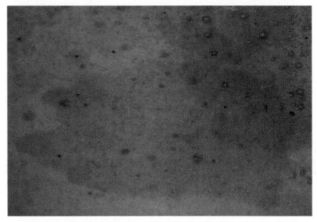

Figure 36-3: Café au lait spots in a patient with neurofibromatosis type 1. (Accrochoc at fr.wikipedia; CC BY-SA [http://creativecommons.org/licenses/by-sa/3.0/])

TABLE 36-2   Meningitis

AGE	MICROBIOLOGY (TOP TO BOTTOM, MOST TO LEAST COMMON)	MANAGEMENT
0–1 mo	• Group B streptococci • *Escherichia coli* • Listeria	Ampicillin + aminoglycoside (gentamicin) + third-generation cephalosporin (cefotaxime)
1 mo–18 yr	• Neisseria meningitidis • Streptococcus pneumoniae • Haemophilus influenzae	Vancomycin + ceftriaxone +/– dexamethasone
18–50 yr	• S. pneumoniae • N. meningitidis • H. influenzae	

Causative agent differs depending on age of child. Ceftriaxone is avoided as part of empiric therapy in neonates due to risk of hyperbilirubinemia. Dexamethasone is added for cases caused by *S. pneumoniae*.

TABLE 36-3 Table of Lumbar Puncture Cerebrospinal Fluid Analysis

	CELLS	GLUCOSE	PROTEIN	OPENING PRESSURE
Bacterial	PMNs	Decreased	Increased	Increased
Viral	Lymphocytes	Normal	Normal	Normal
Tuberculosis	Lymphocytes	Decreased	Increased	Increased

- Causes: VITAMINs
  - <u>V</u>ascular
    - Vasculitis
    - Stroke
  - <u>I</u>nfectious
    - Meningitis
    - Encephalitis
    - Brain abscess
  - <u>T</u>rauma
  - <u>A</u>utoimmune
  - <u>M</u>etabolic
    - Hypo/hypernatremia
    - Hypo/hyperglycemia
    - Hyper/hypocalcemia
    - Hypomagnesemia
    - Uremia
    - Hyperammonemia
    - Hypoxia
    - Thyroid storm
  - <u>I</u>diopathic
  - <u>N</u>eoplastic
  - <u>P</u>sychiatric (cessation of anticonvulsants)
- Signs and symptoms
  - Loss of consciousness +/− loss of tone
  - Lip smacking, arm jerking, blinking
  - Generalized tonic-clonic contractions
  - Postictal state (confusion)
  - +/− tongue biting
  - +/− bladder/bowel incontinence
- Diagnostics
  - Evaluate for reversible causes of seizure
  - Electroencephalography: identifies seizure type and foci (Table 36-4)
- Management
  - Treat and reverse underlying etiology
  - IV benzodiazepine for intractable seizures
  - Long-term antiepileptics reserved for epilepsy (recurrent seizures without any identifiable reversible etiology)

Febrile seizures have no increased risk of epilepsy except in the following cases:
  I. Seizure lasting >15 min
  II. Focal features
  III. Recurs within 24 hr
  IV. Abnormal development
  V. Family history of epilepsy

TABLE 36-4   Key Features and Management of Specific Types of Seizures

TYPE OF SEIZURE	KEY FEATURES	MANAGEMENT
Absence seizure	• Expressionless, frequent blinking • May be confused as "daydreaming" • Loss of consciousness without loss of tone • EEG: 3-Hz spike and wave discharge	• Ethosuximide • Resolves by adolescence
West syndrome (infantile spasms)	• Infantile spasms • Regression of psychomotor development • EEG: hypsarrhythmia	• ACTH • Vigabatrin
Juvenile myoclonic epilepsy	• Early-morning jerky movements • Common in adolescents	• Valproic acid
Febrile seizure	• Generalized tonic-clonic seizure lasting <10 min associated with high fever • Most common childhood seizure type (6 mo–6 yr of age) • Often have positive family history of febrile seizures	• Symptomatic management • Clinical diagnosis, additional testing not indicated

ACTH, Adrenocorticotropic hormone; *EEG*, electroencephalography.

HYDROCEPHALUS

Definition: increased CSF fluid within the cerebral ventricles secondary to impaired CSF flow or reabsorption resulting in increased intracranial pressure and expansion of the ventricles (Figs. 36-4, 36-5, and 36-6)
   Types of hydrocephalus
• Communicating: normal CSF flow, impaired CSF reabsorption or increased CSF production; commonly due to damaged arachnoid villi granulations secondary to blood or meningitis
• Noncommunicating: impaired CSF flow, normal CSF reabsorption; commonly due to physical obstruction such as abnormal brain anatomy or brain tumor
• Ex vacuo: normal CSF flow, normal CSF absorption; falsely appearing enlarged ventricles secondary to brain atrophy
Dandy Walker Malformation
– Cystic expansion of the fourth ventricle
– Agenesis of the posterior cerebellar vermis
– Enlarged posterior fossa, noncommunicating hydrocephalus
– Prominent occiput, cerebellar ataxia, delayed motor development
Arnold-Chiari Malformation
– Pathophysiology: herniation of cerebellar tonsils through the foramen magnum causing displacement of the caudal brainstem
– Signs and symptoms
  • Neck pain, occipital headache
  • Cerebellar ataxia
  • Vertigo
– Diagnostics
  • MRI brain (cerebellar tonsillar herniation, noncommunicating hydrocephalus)
  • Degree of herniation on MRI classifies Arnold-Chiari subtype
– Associations
  • Syringomyelia
  • Myelomeningocele
  • Neurofibromatosis
– Management
  • Mild symptoms: conservative management
  • Severe symptoms, neurologic deficits: surgical decompression
– Complications
  • Cranial nerve paralysis
  • Apnea
Intraventricular Hemorrhage
– Pathophysiology: subependymal germinal matrix capillary fragility resulting in increased risk of intracranial hemorrhage and impaired autoregulation of cerebral blood flow
– Risk factors
  • Prematurity
  • Low birthweight (<1500 g)
  • Maternal cocaine use

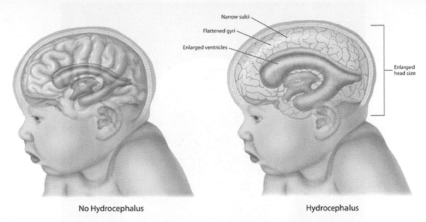

Figure 36-4: Illustration of the effects of hydrocephalus. (Image courtesy of the CDC.)

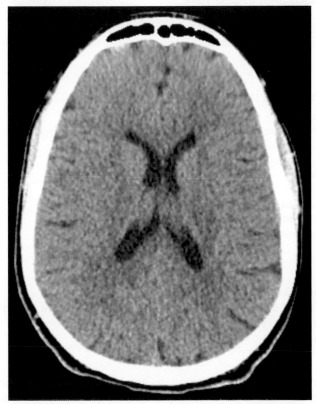

Figure 36-5: Normal computed tomography head. (Image courtesy of Mikael Häggström, M.D [CC0])

- Signs and symptoms
  - Rapidly increasing head circumference
  - Bulging fontanelles
  - Lethargy, irritability, hypotonia
  - Vomiting
- Diagnostics: serial head ultrasounds
- Management: prevention of preterm labor and delivery with corticosteroids
- Complications
  - Communicating hydrocephalus (blood irritates the arachnoid villi impairing CSF absorption)
  - Neurodevelopmental delay (cerebral palsy)
  - Seizures

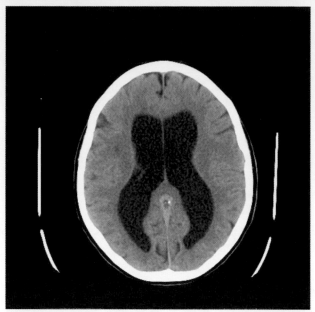

Figure 36-6: Hydrocephalus on computed tomography head. (Imagea courtesy of Lucien Monfils.)

SPINAL CORD ABNORMALITIES

Spinal Muscular Atrophy
- Pathophysiology: defective survivor motor neuron (SMN) gene resulting in apoptosis of motor neuroblasts and degeneration of lower motor neurons
- Signs and symptoms
  - Progressive hypotonia
  - Generalized weakness
  - Flaccid paralysis, absent deep tendon reflexes, fasciculations
  - Feeding difficulties, choking
  - Respiratory failure (most common cause of death)
- Diagnostics
  - SMN gene mutation
  - Muscle biopsy
  - Management: supportive, death at 2 years

Neural tube defects occur due to incomplete closure of the anterior or posterior neuropores during weeks 3–4 of pregnancy resulting in vertebral, spinal cord, or brain abnormalities (Table 36-5; Fig. 36-7). Associated with inadequate folate.

BRAIN TUMORS

Key principles: all present with some combination of chronic worsening headache that wakes patient up at night, vomiting, visual disturbances, seizures, papilledema, altered mental status, and gait disturbances. Each tumor has specific features or associations that can differentiate it from other tumors; however, in clinical practice histopathologic evaluation is the only means of definitive diagnosis (Table 36-6).

TABLE 36-5   Neural Tube Defects

TYPE OF NEURAL TUBE DEFECT	KEY FEATURES
Spina bifida occulta	• Midline lumbosacral vertebral body defect without protrusion of spinal cord elements • Midline tuft of hair
Meningocele	• Posterior vertebral herniation of meninges only
Myelomeningocele	• Posterior vertebral herniation of meninges and spinal cord
Myeloschisis	• Most severe posterior neural tube defect • Entire spinal cord is exposed covered only by semitransparent membrane
Anencephaly	• Failure of anterior neural tube closure resulting in exposed brain tissue and degeneration • Incompatible with life

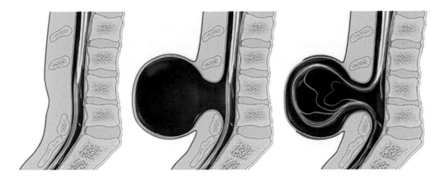

Spina bifida occulta   Meningocele   Myelomeningocele

Figure 36-7: Image of the types of spina bifida. (Image courtesy of the CDC.)

TABLE 36-6   Types of Pediatric Brain Tumors

TYPE OF MALIGNANCY	LOCATION	KEY FEATURES
Astrocytoma	Posterior fossa, cerebellum	• Most common cause of brain tumor in children • Contain cystic and solid components on imaging; differentiates it from medulloblastoma, which only has solid components
Ependymoma	Fourth ventricle	• Overgrowth of cells lining the ventricles results in signs and symptoms of obstructive hydrocephalus • Common cause of spinal cancer resulting in extramedullary spinal compression
Medulloblastoma	Cerebellum	• Neuroectodermal tumor • Drop metastases to the spinal cord • Associated with Turcot syndrome: familial predisposition to colon cancer
Hemangioblastoma	Cerebellum	• Associated with von Hippel-Lindau syndrome; these patients also have increased risk of renal cell carcinoma, retinal angiomas, pheochromocytoma, pancreatic neuroendocrine tumors • Can produce erythropoietin resulting in secondary polycythemia
Craniopharyngioma	Sella turcica	• Calcification on imaging • Childhood central nervous system tumor that is commonly supratentorial • Derived from remnants of Rathke pouch

CHAPTER 37
Head, Eyes, Ears, Nose, and Throat

HEAD

There are three subtypes of postdelivery head swelling differentiated based on the timing, clinical history, and whether it crosses sutures (Table 37-1; Fig. 37-1).

EYES

Retinitis differential diagnosis
- Toxoplasma: hydrocephalus, generalized intracranial calcifications
- Cytomegalovirus (CMV): periventricular calcifications, sensorineural hearing loss
- Syphilis: mucopurulent rhinitis, desquamating palms and soles, osteochondritis, saber shins, saddlenose
- Varicella: scarring skin lesions, limb deformities

Eye redness in the first 2 days of life is important to recognize to prevent irreversible visual deficits (Table 37-2).

Strabismus

Chemical conjunctivitis is becoming increasingly uncommon due to use of erythromycin eyedrops rather than silver nitrate. Chlamydia ophthalmia may be complicated by trachoma; characterized by follicular conjunctivitis, eyelid scarring, eyelash inversion, and blindness; represents the most common cause of blindness worldwide.

- – Definition: misalignment of the eyes
- – Pathophysiology: image is suppressed in the deviated eye resulting in permanent cortical blindness of the suppressed eye
- – Signs and symptoms
  - Diplopia

Trilateral retinoblastoma = bilateral retinoblastoma + pineal gland tumor

  - Abnormal red reflex
  - Ptosis
  - Decreased visual acuity
- – Diagnostics
  - Hirschberg corneal light reflex
  - Cover-uncover test: cover the good eye, which should result in correction of misaligned eye
  - Brighter red reflex in deviated eye
- – Management
  - Eye patch over the "good" eye to prevent misalignment of the "bad" eye
  - Surgical correction of misalignment for refractory cases
- – Complications: amblyopia

Retinoblastoma
- – Epidemiology: most common primary malignant intraocular tumor
- – Pathophysiology: retinoblastoma gene mutation resulting in inactivation of retinoblastoma suppressor gene
- – Signs and symptoms
  - Leukocoria (Fig. 37-2)
  - Strabismus

TABLE 37-1   Postdelivery Head Swelling Complications Associated With Difficult-to-Deliver Macrosomic Babies Requiring Instrumental Delivery

Cephalohematoma	• Presents a few days after delivery • Subperiosteal hemorrhage that does not cross suture lines • Jaundice • Spontaneously resorbed within weeks
Caput succedaneum	• Presents immediately after birth • Diffuse scalp edema • Crosses suture lines
Subgaleal/subaponeurotic hemorrhage	• Associated with vacuum delivery • Shearing of the emissary veins • May present with hypovolemic shock as infants may lose significant blood volume between galeal aponeurosis and periosteum • Feels similar to cephalohematoma that crosses suture lines

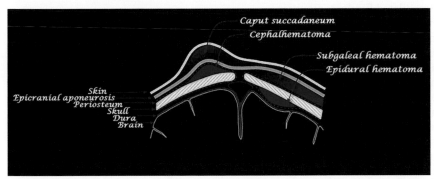

Figure 37-1: Diagram of the infant scalp showing the locations of the common scalp hematomas in relation to the layers of the scalp. (Image and caption courtesy of AMH Sheikh; CC BY-SA 3.0 [http://creativecommons.org/licenses/by-sa/3.0/])

TABLE 37-2   Ophthalmia Neonatorum Differential Diagnosis

	ONSET	SIGNS AND SYMPTOMS	TREATMENT
Chemical	First 24 hr of life	• Conjunctival injection	• Self-limited
Neisseria gonorrhea	Within 2–5 days	• Thick, purulent conjunctival discharge • Corneal ulceration or perforation	• Prevention: erythromycin eyedrops at birth • Intramuscular ceftriaxone + saline irrigation
Chlamydia trachomatis	Within 1–2 wk	• Eyelid edema • Watery, serosanguineous conjunctival discharge • Tarsal conjunctivae	• Oral erythromycin (may prevent subsequent chlamydia pneumonia) + saline irrigation

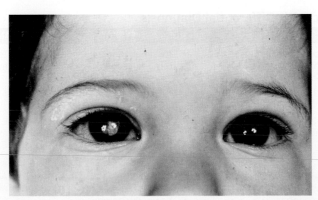

Figure 37-2: Leukocoria in a patient with retinoblastoma. (Image courtesy of the National Cancer Institute.)

- Ocular pain
- Glaucoma
  - Diagnostics
    - Orbital computed tomography (CT)/ultrasound: intraocular calcifications
    - Avoid biopsy due to risk of seeding vitreous fluid
  - Management
    - Large tumors: enucleation
    - Small tumors: external beam radiation (may result in secondary tumors)

Retinopathy of Prematurity
- Risk factors
  - Premature infant
  - Low birthweight
  - Hyperoxia
  - Neonatal respiratory distress syndrome
- Pathophysiology: progressive proliferation and neovascularization of retinal vessels secondary to hyperoxia
- Diagnostics: dilated fundoscopic exam
- Management
  - Minimize supplemental O2 exposure
  - Frequent ophthalmologic examinations every 1–2 weeks to evaluate for retinal vessel maturation
  - Retinal cryotherapy, laser photocoagulation
  - Screening for low birthweights and premature infants
- Complications
  - Myopia
  - Retinal detachment
  - Amblyopia

Retinitis Pigmentosa
- Congenital disorder resulting in degeneration of photoreceptors
- Characterized by nyctalopia, peripheral vision loss, photopsia
- Often associated with other genetic syndromes

Conjunctivitis can be divided into three main etiologies: bacterial, viral, and allergic. These are differentiated based on the type of discharge and laterality (Table 37-3).

Differentiating periorbital from orbital cellulitis is important as the former can be treated with outpatient oral antibiotics and the latter requires inpatient broad-spectrum IV antibiotics with careful evaluation for associated complications (Table 37-4).

EARS
Otitis Media
- Epidemiology: more common in children due to narrower eustachian tube predisposing to obstruction and subsequent infection
- Definition: infection/inflammation of the middle ear space (Fig. 37-4)
- Microbiology
  - Streptococcus pneumoniae
  - Haemophilus influenzae
  - Moraxella catarrhalis
  - Viral

TABLE 37-3 Conjunctivitis Differential Diagnosis

	CAUSES	SIGNS AND SYMPTOMS	MANAGEMENT
Bacterial	• Streptococcus pneumoniae • Nontypeable Haemophilus influenzae • Moraxella catarrhalis • Staphylococcus aureus	• Unilateral, mucopurulent discharge • Early-morning eyelid closure	• Topical fluoroquinolone or macrolide
Viral	• Adenovirus • Enterovirus	• Concurrent upper respiratory tract infection • Hyperemic conjunctiva • Bilateral watery discharge	• Conservative management • Good handwashing
Allergic	• Grass • Pollen • Seasonal change	• Itchiness • Previous history • Watery discharge	• Avoid exposure • Antihistamines

TABLE 37-4   Periorbital Versus Orbital Cellulitis

	PERIORBITAL CELLULITIS	ORBITAL CELLULITIS
Definition	• Infection prior to the orbital septum	• Infection involving and posterior to the orbital septum
Microbiology	• *Streptococcus pneumoniae* • *Haemophilus influenzae* • *Neisseria meningitidis* • *Staphylococcus aureus* • Preceded by upper respiratory infection (URI)	
Signs and symptoms	• Periorbital erythema/edema (Fig. 37-3) • Conjunctival injection	• Similar symptoms as periorbital cellulitis plus the following: • Ophthalmoplegia • Pain with extraocular movement • Proptosis • Visual deficits
Diagnostics	• Clinical	• Clinical • Computed tomography scan of the orbits (evaluate for complications such as cavernous sinus thrombosis, subperiosteal abscess)
Management	• Oral antibiotics covering URI organisms: • TMP-SMX or clindamycin • PLUS • Amoxicillin or amoxicillin-clavulanate or cefpodoxime or cefdinir	• Broad-spectrum IV antibiotics (vancomycin + ceftriaxone or cefotaxime)
Complications	• Uncommon, may extend into orbital cellulitis if left untreated	• Meningitis • Brain abscess • Blindness

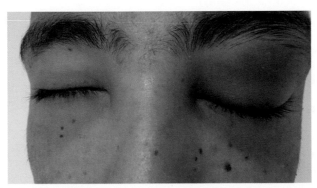

Figure 37-3: Patient with left periorbital erythema, edema, and pain without ophthalmoplegia consistent with preseptal cellulitis.

- Signs and symptoms
  - Fever, chills
  - Otorrhea
  - Ear pain/tugging
  - Decreased hearing
- Diagnostic: clinical + otoscopy
  - Pneumatic otoscopy: identifies presence of middle ear effusion based on abnormal movement of the tympanic membrane
  - Bulging tympanic membrane
  - Perforated tympanic membrane
- Management
  - Acute
    - Amoxicillin: initial treatment
    - Amoxicillin-clavulanate or cephalosporins or levofloxacin if no initial response or recent exposure to beta-lactam therapy
    - Macrolides: for penicillin allergic

Otitis Media

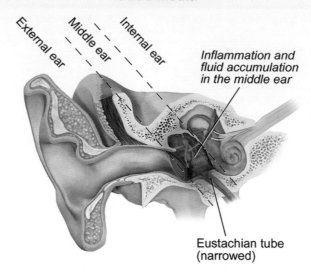

External ear | Middle ear | Internal ear

Inflammation and fluid accumulation in the middle ear

Eustachian tube (narrowed)

Figure 37-4: Anatomy and pathophysiology of otitis media.

- Recurrent
  - Tympanocentesis: sample middle ear to identify exact microbiologic etiology
  - Tympanostomy tubes for more than four episodes of otitis media within the last 12 months or three episodes within the last 6 months
- Complications
  - Meningitis
  - Mastoiditis
  - Facial nerve palsy
  - Cholesteatoma

Otitis Externa (Swimmer's Ear)
- Risk factors
  - Excessive wetness of the ear canal
  - Trauma
- Microbiology
  - Pseudomonas (most common cause)
  - *Staphylococcus aureus* (second most common cause)
- Signs and symptoms
  - Ear pain with manipulation of the outer ear
  - Conductive hearing loss
  - Edema, erythema, otorrhea
  - Preauricular lymphadenopathy
- Diagnostics
  - Clinical
  - CT scan if there is suspicion of temporal bone invasion
- Management
  - Mild cases: topical acetic acid
  - Moderate to severe cases: topical antibiotics
    - Fluoroquinolones: first line
    - Alternatives: aminoglycosides, neomycin
- Prevention: alcohol wipes after getting wet, earplugs
- Complications: malignant otitis externa (treat with IV antipseudomonal antibiotics)

NOSE
Choanal Atresia
- Definition: presence of bony septum impairing passage between nose and pharynx secondary to incomplete canalization
- Signs and symptoms

- Cyanosis worsened by feeding (obligate mouth-breathers) and improved by crying
- Inability to pass catheter into nasopharynx
  - Diagnosis: CT scan to delineate anatomy
  - Associations: CHARGE syndrome (coloboma, heart defects, choanal atresia, growth retardation, genitourinary abnormalities, ear abnormalities)
  - Management: surgical or endoscopic repair

Epistaxis differential diagnosis
  - Digital trauma (most common cause)
  - Disorders of hemostasis (von Willebrand factor deficiency, Bernard-Soulier, Glanzmann thrombasthenia)
  - Thrombocytopenia
  - Nasopharyngeal tumors

Dacryostenosis/Dacryocystitis
- Pathophysiology: failure of canalization of the nasolacrimal duct
- Signs and symptoms
  - Chronic, excessive lacrimation (epiphoria)
  - Discharge of mucoid material from the lacrimal sac
  - Erythema, tenderness of medial canthus
- Diagnostics: clinical
- Management
  - Most cases resolve spontaneously
  - Warm compresses, nasolacrimal massage
  - Topical antibiotics if infection present

THROAT
Pharyngitis
- Microbiology
  - Viral
    - Epstein-Barr virus (EBV)
    - CMV
    - Coxsackievirus
  - Bacterial
    - *Streptococcus pyogenes* (group A beta-hemolytic Streptococcus)
    - *Corynebacterium diphtheriae*
- Signs and symptoms
  - Tonsillar exudates, soft palate petechiae (Fig. 37-5)
  - Strawberry tongue
  - Tender, anterior cervical lymphadenopathy
  - Fevers, chills
  - Upper respiratory infection (URI) symptoms: more common with viral causes
- Diagnostics
  - Clinical
  - Rapid Streptococcus antigen test +/− throat culture
- Management
  - Viral: symptomatic management
  - Bacterial
    - *S. pyogenes:* penicillin or amoxicillin: prompt treatment prevents development of acute rheumatic fever and suppurative complications
    - Diphtheria: macrolide or penicillin + antitoxin
  - Tonsillectomy indications
    - Multiple, recurrent, severe infections (>7 episodes in 1 year)
    - Airway obstruction
- Complications
  - Group A Streptococcus
    - Acute rheumatic fever: prevented by prompt treatment of pharyngitis
    - Poststreptococcal glomerulonephritis
    - Pediatric autoimmune neuropsychiatric disorders with Streptococcus (PANDAS)
    - Suppurative complications
      ○ Otitis media
      ○ Peritonsillar/retropharyngeal abscess
  - EBV: airway obstruction (treat with corticosteroids if impending airway obstruction or signs of respiratory distress)

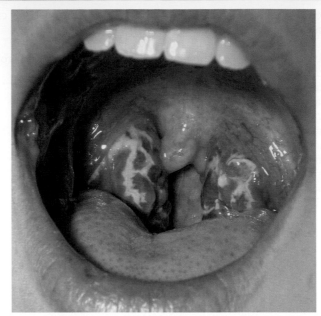

Figure 37-5: Streptococcal pharyngitis with erythematous pharynx, tonsillar enlargement, and exudates.

Pharyngitis-Associated Infections

CENTOR criteria: used to triage patients suspected of group A beta-hemolytic Streptococcus pharyngitis and determine course of treatment or testing. Unreliable in preadolescents. One point for each of the following signs or symptoms. Score >3 should necessitate rapid strep test. Score >4 should necessitate empiric antibiotics.
1. Cough (absence)
2. Exudates (tonsillar)
3. Nodes (cervical lymphadenopathy)
4. Temperature (>38°C)
5. <14 OR >44 – 1 point

– Coxsackievirus
  • Herpangina: small vesicles located in posterior pharynx
  • Hand-foot-mouth disease: vesicles located on hand, foot, and mouth; tend to ulcerate and become painful
  • Acute lymphonodular pharyngitis: nodules located on posterior pharynx with associated lymphadenopathy
– Group A Streptococcus
  • Scarlet fever
    ▪ Secondary to streptococcal pyogenic exotoxins (A, B, C)
    ▪ Circumoral pallor due to erythematous cheeks
    ▪ Papular erythematous rash with sandpaper-like texture
    ▪ Desquamation of the skin involving the palms and soles
    ▪ Strawberry tongue
    ▪ Pastia lines in intertriginous areas
    ▪ Develop immunity to that toxin after exposure; therefore patients can develop scarlet fever up to three times with exposure to each of the different toxins

Retropharyngeal abscesses are highly uncommon after 5 yr of age as the retropharyngeal lymph nodes involute around age 3–4 yr.
Anterior space abscess: bulge medial to the tonsils and lateral pharyngeal wall; swelling along the angle of the mandible results in significant trismus.
Posterior space abscess: swelling more prominent at the level of the hyoid bone; results in minimal trismus.

– Adenovirus: pharyngoconjunctival fever
– CMV: infectious mononucleosis
  • Signs and symptoms
    ▪ Nonspecific prodrome (fever, headache, myalgias, abdominal pain, sore throat, pharyngitis)
    ▪ Generalized lymphadenopathy (posterior cervical, submandibular, epitrochlear)

- Splenomegaly, possible hepatomegaly
- Maculopapular rash after treatment with ampicillin or amoxicillin (immune-mediated vasculitic rash)
  - Diagnostics
    - Heterophile antibodies (monospot test)
    - Atypical lymphocytosis on peripheral smear
  - Management
    - Symptomatic therapy
    - Avoid contact sports in cases of splenomegaly
    - Steroids for management of complications (airway obstruction due to enlarged tonsils, autoimmune hemolytic anemia)

> Steeple sign is also seen in croup.

– Herpes simplex virus: vesicles located on the anterior pharynx

Retropharyngeal Abscess

– Definition: infection between the posterior pharyngeal wall and prevertebral fascia
– Signs and symptoms
  - Neck pain and stiffness
  - Odynophagia/dysphagia
  - Muffled voice
  - Enlargement of posterior pharyngeal wall
– Diagnostics
  - Neck x-ray: widening of the prevertebral strip (Fig. 37-6)
  - CT scan: ring enhancement with central lucency, anterior airway displacement
– Management
  - Incision and drainage
  - IV antibiotics
    - Third-generation cephalosporin
    - PLUS
    - Ampicillin-sulbactam or clindamycin
– Complications
  - Airway compromise, aspiration pneumonia
  - Posterior mediastinitis

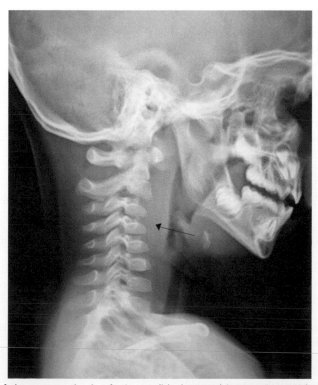

Figure 37-6: Widening of the prevertebral soft tissues *(black arrow)* in a patient with retropharyngeal abscess. (Image courtesy of James Heilman, MD.)

- Sepsis, thrombophlebitis
- Erosion of carotid sheath
- Vertebral osteomyelitis

Peritonsillar Abscess
- Signs and symptoms
  - Dysphasia
  - Trismus: painful spastic contractions of the jaw
  - Asymmetric tonsillar enlargement with associated displacement of the uvula away from the affected side
  - "Hot potato" voice
  - Pooling of saliva
- Diagnostics: clinical
- Management
  - Incision and drainage

> Lemierre syndrome: septic thrombophlebitis of the internal jugular vein, which commonly occurs as a complication of oropharyngeal abscesses. Can result in septic emboli being thrown into the lungs. Diagnose with Doppler of the internal jugular vein. Treated with IV antibiotics and anticoagulation.

  - Antibiotics covering group A beta-hemolytic strep and respiratory anaerobes

Bacterial Tracheitis
- Microbiology: *S. aureus* (most common cause)
- Signs and symptoms
  - Preceding viral URI
  - Rapid-onset high fever, chills
  - Brassy cough
  - Stridor, choking
  - Dysphagia, odynophagia
  - Respiratory distress
- Diagnostics
  - Neck x-ray: subglottic tracheal narrowing (steeple sign)
  - Bronchoscopy (may also be therapeutic to remove infectious debris)
- Management: antistaphylococcal antibiotics +/− airway management if indicated

Epiglottitis
- Microbiology
  - Haemophilus influenza type B (if unimmunized)
  - Staphylococcus/Streptococcus spp.
- Signs and symptoms
  - High fever
  - Muffled voice, drooling
  - Inspiratory stridor
  - Dysphagia, odynophagia
  - Hyperextended neck, tripod position
  - Toxic appearing
- Diagnostics
  - Ensure airway protection prior to diagnostic workup
  - Visualization of edematous and erythematous epiglottis during direct laryngoscopy guided intubation
  - Epiglottic, blood cultures
  - Lateral neck radiographs: "thumbprint" sign; should not delay airway protection
- Management
  - Avoid excessive stimulation during physical exam (may worsen respiratory distress)
  - IV antibiotics: third-generation cephalosporin + antistaphylococcal/streptococcal
  - Rifampin prophylaxis for unimmunized household contacts if caused by H. influenzae

Laryngitis
- Most commonly due to viral infection; other causes include diphtheria, Bordetella, and gastroesophageal reflux disease
- Present with hoarseness, sore throat, rhinorrhea
- Often preceded by URI
- Clinical diagnosis, conservative management

Tracheomalacia
- Abnormal collapse of the tracheal airways
- May be primary (inflammation/infection of proximal airways) or secondary (extrinsic compression from mediastinal mass)
- Wheezing worsens with activity and URIs, otherwise infant is healthy and doing well

Laryngomalacia
- Most common laryngeal airway anomaly
- Most common cause of stridor in infants and children.
- Starts in neonates, loudest at 4–8 months, resolves by 1 year
- Secondary to laxity of supraglottic structures resulting in collapse and inspiratory stridor
- Differentiated from tracheomalacia based on presence of inspiratory stridor worsened by activity, supine, and URIs
- Clinical diagnosis, may require confirmation by flexible laryngoscopy
- Conservative management as most cases are self-limiting, supraglottoplasty in severe cases

Thyroglossal Duct Cyst
- Remnant of embryologic tract when thyroid gland descends from the base of the tongue into its place behind the hyoid bone
- Midline neck mass that moves with swallowing and tongue protrusion
- Cyst may become infected
- May have ectopic thyroid tissue
- Treatment is surgical removal if it becomes infected

NEONATAL DISORDERS

Neonatal Respiratory Distress Syndrome
- Pathophysiology: inadequate surfactant production from immature alveoli resulting in diffuse lung collapse and noncardiogenic pulsmonary edema
- Risk factors
  - Prematurity (<34 weeks)
  - Very low birthweight (<1500 g)
  - Maternal diabetes (high insulin prevents maturation of sphingomyelin)
  - Cesarean section
- Signs and symptoms
  - Tachypnea, accessory muscle inspiration, nasal flaring
  - Cyanosis
  - Hypoxemia
- Diagnostics
  - Chest x-ray
    - Diffuse whiteout of the lungs (Fig. 38-1)
    - Air bronchograms
    - Low lung volumes
  - Clinical
- Management
  - Respiratory support: nasal cannula, continuous positive airway pressure (CPAP)
  - Tocolytics to delay labor and avoid prematurity
  - Antenatal glucocorticoids: aids in lung maturity, stimulates fetal surfactant synthesis
  - Exogenous surfactant (lucinactant)
- Complications
  - Bronchopulmonary dysplasia
  - Retinopathy of prematurity

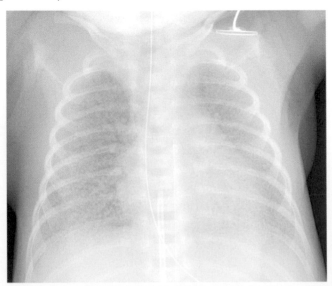

Figure 38-1: Chest x-ray in a patient with neonatal respiratory distress syndrome showing diffuse whiteout of bilateral lung fields. (Image courtesy of Mikael Häggström, MD.)

Transient Tachypnea of the Newborn
- Tachypnea in a newborn term birth following rapid delivery or cesarean section
- Secondary to retained alveolar fluid resulting in mild pulmonary edema
- Chest x-ray shows fluid in the fissures and bilateral perihilar streaking
- Self-limiting, resolves within 48 hours

Meconium Aspiration
- Risk factors: postterm infants born through meconium-stained amniotic fluid
- Pathophysiology: fetal distress results in passage of meconium (may be in utero or with first postnasal inspiration) → meconium is inhaled → obstructs the airway resulting in fetal respiratory distress
- Signs and symptoms
  - Respiratory distress
  - Hypoxemia
  - Cyanosis
- Diagnostics
  - Clinical: history of meconium passage
  - Chest x-ray
    - Diaphragmatic flattening
    - Hyperinflation
    - Patchy infiltrates
- Management: respiratory support
  - CPAP
  - Extracorporal membranous oxygenation
  - Inhaled nitric oxygen
  - Endotracheal intubation plus airway suctioning for nonvigorous infants
- Complications
  - Aspiration pneumonitis/pneumonia
  - Persistent pulmonary hypertension of the newborn

Surfactant functions to decrease alveolar surface tension and prevent alveolar collapse.

AIRWAY DISEASE

Croup (Laryngotracheobronchitis)
- Epidemiology: infants 3 months to 3 years
- Definition: infection and inflammation of the subglottic structures (larynx, trachea, bronchi)
- Microbiology
  - Parainfluenza: most common cause
  - Influenza
- Signs and symptoms
  - Preceding upper respiratory infection (URI) symptoms: fever, sore throat, rhinorrhea
  - Barking, seal-like cough
  - Hoarseness
  - Inspiratory stridor
  - Symptoms worse at night
- Diagnostics
  - Clinical
  - Anteroposterior neck radiographs: steeple sign (subglottic narrowing) (Fig. 38-2)
- Management
  - Mild cases: symptomatic management +/− humidified oxygen
  - Moderate to severe cases: corticosteroids +/− racemic epinephrine (stridor at rest) – Both decrease subglottic edema

Spasmodic croup is related to hypersensitivity reaction with acute onset of stridor. Self resolves without treatment.

Bronchiolitis
- Epidemiology: <2 years old
- Definition: infection and inflammation of the bronchiole secondary to lower respiratory viral infection
- Risk factors
  - Winter
  - Daycare attendance
  - Lack of breastfeeding
  - Tobacco exposure

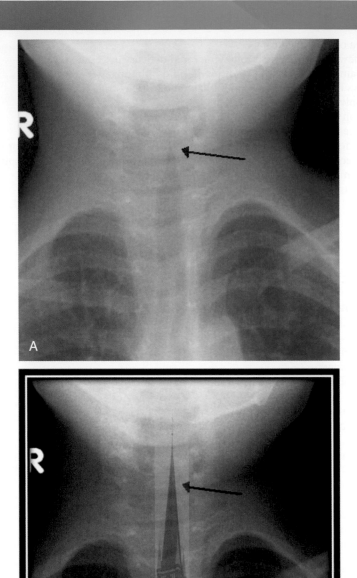

Figure 38-2: Anteroposterior neck x-ray demonstrating (A) the steeple sign in a patient with croup. (B) The steeple sign can also be seen in patients with bacterial tracheitis. Black arrows demonstrating site of narrowing of the subglottic trachea. (Image courtesy of Frank Gaillard / CC BY-SA.)

- Microbiology
  - Respiratory syncytial virus (RSV): most common cause
  - Parainfluenza
- Signs and symptoms
  - URI symptoms (fever, cough, rhinorrhea, nasal congestion)
  - Tachypnea
  - Wheezing
- Diagnostics
  - Clinical
  - Chest x-ray: hyperinflation, patchy infiltrates
- Complications
  - Apnea (more common in young infants, history of prematurity)
  - Recurrent wheezing

- Management
  - Supportive care
  - Avoid tobacco exposure
  - Advise handwashing and breastfeeding
  - +/− nebulized hypertonic saline in hospitalized infants
  - Palivizumab (RSV monoclonal antibody): given prophylactically during RSV peak season for those at high risk of complications or hospitalization (chronic lung disease, hemodynamically significant congenital heart disease, history of prematurity <29 weeks)

Acute Bronchitis
- Causes
  - Viral URI
  - URI organisms (*Streptococcus pneumoniae, Haemophilus influenzae*, Moraxella)
- Signs and symptoms
  - Productive cough
  - Mild hemoptysis
  - Dyspnea, chest discomfort
  - Wheezes, crackles
- Diagnostics
  - Clinical
  - Chest x-ray to rule out pneumonia: will show mild congestive changes, no opacities or consolidation
- Management
  - Supportive care
    - Nonprescription analgesics
    - Cough suppressant (dextromethorphan, guaifenesin)
    - Bronchodilators
  - Antibiotics are generally not recommended; if required in special circumstances (pertussis, limit spread of infection), macrolides are first line

Asthma
- Definition: airway hyperreactivity resulting in bronchoconstriction and obstructive lung disease
- Risk factors
  - Family history, males
  - Allergies, atopy
  - Lack of breast milk
- Triggers
  - Gastroesophageal reflux disease (nighttime asthma)
  - URI
  - Pollen, dander
  - Drugs: aspirin, beta blockers, smoking
  - Cold weather, exercise
- Signs and symptoms
  - Wheezing, dyspnea, tachypnea
  - Cough, chest pain
  - Improvement of symptoms with bronchodilators
  - Pulses paradoxus, absent breath sounds and wheezing, cyanosis: seen in severe cases
- Diagnostics
  - Clinical: severity determined based on the frequency of symptoms (intermittent, mild, moderate, severe), presence of nighttime symptoms, and effect on daily activities
  - Pulmonary function tests (PFTs)
    - Obstructive lung pattern
      - Reversible airway obstruction with improvement of FEV_1 >12% upon administration of bronchodilators: differentiates asthma from chronic obstructive pulmonary disease (COPD)
  - Methacholine challenge: used to diagnose patients that describe history of asthma with normal PFTs and currently asymptomatic
    - Decrease of FEV_1 >20% upon administration is diagnostic
  - Arterial blood gas (ABG)
    - Respiratory alkalosis
    - Normal pH or respiratory acidosis may be indicative of respiratory fatigue and worsening asthma exacerbation
  - Peak expiratory flow: used to determine severity of asthma exacerbation and how far patient is from baseline; home device that allows patient to self-triage (home vs emergency department [ED]) based on present symptoms

- Management
  - Avoid exacerbating factors
  - Pharmacologic: step-up management with each treatment added onto the previous treatment regimens (Fig. 38-3)
    - Step 1: short-acting beta agonists (SABAs): albuterol, levalbuterol
      - Used for acute exacerbations and patients with intermittent asthma
    - Step 2: low-dose inhaled corticosteroids (fluticasone, budesonide)
      - First-line treatment for chronic asthma
      - Side effects: oral thrush (rinse mouth after use)
    - Step 3: low dose of inhaled corticosteroids (ICS) plus long-acting beta agonists (LABA; i.e., salmeterol, formoterol) or medium-dose ICS
    - Step 4: medium dose of inhaled corticosteroid and LABA
    - Step 5: maximum dose of inhaled corticosteroids plus LABA
      - Consider omalizumab in patients with high levels of immunoglobulin E (IgE)
    - Step 6: oral corticosteroids
      - If patient is not responding to step-up management, ensure that patient is administering medication in the proper manner
    - Alternatives
      - Leukotriene antagonist: montelukast, zafirlukast
      - Theophylline
        - Phosphodiesterase inhibitor with narrow therapeutic index
        - Side effects: arrhythmias, neurotoxicity
      - Zileuton
      - Cromolyn sodium prevents mast cell degranulation
      - Magnesium sulfate: used in severe asthma exacerbations in the ED in patients unresponsive to initial treatment
  - Thermoplasty: removes smooth muscle hyperplasia in bronchial airways

Omalizumab mechanism of action: monoclonal antibody that binds IgE in the serum.
Long-acting beta agonist side effects: tremors, arrhythmias.

Management of asthma exacerbation
- Severity determined based on difference of peak expiratory flow (PEF) from patient baseline and ABG
- Administer SABA, corticosteroids, oxygen
- Monitor response to treatments based on PEF, pulse oximetry, and presence of wheezing
- Never use LABA in acute exacerbations as it increases mortality
- Decision whether to admit patient from the ED with asthma exacerbation is dependent upon degree of response

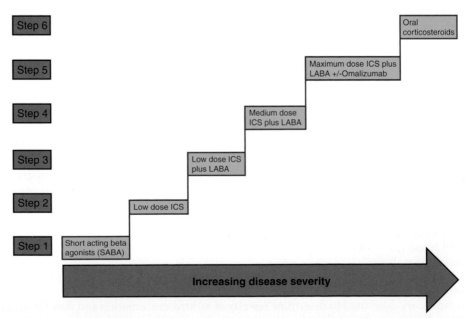

Figure 38-3: Summary of asthma step-up therapy. Every medication is added to the regimen from the previous step. *ICS*, Inhaled corticosteroid; *LABA*, long-acting beta agonist.

- Good response: discharge from the ED
- Poor or worsening response: admit to the floors or intensive care unit
- Consider mechanical ventilation or noninvasive positive-pressure ventilation (bilevel positive airway pressure) in patients who develop respiratory fatigue, normalizing pH, altered mental status, "silent chest" with absent wheezing and breath sounds

Additional considerations and notes when managing asthma patients:
- Consider referring patient to pulmonologist at step 3 or 4
- Most patient's asthma symptoms will significantly decrease or resolve by adolescence
- Avoid use of beta blockers (especially nonspecific beta blockers) unless necessary in patients with chronic asthma
- Ensure vaccination against pneumococcal and influenza

> Aspirin-induced asthma/respiratory disease: aspirin inhibits cyclooxygenase, which results in shunting of the arachidonic acid system down the leukotriene pathway increasing leukotriene levels, which have bronchoconstrictive effects.

GENETIC PULMONARY SYNDROMES

Cystic Fibrosis
- Definition: autosomal recessive genetic disorder affecting whites most commonly due to deletion of phenylalanine at the 508 position
- Pathophysiology: defective chloride channels prevent movement of chloride ions across membranes resulting in thick secretions
- Signs and symptoms
  - Pulmonary
    - Recurrent pneumonia with *Staphylococcus aureus* (<20 years old) and *Pseudomonas* (>20 years old)
    - Bronchiectasis, chronic bronchitis
    - Allergic bronchopulmonary aspergillosis
    - Nasal polyps
  - Gastrointestinal
    - Recurrent pancreatitis, steatorrhea, fat-soluble vitamin deficiencies (A, D, E, K)
    - Meconium ileus in newborns, rectal prolapse
    - Jaundice, biliary cirrhosis
    - Failure to thrive
  - Genitourinary
    - Decreased fertility in females (thick cervical mucus)
    - Infertility in males (absence of vas deferens)
- Diagnostics: clinical and evidence of *CFTR* dysfunction
  - Increased sweat chloride concentration
  - Newborn screen: increased immunoreactive trypsinogen
  - Abnormal nasal potential difference
- Management: mostly symptomatic, no present cure
  - Pneumonia: antibiotics covering *S. aureus* and *Pseudomonas* (Fig. 38-4)
  - Pancreatic insufficiency, steatorrhea: pancreatic enzyme replacement
  - Pulmonary secretions
    - Chest physiotherapy
    - Albuterol/saline
    - Mucolytics (N-acetylcysteine), DNase
  - Ivacaftor: CFTR modulator that treats cystic fibrosis patients with G551D mutation by restoring function of the defective protein

Further management of cystic fibrosis
- Administer all routine vaccines, including pneumococcal and yearly influenza
- Azithromycin: slows decline of lung function
- High-dose ibuprofen: antiinflammatory benefits
- Lung transplantation: for severe cystic fibrosis lung disease

Alpha-1 Antitrypsin Deficiency
- Definition: codominance inherited disorder affecting the lungs and liver in young patients with minimal to nonexistent smoking or alcohol history
- Pathophysiology
  - Alpha-1 antitrypsin prevents breakdown of elastin by elastase in the lungs
  - Deficiency of alpha-1 antitrypsin results in unopposed elastase activity in the alveoli
  - Alpha-1 antitrypsin proteins buildup in the liver → hepatocellular dysfunction

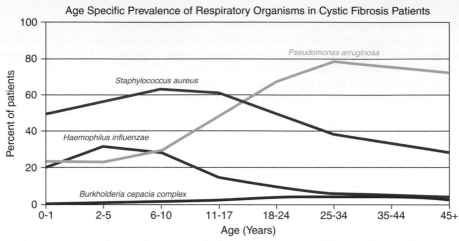

Figure 38-4: Prevalence of respiratory infections in patients with cystic fibrosis, by age.

- Signs and symptoms
  - Pulmonary
    - Dyspnea, cough, wheezing
    - COPD
    - Panacinar emphysema affecting predominantly the lower lobes
  - Gastrointestinal
    - Jaundice, hyperbilirubinemia
    - Cirrhosis, hepatocellular carcinoma
- Diagnostics
  - Alpha-1 antitrypsin levels
  - PAS positive and diastase resistant globules in the liver
- Management
  - Avoid smoking and occupational exposure
  - Enzyme replacement in severe cases
  - Liver/lung transplant

Primary Ciliary Dyskinesia (Kartagener Syndrome)

Smoking increases the number of inflammatory cells (polymorphonuclear neutrophils, macrophages) that release elastase accelerating the loss of elastin in the alveoli. In addition, smoking inhibits alpha-1 antitrypsin.

- Definition: autosomal recessive disorder affecting the lungs, heart, genitourinary system, and other organ systems that rely on cilia for proper function
- Pathophysiology: dynein arms defect resulting in immotile cilia
- Signs and symptoms
  - Pulmonary: impaired clearance of secretions
    - Recurrent pneumonia, sinusitis, otitis media
    - Bronchiectasis
    - Nasal polyps
  - Cardiac: impaired cardiac looping during embryonic phase
    - Dextrocardia (part of situs inversus) (Fig. 38-5)
    - Transposition of the great vessels
  - Genitourinary: impaired beating cilia resulting in decreased fertility
    - Males
      - Immotile sperm prevent sperm from reaching egg
      - Epispadias
    - Females: increased risk of ectopic pregnancy as egg is less able to travel down the fallopian tube, and therefore more likely to be fertilized and implant in the fallopian tubes
  - Gastrointestinal: pyloric stenosis
- Diagnostics
  - Screening: low nasal nitric oxide level
  - Definitive: visualization of ciliary defects with transmission electron microscopy after nasal or bronchial biopsy
- Management: symptomatic, most patients have a normal active life span

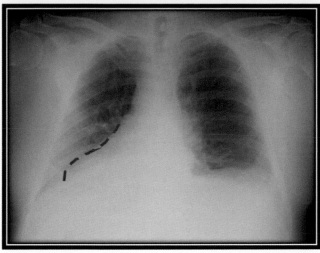

Figure 38-5: Dextrocardia in a patient with Kartagener syndrome. Dotted line demonstrating outline of the heart border with convexity towards the right rather than left.

TABLE 38-1 Pediatric Pneumonia

PEDIATRIC ETIOLOGIES OF PNEUMONIA	KEY FEATURES	TREATMENT
Viral	• Upper respiratory infection symptoms (fever, nasal congestion, rhinorrhea) • Cough, dyspnea • Interstitial infiltrates	• Supportive
Chlamydia trachomatis	• Presents at 1–3 mo of age • Preceding history of conjunctivitis • Staccato cough • Eosinophilia	• Macrolides
Mycoplasma pneumoniae	• Referred to as "walking" pneumonia • Common cause of adolescent pneumonia • Interstitial infiltrates • Positive cold agglutinins	• Macrolides • Tetracyclines • Fluoroquinolones
Bordetella pertussis	• Unimmunized • "Whooping" cough • Robust lymphocytosis; may be confused for acute lymphocytic leukemia	• Macrolides + vaccination
Streptococcus pneumoniae	• Most common bacterial etiology • Fever, chills • Lobar consolidation	• Amoxicillin

PNEUMONIA

Pediatric pneumonia has similar microbiologic etiologies and signs and symptoms as adult pneumonia. *S. pneumoniae* represents the most common bacterial cause etiology. Viral pneumonia is the most common cause overall (Table. 38-1).

MISCELLANEOUS

Foreign Body Aspiration
- Epidemiology: infant 6 months to 6 years
- Definition: ingestion of small object resulting in airway compromise, often unwitnessed
- Signs and symptoms: depends on location of foreign body
  - Extrathoracic (laryngotracheal)
    - Sudden onset choking/coughing
    - Inspiratory stridor
    - Vomiting
  - Intrathoracic (bronchial)
    - Atelectasis
    - Recurrent pneumonia
    - Localized wheezing
    - Chronic cough
- Diagnostics

- Chest x-ray
  - Look for radiopaque objects
  - Evaluate with inspiratory/expiratory and decubitus radiographs
- Bronchoscopy: also therapeutic with ability to retrieve foreign object
– Management
- Secure airway
- Age with object expulsion by encouraging cough
- Bronchoscopy for retrieval of foreign object

Pulmonary hypoplasia of the newborn: occurs secondary to external compression (congenital diaphragmatic hernia) or lack of in utero stimulus (oligohydramnios, Potter sequence)

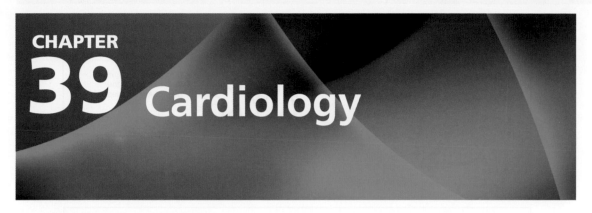

CONGENITAL HEART DISEASES
Key principles
- Prenatally, right-left heart connections exist to allow blood flow to bypass high pulmonary vascular resistance (Fig. 39-1)
- After birth, pulmonary vascular resistance decreases, right-left heart connections close, resulting in postnatal development of cardiovascular system (Fig. 39-2)
- Persistent septal defects tend to be left to right shunts postnatal due to higher left-sided pressures (Table 39-1)
- Left to right shunts may become right to left shunts as increased blood flow results in pulmonary hypertension and reversal of pressure gradient
- Septal defect predisposes to failure to thrive, congestive heart failure, frequent respiratory infections, endocarditis, and paradoxic embolism
- Cyanotic congenital heart defects are ductus dependent to allow oxygenated blood to reach systemic circulation (Table 39-2)
- Congenital heart diseases are identified on echocardiogram (Fig. 39-3)

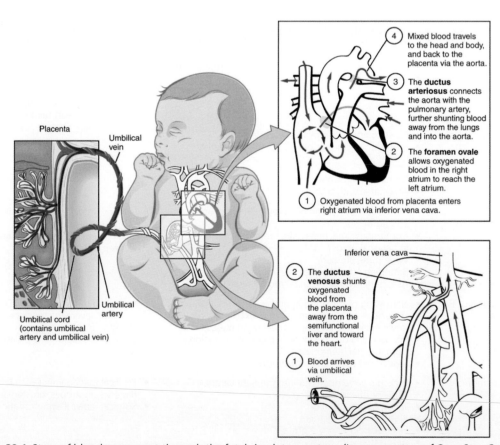

Figure 39-1: Steps of blood movement through the fetal circulatory system. (Image courtesy of OpenStax College.)

373

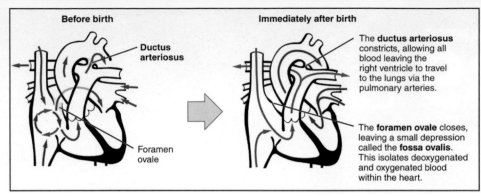

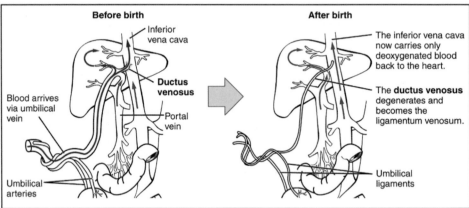

Figure 39-2: Illustration of the neonatal circulatory system immediately before and after birth. (Image courtesy of OpenStax College.)

TABLE 39-1   Acyanotic Congenital Heart Disease

CONGENITAL HEART DEFECT	KEY FEATURES	MANAGEMENT
Atrial septal defect (ASD)	• Wide, fixed splitting S2 • Systolic ejection murmur at upper left sternal border • Asymptomatic	• Conservative management, spontaneous closure for small asymptomatic defects • Surgical closure for large defect, pulmonary hypertension, arrhythmias, heart failure
Ventricular septal defect (VSD)	• Most common congenital heart defect • Holosystolic murmur over the left lower sternal border	
Atrioventricular canal	• Combination of ASD and VSD • Associated with trisomy 21	
Patent ductus arteriosus (PDA)	• Allows for connection between pulmonary artery and aorta • Continuous "machinery-like" murmur over the upper left sternal border • Wide pulse pressure • Bounding arterial pulses • Associated with congenital rubella infection	• Isolated defect: indomethacin to stimulate closure • Ductus dependent: prostaglandin to keep open
Coarctation of the aorta	• Narrowing of the aorta after the left subclavian artery • Hypertensive upper extremities (pink), hypotensive lower extremities (cyanotic, decreased pulses) • Rib notching on chest x-ray (collateral circulation from internal memories) • Associated with Turner syndrome	• Prostaglandin to maintain PDA open for severe ductus dependent coarctation • Surgical or balloon angioplasty repair
Ebstein anomaly	• Tricuspid valve displaced into the right ventricle • Triple or quadruple gallop • Tricuspid regurgitation • Right atrial enlargement • Electrocardiography: right axis deviation, tall P waves • Associated with maternal lithium use	• Medical management with loop diuretics, inotropes, prostaglandin • Surgical repair if symptomatic

TABLE 39-1   Acyanotic Congenital Heart Disease—(*continued.*)

CONGENITAL HEART DEFECT	KEY FEATURES	MANAGEMENT
Aortic stenosis	• Systolic ejection murmur at base • Most commonly due to a bicuspid aortic valve (associated with Turner syndrome) • Severe cases present with congestive heart failure	• Balloon valvuloplasty or surgical replacement if symptomatic
Pulmonic stenosis	• Systolic ejection murmur at the upper left sternal border • Most commonly asymptomatic, congestive heart failure in severe cases • Prominent pulmonary arteries on chest x-ray	• Prostaglandin to maintain PDA in severe cases while pending definitive treatment • Balloon valvuloplasty in severe or symptomatic cases

TABLE 39-2   Cyanotic Congenital Heart Disease

CONGENITAL HEART DEFECT	KEY FEATURES	MANAGEMENT
Tetralogy of Fallot	• Pulmonic stenosis • Right ventricular hypertrophy • Overriding aorta (aorta overlying ventricular septal defect [VSD]) • VSD • Chest x-ray: "boot-shaped" heart • Cyanosis dependent on degree of right to left shunting • Increased systemic vascular resistance (valsalva, squatting, knee-chest position, systemic hypertension) decreases right to left shunting and improves cyanosis • Decreased systemic vascular resistance (hypotension, exercise, dehydration, crying) increases the right to left shunting and worsens cyanosis	• Prostaglandin • Beta blocker • Surgical repair
Transposition of the great vessels	• Separate pulmonary and systemic circulation • VSD • Single S2 • Chest x-ray: "egg on a string" • Associated with uncontrolled maternal diabetes, DiGeorge syndrome	• Prostaglandin to maintain patent ductus arteriosus connection between separate pulmonary and systemic circulation • Balloon atrial septostomy (maintains patent foramen ovale [PFO] prior to definitive surgical repair) • Surgical repair
Truncus arteriosus	• Aorta and pulmonary artery originate from common trunk • Mixing of oxygenated and deoxygenated blood results in mild cyanosis • VSD • Diastolic murmur at apex • Systolic ejection murmur along the left sternal border • Associated with DiGeorge syndrome	• VSD repair • Graft separating aorta and pulmonary artery
Total anomalous pulmonary venous return	• Pulmonary veins drain into systemic circulation → mixing of oxygenated and deoxygenated blood entering right atrium → mild cyanosis • Pulmonic ejection murmur at left sternal border • Chest x-ray: "snowman" appearance	• Surgical repair
Tricuspid atresia	• Interatrial connection (atrial septal defect, PFO) present to allow for right to left shunting • Left atrial dilation + left ventricular hypertrophy • Electrocardiography: deviation, small or absent R waves in precordial leads	• Multistage surgical repair

Understanding the normal fetal circulatory system and the transitions that occur after birth will aid in understanding the cyanotic and acyanotic congenital heart disease.

Benign murmurs
1. Murmurs are common in neonates and infants due to persistent septal defect
2. Most commonly asymptomatic
3. Systolic, grade 2/6 or less
4. No other precipitating factor (fever, anemia, infection)
5. No other diagnostic testing required if infant is otherwise doing well

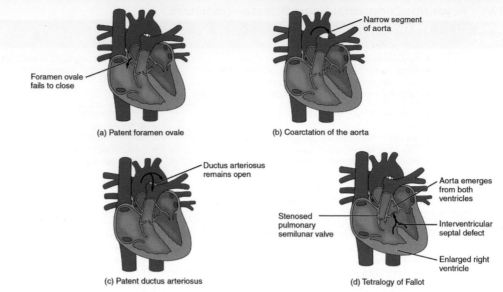

Figure 39-3: Illustration of various congenital heart defects. (Image courtesy of OpenStax College.)

VASCULAR, VALVULAR, ARRHYTHMIAS, AND HYPERTENSION

Kawasaki Disease
– Definition: small to medium vessel vasculitis that involves the coronary arteries
– Epidemiology
  • Most common cause of acquired heart disease in children (<5 years old) in the United States
  • Increased incidence in children of Asian descent

> Live vaccine administration should be delayed for 11 months after administration of IV immunoglobulin due to potential interference with developing a robust immune response.

– Signs and symptoms (Fig. 39-4)
  • Diagnostic symptoms
    ▪ Fever lasting >5 days (typically nonresponsive to antipyretics)
    ▪ Bilateral nonexudative conjunctivitis
    ▪ Strawberry tongue, swollen cracked lips
    ▪ Polymorphous rash

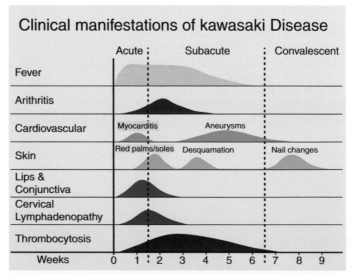

Figure 39-4: Time course and clinical manifestations of Kawasaki disease. (Image courtesy of Maen K Househ.)

- Cervical adenopathy >1.5 cm
- Peripheral erythema and edema, desquamating fingertips
  - Nondiagnostic, supportive features
    - Coronary artery aneurysms, myocarditis
    - Sterile pyuria
    - Gallbladder hydrops
    - Aseptic meningitis
    - Arthralgias
    - Anterior uveitis
- Diagnostics: fever PLUS four of five diagnostic features
- Management
  - Aspirin plus IV immunoglobulin: decreases incidence of coronary artery aneurysms
  - Baseline echocardiogram followed by repeat at 6–8 weeks to evaluate for presence of coronary artery aneurysms

Acute Rheumatic Fever
- Epidemiology: most common cause of acquired heart disease worldwide
- Pathophysiology: autoimmune molecular mimicry response following group A Streptococcus (Streptococcus pyogenes) pharyngitis resulting in inflammation of the heart, joints, brain, and skin
- Signs and symptoms: JONES major criteria
  - Joints: migratory polyarthritis
  - Cardiac
    - Mitral regurgitation, later mitral stenosis following recurrent infections
    - Myocarditis
  - Nodules: firm, painless subcutaneous nodules along the extensor surfaces
  - Erythema marginatum (evanescent, pinkish red nonpruritic rash involving the trunk)
  - Syndeham chorea
    - Involuntary purposeless movements, emotional disturbances
    - Inflammation of the basal ganglia and caudate nuclei
  - Minor criteria
    - Fever, leukocytosis
    - Arthralgias
    - Elevated erythrocyte sedimentation rate, prolonged PR interval
- Diagnostics
  - Recent streptococcal infection plus two major criteria or one major plus two minor
  - Antistreptolysin O titers
  - AntiDNAse antibodies
- Management
  - Eradication of group A Streptococcus infection: intramuscular penicillin
  - Secondary prophylaxis
    - Intramuscular penicillin every 3–4 weeks depending on the severity of heart disease
    - Decreases recurrence of future infections and prevents worsening of heart disease
    - Arthritis, inflammation control: nonsteroidal antiinflammatory drugs

Group A Streptococcus infection involving the skin does not cause rheumatic fever, only glomerulonephritis.

Hypertension
- Causes: most commonly secondary hypertension; however, increasing incidence of essential hypertension due to childhood obesity
  - Cardiac
    - Essential hypertension: most common in adolescents
    - Coarctation of the aorta
  - Renal
    - Renal artery stenosis
    - Vasculitis
    - Liddle syndrome
    - Wilms tumor
    - Polycystic kidney disease
  - Endocrine
    - Hyperthyroidism
    - Cushing syndrome

- - Pheochromocytoma
  - Neuroblastoma
  - Congenital adrenal hyperplasia
- Signs and symptoms: asymptomatic, unless patient is experiencing hypertensive emergency
- Diagnostics
  - Blood pressure >95th percentile for age
  - Thorough physical examination and laboratory workup to evaluate secondary hypertension etiology
- Management
  - Treat underlying secondary cause
  - Lifestyle modifications
- Complications: hypertensive emergency (severe hypertension with end-organ damage)

Prolonged QT Syndrome

- Causes
  - Potassium channelopathy (Romano-Ward, Jervell and Lange-Nielsen syndrome)
  - Medications (more common in adults)
    - Macrolides, antifungals
    - Tricyclic antidepressants, selective serotonin reuptake inhibitors
- Signs and symptoms
  - Recurrent syncope
  - Palpitation
  - Sudden cardiac death
  - Sensorineural deafness (Jervell and Lange-Nielsen syndrome)
- Diagnostics
  - Electrocardiography: corrected QT interval >470 ms
  - Genetic testing (may have family history of sudden cardiac death)
- Management
  - Avoid dehydration, excessive exercise
  - Asymptomatic: beta blocker (propranolol, nadolol)
  - Symptomatic: beta blocker plus implantable cardioverter defibrillator
- Complications: Torsades de Pointes

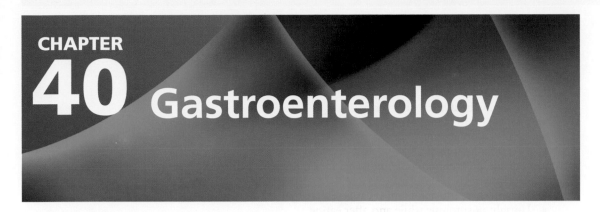

ESOPHAGUS

Gastroesophageal Reflux Disease (GERD)

– Epidemiology: common asymptomatic entity in infants, affecting >50%
– Pathophysiology (Fig. 40-1)
  • Laxity of lower esophageal sphincter resulting in reflux of gastric contents into the esophagus
  • Shorter esophagus
  • Increased time spent in supine position
– Signs and symptoms
  • Physiologic
    ▪ Asymptomatic
    ▪ Postprandial regurgitation ("spitting up," "happy spitters")

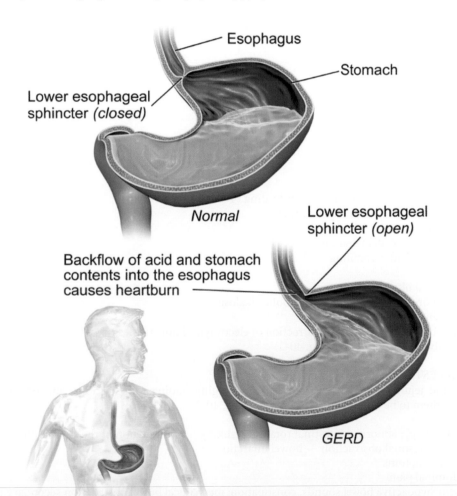

Gastroesophageal Reflux Disease (GERD)

Figure 40-1: Pathophysiology of gastroesophageal reflux disease.

- Pathologic
  - Failure to thrive
  - Feeding refusal, irritability
  - Sandifer syndrome: severe GERD plus torticollis with arching of the back
- Diagnostics
  - Clinical
  - Other testing in atypical or severe cases
    - Esophageal pH monitoring
    - Barium esophagram
    - Upper endoscopy
- Management: interventions only indicated for GERD with pathologic symptoms
  - Conservative
    - Reassurance, education: most cases resolve by 1 year
    - Upright positioning while and after eating
    - Frequent small meals
    - Thickened feeds
  - Medical
    - H2 blockers, proton pump inhibitors
    - Prokinetics for delayed gastric emptying: erythromycin, metoclopramide
  - Surgical: Nissen fundoplication
- Complications
  - Esophageal strictures
  - Barrett esophagus
  - Recurrent pneumonitis/laryngitis/wheezing

In contrast, nonbilious vomiting in tracheoesophageal fistula occurs after first feeds.

STOMACH

Pyloric Stenosis
- Risk factors
  - Firstborn
  - Males
  - Erythromycin
  - Formula feeding
- Signs and symptoms
  - Nonbilious projectile vomiting after feeding (4–8 weeks after birth)
  - Olive-shaped, palpable epigastric mass
  - Peristaltic waves
  - Failure to thrive, dehydration
  - Eager to feed after vomiting
- Diagnostics
  - Abdominal ultrasound
  - Hypochloremic, hypokalemic metabolic alkalosis
- Management
  - Initial: IV fluid resuscitation, correction of electrolyte abnormalities
  - Definitive: pyloromyotomy (Fig. 40-2)

SMALL INTESTINE

Duodenal and jejunal atresia have characteristic imaging findings, associations, and pathophysiology, which allow them to be differentiated (Table 40-1; Fig. 40-3).

Malrotation
- Pathophysiology: abnormal intestinal rotation resulting in compression of the superior mesenteric arteries → intestinal obstruction → bowel infarction
- Signs and symptoms
  - Abdominal pain
  - Absent/hypoactive bowel sounds, constipation: mechanical bowel obstruction secondary to development of peritoneal bands (Ladd bands)
  - Anorexia
  - Bloody, dark stools

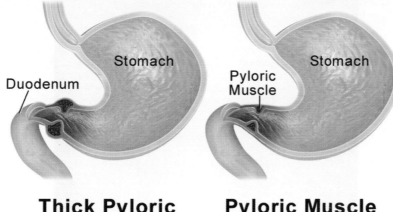

Thick Pyloric Muscle Before Surgery

Pyloric Muscle After Surgery

Figure 40-2: Pyloric stenosis before and after pyloromyotomy.

TABLE 40-1   Duodenal Versus Jejunal Atresia

	DUODENAL ATRESIA	JEJUNAL ATRESIA
Pathophysiology	• Failure of duodenal lumen to recanalize at 8–10 wk gestation	• Mesenteric vascular accident in utero (maternal use of vasoconstrictive medications: cocaine, tobacco, nasal decongestants)
Signs and symptoms	• Bilious vomiting following first feeds • Feeding refusal • Polyhydramnios	• Bilious vomiting • Abdominal distention
Diagnostics	• Abdominal x-ray: "double bubble" sign • Upper gastrointestinal (GI) study	• Abdominal x-ray: multiple air-fluid levels, "triple bubble" sign • Upper GI study
Associations	• VACTERL syndrome • Down syndrome	• None
Management	• Stabilization: IV fluids, bowel rest • Definitive: surgical correction	

– Diagnostics: upper gastrointestinal (GI) study with small bowel follow-through (demonstrates malrotated intestines: ligament of Treitz on the right side of the abdomen)
– Management
  • Intestinal obstruction: gastric decompression, bowel rest, IV fluids
  • Intestinal infarction: exploratory laparotomy with resection of infarcted bowel segments
The presence of bilious versus nonbilious vomiting and the onset of symptoms can help localize the site of pathology (Table 40-2).
Intussusception
– Epidemiology: 6–24 months old
– Pathophysiology: telescoping of the proximal intestinal segment (lead point) into a more distal segment → intestinal obstruction → ischemia and necrosis (Fig. 40-4)
– Causes: any of the following can act as a lead point and increase the risk of intussusception
  • Peyer patches hyperplasia (viral infection, lymphoma)
  • Meckel diverticulum
  • Intestinal polyp/tumor
– Signs and symptoms
  • Episodic, colicky abdominal pain
  • Vomiting, lethargy
  • Sausage-shaped right upper quadrant mass
  • Empty right lower quadrant
  • "Currant jelly" stool: indicative of intestinal ischemia

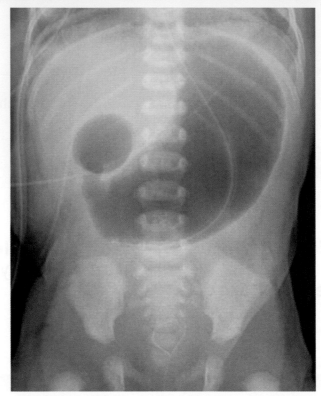

Figure 40-3: Abdominal x-ray showing dilated stomach and proximal duodenum with atretic distal segment consistent with "double bubble" sign in a patient with duodenal atresia.

TABLE 40-2   Differential of Bilious Versus Nonbilious Vomiting and Their Onset

	BILIOUS	NONBILIOUS	ONSET
Tracheoesophageal fistula		+	After first feed
Pyloric stenosis		+	4–8 wk after birth
Duodenal/jejunal atresia	+		After first feed
Hirschsprung disease	+		Weeks–months

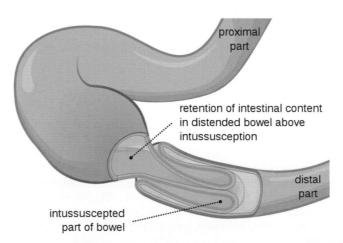

Figure 40-4: Diagrammatic representation of intussusception demonstrating telescoping of the proximal segment of bowel into a more distal portion and resulting in bowel obstruction.

- Diagnostics
  - Abdominal x-ray: evaluate for perforation and/or obstruction
  - Air contrast enema: "coil spring" sign
  - Abdominal ultrasound: "target" sign

- Management
  - Air/contrast enema: both diagnostic and therapeutic
  - Surgery if obstruction is unrelieved by enema

Other intussusception facts:
- Rotavirus immunization is contraindicated in patients with history of intussusception
- Intussusception most commonly occurs at the ileocolic junction
- Intussusception is associated with Henoch-Schönlein purpura vasculitis

Meckel Diverticulum
- Pathophysiology
  - Ectopic gastric/pancreatic tissue most commonly located in the small intestine resulting in intestinal erosion
  - Remnant of vitelline duct (incomplete obliteration in utero)
  - True diverticulum with intestinal outpouching
- Signs and symptoms
  - Asymptomatic: most common
  - Painless hematochezia
- Diagnostic: technetium 99 m pertechnetate scan (Meckel scan): localizes heterotopic gastric tissue
- Management: diverticulectomy
- Complications
  - Intussusception
  - Intestinal obstruction
  - Volvulus
  - Iron deficiency anemia

Meckel diverticulum rule of 2s:
- 2% of the population
- 2 feet from ileocecal valve
- 2 inches long
- 2 types of ectopic tissue (gastric, pancreatic)
- 2 years old
- Males 2:1

PANCREAS
Nesidioblastosis (Congenital Hyperinsulinism)
- Pathophysiology: hyperinsulinism secondary to beta cell hyperplasia
- Signs and symptoms
  - Jitteriness, lethargy
  - Episodic hypothermia
  - Convulsions
  - Macrosomia in utero
- Diagnostics
  - Persistent hypoglycemia in infants and neonates
  - Glucagon challenge test: inadequate increase in blood glucose after administration of glucagon
  - Molecular/genetic testing
- Management
  - Medical
    - Diazoxide
    - Frequent feedings
  - Surgical: partial pancreatectomy

HEPATOBILIARY
Jaundice
- Yellowing of the skin and sclera secondary to elevated bilirubin levels
- Problems related to intravascular hemolysis of red blood cells (RBCs) or hepatobiliary mechanisms (impaired conjugation, biliary transport)
- Normal enterohepatic circulation (Fig. 40-5)
- Unconjugated bilirubin is formed from breakdown of RBCs (Table 40-3)

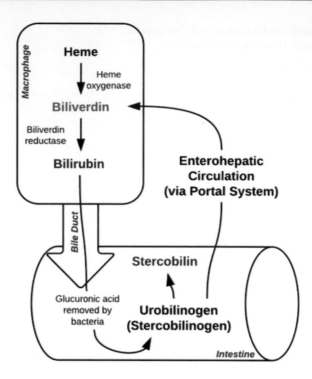

Figure 40-5: Diagrammatic representation of heme breakdown and bilirubin metabolism. (Image courtesy of Johndheathcote; CC BY-SA 3.0 [https://creativecommons.org/licenses/by-sa/3.0])

TABLE 40-3   Causes of Unconjugated Hyperbilirubinemia

	PATHOPHYSIOLOGY	KEY FEATURES	MANAGEMENT
Gilbert syndrome	Mildly decreased UDP-glucuronosyltransferase	• Typically, asymptomatic • Intermittent mild jaundice • Mild, unconjugated hyperbilirubinemia during stress (fasting, infection, surgery)	• Reassurance
Crigler-Najjar syndrome	Absent UDP-glucuronosyltransferase activity	• Unconjugated hyperbilirubinemia • Kernicterus (deposition of bilirubin into the basal ganglia and brainstem resulting in neurologic manifestations: seizures, delayed development, hearing loss, choreoathetosis)	• Phototherapy: asymptomatic, bilirubin 6–12 mg/dL • Exchange transfusion: bilirubin encephalopathy, failed phototherapy • Liver transplant
Dubin-Johnson syndromeRotor syndrome	Impaired biliary transport of conjugated bilirubin	• Typically, asymptomatic • Conjugated hyperbilirubinemia • Black liver (Rotor syndrome)	• Reassurance

- Unconjugated bilirubin is transported to the liver via albumin to be conjugated by the enzyme UDP-glucuronosyltransferase
- Conjugated bilirubin is excreted into intrahepatic biliary ducts to be stored in the gallbladder
- Bile from the gallbladder is released through the cystic duct, common bile duct into the duodenum in response to food to aid in digestion
- Bile travels down the small intestine and is reabsorbed at the terminal ileum to allow recycling of bile through the enterohepatic circulation

Biliary Atresia
- Epidemiology: 2–8 weeks old
- Pathophysiology: fibrosis and sclerosis of the biliary system impairing extrahepatic biliary transport
- Signs and symptoms
  - Progressively, worsening jaundice
  - Pale stools (bile unable to reach the gut)
  - Dark urine (conjugated bilirubin excreted through the urine)

- Hepatomegaly
- Splenomegaly (portal hypertension)
– Diagnostics
  - Direct hyperbilirubinemia
  - Abdominal ultrasound: absent/abnormal gallbladder
  - Phenobarbital (stimulates bile flow) followed by hepatobiliary iminodiacetic acid scan: lack of bile reaching the duodenum is suggestive of biliary atresia
  - Intraoperative cholangiogram: confirmatory
  - Management
  - Surgical repair (Kasai procedure: portoenterostomy) prior to development of biliary cirrhosis to reestablish bile flow
  - Liver transplant: definitive treatment
– Complications: biliary cirrhosis

Metabolic
Reye Syndrome
– Acquired mitochondrial hepatopathy secondary to use of aspirin during viral infection
– Nausea, vomiting, hepatomegaly, seizure, cerebral edema
– Transaminitis, hyperammonemia, coagulopathy, hypoglycemia
– Treatment is supportive
Wilson Disease (Hepatolenticular Degeneration)
– Epidemiology: autosomal recessive disorder, presents in early adolescence or adulthood
– Pathophysiology: disorder of copper metabolism (decreased levels of copper transport protein ceruloplasmin) → elevated free copper levels → systemic copper organ deposition (liver, basal ganglia) resulting in oxidative damage
– Signs and symptoms
  - Neuropsychiatric
    - Depression, hallucinations, psychosis
    - Tremors, ataxia, dysarthria
    - Seizures
  - GI
    - Abdominal pain, hepatomegaly
    - Jaundice
    - Cirrhosis
  - Musculoskeletal: pseudogout
  - Hematologic: Coombs-negative hemolytic anemia
  - Renal
    - Type 2 renal tubular acidosis, Fanconi syndrome
    - Nephrolithiasis
  - Eyes
    - Kayser-Fleischer rings (greenish brown rings around the cornea representing copper deposition in Descemet membrane) (Fig. 40-6)
    - Cataracts

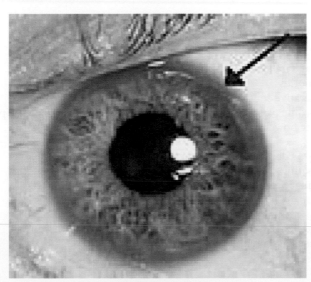

Figure 40-6: Kayser-Fleischer rings in a patient with Wilson disease.

– Diagnostics
  • Slit-lamp examination
  • Decreased ceruloplasmin levels
  • Increased urinary copper after administration of penicillamine
  • Liver biopsy: increased hepatic copper (>250 mcg/g dry weight)
– Management: copper excretion
  • Copper chelators: penicillamine, trientine
  • Zinc (interferes with intestinal absorption)

Menke disease: X-linked recessive defect of copper transport. Presents with "kinky" hair, developmental delay, failure to thrive, seizures, low ceruloplasmin, serum copper, and tissue copper.

LARGE INTESTINE

Necrotizing Enterocolitis
– Risk factors
  • Prematurity (immature GI tract)
  • Very low birthweight
  • Congenital heart disease (decreased perfusion to GI tract increases risk for enteric bacterial translocation)
  • Enteral feeding (act as source for bacterial proliferation)
– Signs and symptoms
  • Fever, lethargy
  • Abdominal distention
  • Abdominal wall erythema
  • Poor feeding, bilious vomiting
  • Bloody bowel movements
– Diagnostics
  • Abdominal x-ray
    ▪ Pneumatosis intestinalis
    ▪ Portal vein gas
    ▪ +/− free air under the diaphragm
  • Supporting features
    ▪ Thrombocytopenia
    ▪ Disseminated intravascular coagulation
    ▪ Metabolic acidosis
– Management
  • Gastric decompression
  • Broad-spectrum IV antibiotics
  • Stop enteric feeds, initiate parenteral nutrition
  • +/− surgery if there are signs of perforation or bowel necrosis

Diarrhea

Diarrhea
– Causes
  • Infectious: bacterial, viral, parasitic (Table 40-4)
  • Medications: antibiotics
  • Inflammatory: ulcerative colitis, Crohn disease
  • Malabsorption: chronic pancreatitis, lactose intolerance, celiac disease, Whipple disease
  • Psychiatric: irritable bowel syndrome
– Signs and symptoms
  • Increase frequency or decreased consistency of bowel movement
  • Watery, bloody, floating
  • Dehydration, anemia, hemoconcentration
– Diagnostics
  • Clinical
  • Electrolyte derangements: hypokalemic, nonanion gap metabolic acidosis
– Management: fluid resuscitation and treat underlying etiology

TABLE 40-4   Infectious Causes of Diarrhea and Their Associations

ETIOLOGY	ASSOCIATIONS	TREATMENT
Rotavirus, norovirus	• Watery diarrhea • Vomiting • Common in pediatrics (rotavirus)	• Supportive
Bacillus cereus	• Fried rice • Acute onset • Vomiting	
Staphylococcus aureus	• Potato salad, mayonnaise • Acute onset • Vomiting	
Shigella	• Uncooked beef • Hemolytic uremic syndrome	
Giardia	• Campers, hikers	• Metronidazole
Clostridium difficile	• Recent antibiotic use • Pseudomembranous colitis	• Oral vancomycin or fidaxomicin • Metronidazole
C. botulinum	• Unpasteurized honey (infants) • Canned foods • Flaccid paralysis	• Antitoxin
Campylobacter	• Guillain-Barré syndrome • Pseudoappendicitis • Chickens, turtles	• Supportive • Antibiotics in severe cases or immunocompromised: fluoroquinolones
Salmonella	• Chickens, raw eggs • Gallbladder colonization	
Entamoeba histolytica	• Travel to Africa, South America, Southeast Asia • Bloody diarrhea • Liver abscess	• Metronidazole, paromomycin
Trichinella	• Undercooked pork • Myalgias, periorbital edema, eosinophilia	• Albendazole, mebendazole
Taenia solium	• Undercooked pork • Cysts in muscles (cysticercosis) or brain (neurocysticercosis)	• Praziquantel • Albendazole + steroids for central nervous system infection

TABLE 40-5   Celiac Disease Versus Tropical Sprue

	CELIAC DISEASE	TROPICAL SPRUE
Key manifestations	• Chronic diarrhea, weight loss • Iron deficiency anemia, fat-soluble vitamin deficiencies • Dermatitis herpetiformis (subepidermal microabscesses at the tip of the dermal papillae) on extensor surfaces such as elbows, knees, and buttocks: specific for celiac disease • D-xylose test: lower urinary and venous D-xylose levels • Less common: transaminitis, arthritis, neurologic symptoms	
Diagnosis	• Serology: immunoglobulin A (IgA) antiendomysial, IgA antitransglutaminase antibodies • Serology may be falsely negative in patients with IgA deficiency, in these cases check for IgG • Esophagogastroduodenoscopy (EGD) with biopsy: atrophy and effacement of small intestinal villi	• EGD with biopsy: blunted villi with increased inflammatory cells in the lamina propria
Treatment	• Gluten-free diet • Dapsone for dermatitis herpatiformis	• Tetracycline + folic acid for 3–6 mo
Complications	• Increased risk for T-cell lymphoma	

Malabsorption Syndromes

Malabsorption syndromes may be genetic or acquired and results in decreased absorption in a particular bowel segment (Table 40-5).

Lactose Intolerance

– Epidemiology: African, Asian, Latino, Native American descent

- Pathophysiology
  - Primary: lactase enzyme deficiency along the intestinal brush border whose concentration steadily declines as we age
  - Secondary: postinfectious gastroenteritis, which destroys the intestinal brush border resulting in temporary lactose intolerance until intestinal villi and lactase enzyme are regenerated
- Signs and symptoms: occur only after ingestion of lactose containing products
  - Abdominal discomfort/cramping
  - Bloating
  - Watery diarrhea
  - Flatulence
  - No systemic symptoms or lab abnormalities
- Diagnostics
  - Clinical
  - Lactose hydrogen breath test: increased levels after ingestion of lactose
  - Elevated stool osmolar gap in otherwise healthy patient with diarrhea
- Management
  - Avoidance of lactose (milk, ice cream, cheese)
  - Lactase supplements before lactose ingestion

COLON CANCER–RELATED SYNDROMES

Inflammatory bowel disease can be due to ulcerative colitis or Crohn disease, both of which have an increased predilection for developing colon cancer; however, a high risk is associated with ulcerative colitis due to its predilection for the rectum and colon (Table 40-6).

TABLE 40-6 Inflammatory Bowel Disease—Ulcerative Colitis Versus Crohn Disease

	ULCERATIVE COLITIS (UC)	CROHN'S DISEASE
Epidemiology	• Bimodal distribution: age 15–40, age 50–80	• Second and third decade of life
Signs and symptoms	• Chronic bloody diarrhea, rectal pain, tenesmus, incontinence • Serology: ANCA positive, elevated inflammatory markers, leukocytosis, anemia	• Chronic watery diarrhea, abdominal pain, nausea, vomiting • Serology: ASCA positive, elevated inflammatory markers, leukocytosis, anemia
Colonoscopy	• Continuous mucosal inflammation starting in the rectum and extending proximally • Pseudopolyps	• Skip lesions: areas of transmural inflammation separated by normal intestine • May involve any part of the gastrointestinal tract; most commonly involves terminal ileum
Biopsy	• Crypt abscesses	• Transmural granulomas
Complications	• Toxic megacolon	• Fistulas (enteroenteric, enterocystic, intravaginal) • Abscesses • Obstruction
Extraintestinal manifestations	• Erythema nodosum • Pyoderma gangrenosum • Primary sclerosing cholangitis • Arthritis, uveitis, spondyloarthritis	• Nephrolithiasis (increased oxalate absorption) • Subacute combined degeneration (B12 deficiency, terminal ileitis) • Gallstones (lack of bile acid reabsorption and cholesterol supersaturation) • Arthritis, uveitis, spondyloarthritis
Treatment	• Acute exacerbation: steroids • Maintenance therapy: mesalamine, sulfasalazine • Surgery is curative and indicated for disease refractory to medical management	• Acute exacerbation: steroids • Maintenance therapy: anti-TNF agents (infliximab, etanercept), immunomodulators (azathioprine, mercaptopurine) • Surgery for the management of complications such as fistulas, strictures, bowel obstruction
Risk of colon cancer	• Increased after 8–10 yr of colonic involvement • Follow-up with colonoscopy every 1–3 yr after having UC for 8–10 yr • Presence of primary sclerosing cholangitis further increases risk	• Increased risk only if there is colonic involvement

ANCA, Antineutrophil cytoplasmic antibodies; *ASCA,* anti-Ssaccharomyces cerevisiae antibodies; *TNF,* tumor necrosis factor.

Peutz-Jeghers Syndrome
- Associated with abnormal serine-threonine tumor suppressor gene
- Genetic syndrome characterized by mucocutaneous hyperpigmentation and hamartomatous polyps
  - Hyperpigmented lips, buccal mucosa, and perioral region (Fig. 40-7)
  - Hamartomatous intestinal polyposis (no increased risk of malignancy from polyps)
  - GI bleeding, small bowel obstruction, intussusception
  - Increased risk of breast, pancreas, stomach, colon cancer

CONSTIPATION

Constipation is defined as decreased frequency or consistency of stool compared to the individual's baseline. In pediatrics, this includes a wide differential ranging from mechanical to functional etiologies (Table 40-7).

Lactose intolerance is the most common cause of diarrhea.

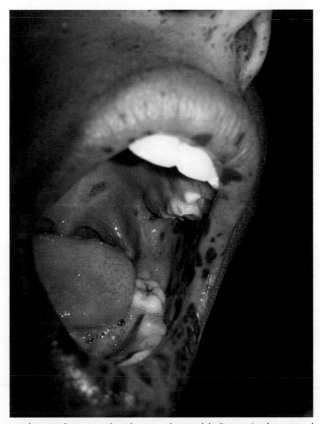

Figure 40-7: Mucocutaneous hyperpigmentation in a patient with Peutz-Jeghers syndrome. (Image courtesy of Abdullah Sarhan; CC BY-SA 4.0 [https://creativecommons.org/licenses/by-sa/4.0])

TABLE 40-7 Meconium Ileus Versus Meconium Plugs

	MECONIUM PLUGS	MECONIUM ILEUS
Definition	• Functional obstruction of the lower colon resulting in failure to pass meconium	• Failure to pass first stool (meconium) within the first 24 hr secondary to thickened meconium
Diagnostics	• Abdominal x-ray: intestinal distention	• Abdominal x-ray: same as meconium plug plus "soap bubble" appearance • Contrast enema: microcolon
Associations	• Hirschsprung disease • Infants of diabetic mother • Mothers who received magnesium sulfate • Small left colon syndrome	• Cystic fibrosis (may be first presenting symptom)
Management	• Enema: both diagnostic and therapeutic	

Hirschsprung Disease
– Pathophysiology: lack of migration of neural crest cells → aganglionic bowel segment → absence of bowel autonomic innervation
– Signs and symptoms
  • Meconium ileus/plug
  • Abdominal distention
  • Bilious vomiting
  • "Blast" sign: expulsion of stool on digital rectal exam
  • Chronic constipation (seen in older infants, adolescents)
– Associations: trisomy 21
– Diagnostics
  • Barium enema: dilated proximal with narrowing of distal segment
  • Rectal suction biopsy: absence of ganglia
– Management: resection of aganglionic segment

Miscellaneous
Foreign Body Ingestion
– Most common in infants and toddlers, increased risk in children with intellectual disability
– Presents with vomiting, choking, feeding difficulty/aversion
– Coins are the most ingested foreign object
– If the coin is visualized within the esophagus or patient is symptomatic, then it should be removed via endoscopy; if the patient is asymptomatic, then the child can be observed to allow spontaneous passage of coin
– Hazardous objects that pose a risk of intestinal perforation, ischemia, and obstruction include sharp objects, batteries, magnets; they should be removed via immediate endoscopy
Congenital Diaphragmatic Hernia
– Defects in the diaphragm allowing protrusion of abdominal viscera into the thoracic cavity causing extrinsic compression of the lungs and pulmonary hypoplasia
– Presents with respiratory distress, scaphoid abdomen
– Chest x-ray shows dilated loops of bowel in the chest (Fig. 40-8)
– Secure airway, gastric decompression, followed by surgical repair

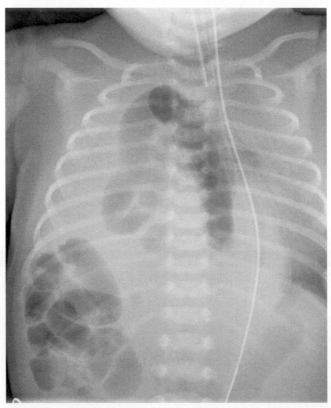

Figure 40-8: Chest x-ray demonstrating bowel loops in the thoracic cavity consistent with right-sided congenital diaphragmatic hernia.

CHAPTER 41 Genitourinary

This section is organized from proximal to distal pathologies starting with the kidneys, followed by the ureters, bladder, and lastly the urethra.

KIDNEYS

Autosomal Recessive Polycystic Kidney Disease
- Signs and symptoms
  - Flank masses
  - Oligohydramnios
  - Pulmonary hypoplasia: decreased amniotic fluid production results in decreased amniotic fluid to stimulate lung expansion
  - Hypertension
  - Liver cysts, cirrhosis
- Diagnostics: renal ultrasound (enlarged, polycystic kidneys)
- Management: renal replacement therapy followed by renal transplant

Alport Syndrome
- Pathophysiology: X-linked inherited defect in type IV collagen
- Signs and symptoms
  - Progressive blindness (anterior lenticonus)
  - Sensorineural hearing loss
  - Hematuria, proteinuria, hypertension
- Diagnostics: renal biopsy with electron microscopy
  - Thickened/thin capillary loops
  - Splitting of the glomerular basement membrane
- Management: renal replacement therapy followed by renal transplant

Wilm Tumor
- Epidemiology
  - Most common childhood renal tumor
  - Commonly presents in children <5 years old
- Signs and symptoms
  - Abdominal mass that does not cross midline
  - Hypertension
  - Hematuria
  - Fever, weight loss, night sweats
- Associations
  - Beckwith-Wiedemann syndrome
  - Macroglossia
  - Hemihypertrophy
  - Organomegaly
  - WAGR syndrome
    - Wilms tumor
    - Aniridia
    - Genitourinary abnormalities
    - Mental retardation
- Diagnostics
  - Abdominal computed tomography (CT)/magnetic resonance imaging
  - Tissue biopsy
- Management: staging +/− surgical resection +/− chemoradiation

Potter sequence: in utero renal agenesis → decrease amniotic fluid production → decreased lung expansion (pulmonary hypoplasia) and flat facies (extrinsic compression against the uterine wall)

URETERS

Vesicoureteral Reflux (VUR)
– Definition: reflux of urine from the bladder into the ureters and kidneys
– Causes: abnormal ureterovesicular insertion (abnormal or absent submucosal tunnel between the mucosa and detrusor muscle)
– Classification (Fig. 41-1)
  • Grade I: reflux into distal ureter
  • Grade II: renal pelvis and calyces without dilation
  • Grade III: renal pelvis and calyces with dilation
  • Grade IV: renal pelvis and calyces with increased dilation and ballooning of the calyces
  • Grade V: entire renal collecting system with tortuosity of the ureters
– Diagnostics: voiding cystourethrogram
– Management
  • Low grade (grade II or less): conservative management as most children tend to outgrow VUR
  • Symptomatic, high grade (grade III or higher)
    ▪ Prophylactic antibiotics: TMP-SMX or nitrofurantoin
    ▪ Referral to a pediatric urologist in severe cases for correction of anatomic abnormality

Wilms tumor is a palpable abdominal mass that does not cross midline, in contrast to neuroblastoma, which does cross midline.

– Complications
  • Recurrent urinary tract infections (UTIs), pyelonephritis
  • Renal scarring
  • Reflux neuropathy

Cystinuria
– Epidemiology: pediatric cause of nephrolithiasis
– Risk factors
  • Dibasic amino acid transport abnormality
  • Family history (autosomal recessive inheritance)
– Signs and symptoms
  • Colicky flank pain radiates to the groin
  • Hematuria
  • Dysuria
– Diagnostics
  • Positive urinary cyanide nitroprusside test
  • Stone analysis: hexagonal crystals
  • Urinalysis: blood, red blood cells
  • Noncontrast CT abdomen
– Management
  • Increase fluid intake
  • Pain control
  • Tiopronin or penicillamine for refractory cases

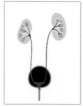 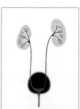 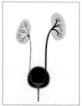 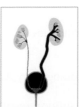 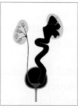

Figure 41-1: Illustration of grade I to grade V vesicoureteral reflux, from left to right. (Image courtesy of ColnKurtz; CC BY-SA 4.0 [https://creativecommons.org/licenses/by-sa/4.0])

BLADDER
Cystitis
- Risk factors
  - Female (shorter distance from anus to urethra)
  - Anatomic abnormalities (vesicoureteral reflux, posterior urethral valves)
  - Uncircumcised boys <1 year old
  - Polycystic kidney disease
- Pathophysiology: ascending bacterial infection through the urethra
- Microbiology
  - Escherichia coli: most common
  - Klebsiella
  - Staphylococcus saprophyticus
  - Enterococcus
- Signs and symptoms
  - Neonates/infants: fever, vomiting, irritability
  - Older children: similar to adults
    - Burning, frequency, urgency
    - Suprapubic pain
    - +/− hematuria, fever
- Diagnostics
  - Obtain urinalysis
    - Infant/neonates: suprapubic aspiration
    - Older children: clean-catch urine sample
  - Urinalysis: positive nitrites and leukocyte esterase, numerous white blood cells
  - Urine culture
  - Renal ultrasound +/− voiding cystourethrography (VCUG) for recurrent UTIs, <2 years old, febrile UTI, family history of renal or urologic disorders
- Management: empirically cover gram-negative rods (most commonly *E. coli*)
  - Outpatient
    - Otherwise well appearing, tolerating oral intake
    - Cephalosporin +/− ampicillin (if enterococcus is suspected)
  - Inpatient
    - Toxic-appearing, vomiting, suspected pyelonephritis
    - IV cephalosporin + aminoglycoside
- Complications: pyelonephritis (toxic appearing, costovertebral angle tenderness)

URETHRA
Posterior Urethral Valves
- Abnormal folds of tissue in the distal urethra causing bladder outlet obstruction
- Most common cause of obstructive uropathy in young boys
- Presents with oligohydramnios, suprapubic fullness, weak urinary stream, and recurrent UTIs
- Renal ultrasound will show bilateral hydronephrosis
- Diagnosis confirmed with VCUGs and cystoscopy
- Treatment is valve ablation

CHAPTER 42 Endocrinology

PITUITARY

Kallmann Syndrome
- Pathophysiology: hypothalamic hypogonadism → gonadotropin-releasing hormone (GnRH) deficiency → decreased follicle-stimulating hormone (FSH) and luteinizing hormone (LH) → delayed secondary sex characteristics
- Clinical features
  - Anosmia due to involvement of olfactory bulb
  - Lack of secondary sexual characteristics
    - Decreased testicular volume
    - Absent breast development
    - Lack of pubic and axillary hair
    - Decreased libido
  - Renal agenesis, congenital heart defects, adrenocortical insufficiency
- Management: GnRH replacement

Diabetes Insipidus
- Causes
  - Central
    - Pituitary tumor
    - Trauma, resection of pituitary stalk
    - Infarction, infection
    - Infiltrative diseases
      - Hemochromatosis, sarcoidosis
      - Langerhans histiocytosis X
      - Lymphocytic hypophysitis
  - Nephrogenic
    - Medications
      - Lithium
      - Demeclocycline, foscarnet, amphotericin B
      - Cidofovir
    - Hypokalemia, hypercalcemia
    - Tubulointerstitial renal disease
    - Mutation in ADH receptor or aquaporin gene
- Pathophysiology: deficiency (central) or resistance (nephrogenic) of antidiuretic hormone (ADH) resulting in excess loss of free water
- Signs and symptoms
  - Polyuria (>5 L daily), polydipsia
  - Central nervous system (CNS) manifestations secondary to hyponatremia if unable to keep up with free water loss
    - Altered mental status, confusion
    - Headaches, cerebral edema
    - Seizures
- Diagnostics: water deprivation test (monitor urine osmolality to determine true diabetes insipidus vs psychogenic polydipsia) (Table 42-1)
  - Psychogenic polydipsia: urine osmolality appropriately increases as free water is reabsorbed during water deprivation test

TABLE 42-1   Summary of Urine Deprivation Test Results

	URINE OSMOLARITY IN RESPONSE TO WATER DEPRIVATION	URINE OSMOLARITY IN RESPONSE TO DDAVP
Psychogenic polydipsia	Increased	Increased
Central diabetes insipidus	Dilute	Increased
Nephrogenic diabetes insipidus	Dilute	Dilute

- Diabetes insipidus: urine osmolality remains inappropriately dilute
  - To differentiate central (deficiency of ADH) vs nephrogenic (resistance to ADH), DDAVP is administered
    - Urine osmolality appropriately increases in central diabetes insipidus after DDAVP administration as you are supplementing ADH deficiency
    - Urine osmolality remains inappropriately dilute in nephrogenic diabetes insipidus due to lack of response to ADH
- Management
  - Central: ADH replacement (DDAVP)
  - Nephrogenic
    - Treat or stop offending agent
    - HCTZ: increased excretion of sodium resulting in increased reabsorption of sodium and water in the proximal tubules
    - Triamterene, amiloride
    - Nonsteroidal antiinflammatory drugs
- Complications: cerebral edema (secondary to rapid overcorrection)

Gigantism
- Excessive prepubertal growth hormone (prior to closure of epiphyseal plates) resulting in increased growth of long bones and tall stature
- Increased insulin-like growth factor 1 levels
- Management via transsphenoidal resection of pituitary adenoma
  - Alternatives if the patient is not a surgical candidate include radiation or medical management (octreotide, bromocriptine)

THYROID

Hypothyroidism
- Causes
  - Hashimoto thyroiditis (chronic lymphocytic; autoimmune thyroiditis): most common cause of hypothyroidism
  - Medications: amiodarone, lithium
- Signs and symptoms
  - Myopathy, weakness
  - Fatigue, lethargy, depression
  - Bradycardia
  - Decreased deep tendon reflexes, carpal tunnel syndrome
  - Cold intolerance, weight gain
  - Dry skin, lateral eyebrow hair loss
  - Nonpitting edema
  - Constipation, decreased appetite
  - Menorrhagia
- Diagnostics
  - Primary hypothyroidism: high TSH, low T4
  - Secondary hypothyroidism: low TSH, low T4
  - Hashimoto thyroiditis (chronic lymphocytic; autoimmune thyroiditis): antithyroid peroxidase, antimicrosomal antibodies
  - Supporting labs
    - Normocytic anemia
    - Euvolemic hyponatremia
    - Dyslipidemia
- Management: thyroid hormone replacement
- Complications: myxedema coma

Cretinism
- Inadequate thyroid hormone during fetal and neonatal development
- Results in significant intellectual disability and growth delay

Myxedema Coma
- Caused by prolonged, untreated hypothyroidism
- Precipitated by infection, cold exposure, medication (narcotics), trauma
- Signs and symptoms
  - Altered mental status, stupor, delirium, hypothermia
  - Hypoventilation, bradycardia, hypotension
  - Hypoglycemia, hyponatremia
  - Diffuse nonpitting edema
- Management
  - IV T3/T4 + stress dose steroids (hydrocortisone)
  - Supportive care

PARATHYROID DISORDERS
Function of parathyroid hormone (PTH) in calcium metabolism (Fig. 42-1)
- PTH is secreted by the parathyroid glands located posterior to the thyroid glands
- PTH is secreted in response to hypocalcemia and works at the kidneys and bone to maintain calcium homeostasis
- Functions at the distal convoluted tubules to increase calcium reabsorption and phosphate excretion
- Stimulates 1-alpha hydroxylase in the kidneys to convert 25-hydroxylase to 1,25-hydroxylase (active form of vitamin D)
- Functions at the bone by stimulating osteoclasts and bone resorption
Hypoparathyroidism
- Causes
  - Complication of thyroidectomy
  - DiGeorge syndrome
  - Polyglandular autoimmune syndrome type I
- Key manifestations: related to hypocalcemia
  - Chvostek sign (tingling along with facial nerve distribution when percussing the zygoid bone below the ear)
  - Trousseau sign (carpopedal spasms upon inflation of blood pressure cuff)
  - Perioral numbness and tingling
  - Anxiety, irritability, seizures
  - Prolonged QT
  - Early cataracts
- Diagnostics
  - Low PTH
  - Low calcium, high phosphate
  - Low 1,25-vitamin D
- Management: calcium and vitamin D replacement
Pseudohypoparathyroidism
- Mutation of *GNAS-1* gene resulting in resistance of tissues to PTH
- Biochemical testing
  - Elevated PTH
  - Elevated phosphate, low calcium
- Associated with Albright hereditary osteodystrophy (short stature, shortened fourth metacarpal, obesity, developmental delay)

ADRENAL GLAND
Neuroblastoma
- Epidemiology: primarily affects <2 years old, majority of cases present by 5 years old
- Pathophysiology: N-myc oncogene mutation
- Definition: malignancy of immature neural crest cells along the sympathetic nervous system, most commonly occurring in the adrenal glands
- Signs and symptoms
  - Palpable abdominal mass that crosses the midline
  - Horner syndrome (involvement of superior cervical ganglion)
  - Peripheral neuropathy

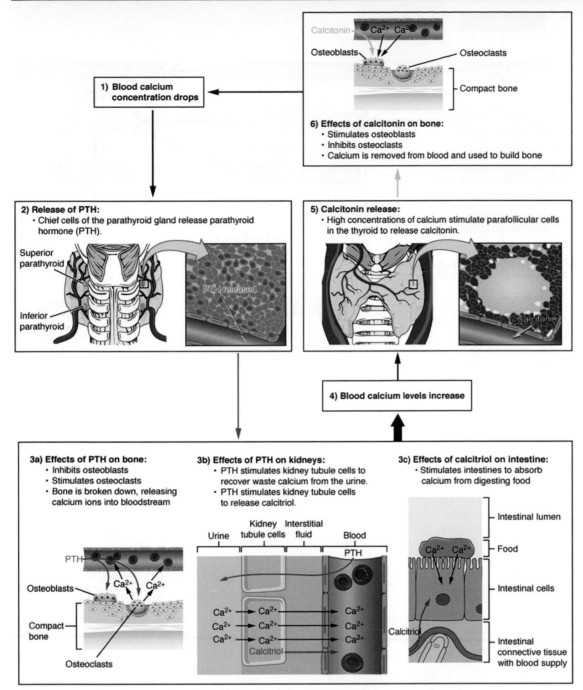

Figure 42-1: Diagrammatic representation of parathyroid hormone and calcium homeostasis.

- Proptosis
- Opsoclonus myoclonus ("dancing eyes and feet")
- Hypertension
- Diagnostics
  - Elevated homovanillic acid, vanillylmandelic acid level
  - Computed tomography/magnetic resonance imaging (MRI) abdomen and pelvis: calcification and hemorrhages of suprarenal mass
  - Bone marrow biopsy
- Management: staging (commonly metastatic upon initial presentation) +/– surgery +/– chemoradiation

Congenital Adrenal Hyperplasia

- Pathophysiology: autosomal recessive adrenal enzyme deficiency (most commonly 21-hydroxylase) → inadequate cortisol, aldosterone, or sex steroids → increased adrenocorticotropic hormone from the anterior pituitary due to lack of negative feedback → adrenal hyperplasia and shunting production of adrenal hormones through alternative and functional enzymatic pathways

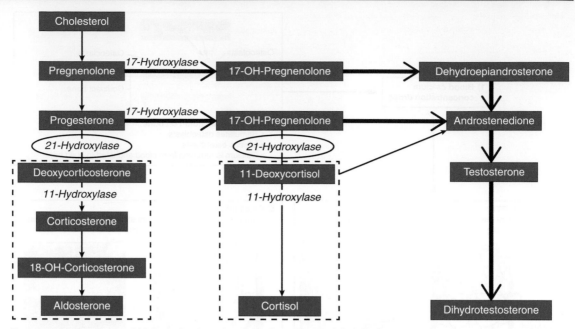

Figure 42-2: Corticosteroid biosynthesis pathway in the adrenal gland. Deficiency of one enzyme results in shunting and increased production through an alternative pathway. (StarBuG; CC BY-SA 3.0 [https://creativecommons.org/licenses/by-sa/3.0])

- Signs and symptoms: depends on subtype and enzymatic deficiency (Fig. 42-2)
  - Classic (21-hydroxylase deficiency)
    - Salt wasting (hyponatremia, dehydration)
    - Hyperkalemia
    - Female virilization
  - Nonclassic (21-hydroxylase deficiency)
    - Premature adrenarche
    - Precocious puberty
    - Clitoromegaly
    - Premature acne
    - Normal electrolytes
  - 11-hydroxylase deficiency
    - Hypertension (11-deoxycorticosterone precursor has mineralocorticoid-like activity)
    - Hypokalemia
- Diagnostics
  - 21-hydroxylase deficiency: elevated 17-hydroxyprogesterone
  - 11 hydroxylase deficiency: elevated 11-deoxycortisol, 11-deoxycorticosterone
- Management
  - Hydrocortisone
  - Fludrocortisone (if aldosterone deficient)

3-beta hydroxysteroid dehydrogenase deficiency: deficiency of all steroid hormones; presents with irritability, feeding difficulties, hypotension, hyperkalemia, hyponatremia, and ambiguous genitalia

5-alpha reductase deficiency: prevents conversion of testosterone to dihydrotestosterone; impaired male virilization of the external genitalia (penis, prostate, scrotum); normal internal urogenital system (epididymis, vas deferens, ejaculatory ducts), as the development of these organs is driven by testosterone

PUBERTY

Puberty timeline: last 3–4 years in both males and females, starts ~2 years earlier in females than males (Figs. 42-3, 42-4, and 42-5)

Aromatase deficiency: prevents conversion of androgens to estrogen; deficiency of aromatase in the placenta can result in fetal androgens crossing the placenta and causing maternal virilisation

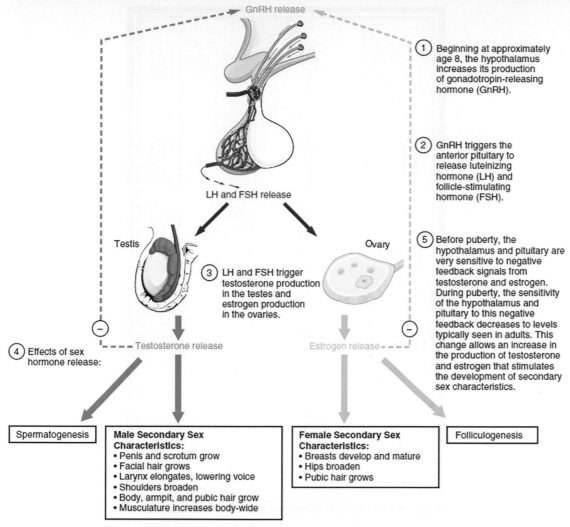

① Beginning at approximately age 8, the hypothalamus increases its production of gonadotropin-releasing hormone (GnRH).

② GnRH triggers the anterior pituitary to release luteinizing hormone (LH) and follicle-stimulating hormone (FSH).

③ LH and FSH trigger testosterone production in the testes and estrogen production in the ovaries.

④ Effects of sex hormone release:

⑤ Before puberty, the hypothalamus and pituitary are very sensitive to negative feedback signals from testosterone and estrogen. During puberty, the sensitivity of the hypothalamus and pituitary to this negative feedback decreases to levels typically seen in adults. This change allows an increase in the production of testosterone and estrogen that stimulates the development of secondary sex characteristics.

GnRH release

LH and FSH release

Testis

Ovary

Testosterone release

Estrogen release

Spermatogenesis

Male Secondary Sex Characteristics:
• Penis and scrotum grow
• Facial hair grows
• Larynx elongates, lowering voice
• Shoulders broaden
• Body, armpit, and pubic hair grow
• Musculature increases body-wide

Female Secondary Sex Characteristics:
• Breasts develop and mature
• Hips broaden
• Pubic hair grows

Folliculogenesis

Figure 42-3: Normal pubertal initiation and development. (Image courtesy of OpenStax College; CC BY 3.0 [https://creativecommons.org/licenses/by/3.0])

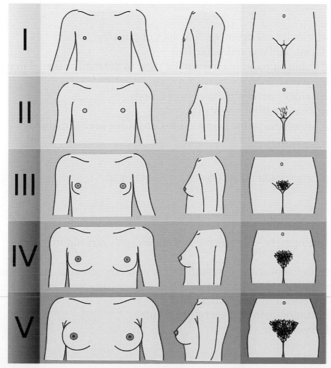

I

II

III

IV

V

Figure 42-4: Female stages of Tanner development based on breast and pubic hair development. (Images courtesy of Michał Komorniczak; CC BY-SA 3.0 [https://creativecommons.org/licenses/by-sa/3.0])

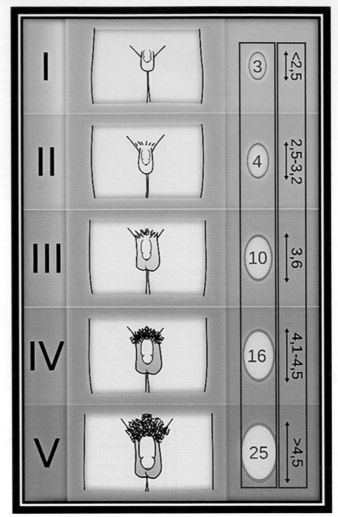

Figure 42-5: Male stages of Tanner development based on pubic hair, testicular volume in mL (numbers in ovals), and testicular length in cm. (Images courtesy of Michał Komorniczak; CC BY-SA 3.0 [https://creativecommons.org/licenses/by-sa/3.0])

- Males
  - 11–12 years old: testicular enlargement, first sign of puberty
  - 12–13 years old: facial, axillary, and pubic hair
  - Tanner staging of pubic hair and male genitalia used to determine sexual maturity
- Females
  - 9–10 years old: thelarche (development of breast buds)
  - 12–13 years old: menarche (first menstrual cycle)
  - Tanner staging of breast and pubic hair used to determine sexual maturity

---

Isolated adrenarche, menarche, thelarche require no additional intervention or workup.

Precocious Puberty
- Definition: sexual development <8 years old in females, <9 years old in males
- Causes
  - Idiopathic (premature activation of hypothalamic pituitary gonadal axis): most common cause
  - Nonclassic congenital adrenal hyperplasia
  - Leydig cell tumor (testosterone-secreting tumor)
  - Ovarian germ cell tumor (estrogen-secreting tumor)
  - McCune-Albright syndrome
  - Hypothyroidism

- Diagnostics: differentiate between central vs peripheral causes
  - Advanced bone age
  - Central
    - Elevated FSH and LH
    - MRI brain: evaluate for CNS lesion stimulating the hypothalamic-pituitary-adrenal (HPA) axis
  - Peripheral
    - Decreased FSH and LH
    - GnRH stimulation test: high LH indicates peripheral cause, low LH indicates central cause
    - Imaging of ovaries, testicle, and adrenal gland to look for peripheral source
- Management
  - Central: GnRH analog
  - Peripheral: treat underlying etiology

Presence of Tanner stage II <8 years old in females, and <9 years old in females is defined as precocious puberty

Delayed Puberty
- Definition: lack of sexual development by age 14 years in males, lack of breast tissue by age 13 years or menarche by age 16 years in females
- Causes
  - Delayed activation of HPA axis: most common
  - Hypopituitarism
  - Genetic syndromes (Kallmann syndrome, Turner syndrome, Prader-Willi)
  - Chronic disease/infection
  - Hypothyroidism: can also cause precocious puberty
  - Gonadal dysfunction
- Diagnostics: depends on other signs and symptoms (Fig. 42-6)
- Management: treat reversible etiologies

DIABETES MELLITUS
Diabetes Mellitus
- Risk factors
  - Family history
  - Obesity
  - Gestational diabetes
  - Hereditary hemochromatosis
- Subtypes
  - Type I
  - Type II
- Pathophysiology (Fig. 42-7)
  - Type I: autoimmune destruction of insulin-producing pancreatic beta cells
  - Type II: insulin resistance secondary to excess adipose resulting in burnout of pancreatic beta cells
- Signs and symptoms
  - Asymptomatic (most common)
  - Polyuria, polydipsia, polyphagia

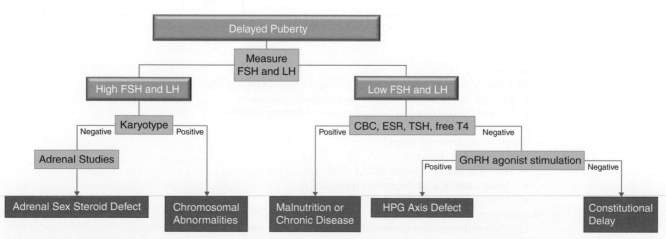

Figure 42-6: Flow chart depicting the diagnostic workup and evaluation of delayed puberty. (Image courtesy of Poodle0011; CC BY-SA 4.0 [https://creativecommons.org/licenses/by-sa/4.0])

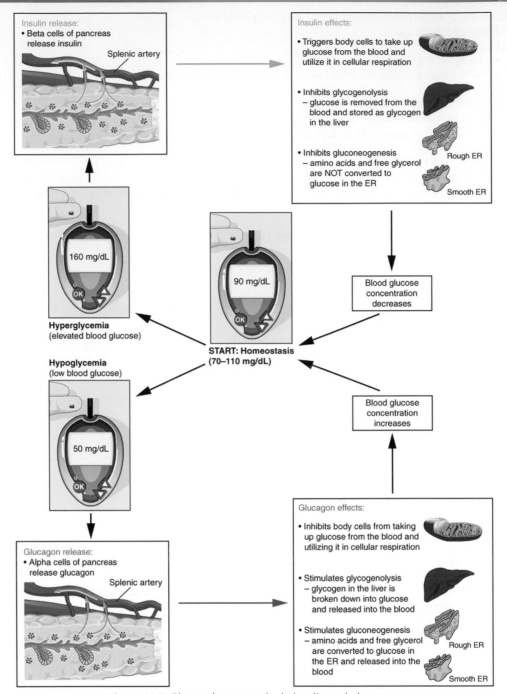

Figure 42-7: Glucose homeostasis via insulin and glucagon.

- Diagnostics
  - Any one of the three can be used to diagnose diabetes mellitus
    - Fasting blood sugar >125 on two separate occasions
    - Glucose >200 mg/dL plus symptoms of hyperglycemia
    - Hemoglobin A1c >6.5%
  - Supporting autoantibodies
    - Antiinsulin (IAA)
    - Antiislet cell cytoplasm (ICA)
    - Antiglutamic acid decarboxylase (GAD)
    - Antityrosine phosphatase (IA2)
- Management
  - Lifestyle changes: low carbohydrate diet, exercise, weight loss
  - Pharmacotherapy (Table 42-2)

TABLE 42-2 Diabetes Mellitus Pharmacotherapy

DRUG	MECHANISM OF ACTION	SIDE EFFECTS
Metformin (first line)	• Inhibits gluconeogenesis • Increases insulin sensitivity	• Gastrointestinal (GI) disturbances • Rarely, lactic acidosis in renal dysfunction • B12 deficiency
Sulfonylureas (glyburide, glipizide)	• Stimulate release of insulin from the pancreas	• Hypoglycemia • Weight gain
GLP-1 analogues (exenatide, liraglutide)	• Increase insulin and decrease glucagon release from the pancreas • Decreases gastric motility	• Administered as an injection • Weight loss • Caution in patients with medullary thyroid cancer or MEN II syndrome
DPP-4 inhibitors (sitagliptin, linagliptin, saxagliptin)	• Prevent breakdown of GLP-1 analogues (incretin mimetics) prolonging their effect	• GI disturbances • Nasopharyngitis
Thiazolidinediones (rosiglitazone, pioglitazone)	• Increases insulin sensitivity through transcription regulators	• Weight gain • Fluid retention (increased risk of congestive heart failure exacerbation) • Hepatotoxicity • Fractures, osteoporosis
SGLT2 inhibitors (canagliflozin, dapagliflozin)	• Blocks sodium-glucose cotransporter at the proximal convoluted tubule	• Mycotic urinary infections • Glucosuria • Euglycemic diabetic ketoacidosis
Alpha-glucosidase inhibitors (acarbose, miglitol)	• Blocks enzyme at intestinal brush border resulting in delayed carbohydrate breakdown absorption	• Abdominal cramping, flatulence

TABLE 42-3 Insulin Subtypes

TYPES OF INSULIN	ONSET	DURATION OF ACTION
Short acting (aspart, lispro)	15–45 min	3–5 hr
Medium acting (NPH)	3 hr	18–26 hr
Long-acting (glargine, detemir)	2–3 hr	24 hr
70/30 mixture (70% NPH, 30% aspart)	30 min	14 hr

- Oral antihyperglycemic: preferred for mild cases (hemoglobin A1c <9%) as these can only lower hemoglobin A1c by 2%
- Insulin: indicated for the following cases as it can lower hemoglobin A1c by 4% to 5% (Table 42-3)
  ○ Uncontrolled diabetes (hemoglobin A1c >9%)
  ○ Symptomatic hyperglycemia
  ○ Type I diabetics
  ○ Failure of oral antihyperglycemics
- Complications: related to long-term uncontrolled diabetes and can be managed/prevented with strict glycemic control (hemoglobin A1c <7%); require periodic reassessment (every 6–12 months) to monitor and prevent progression to end-stage complications (blindness, end-stage renal disease)

Complications of Diabetes
- Microvascular damage (microangiopathy)
  • Retinopathy
    ▪ Epidemiology: most common cause of blindness in US adults
    ▪ Types
      ○ Nonproliferative
      ○ Proliferative
    ▪ Signs and symptoms: seen on fundoscopy
      ○ Exudates, hemorrhage
      ○ Macular edema, cotton wools spots
      ○ Neovascularization
    ▪ Management
      ○ Nonproliferative: strict glycemic control
      ○ Proliferative: laser photocoagulation
      ○ Regular ophthalmologist follow-up

- Nephropathy (nephrotic syndrome, chronic kidney disease)
    - Pathophysiology: intercapillary glomerulosclerosis initially results in increased glomerular filtration rate (GFR) (later followed by decreased GFR after prolonged hyperfiltration injury), increased basement membrane thickening and permeability
    - Histopathology: diffuse glomerulosclerosis, nodular glomerulosclerosis (Kimmelstiel-Wilson nodules), mesangial expansion
    - Management: angiotensin-converting enzyme inhibitor or angiotensin receptor blocker initiation once microalbuminuria (30–300 mg protein per 24 hours) is detected to decrease intraglomerular and systemic hypertension (130/80)
- Neuropathy
    - Autonomic neuropathy
        - Gastroparesis
            - Pathophysiology: decreased gastric emptying time and contractility secondary to vagus nerve dysfunction
            - Signs and symptoms
                - Nausea, vomiting
                - Abdominal pain, early satiety, bloating, constipation
                - Anorexia, hiccups, dyspepsia
                - Recurrent hypoglycemia
            - Diagnostics: gastric emptying study
            - Management
                - Lifestyle modifications: small frequent, high-fiber meals
                - Promotility agents
                - Acute: erythromycin (motilin receptor agonist; limited by tachyphylaxis)
                - Chronic: metoclopramide (D2 receptor antagonist; prokinetic, antiemetic)
        - Overflow incontinence
            - Pathophysiology
                - Dysfunction of parasympathetic nerves supplying bladder smooth muscle (detrusor) resulting in decreased contractility and increased postvoidal urine
                - Passage of urine only when bladder pressure exceeds external urethral sphincter pressure; urine stream stops once pressures equilibrate
            - Signs and symptoms
                - Lower abdominal fullness
                - Suprapubic tenderness
                - Recurrent urinary tract infections
            - Diagnostics: voiding cystourethrogram
            - Management: bethanechol or intermittent catheterization
        - Postural hypotension
        - Impotence
    - Peripheral neuropathy
        - Signs and symptoms
            - Stocking-glove distribution (distal sensorimotor neuropathy involving bilateral hands and feet) numbness and tingling
            - Decreased vibratory sensation, proprioception
            - Charcot arthropathy
            - Initially painful, later becomes painless
            - Chronic nonhealing lower extremity words
        - Diagnostics: monofilament testing
        - Management:
            - Neuropathic pain
                - Gabapentin, pregabalin
                - Duloxetine, tricyclic antidepressants
                - Carbamazepine
            - Chronic lower extremity wounds: regular podiatrist follow-up, wound care, IV antibiotics if osteomyelitis +/− amputation
    - Cranial nerve neuropathy
        - Secondary to ischemia involving vasculature supplying nerves (most commonly cranial nerve III, IV, or VI)
        - Large nerves also affected (peroneal, radial)
- Diabetic ketoacidosis (DKA)
    - Epidemiology: most commonly in type I diabetics
    - Causes

- Insulin noncompliance or inadequate amount
- Acute illness (infection, acute coronary syndrome)
- Trauma, surgery
  - Pathophysiology
    - Lack of insulin or insulin unresponsiveness results in starvation state as cells are deprived of glucose for adenosine triphosphate (ATP) production
    - Cells switch to fatty acid metabolism for energy resulting in production of ketones as a byproduct
  - Signs and symptoms
    - Polyuria, polydipsia: secondary to hyperglycemia-induced osmotic diuresis
    - Anorexia, nausea, vomiting, abdominal pain
    - Kussmaul respirations (rapid deep breathing), fruity acetone breath
    - Hypotension, tachycardia, dry mucous membranes
    - Altered mental status, confusion, coma
  - Diagnostics
    - Elevated blood glucose >400
    - Elevated serum ketones, acetone, beta-hydroxybutyrate
    - Elevated anion gap metabolic acidosis
    - Supporting labs
      - Hyperkalemia (however, decreased total body potassium stores)
      - Pseudohyponatremia
  - Management: goal of therapy is to close the anion gap
    - Aggressive IV fluids
    - IV insulin infusion
    - Supplemental potassium and glucose: prevent insulin-induced hypokalemia and hypoglycemia
    - Replace electrolytes as needed
    - Correct precipitating cause
    - Bridge IV to subcutaneous insulin once anion gap is closed, glucose <200, or able to eat
- Hyperosmolar hyperglycemic nonketotic syndrome
  - Similar causes, signs and symptoms, and treatment as indicated
  - Occurs more commonly in type II diabetics
  - Blood glucose >800 without ketoacidosis
  - Strict glycemic control resulting in prevention of macrovascular complications (stroke, myocardial infarction) has not been established.
  - Hyperkalemia in diabetic ketoacidosis occurs secondary to cellular hydrogen-potassium exchange pump (hydrogen in, potassium out) to correct acidosis.
  - Low levels of insulin in type II diabetics prevent transition to fatty acid metabolism and ketoacidosis

Strict glycemic control resulting in prevention of macrovascular complications (stroke, myocardial infarction) has not been established.
  Hyperkalemia in diabetic ketoacidosis occurs secondary to cellular hydrogen-potassium exchange pump (hydrogen in, potassium out) to correct acidosis.

Facts about insulin:
- Hormone produced by pancreatic islet beta cells; simultaneously secreted with C-peptide
- Released in response to hyperglycemia
- Functions by driving glucose into cells to be used for ATP production
- Activate lipoprotein lipase in adipose to decrease triglyceride levels and treat significant hypertriglyceridemia (>1000)
- Stimulates sodium-potassium ATPase to cause intracellular shifts of potassium and temporarily treat hyperkalemia

Hypoglycemia
- Causes
  - Excess insulin administration
  - Sulfonylurea abuse
  - Insulinoma
  - Decreased by mouth intake (alcoholism, malnutrition)
  - Sepsis
  - Cortisol deficiency
  - Glycogen storage diseases

TABLE 42-4 Differentiating Causes of Hypoglycemia

	C-PEPTIDE	SULFONYLUREA SCREEN
Insulinoma	Elevated	Negative
Sulfonylurea abuse	Elevated	Positive
Surreptitious insulin	Decreased	Negative

- Signs and symptoms
  - Palpitations, tremulousness, diaphoresis
  - Confusion, altered mental status, seizure, coma
  - Whipple triad
    - Hypoglycemia when fasting
    - Hypoglycemic symptoms concurrent with low glucose
    - Hypoglycemic symptoms relieved by glucose administration
- Diagnostics (Table 42-4)
  - Serum or fingerstick glucose <70 or symptoms of hypoglycemia
  - C-peptide levels: distinguishes surreptitious insulin use vs true hyperinsulinemia causing hypoglycemia
    - If elevated, indicates endogenous hyperinsulinemia (insulinoma, sulfonylurea abuse)
    - If decreased, indicates exogenous hyperinsulinemia (excessive insulin intake)
  - Sulfonylurea screen
- Management: glucose replacement
  - Vitamin B1 prior to administration of glucose to prevent Wernicke encephalopathy
  - High sugar foods if patient able to take orally
  - IV D50
  - IM glucagon

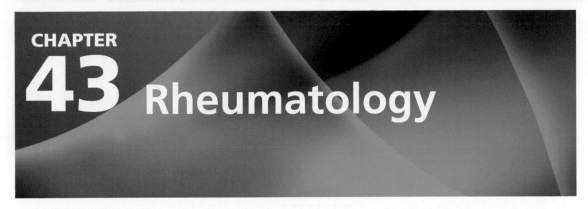

CHAPTER 43 Rheumatology

FRAGILE BONES

Rickets
- Definition: inadequate bone mineralization most commonly secondary to vitamin D deficiency
- Causes: vitamin D deficiency
  - Vitamin D dependent rickets (1-alpha hydroxylase deficiency)
  - Vitamin D independent rickets (renal phosphorus wasting, X-linked dominant inheritance)
  - Inadequate sunlight exposure
  - Inadequate nutritional intake
  - Malabsorption syndromes (cystic fibrosis, celiac disease)
  - Impaired vitamin D activation (hepatic, renal dysfunction)
  - Anticonvulsants
- Signs and symptoms
  - Failure to thrive
  - Frequent fractures
  - Bowing of the legs
  - Hypocalcemia (tetany, carpopedal spasm)
  - Prominent costochondral junction (rachitic rosary)
  - Frontal bossing
  - Craniotabes (depression of skull bones on palpation)
- Diagnostics
  - Wrist radiograph
    - Widening of the epiphyseal plate
    - Growth plate cupping, spurring, and stippling (Fig. 43-1)

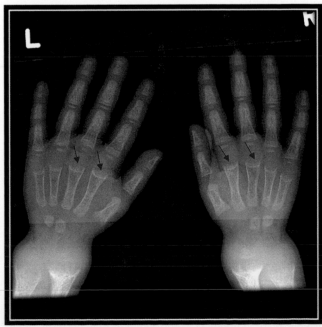

Figure 43-1: Epiphyseal cupping *(red arrows)* in a patient with rickets disease. (Image courtesy of Frank Gaillard; CC BY-SA 4.0 [https://creativecommons.org/licenses/by-sa/4.0])

- Laboratory studies
  - Low vitamin D
  - Elevated parathyroid hormone
  - Low phosphorus
  - Low/normal calcium
- Management
  - Vitamin D replacement
  - Phosphorus replacement for vitamin D resistant rickets

Osteogenesis Imperfecta
- Pathophysiology: impaired type I collagen synthesis → impaired bone formation → increased risk of fractures
- Signs and symptoms
  - Frequent fractures from minimal trauma (may be taken for child abuse)
  - Blue sclera (thinning of the sclera allowing for visualization of underlying choroidal veins) (Fig. 43-2)
  - Dentinogenesis imperfecta (translucent teeth)
  - Osteoporosis
  - Easy bruisability
  - Early deafness
  - Short stature
- Diagnostics
  - Rule out child abuse
  - Collagen biochemical studies
- Management: treatment of complications, no cure

Four subtypes of osteogenesis imperfecta range from incompatible with life (type II) to less severe, but still symptomatic (type I).

BONE TUMORS

Osteosarcoma
- Epidemiology: most common primary bone tumor in young adults and adolescents most commonly affecting the distal femur (metaphysis of long bones)
- Risk factors
  - Paget disease of the bone
  - Prolonged use of teriparatide
  - Chemoradiation
  - Retinoblastoma gene mutation
- Signs and symptoms
  - Bone pain, muscle aches
  - Tender soft tissue mass
  - Pathologic fractures
- Diagnostics
  - Imaging (magnetic resonance imaging/computed tomography [CT])
    - Periosteal elevation (Codman triangle)
    - Spiculated "sunburst" pattern

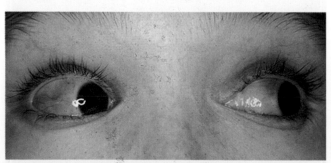

Figure 43-2: Characteristic blue sclera in a patient with osteogenesis imperfecta. (Image courtesy of Herbert L. Fred, MD and Hendrik A. van Dijk; CC BY-SA 3.0 [https://creativecommons.org/licenses/by-sa/3.0])

- Staging: CT chest (lung is common site of metastasis)
- Biopsy
- Elevated lactate dehydrogenase, alkaline phosphatase
– Management
- Surgical resection
- Chemotherapy: methotrexate-based regimen (cisplatin + doxorubicin)

Ewing Sarcoma
– Commonly affects young boys and adolescents
– Malignant anaplastic small blue cell tumor arising from diaphysis of long bones
– Onionskin pattern on x-ray (Fig. 43-3)
– 11:22 translocation

JOINT DISORDERS
Septic Arthritis
– Definition: infection involving joint space (synovial membrane)
– Pathophysiology: hematogenous spread (children) or direct invasion (adults) from overlying skin/soft tissue infection
– Microbiology
- *Staphylococcus aureus:* most common cause
- *Neisseria gonorrhoeae:* young sexually active, neonates
- *Streptococcus pneumoniae:* splenic dysfunction
- Gram negative: gastrointestinal infection, immunocompromised
- *Borrelia burgdorferi* (Lyme disease): bull's-eye rash, hiking, tick bite
– Signs and symptoms
- Infants/neonates
  - Fever, irritability
  - Limp, refusal to walk
- Pain with range of motion
- Painful, erythematous joint
- Palpable effusion

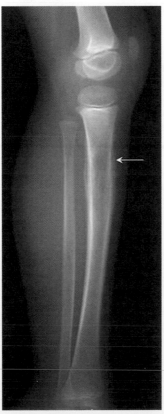

Figure 43-3: Periosteal reaction and onionskin pattern (white arrow) in a patient with Ewing sarcoma. (Image courtesy of Michael Richardson, MD; CC BY-SA 3.0 [http://creativecommons.org/licenses/by-sa/3.0/])

- Diagnostics
  - Arthrocentesis: always initial step in a patient with painful, erythematous joint; obtain culture and sensitivities
    - Opaque, purulent fluid
    - >50,000 red blood cells, >75% polymorphonuclear cells, positive Gram stain and culture
  - Polymerase chain reaction if gonococcal arthritis is suspected
  - Radiographs/ultrasound: joint effusion
- Management
  - Joint washout
  - Empiric treatment with vancomycin (gram-positive methicillin-resistant *S. aureus* coverage) +/− third- or fourth-generation cephalosporin (gram-negative coverage)

Transient Synovitis
- Definition: inflammation of the joint space
- Microbiology: viral
- Signs and symptoms
  - Prodromal upper respiratory tract infection
  - Mild joint pain
  - Mildly restrictive range of motion
  - +/− fever
- Diagnostics: rule out septic arthritis
  - Normal white blood cells
  - Normal inflammatory markers (erythrocyte sedimentation rate [ESR], C-reactive protein [CRP])
  - Normal radiographs
  - Sterile arthrocentesis (however, not needed if there is no other supporting laboratory findings)
- Management
  - Nonsteroidal antiinflammatory drugs (NSAIDs)
  - Bed rest
  - Avoid weight bearing until resolution of symptoms

MUSCULAR DISORDERS

Duchenne Muscular Dystrophy
- Pathophysiology: deletion or mutation in the dystrophin gene resulting in degeneration of muscle fibers
- Signs and symptoms
  - Progressive muscle weakness
  - Inability to walk by adolescence
  - Gower sign ("climbing up" thighs due to weakness of proximal thigh and pelvic muscles to stand up)
  - Calf pseudohypertrophy (replacement of calf muscles by fatty infiltration)
  - Cardiac/respiratory failure: most common cause of death
- Diagnostics
  - Elevated creatine kinase
  - Muscle biopsy: muscle fiber degeneration fibrosis
  - Gene testing: dystrophin gene deletion
  - Immunohistochemistry: absent or decreased for dystrophin
- Management: symptomatic, no cure
  - Steroids may be helpful
  - Physical/occupational therapy

Becker muscular dystrophy: similar presentation and pathophysiology to Duchenne muscular dystrophy, overall, less severe

Cerebral Palsy
- Pathophysiology: prenatal insult to the brain resulting in intellectual and motor disability
- Risk factors
  - Prematurity
  - Intrauterine infection
  - Maternal drug abuse
  - Intrauterine growth restriction
  - Antepartum hemorrhage

– Signs and symptoms
  • Spastic paresis
  • Intellectual disability
  • Epilepsy
  • Strabismus
– Diagnostics: clinical
– Management: symptomatic, no cure
  • Antispasmodic
  • Physical/occupational therapy
  • Speech therapy
  • Treatment of associated comorbidities
– Prophylaxis: intrapartum magnesium prior to 32 weeks decreases risk of cerebral palsy

SYSTEMIC DISORDERS

Henoch-Schönlein Purpura
– Pathophysiology: immune-mediated vasculitis secondary to deposition of immunoglobulin A immune complexes
– Signs and symptoms
  • Gastrointestinal: abdominal pain, bloody diarrhea, intussusception
  • Musculoskeletal: arthralgias, myalgias
  • Renal: hematuria, proteinuria
  • Cutaneous: lower extremity palpable purpura (Fig. 43-4)
– Diagnostics
  • Clinical
  • Biopsy: leukocytoclastic vasculitis
  • Normal complement levels
– Management
  • Supportive care, most cases resolve spontaneously
  • Steroids for severe refractory cases

Systemic Lupus Erythematosus (SLE)
– Epidemiology: primarily affects middle-aged women with personal or family history of other autoimmune disease (rheumatoid arthritis, Sjögren, scleroderma)
– Definition: systemic, multiorgan autoimmune disorder
– Key manifestations (Fig. 43-5)
  • Cutaneous
    ▪ Photosensitivity malar rash (Fig. 43-6)
    ▪ Painless oral ulcers
    ▪ Discoid rash
    ▪ Raynaud phenomenon

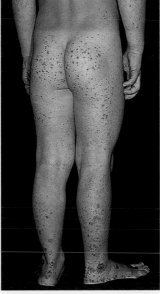

Figure 43-4: Lower extremity palpable purpura of Henoch-Schönlein purpura.

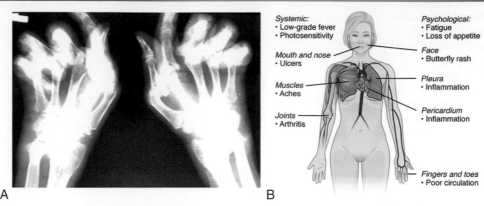

Figure 43-5: (A) Radiographs of the wrist and hand in a patient with systemic lupus erythematosus demonstrating ulnar deviation of the metacarpophalangeal joints without erosive changes. (B) Diagrammatic representation of the symptoms of systemic lupus erythematosus, system by system.

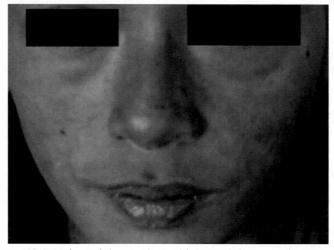

Figure 43-6: Malar rash in a patient with systemic lupus erythematosus.

Drug-induced SLE (SHIPPE): sulfasalazine, hydralazine, isoniazid, procainamide, phenytoin, etanercept

Drug-induced lupus does not have central nervous system or renal manifestations; associated with antihistone antibodies, which are highly specific.

Anti-Ro and anti-La associated with neonatal lupus; these babies present with complete heart block requiring pacing at birth.

- Musculoskeletal
  - Avascular necrosis of the hip
  - Migratory, symmetric arthritis/arthralgias
- Hematologic/immunologic
  - Autoimmune thrombocytopenia, hemolytic anemia, leukopenia: type 2 hypersensitivity reaction
  - Anemia of chronic disease
  - Diffuse lymphadenopathy
  - Antiphospholipid syndrome (anticardiolipin, lupus anticoagulant, anti-beta-2 glycoprotein antibody)
- Serology
  - Antinuclear antibody (ANA; highly sensitive)
  - Anti-dsDNA (highly specific), anti-Smith (highly specific)
  - Hypocomplementemia (low C3/C4)
  - Elevated inflammatory markers (ESR, CRP)
- Renal
  - Rapidly progressive glomerulonephritis (crescenteric glomerulonephritis)
  - Membranous nephropathy

- Neurologic
  - Cerebritis
  - Stroke (secondary to vasculitis)
  - Seizures
  - Cognitive deficits
- Pulmonary
  - Pleuritis
  - Pleurisy
  - Interstitial lung disease
  - Pleural effusion
- Cardiac
  - Liebman-Sacks endocarditis
  - Pericarditis, pericardial effusion
  - Early atherosclerosis/coronary artery disease
  - Myocarditis
- Diagnostics: 4 of 11 diagnostic criteria (SOAP BRAIN MD)
- Management
  - Acute flare: glucocorticoids
  - Chronic disease:
    - Mild disease: hydroxychloroquine, NSAIDs
    - Moderate disease: methotrexate, azathioprine
    - Severe disease (life-threatening renal or central nervous system [CNS] disease): steroid-sparing agents (cyclophosphamide, mycophenolate)
  - Steroids also used for lupus with renal, CNS, and hematologic manifestations

SOAP BRAIN MD lupus diagnostic criteria:
- Serositis
- Oral ulcers
- Arthralgias, arthritis
- Photosensitivity rash
- Blood dyscrasias (anemia, thrombocytopenia, leukopenia)
- Renal
- Antinuclear antibody+
- Immunologic (anti-dsDNA, anti-Smith)
- Neurologic
- Malar rash
- Discoid rash

Juvenile Idiopathic Arthritis
- Epidemiology: 1–3 years old, females
- Definition: idiopathic synovitis of peripheral joints
- Subtypes
  - Pauciarticular
  - Polyarticular
  - Systemic (Still disease)
- Signs and symptoms
  - Arthritic manifestations
    - Morning stiffness
    - Muscle atrophy
    - Decreased range of motion
  - Extraarticular manifestations
    - Fever of unknown origin
    - Salmon-colored rash on trunk and extremities
    - Uveitis
    - Lymphadenopathy
    - Hepatosplenomegaly
    - Serositis
- Diagnostics
  - Clinical criteria
    - Fever >2 weeks
    - Arthritis >6 weeks
    - Symmetric arthritis involving more than one joint

- Supporting labs
  - Anemia of chronic disease
  - Elevated ESR, CRP
  - Thrombocytosis
  - ANA, rheumatoid factor positive
- Management
  - Mild disease: NSAIDs
  - Moderate to severe disease: methotrexate, tumor necrosis factor inhibitors

Juvenile Dermatomyositis/Polymyositis
- Definition: autoimmune inflammatory myopathy resulting in muscle damage and characteristic cutaneouas manifestations
- Signs and symptoms
  - Fever, malaise, lethargy
  - Muscle aches, weakness
  - Symmetric proximal myopathy (difficulty getting up from seated position, raising arms above shoulder level)
  - No neurologic deficits
  - Cutaneous (associated with dermatomyositis)
    - Gottron papules (patchy, erythematous rash involving dorsum of hand) (Fig. 43-7)
    - Heliotrope rash (purplish discoloration around periorbital region) (Fig. 43-8)
    - Shawl sign (rash involving upper neck, back, chest, and shoulders)
    - Mechanics hand (dark, dirty-appearing hands with cracks and fissures)
- Diagnostics
  - Elevated creatine phosphokinase, aldolase
  - Muscle biopsy: mononuclear infiltrate and necrosis
- Management
  - Glucocorticoids: initial treatment

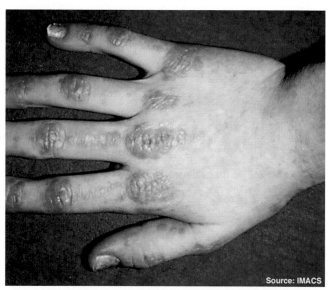

Figure 43-7: Gottron papules in a patient with dermatomyositis.

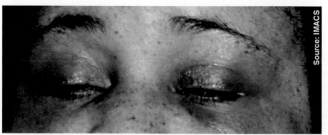

Figure 43-8: Heliotrope rash in a patient with dermatomyositis.

- Steroid-sparing agents for steroid unresponsive
  - Methotrexate
  - Cyclosporine

Juvenile dermatomyositis presents with similar cutaneous manifestations as the adult version; however, less visceral involvement, no associated increase risk of visceral malignancy, and no characteristic autoantibodies.

CHAPTER 44
Hematology and Oncology

BASICS OF HEMATOLOGY

Understanding the origins and functions of the different cell lines allows for better mastery of the various blood dyscrasia and their associated symptomatology (Figs. 44.1 and 44.2).

ANEMIA

General principles of anemia
- Definition: deficiency of red blood cells: <13 g/dL in men and <12 g/dL in women
- Pathophysiology: secondary to production abnormalities, destruction disorders, or bleeding (Fig. 44.3)
- Signs and symptoms
  - Palpitations, tachycardia, chest pain, dyspnea on exertion/rest
  - Lightheadedness, dizziness, orthostatic hypotension
  - Fatigue, lethargy
  - Pallor, pale conjunctiva
- Diagnostics
  - Mean corpuscular volume (MCV): average size of red blood cells (RBCs); normal range 80–100
  - Red cell distribution width: variation in size between RBCs; higher values indicate greater size heterogeneity between RBCs
  - Reticulocyte count: precursor of RBCs that will mature into erythrocytes within 24 hours; indicator of bone marrow response to anemia
  - Lactate dehydrogenase (LDH), haptoglobin, indirect bilirubin: indicators of hemolytic anemia; LDH and indirect bilirubin elevated, haptoglobin levels decreased
  - Bone marrow biopsy: evaluate production abnormalities of anemia
  - Peripheral smear

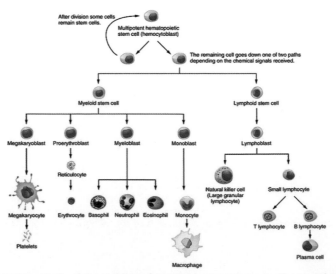

Figure 44.1: Hematopoeiosis of the cell lines from the bone marrow to the peripheral circulation.

Formed element	Major subtypes	Numbers present per microliter (μL) and mean (range)	Appearance in a standard blood smear	Summary of functions	Comments
Erythrocytes (red blood cells)		5.2 million (4.4–6.0 million)	Flattened biconcave disk; no nucleus; pale red color	Transport oxygen and some carbon dioxide between tissues and lungs	Lifespan of approximately 120 days
Leukocytes (white blood cells)		7000 (5000–10,000)	Obvious dark-staining nucleus	All function in body defenses	Exit capillaries and move into tissues; lifespan of usually a few hours or days
	Granulocytes including neutrophils, eosinophils, and basophils	4360 (1800–9950)	Abundant granules in cytoplasm; nucleus normally lobed	Nonspecific (innate) resistance to disease	Classified according to membrane-bound granules in cytoplasm
	Neutrophils 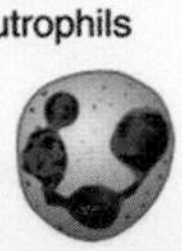	4150 (1800–7300)	Nuclear lobes increase with age; pale lilac granules	Phagocytic; particularly effective against bacteria. Release cytotoxic chemicals from granules	Most common leukocyte; lifespan of minutes to days
	Eosinophils 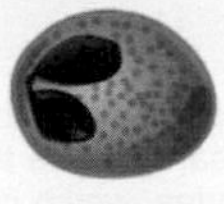	165 (0–700)	Nucleus generally two-lobed; bright red-orange granules	Phagocytic cells; particularly effective with antigen- antibody complexes. Release antihistamines. Increase in allergies and parasitic infections	Lifespan of minutes to days
	Basophils 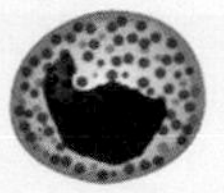	44 (0–150)	Nucleus generally two-lobed but difficult to see due to presence of heavy, dense, dark purple granules	Promotes inflammation	Least common leukocyte; lifespan unknown
	Agranulocytes including lymphocytes and monocytes	2640 (1700–4950)	Lack abundant granules in cytoplasm; have a simple-shaped nucleus that may be indented	Body defenses	Group consists of two major cell types from different lineages
	Lymphocytes 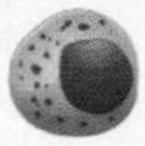 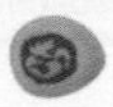	2185 (1500–4000)	Spherical cells with a single often large nucleus occupying much of the cell's volume; stains purple; seen in large (natural killer cells) and small (B and T cells) variants	Primarily specific (adaptive) immunity: T cells directly attack other cells (cellular immunity); B cells release antibodies (humoral immunity); natural killer cells are similar to T cells but nonspecific	Initial cells originate in bone marrow, but secondary production occurs in lymphatic tissue; several distinct subtypes; memory cells form after exposure to a pathogen and rapidly increase responses to subsequent exposure; lifespan of many years
	Monocytes 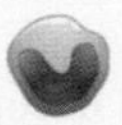	455 (200–950)	Largest leukocyte with an indented or horseshoe-shaped nucleus	Very effective phagocytic cells engulfing pathogens or worn out cells; also serve as antigen-presenting cells (APCs) for other components of the immune system	Produced in red bone marrow; referred to as macrophages after leaving circulation
Platelets 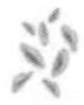		350,000 (150,000–500,000)	Cellular fragments surrounded by a plasma membrane and containing granules; purple stain	Hemostasis plus release growth factors for repair and healing of tissue	Formed from megakaryocytes that remain in the red bone marrow and shed platelets into circulation

Figure 44.2: Number, appearance, and function of the various hematologic cell types.

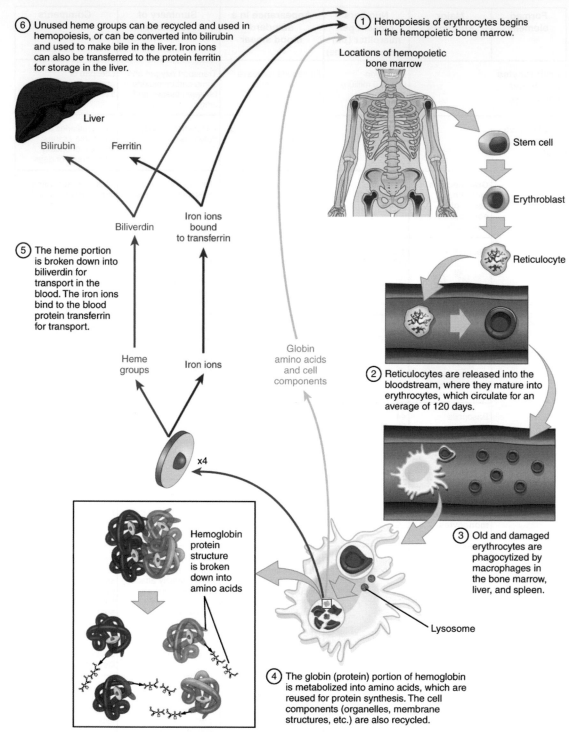

6) Unused heme groups can be recycled and used in hemopoiesis, or can be converted into bilirubin and used to make bile in the liver. Iron ions can also be transferred to the protein ferritin for storage in the liver.

Liver

Bilirubin   Ferritin

Biliverdin

Iron ions bound to transferrin

5) The heme portion is broken down into biliverdin for transport in the blood. The iron ions bind to the blood protein transferrin for transport.

Heme groups   Iron ions

1) Hemopoiesis of erythrocytes begins in the hemopoietic bone marrow.

Locations of hemopoietic bone marrow

Stem cell

Erythroblast

Reticulocyte

2) Reticulocytes are released into the bloodstream, where they mature into erythrocytes, which circulate for an average of 120 days.

3) Old and damaged erythrocytes are phagocytized by macrophages in the bone marrow, liver, and spleen.

Lysosome

Globin amino acids and cell components

Hemoglobin protein structure is broken down into amino acids

4) The globin (protein) portion of hemoglobin is metabolized into amino acids, which are reused for protein synthesis. The cell components (organelles, membrane structures, etc.) are also recycled.

Figure 44.3: Figure depicting a normal red blood cell (RBC) life cycle. Anemia results in disruption of this process resulting in decreased RBC life span. (Image courtesy of OpenStax College.)

– Management
  • Treat underlying cause
  • Transfusion if necessary (Fig. 44.4)
    ▪ Hemoglobin <7
    ▪ Hemoglobin <8 with preexisting coronary artery disease
    ▪ Hemoglobin <10 with symptoms

Painful vasoocclusive crises are typically caused by hypoxia, infections, dehydration, and acidosis.

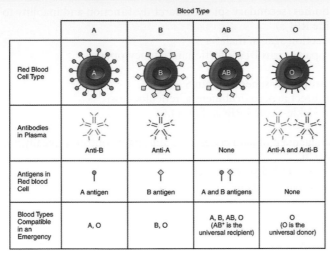

Blood Type

	A	B	AB	O
Red Blood Cell Type				
Antibodies in Plasma	Anti-B	Anti-A	None	Anti-A and Anti-B
Antigens in Red blood Cell	A antigen	B antigen	A and B antigens	None
Blood Types Compatible in an Emergency	A, O	B, O	A, B, AB, O (AB⁺ is the universal recipient)	O (O is the universal donor)

Figure 44.4: Table comparing blood types and blood compatibility.

Hemolytic Anemia

Principles of hemolytic anemia: hemolytic anemias can be differentiated into intravascular vs extravascular hemolysis; intravascular hemolysis as the name suggests results in hemolysis within the blood vessels resulting in indirect hyperbilirubinemia, elevated LDH, and low haptoglobin. Haptoglobin is a protein that binds to free hemoglobin in the blood so that hemoglobin can be removed by the reticuloendothelial system (spleen, liver). Therefore haptoglobin levels will be low during intravascular hemolysis as it is utilized to bind free hemoglobin. In extravascular hemolysis, abnormal RBCs are phagocytosed by the reticuloendothelial system without release of intracellular RBC contents.

Sickle Cell Disease
– Pathophysiology: chronic hemolytic anemia due to beta-globin gene mutation at position 6 resulting in a valine for glutamic substitution and recurrent vasoocclusive crises
– Key manifestations
  • Neurologic: stroke, retinopathy
  • Cardiac
    ▪ Hyperdynamic changes, high output heart failure
    ▪ Systolic flow murmur
  • Pulmonary
    ▪ Acute chest syndrome (cough, shortness of breath)
    ▪ Pulmonary embolism, pulmonary hypertension
  • Gastrointestinal
    ▪ Bilirubin gallstones
    ▪ Autosplenectomy (autoinfarction)
    ▪ Acute abdomen
    ▪ Splenic sequestration crisis: acute splenomegaly, drop in hemoglobin, diffuse reticulocytosis, hypovolemic shock; treat with exchange transfusion and splenectomy
  • Rheumatologic
    ▪ Osteomyelitis: increased incidence of Salmonella osteomyelitis; however, osteomyelitis from *Staphylococcus aureus* is the most common cause overall
    ▪ Avascular necrosis of femoral head
    ▪ Dactylitis
    ▪ Growth delay
  • Renal
    ▪ Hematuria, recurrent urinary tract infections, papillary necrosis
    ▪ Diabetes insipidus
    ▪ Distal renal tubular acidosis
    ▪ Membranoproliferative glomerulonephritis, focal segmental glomerulosclerosis
  • Dermatologic: dermal occlusions, nonhealing skin ulcers
  • Hematologic
    ▪ Sepsis: secondary to encapsulated organisms (*Streptococcus pneumoniae*, Neisseria, Haemophilus) after splenic autoinfarction
    ▪ Priapism

- Howell-Jolly bodies (secondary splenic infarct/dysfunction and inability to remove nuclear remnants inside RBCs)
- Increased protection against malaria
  - Aplastic crisis: parvovirus B19 infection, reticulocytopenia
- Diagnostics
  - Hemoglobin electrophoresis: hemoglobin S >50%
  - Elevated LDH, indirect hyperbilirubinemia, reticulocytosis
  - Peripheral smear: sickle-shaped RBCs (Fig. 44.5)
- Management
  - Symptomatic management of pain crises: IV fluids, pain control (typically requires opioids), supplemental oxygen
  - Penicillin prophylaxis until 5 years of age
  - Low threshold to initiate antibiotics
  - Pneumococcal, Neisseria, influenza vaccination
  - Folate supplementation
  - Hydroxyurea: prevents recurrent sickle cell crisis
  - Exchange transfusion: stroke, acute chest syndrome, symptomatic anemia, reticulocytopenia, splenic sequestration crisis

---

Diffuse reticulocytosis vs reticulocytopenia is a key differentiator between splenic sequestration crisis and aplastic crisis.

Hydroxyurea: inhibits ribonucleotide reductase and increases hemoglobin F levels to prevent recurrent pain crises; also used in chronic myeloid leukemia. Common side effect is bone marrow suppression.

Sickle cell trait: ~50% hemoglobin S, 50% hemoglobin A on electrophoresis; asymptomatic; may have painless hematuria, isosthenuria; no intervention required.
Hemoglobin SC: ~50% hemoglobin S, 50% hemoglobin C; similar signs and symptoms as sickle cell disease; however, with less frequency and severity.

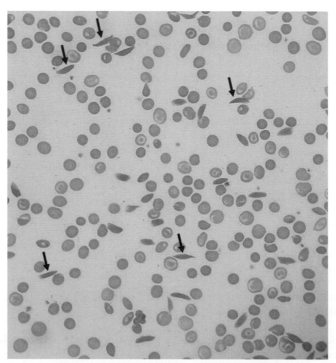

Figure 44.5: Sickled cells on peripheral smear.

Hereditary Spherocytosis
– Pathophysiology
  • Autosomal dominant extravascular hemolytic anemia characterized by ankyrin gene RBC membrane defect resulting in spectrin deficiency
  • Abnormal scaffolding proteins results in less deformable RBCs and increased splenic sequestration
– Key manifestations
  • Anemia, jaundice
  • Bilirubin gallstones, acute cholecystitis, splenomegaly
  • Parvovirus B19 aplastic anemia
– Diagnostics
  • Increased osmotic fragility on acidified glycerol lysis test
  • Eosin-5-maleimide binding test (flow cytometry)
  • Elevated mean corpuscular hemoglobin concentration: cellular dehydration, membrane loss
  • Peripheral smear: spherocytes (Fig. 44.6)
– Management: symptomatic
  • Transfusion as needed
  • Folate supplementation
  • Splenectomy as last resort

Hereditary spherocytosis is a Coombs-negative hemolytic anemia. Autoimmune hemolytic anemia is Coombs positive. Previously used osmotic fragility test has poor sensitivity for diagnosing hereditary spherocytosis.

Spherocytes are seen in several other disorders (autoimmune hemolytic anemia, G6PD deficiency) and are nonspecific for hereditary spherocytosis.

Glucose-6-Phosphate Dehydrogenase (G6PD Deficiency)
– Epidemiology: African, Mediterranean descent
– Definition: hemolytic anemia secondary to decreased G6PD after exposure to hemolytic triggers (infection, sulfa drugs, antimalarials, fava beans)
– Pathophysiology: deficiency of G6PD dehydrogenase → decreased RBC NADPH → decreased glutathione production (antioxidant) → increased RBC radical damage
– Signs and symptoms
  • Abdominal pain
  • Nausea, vomiting
  • Jaundice
  • Fever
  • Dark urine (hemoglobinuria)
– Diagnostics
  • Elevated LDH, low haptoglobin
  • Peripheral smear: bite cells, Heinz bodies

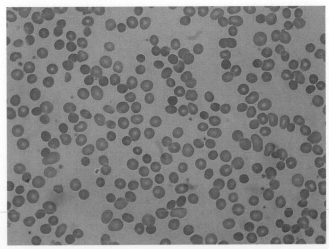

Figure 44.6: Peripheral blood smear in a patient with hereditary spherocytosis showing spherocytes.

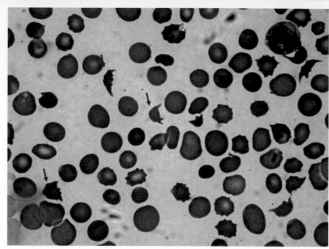

Figure 44.7: Schistocytes (red arrows) in a patient with hemolytic anemia. May be seen with any of the causes of hemolytic anemia discussed in this section.

- • Reticulocytosis
  - • RBC G6PD levels after hemolytic crisis
  - Management
    - • Symptomatic management
    - • Avoid hemolysis triggers

Hemolytic Uremic Syndrome (HUS)
- Epidemiology: children 5–10 years old
- Pathophysiology: infection by Shiga toxin–producing *Escherichia coli* 0157:H7 from undercooked beef
- Signs and symptoms
  - • Anemia, jaundice
  - • Bloody diarrhea
  - • Fevers, chills
- Diagnostics: clinical
  - • Acute kidney injury
  - • Complete blood count (CBC): normocytic anemia, thrombocytopenia
  - • Peripheral smear: schistocytes (Fig. 44.7)
  - • Elevated LDH, indirect hyperbilirubinemia, reticulocytosis
- Management: supportive; most cases resolve spontaneously

Thrombotic Thrombocytopenic Purpura (TTP)
- Epidemiology: hereditary form is more common in children, and acquired form more common in adults
- Pathophysiology
  - • Decreased ADAMTS13 activity (plasma protease) secondary to autoantibody leading to inability to break down von Willebrand factor (vWF) multimers → development of diffuse small vessel thrombi, which consume platelets and shear RBCs
  - • ADAMTS13 functions to cleave vW multimers from endothelial surface
- Signs and symptoms: classic pentad of symptoms (FAT RN)
  - • <u>F</u>ever
  - • Microangiopathic hemolytic <u>a</u>nemia
  - • <u>T</u>hrombocytopenia
  - • <u>R</u>enal insufficiency
  - • <u>N</u>eurologic symptoms (altered mental status, seizures)
- Diagnostics: do not need all five symptoms to make diagnosis, only requirement is evidence of hemolytic anemia and thrombocytopenia
  - • Peripheral smear: schistocytes
  - • Decreased ADAMTS13 levels
  - • Elevated hemolysis markers (elevated LDH, indirect hyperbilirubinemia)
- Management: plasmapheresis +/− glucocorticoids

Malaria
- Microbiology

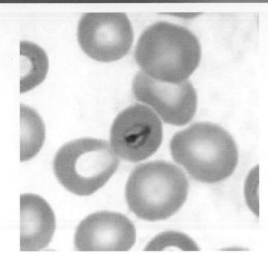

Figure 44.8: Intraerythrocytic parasite in a patient with malaria on Giemsa stain.

- • Intraerythrocytic infection caused by Plasmodium parasite
- • Transmitted by Anopheles mosquito; infects RBCs and hepatocytes depending on the species
- Species
  - • Plasmodium falciparum: most lethal
  - • P. vivax, P. ovale: remains dormant in the liver
  - • P. malaria: associated with nephrotic syndrome
- Signs and symptoms
  - • Cyclic fevers, chills, pallor
  - • Headaches, myalgias
  - • Abdominal pain, splenomegaly, diarrhea, nausea, vomiting
- Diagnostics: clinical and laboratory
  - • Peripheral smear (Fig. 44.8)
    - ▪ Banana-shaped gametocytes
    - ▪ Intraerythrocytic parasites on Giemsa stain
  - • Elevated liver function tests (LFTs; only in *P. vivax* and *P. ovale* infection)
  - • Hemolysis markers (elevated LDH, low haptoglobin, reticulocytosis)
  - • Anemia, thrombocytopenia
- Management
  - • Intrahepatic (vivax, ovale): primaquine
  - • Intraerythrocytic (all species): depends on region and resistance patterns
    - ▪ Chloroquine, hydroxychloroquine
    - ▪ Artemether
    - ▪ Mefloquine
    - ▪ Quinine
- Complications
  - • Stroke, visual disturbances, seizures
  - • Hematuria, renal failure
  - • Pulmonary edema
- Prophylaxis
  - • Lifestyle modifications: long-sleeve clothing, insect repellent
  - • Pharmacologic: choice depends on side effect profile
    - ▪ Mefloquine
    - ▪ Chloroquine
    - ▪ Doxycycline
    - ▪ Atovaquone-proguanil

Partial immunity against malaria in patients with hemoglobinopathies

Malaria is endemic to South America, Africa, South Euthanasia. Most common cause of malaria in the United States is from travelers returning from endemic areas without appropriate prophylaxis.

Babesiosis
- Microbiology

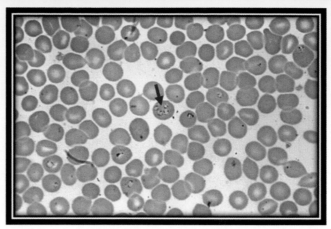

Figure 44.9: Intraerythrocytic rings (red arrow) in a patient with babesiosis.

- • Tickborne illness caused by *Babesia microti*
- • Associated with Exodes tick (also transmits Lyme disease, human granulocytic anaplasmosis)
- – Signs and symptoms: similar to malaria
- – Diagnostics
  - • Peripheral smear: intraerythrocytic rings ("Maltese cross") (Fig. 44.9)
  - • Anemia, thrombocytopenia
  - • Hemolysis markers (LDH, haptoglobin, reticulocytosis)
  - • Elevated LFTs
- – Management
  - • Azithromycin + atovaquone: first line
  - • Severe cases: quinine + clindamycin in severe cases
- – Complications
  - • Acute respiratory distress syndrome, congestive heart failure
  - • Disseminated intravascular coagulopathy (DIC)
  - • Splenic rupture

Microcytic Anemia
Iron metabolism/homeostasis
- • Absorbed in the proximal intestine (duodenum) through divalent metal transporters
- • Absorption is regulated by hepcidin, which is a protein produced by the liver, which prevents excessive iron absorption. Deficiency of hepcidin results in unopposed iron absorption and iron overload (hemochromatosis). Excess hepcidin is produced in inflammatory or infectious states preventing iron absorption and iron deficiency.
- • After absorption through divalent metal transporters, iron is transported through the blood by transferrin proteins and stored intracellularly as ferritin.

Iron Deficiency Anemia
- – Causes
  - • Blood loss (gastrointestinal, menorrhagia, antiplatelets, anticoagulants)
  - • Insufficient dietary intake (lack of animal protein)
  - • Increased requirements (infants, adolescents)
  - • Malabsorption (celiac disease, small bowel resection, inflammatory bowel disease)
- – Signs and symptoms
  - • Fatigue, malaise
  - • Pallor
  - • Palpitations, chest pain, dyspnea
  - • Lightheadedness, dizziness
  - • Pica, ice craving
  - • Restless leg syndrome
- – Diagnostics
  - • Low MCV
  - • Elevated RBC distribution width
  - • Reactive thrombocytosis
  - • Iron studies
  - • Peripheral smear: hypochromic, microcytic RBCs (Fig. 44.10)

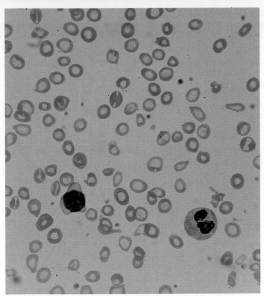

Figure 44.10: Peripheral smear in a patient with deficiency anemia showing microcytosis, hypochromasia, aniso-cytosis, and poikilocytosis.

– Management: oral or IV iron replacement

Additional notes regarding iron:
1. Monitor for allergic reaction when administering IV iron transfusion.
2. Iron replacement is sometimes given with vitamin C to increase absorption as vitamin C is a reducing agent converting Fe^{3+} to Fe^{2+}.
3. Side effects of oral iron replacement include nausea, constipation, dark stools.

Lead inhibits ferrochelatase and ALA dehydratase resulting in defective heme synthesis.
Basophilic stippling is also seen in sideroblastic anemia, thalassemia, sickle cell disease.

Basics of hemoglobin: hemoglobin is a peptide tetramer that requires two alpha-globin groups and two nonalpha blood globin groups (beta, gamma, or delta) to form hemoglobin.
- Normal adult hemoglobin (HbA) = 2 alpha + 2 beta
- Fetal hemoglobin (HbF) = 2 alpha + 2 gamma
- Deficiency of either alpha- or beta-globin results in formation of abnormal tetramers; these abnormal hemoglobin result in decreased RBC life span (Table 44.1)

Lead Poisoning
– Causes
- Ingestion from lead-painted older houses: most commonly in children
- Occupational exposure (batteries, plumbing, painting, construction): most commonly in adults
– Signs and symptoms
- Neurologic
  - Headache, irritability
  - Encephalopathy
  - Peripheral neuropathy
- Gastrointestinal
  - Nausea, vomiting
  - Abdominal pain, constipation
- Hematologic: microcytic sideroblastic anemia
- Lead line: pigmentation of gum-tooth line
– Diagnostics
- Elevated venous lead level
- Elevated zinc protoporphyrin
- X-ray fluorescence: detects lead lines in bone
- Peripheral smear: basophilic stippling
- Iron studies (Table 44.2)

TABLE 44.1   Alpha- Versus Beta-Thalassemia

	ALPHA-THALASSEMIA	BETA-THALASSEMIA
Pathophysiology	• Defect in alpha-globin production due to deletion in up to 4 alpha-globin genes resulting in formation of beta-globin tetramers	• Defect in beta-globin production due to mutation in up to two beta-globin genes
Signs and symptoms	Depends on number of alpha genes deleted: • One-gene deletion: normal phenotype, no symptoms • Two-gene deletion: mild anemia under stress, mostly asymptomatic • Three-gene deletion: moderate anemia requiring occasional transfusion • Four-gene deletion: fatal in newborns, hydrops fetalis	Depends on number of beta genes mutated: • One-gene mutation: normal phenotype, no symptoms • Two-gene mutation: moderate anemia requiring transfusions, growth retardation, extramedullary hematopoiesis (hepatosplenomegaly, chipmunks facies, crew-cut appearance on head x-ray), jaundice
Diagnostics	Hemoglobin (Hb) electrophoresis: • One- or two-gene deletion: normal • Three-gene deletion: HbH • Four-gene deletion: Hb Barts • Peripheral smear: hypochromic microcytic red blood cells • Hemolysis markers (elevated lactate dehydrogenase, decreased haptoglobin, reticulocytosis)	Hemoglobin electrophoresis: • One-gene mutation: increased HbF, HbA2 • Two-gene mutation: no HbA, increased HbF • Similar peripheral smear and hemolysis markers as alpha-thalassemia
Management	• One- or two-gene deletion: no treatment necessary • Three-gene deletion: transfusions as needed, folate replacement, iron chelators (deferoxamine, deferasirox) to prevent iron overload. Consider splenectomy in severe cases. Allogeneic hematopoietic cell transplantation is potentially curative • Four-gene deletion: no treatment, death in utero	• One-gene mutation: no treatment necessary • Two-gene mutation: similar to 3-alpha gene deletion

Hemoglobinopathies characterized by decreased synthesis or absence of alpha- or beta-globin.

TABLE 44.2   Iron Studies Table

	SERUM IRON	IRON SATURATION	FERRITIN	TOTAL IRON BINDING CAPACITY (TIBC)
Iron deficiency anemia	Decreased	Decreased	Decreased	Increased
Anemia of chronic disease	Decreased	Decreased	Increased	Normal/low
Thalassemia	Normal	Normal	Normal	Normal
Lead poisoning; sideroblastic anemia	Normal	Increased	Increased	Decreased
Hemochromatosis	Increased	Increased	Increased	Decreased

Interpreting iron deficiency iron studies: low serum iron → low iron saturation → increased number of circulating transferrin not bound to iron (increased TIBC) → low intracellular iron stores

- Management: depends on lead levels
  - <45 mcg/dL: no treatment, removal from work exposure
  - >45 mcg/dL: lead chelators
    - EDTA, dimercaprol
    - Succimer (most preferred in children)
    - Penicillamine

Macrocytic Anemia
Folate Deficiency
- Causes
  - Dietary deficiency, goat's milk

- Medications: methotrexate, TMP-SMX, phenytoin
- Chronic hemolysis
- Signs and symptoms: related to anemia
- Diagnostics
  - MCV >100
  - Decreased RBC folate levels
  - Peripheral smear: hypersegmented neutrophils, megaloblastic macrocytic RBCs
  - Elevated LDH, indirect hyperbilirubinemia, decreased reticulocyte
- Management: folate replacement

> Orotic aciduria: congenital disorder of uridine monophosphate synthase deficiency (de novo pyrimidine synthesis pathway) resulting in macrocytic megaloblastic anemia and developmental delay; treat with replacement uridine monophosphate.

Diamond-Blackfan Anemia (Congenital Red Cell Anemia)
- Epidemiology: <1 year old
- Pathophysiology: isolated RBC progenitor cells apoptosis
- Signs and symptoms
  - Anemia
  - Growth delay, short stature
  - Intellectual disability
  - Craniofacial abnormalities (hypertelorism, snub nose)
  - Triphalangeal thumbs
  - Cardiac/renal defects
- Diagnostics
  - Macrocytic anemia
  - Reticulocytopenia
  - Hemoglobin electrophoresis: elevated hemoglobin F
  - Bone marrow biopsy
  - Normal chromosomal studies
- Management
  - Corticosteroids
  - Transfusion as needed

Transient Erythroblastopenia of Childhood
- Similar to Diamond-Blackfan anemia as it presents as pure red cell aplasia; however, without macrocytosis
- Possibly related to postviral infection
- No treatment needed, most cases self-resolving

Fanconi Anemia (Congenital Pancytopenia)
- Epidemiology: 5–10 years old
- Pathophysiology: mutation in DNA repair genes
- Signs and symptoms
  - Musculoskeletal
    - Microcephaly
    - Short stature
    - Absent/hypoplastic thumbs
    - Absent radius
  - HEENT
    - Recurrent middle ear infections
    - Hypertelorism
    - Low-set ears
    - Strabismus
  - Dermatologic: café au lait spots, freckles
  - Renal: horseshoe kidney
  - Reproductive: hypogonadism
- Diagnostics
  - CBC: pancytopenia
    - Macrocytosis
    - Reticulocytopenia
  - Bone marrow biopsy: diffuse hypoplasia
  - Cytogenetic studies: chromosomal breakage when exposed to DNA cross-linking agents
  - Hemoglobin electrophoresis: increased hemoglobin F

– Management
  • Allogeneic hematopoietic cell transplantation
  • Transfusions as needed
– Complications: increased risk of cancers

Holt-Oram syndrome: primarily heart (atrial septal defect) and musculoskeletal (absent radius) defects; no hematologic abnormalities

---

Polycythemia

Polycythemia
– Definition: increased RBC mass, hematocrit >60%
– Causes
  • Cyanotic congenital heart disease (erythropoietin stimulation secondary to chronic hypoxia)
  • Infants of diabetic mothers
  • Malignancy

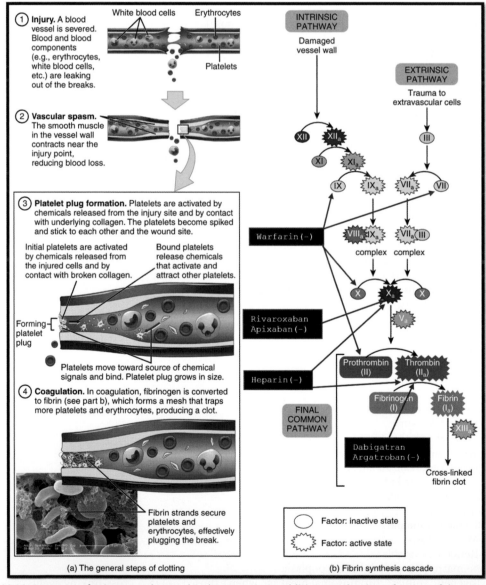

Figure 44.11: Summary of primary and secondary hemostasis. In addition, mechanism of action of drugs commonly used to manipulate the coagulation cascade. (-), inhibits. (a) General steps of clotting involved in primary hemostasis. (b) Fibrin synthesis cascade involved in secondary hemostasis.

- Androgen-producing tumors (ovarian, adrenal)
- Erythropoietin-producing tumors (renal, von Hippel-Lindau syndrome)
- Signs and symptoms
  - Facial plethora
  - Ruddy complexion
  - Thrombosis (secondary to hyperviscosity)
- Diagnostics
  - CBC: hematocrit >60%
  - Elevated erythropoietin levels, may be low in malignancy
- Management: treat underlying etiology

BLEEDING

Primary hemostasis: formation of platelet plugs via platelet adhesion and aggregation (Fig. 44.11)
1. Endothelial injury exposes subendothelial collagen
2. vWF binds subendothelial collagen
3. Platelet glycoprotein 1B binds to vWF (platelet adhesion)
4. Platelets release adenosine diphosphate resulting in expression of glycoprotein IIb/IIIa
5. Fibrinogen binds to glycoprotein IIB/IIIa and links platelets (platelet aggregation)

Secondary hemostasis: activation of clotting factors to convert fibrinogen into fibrin and formation of fibrin clot (see Fig. 44.11)
1. Tissue factor activates extrinsic pathway (factor VII) and clotting cascade
2. Activation of intrinsic pathway begins with factor XII
3. Extrinsic and intrinsic clotting pathways function to activate combined pathway (factor X)
4. Combined pathway converts fibrinogen into fibrin resulting in formation of fibrin clot

Platelet Quantity Disorders

Thrombocytopenia
- Causes
  - Destruction
    - Heparin-induced thrombocytopenia
    - Systemic lupus erythematosus (antibodies against platelets; type 2 hypersensitivity reaction)
    - TTP/HUS
    - DIC
  - Production/suppression
    - Alcohol, chemotherapy, valproate, quinine, interferon, linezolid
    - Bone marrow dysfunction, leukemia
    - Sepsis
    - Viral infections (Epstein-Barr virus, cytomegalovirus, human immunodeficiency virus, hepatitis)
    - Babesia, malaria, Rocky Mountain spotted fever, dengue
    - Nutritional deficiencies (B12, folate, copper)
  - Consumption: splenic sequestration
  - Other causes
    - Wiskott-Aldrich syndrome (immunodeficiency associated with eczema and thrombocytopenia)
    - Pseudothrombocytopenia (platelet clumping)
    - Immune thrombocytopenic purpura (ITP): diagnosis of exclusion
- Signs and symptoms
  - Petechiae, ecchymosis, easy bruising
  - Gingival bleeding
- Diagnostics
  - CBC: platelets <150,000
  - Peripheral smear: elevated megakaryocytes
- Management
  - Treat underlying disorder
  - ITP
    - Prednisone, IV immunoglobulin
    - Splenectomy last resort
  - Platelet stimulators if severe bleeding is present and platelets <30,000
    - Synthetic thrombopoietin: romiplostim, eltrombopag
    - Oprelvekin (interleukin-11)
  - Platelet transfusion if needed under the following circumstances
    - Asymptomatic: <10,000
    - Severe bleeding: <30,000

- Intracranial bleeding or prior to central nervous system (CNS) surgery: <100,000
- Prior to major surgery: <50,000

Platelet Function Disorders

vWF Deficiency
- Epidemiology
  - Most common inherited bleeding disorder
  - Autosomal dominant inheritance
- Subtypes
  - Type I: decreased vWF
  - Type II: defective vWF
  - Type III (most severe): complete deficiency of vW multimers
- Signs and symptoms
  - Epistaxis, gingival bleeding
  - Petechiae, ecchymosis
  - Easy bruising/bleeding
  - Mucosal bleeding (gastrointestinal, genitourinary)
  - Significant bleeding after initiation of aspirin or antiplatelets
- Diagnostics
  - Decreased serum vWF antigen
  - Ristocetin cofactor assay (measures ability vWF binds to glycoprotein IB)
  - Decreased factor VIII activity
  - Slightly elevated partial thromboplastin time (PTT; vWF stabilizes factor VIII)
- Management
  - DDAVP: stimulates release of vWF and factor VIII from Weibel-Palade bodies located in endothelial cells
  - vWF replacement

Bernard-Soulier Syndrome
- Defective glycoprotein 1B resulting in inadequate platelet adhesion
- Mild thrombocytopenia
- Giant platelets
- Bleeding out of proportion to the degree of thrombocytopenia

Glanzmann Thrombasthenia
- Defective glycoprotein IIB/IIIa resulting in inadequate platelet aggregation
- Mucocutaneous bleeding
- Associated with defects in leukocyte function (leukocyte adhesion deficiency)

Inherited Coagulopathies

Hemophilia A/B
- Pathophysiology: X-linked inherited disorder (only affects males) resulting in deficiency of factor VIII (hemophilia A) or IX (hemophilia B)
- Signs and symptoms
  - Muscle hematomas
  - Retroperitoneal bleeds
  - Hemarthroses
  - Early osteoarthritis
- Diagnostics: decreased serum factor VIII or IX
- Management
  - Factor replacement
  - Desmopressin for mild hemophilia A

Acquired Coagulopathies

Vitamin K Deficiency
- Causes
  - Prolonged antibiotic use (destroys vitamin K–producing bacterial flora)
  - Newborns (lack of colonization by vitamin K–producing flora)
  - Malnutrition
  - Fat malabsorption syndromes (cystic fibrosis, celiac disease, inflammatory bowel disease, obstructive biliary disease)
  - Liver disease
  - Warfarin

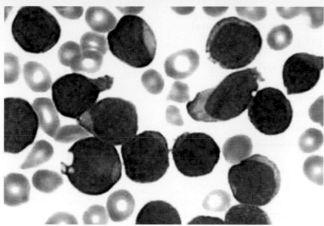

Figure 44.12: Peripheral smear in a patient with acute lymphoblastic leukemia demonstrating multiple lympho-blasts. (Image courtesy of James Grellier - derivative of original work by VashiDonsk at en.wikipedia; CC BY-SA 3.0 [https://creativecommons.org/licenses/by-sa/3.0])

– Signs and symptoms: bleeding
– Diagnostics
  • Elevated prothrombin time (PT)/PTT (PT increases first)
  • Decreased plasma levels of factor II, VII, IX, X, protein C/S
– Management
  • Fresh frozen plasma for severe bleeding
  • Vitamin K replacement for mild to asymptomatic cases

HEMATOLOGIC MALIGNANCIES

Acute Lymphoblastic Leukemia
– Epidemiology: most common malignancy in children
– Definition: hematologic malignancy of B- or T-cell lymphocytic precursors (lymphoblasts)
– Associations
  • Down syndrome
  • Klinefelter syndrome
– Signs and symptoms
  • Anemia, thrombocytopenia, neutropenia
  • Hepatosplenomegaly
  • Lymphadenopathy
  • T-cell leukemia–specific symptoms
    ▪ Neurologic dysfunction (CNS involvement)
    ▪ Testicular mass
    ▪ Anterior mediastinal mass (superior vena cava [SVC] syndrome, tracheal obstruction)
– Diagnostics
  • CBC: leukocytosis with lymphocytic predominance
  • Peripheral smear: >20% lymphoblasts (Fig. 44.12)
  • Markers: CALLA antigen (CD10), TdT positive
  • Flow cytometry: differentiate B-cell vs T-cell leukemia
  • Bone marrow biopsy
– Management: highly responsive to chemotherapy
  • Induction, consolidation, and maintenance chemotherapy
  • CNS prophylaxis due to poor blood brain barrier penetration of chemotherapeutic agents
  • Hematopoietic cell transplantation is curative

Acute Myeloid Leukemia (AML)
– Definition: hematologic malignancy characterized by excessive production of immature granulocyte (>20% blasts forms)
– Associations
  • Trisomy 21
  • Klinefelter syndrome
  • Radiation/toxin exposure
  • Chemotherapy
  • Myelodysplastic syndrome, polycythemia vera

- Subtypes: seven total subtypes
  - AML M3 (acute promyelocytic leukemia)
    - Auer rods on peripheral smear; DIC
    - 15:17 translocation
    - Treated with all-trans-retinoic acid
  - AML M4/M5 (myelocytic leukemia)
    - Mimics meningitis due to CNS involvement
    - Skin and soft tissue nodules
    - Gingival hyperplasia
  - AML M6: PAS-positive blasts
- Signs and symptoms
  - Fatigue, shortness of breath: anemia
  - Easy bruising, bleeding: thrombocytopenia
  - Recurrent infections: malfunctioning granulocytes
  - Hepatosplenomegaly: extramedullary hematopoiesis
  - Lymphadenopathy
  - Bone and joint pain
- Diagnostics
  - CBC: anemia, thrombocytopenia, leukocytosis
  - Peripheral smear: Auer rods, >20% blasts
  - Chromosomal studies, cytogenetics
  - Flow cytometry
  - Myeloperoxidase positive
- Management: induction chemotherapy followed by allogeneic hematopoietic cell transplantation

Chronic myeloid leukemia and chronic lymphocytic leukemia are rarely seen in pediatrics and further discussed in Part 1.

Lymphoma

Basic principles of lymphoma
- Cancer of the lymphatic system
- Has the potential to spread into the blood causing leukemia
- Presents with painless lymphadenopathy plus A symptoms (asymptomatic) or B symptoms (fever, weight loss, night sweats); presence of B symptoms indicate a worse prognosis
- Location of lymphadenopathy results in local compressive symptoms: mediastinal (cough, shortness of breath, SVC syndrome), mesenteric (abdominal pain), retroperitoneal (back pain)
- May invade other organs such as spleen (splenomegaly), liver (hepatomegaly), and bone marrow (bone pain)
- Divided into Hodgkin and non-Hodgkin lymphoma
- Hodgkin lymphoma staging (Ann Arbor system) is determined based on number of lymph nodes involved, location of lymph nodes (above or below the diaphragm), and extralymphatic spread (Fig. 44.13)
- Some lymphoma subtypes are characterized by chromosomal translocation

Lymph nodes may become tender when drinking alcohol.

Hodgkin Lymphoma
- Epidemiology: bimodal distribution, 15–30 years old and >50 years old
- Subtypes
  - Nodular sclerosing: most common

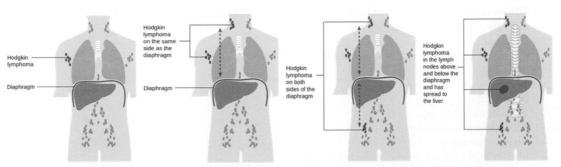

Figure 44.13: Ann Arbor staging of Hodgkin lymphoma, stages 1 to 4 from left to right.

- Mixed cellularity
- Lymphocytic rich: best prognosis
- Lymphocyte depleted: worse prognosis
– Signs and symptoms: painless lymphadenopathy plus A or B symptoms
– Diagnostics
  - Excisional lymph node biopsy: Reed-Sternberg cells (owl's-eye nucleus; CD15, CD30 positive)
  - Elevated LDH
  - Ann Arbor staging
    - Computed tomography (CT) chest abdomen and pelvis
    - Bone marrow biopsy
– Management
  - Localized disease: radiation +/− chemotherapy
  - Advanced disease: chemotherapy
– Complications: related to radiation therapy
  - Increased risk of future solid organ malignancy (lung, breast, thyroid, gastrointestinal, bone)
  - Non-Hodgkin lymphoma
  - Leukemia from chemoradiation

Associated with minimal change disease (nephrotic syndrome), hypervitaminosis D (increased production of 1,25-dihydroxy-vitamin D), Lambert-Eaton syndrome (antibodies against presynaptic voltage-gated calcium channels), Guillain-Barré syndrome

Non-Hodgkin Lymphoma
– Most subtypes present in adults
– Burkitt lymphoma is one of the few pediatric subtypes
  - Associated with 8:14 translocation
  - Presents with rapidly enlarging abdominal/mandibular mass
  - Starry-sky appearance on histology
– Diagnostics
  - Excisional lymph node biopsy: allows for evaluation of entire lymph node architecture
  - Elevated LDH, beta-2 microglobulin
  - Staging
    - CT chest abdomen and pelvis
    - Bone marrow biopsy
– Management: chemotherapy, due to commonly presenting at late stage

Hodgkin lymphoma most commonly presents during localized early stage disease treated with radiation.

VIRAL INFECTIONS

Erythema Infectiosum
– Microbiology: parvovirus B19
– Signs and symptoms: vary depending on the individual affected
  • Young children
    ▪ Bilateral erythematous rash involving the cheeks (slapped-cheek appearance) (Fig. 45.1)
    ▪ Lacy reticular rash
  • Adult/adolescence: arthralgias
  • Hemoglobinopathies: aplastic anemia
  • Fetus: hydrops fetalis
– Diagnostics: clinical
– Management: supportive

Roseola Infantum
– Caused by human herpesvirus (HHV) 6/7
– Rapid high fever followed by erythematous papular rash
– Clinical diagnosis, supportive management

Coxsackievirus Associations
– Herpangina: small vesicles located in posterior pharynx
– Hand-foot-mouth disease:
  • Vesicles located on hand, foot, and mouth
  • Vesicles tend to ulcerate and become painful
– Acute lymphonodular pharyngitis: nodules located on posterior pharynx with associated lymphadenopathy
– Type I diabetes
– Myocarditis

Infectious Mononucleosis
– Risk factors: saliva transmission
– Microbiology: Epstein-Barr virus (EBV)

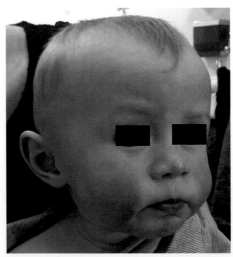

Figure 45.1: Slapped-cheek rash in a patient with erythema infectiosum.

- Signs and symptoms
  - Nonspecific prodrome
  - Fever, headache
  - Myalgias, abdominal pain
  - Sore throat, pharyngitis
  - Generalized lymphadenopathy (posterior cervical, submandibular, epitrochlear)
  - Splenomegaly, possible hepatomegaly
  - Maculopapular rash after treatment with ampicillin or amoxicillin (immune-mediated vasculitic rash)
- Diagnostics
  - Heterophile antibodies (monospot test) positive
  - EBV immunoglobulin M (IgM) antibodies
  - Peripheral smear: atypical lymphocytosis
- Management
  - Symptomatic therapy
  - Avoid contact sports in cases of splenomegaly
  - Steroids for management of complications (airway obstruction due to enlarged tonsils, autoimmune hemolytic anemia)

Epstein-Barr virus cancer associations:
1. Burkitt lymphoma
2. Nasopharyngeal carcinoma
3. Centrall nervous system lymphoma
4. Hodgkin lymphoma

Adenovirus causes pharyngoconjunctival fever.
Rhinovirus causes the common cold.

Many of the more severe childhood diseases are less commonly seen due to widespread vaccination; however, when seen in unvaccinated patients they have a characteristic presentation (Table 45.1).

PARASITIC INFECTIONS
Enterobiasis
- Epidemiology: most common helminth infection in the United States
- Microbiology: Enterobiasis vermicularis (pinworm)
- Risk factors
  - Poor hygiene and handwashing (fecal-oral transmission)
  - School-age children
- Signs and symptoms: anal/vulvar pruritus
- Diagnostics
  - Adhesive tape test at night (females migrate at night to deposit eggs in perianal region): examines for presence of eggs under microscopy
  - Stool ova and parasites (O&P) test
- Management: albendazole or pyrantel pamoate for patient and household contacts
Giardiasis
- Epidemiology: most common parasitic infection overall
- Microbiology: *Giardia intestinalis*
- Risk factors
  - Drinking contaminated stream water
  - Daycare
  - Camping, hiking
- Signs and symptoms
  - Chronic watery, foul-smelling diarrhea
  - Abdominal pain, bloating, flatulence
- Diagnostics: stool O&P
- Management: metronidazole
Cysticercosis
- Microbiology: *Taenia solium*

TABLE 45.1   Diseases Associated With Unvaccinated Children

INFECTION	CLINICAL MANIFESTATIONS	MANAGEMENT
Measles	• Cough, coryza, conjunctivitis • Koplik spots (gray-white spots on buccal mucosa) • Otitis media • Pneumonia • Subacute sclerosing panencephalitis	• Supportive care • Vitamin A
Mumps	• Parotitis • Orchitis • Pancreatitis	• Supportive care
Rubella	• Maculopapular rash starting on face and spreading caudally • Retroauricular, occipital lymphadenitis • Forscheimer spots	• Supportive care
Varicella	• Maculopapular, crusting vesicles • Pneumonia • Guillain-Barré syndrome • Encephalitis, cerebellar ataxia • Ramsey Hunt syndrome • Superimposed group A Streptococci cellulitis	• Acyclovir
Diphtheria	• Pharyngitis with gray-white membrane (potential for airway obstruction) • "Bull" neck • Myocarditis • Encephalitis	• Erythromycin or penicillin • Antitoxin
Tetanus	• Muscle spasms • Diffuse hypertonicity • Trismus (lock jaw) • Respiratory failure	• Metronidazole • Tetanus vaccine +/− immune globulin
Pertussis	• Upper respiratory infection symptoms • Inspiratory "whooping" cough • Posttussive emesis	• Macrolide for patients and close contacts • Respiratory isolation
Polio	• Asymmetric flaccid paralysis • Fasciculation • Respiratory failure	• Supportive care
Haemophilus influenzae type B	• Epiglottitis • Meningitis	• Third-generation cephalosporin • Rifampin prophylaxis for close contacts

- Risk factors
  • Ingestion of undercooked pork
  • Contaminated water
  • Pig farmers
  • Immigrants from Mexico, South America
- Signs and symptoms: depends on location where tapeworms infect
  • Skin: subcutaneous nodules
  • Muscle: myalgias
  • Brain: neurocysticercosis
    ▪ Headache, vomiting
    ▪ Seizures, stroke
- Diagnostics
  • Stool O&P
  • Magnetic resonance imaging brain
    ▪ Enhancing and nonenhancing calcified lesions in the brain with edema
    ▪ Swiss cheese appearance
    ▪ Hydrocephalus
- Management
  • Albendazole +/− steroids
  • Antiepileptics for seizures

Ascariasis
- Microbiology: Ascaris lumbricoides (roundworm)
- Signs and symptoms: secondary to large worm burden and size
  - Abdominal pain/distention
  - Small bowel obstruction
  - Biliary obstruction
  - Loeffler syndrome: hemoptysis plus eosinophilic pneumonitis
- Diagnostics
  - Stool O&P
  - Eosinophilia
- Management: antihelminthic
  - Albendazole
  - Mebendazole
  - Pyrantel pamoate (for pregnant women)

Hookworm
- Microbiology: Ancylostoma/Necator americanus
- Risk factors: walking barefoot (parasite penetrates skin)
- Signs and symptoms
  - Abdominal pain, diarrhea
  - Iron deficiency anemia (chronic blood loss)
  - Intense pruritic rash at the site of skin penetration
  - Green-yellow skin discoloration (chlorosis)
- Diagnostics
  - Stool O&P
  - Eosinophilia
- Management
  - Antihelminthic
    - Albendazole
    - Mebendazole
    - Pyrantel pamoate
  - Iron supplementation

Strongyloidiasis
- Microbiology: strongyloidiasis stercoralis
- Signs and symptoms
  - Abdominal pain, nausea, vomiting
  - Pruritus, urticaria
  - Wheezing, hemoptysis
- Diagnostics
  - Enzyme-linked immunosorbent assay: preferred test
  - Stool O&P
- Management: ivermectin

Trichuris Trichiura
- Infection frequently occurs with Ascaris lumbricoides
- Most commonly asymptomatic
- Symptomatic patients present with mucus/bloody stools, rectal prolapse, eosinophilia
- Treat with mebendazole

Cutaneous Larva Migrans (Creeping Eruption)
- Infection by dog or cat hookworms after encountering contaminated soil
- Serpiginous, erythematous, pruritic tracking skin lesion
- No treatment necessary, self-resolving
- Consider ivermectin or albendazole in severe cases

Strongyloidiasis superinfection may occur in immunocompromised and presents with more severe symptomatology.

CONGENITAL INFECTIOUS SYNDROMES

All congenital infections present with nonspecific symptoms such as jaundice, lymphadenopathy, hepatosplenomegaly, intrauterine growth restriction, and blueberry muffin spots.
  TORCHeS infections:
- Toxoplasma
- Other (varicella-zoster virus [VZV], parvovirus, listeria)
- Rubella

- <u>C</u>ytomegalovirus (CMV)
- <u>H</u>erpes/Human immunodeficiency virus/hepatitis
- <u>S</u>yphilis

Toxoplasmosis
- Microbiology: Toxoplasma gondii
- Risk factors
  - Cat feces
  - Uncooked meat
- Signs and symptoms
  - Chorioretinitis
  - Intracranial calcifications
  - Seizures
  - Microcephaly
- Diagnostics
  - Mother: toxoplasma IgM/IgG
  - Fetus: amniocentesis for toxoplasma DNA polymerase chain reaction (PCR)
- Management
  - Spiramycin: treats maternal disease, without evidence of fetal disease
  - Pyrimethamine/sulfadiazine + leucovorin: treats fetal disease

VZV
- Microbiology: HHV-3 (DNA virus)
- Risk factors: primary maternal varicella infection
- Signs and symptoms
  - Mother
    - Erythematous, vesicular rash
    - Pneumonia
    - Encephalitis
  - Neonate
    - Limb hypoplasia
    - Cicatricial (scarring, zigzag) skin lesions
    - Microcephaly, microphthalmia
    - Seizures, chorioretinitis

Reactivation of varicella-zoster virus resulting in congenital varicella syndrome typically occurs anywhere from 5 days prior to delivery to 2 days postpartum.

- Diagnostics
  - Clinical
  - DNA PCR from vesicular lesions
- Management
  - Maternal
    - Pre/postpregnancy: live attenuated VZV vaccine
    - Postexposure prophylaxis: VZV immunoglobulin
    - Uncomplicated infection: oral acyclovir
    - Isolation from fetus if active lesions are present
  - Neonates: IV acyclovir +/− VZV immunoglobulin (if disease occurs between 5 days prior to delivery and 2 days postpartum)

Parvovirus
- Microbiology: parvovirus B19 (DNA virus)
- Risk factors: primary maternal infection
- Signs and symptoms
  - Mother: self-limiting arthritis
  - Neonatal
    - Hydrops fetalis
    - High-output cardiac failure
    - Anemia (cytotoxic to erythroid progenitor cells), thrombocytopenia
- Diagnostics
  - Maternal parvovirus IgM antibodies
  - Transcranial Doppler: monitor for fetal anemia
- Management: symptomatic
  - Transfuse as needed via percutaneous umbilical blood sampling
  - Drain pleural effusions and ascites

Listeriosis
- Microbiology: *Listeria monocytogenes* (gram-positive rod, tumbling motility)
- Risk factors
  • Deli meats
  • Goat cheese
  • Dairy products
- Signs and symptoms
  • Maternal: mild gastroenteritis
  • Neonate
    ▪ Diffuse granulomas with microabscesses
    ▪ Meningitis
    ▪ Sepsis
    ▪ Chorioamnionitis, spontaneous abortion, placental lesions
- Diagnostics: neonatal cerebrospinal fluid/blood cultures
- Management
  • Mother: supportive care
  • Neonate: IV ampicillin + gentamicin for the neonate

Rubella
- Microbiology: togaviridae (single-stranded RNA virus)
- Risk factors: primary maternal rubella infection
- Signs and symptoms
  • Maternal
    ▪ Rash
    ▪ Arthritis
  • Neonates
    ▪ Patent ductus arteriosus
    ▪ Cataracts
    ▪ Congenital deafness
    ▪ Intellectual disability
- Diagnostics: maternal rubella IgM antibodies
- Management
  • Mother: measles-mumps-rubella live attenuated vaccine before or after pregnancy
  • Neonates: supportive care

CMV
- Epidemiology: most common congenital viral infection
- Microbiology: cytomegalovirus (HHV-5, DNA virus)
- Signs and symptoms
  • Mother: asymptomatic +/− mononucleosis-like syndrome
  • Fetus
    ▪ Periventricular calcifications
    ▪ Hearing loss: most common cause of congenital deafness
    ▪ Chorioretinitis
    ▪ Interstitial pneumonitis
    ▪ Fetal hydrops
- Diagnostics
  • Maternal CMV IgG/IgM antibodies
  • Antenatal ultrasound determines severity of infection
- Management: ganciclovir (reduces neurologic sequelae)

Herpes
- Microbiology: herpes simplex virus (HSV; DNA virus)
- Signs and symptoms
  • Mother
    ▪ Vesicular, erythematous rash
    ▪ Prodromal numbness/tingling
  • Neonate
    ▪ Skin/mucous membranes: vesicular lesions, conjunctivitis
    ▪ Central nervous system
      ○ Meningoencephalitis
      ○ Hydrocephalus
      ○ Lethargy, irritability
    ▪ Pneumonia
    ▪ Hepatitis

- Diagnostics
  - Clinical
  - HSV PCR
- Management: prevent genital herpes at the time of delivery to allow for vaginal delivery and prevent vertical transmission
  - Mother
    - Acyclovir: indicated for the following scenarios
      - Suppressive therapy starting at 36 weeks until time to deliver
      - Primary infection prior to delivery
    - Cesarean section: if active lesions present at time of delivery
  - Neonate
    - Asymptomatic: monitoring +/− prophylactic acyclovir depending on maternal history of HSV and presence of active lesions
    - Symptomatic: IV acyclovir

Syphilis
- Microbiology: *Treponema pallidum* (gram-negative spirochete)
- Risk factors: multiple sexual partners
- Signs and symptoms
  - Neonate to 2 years old
    - Desquamation of palms and soles
    - Snuffles (copious mucopurulent rhinorrhea)
    - Periostitis, osteochondritis
    - Interstitial keratitis, photophobia
    - Nonimmune hydrops fetalis
  - >2 years old:
    - Hutchinson teeth
    - Cranial nerve VIII palsy
    - Saber shins
    - Frontal bossing, saddlenose
    - Rhagades (fissures at the corners of the mouth)
    - Mulberry molar (rounded enamel cusps)
- Diagnostics: antenatal or neonatal testing
  - Venereal Disease Research Laboratory/rapid plasma reagin
  - Antitreponemal antibodies
- Management: penicillin

If syphilis is diagnosed during antenatal testing in mother, treatment is with penicillin regardless of allergies. If mother is allergic to penicillin, treatment is to desensitize mother as alternative treatments (doxycycline) are contraindicated in pregnancy.

CHAPTER 46
Allergy and Immunology

ALLERGIES
Allergic Reactions

Atopic Dermatitis (Eczema)
– Pathophysiology: inflammatory dermatitis in response to environmental agents
– Risk factors
  • Family history
  • Asthma
  • Allergic rhinitis
  • Weather change
– Signs and symptoms
  • Recurrent pruritic rash involving extensor (infants) and/or flexor (older children) surfaces
  • Lichenification (secondary to chronic itching)
  • Hyperpigmentation
  • Dermatographism (wheal and flare reaction when scratching skin with object)
– Diagnostics: clinical
– Management
  • Avoid triggering factors
  • Topical corticosteroids
  • Antihistamines

Allergic Rhinitis
– Pathophysiology: immune-mediated inflammatory response within nasal mucosa in response to inhaled antigens
– Risk factors
  • Atopy, asthma
  • Family history
  • Seasonal change
  • Grass, pollen
– Signs and symptoms
  • Rhinorrhea, sneezing
  • Nasal pruritus, nasal polyp
  • Lacrimation
  • Pale, edematous nasal mucosa
  • Pharyngeal cobblestoning
  • Transverse nasal creases ("allergic salute")
  • Infraorbital edema and discoloration ("allergic shiners")
  • Prominence of lower eyelids (Dennie-Morgan line)
– Diagnosis: clinical
– Management
  • Avoid triggering factors
  • Intranasal glucocorticoids: first line
  • Antihistamines

Hypersensitivity Reactions

There are four main types of hypersensitivity reactions involving different cell types, antigens, and antibodies. These are the basis of the different autoimmune diseases (Fig. 46.1).

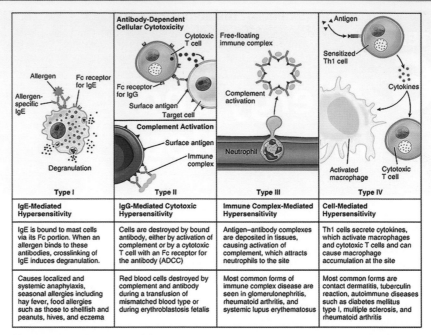

Figure 46.1: Differentiating the types of hypersensitivity reactions based on pathophysiology and etiologies. (Image courtesy of OpenStax College.)

Urticaria
– Pathophysiology: type I hypersensitivity immunoglobulin E (IgE)–mediated reaction resulting in mast cell degranulation of histamine and localized anaphylaxis
– Causes
  • Medications
    ▪ Penicillins
    ▪ Sulfa drugs
    ▪ Nonsteroidal antiinflammatory drugs
    ▪ Anticonvulsants
    ▪ Narcotics, radiocontrast dye: result in direct mast cell activation
  • Foods: peanuts, shellfish
  • Infections: acute hepatitis B, Strongyloides
  • Insect bites/sting
  • Systemic mastocytosis
  • Idiopathic
  • Chronic urticaria triggered by pressure (dermatographism), cold, vibration, and systemic disorders (vasculitis, autoimmune, malignancy)
– Signs and symptoms: prodromal/localized anaphylaxis
  • Sudden onset wheal and flare reaction: well-circumscribed, erythematous plaques with central pallor
  • Severe pruritus
– Diagnostics: clinical
– Management
  • Epinephrine if there are signs of anaphylaxis (respiratory compromise, hypotension)
  • Antihistamines
  • Oral glucocorticoids for severe unresponsive cases
  • Desensitization for unavoidable triggers
Anaphylaxis
– IgE-mediated type I hypersensitivity reaction resulting in systemic vasodilation and bronchoconstriction
– Other symptoms include pruritus, urticaria, and diarrhea
– Associated with many causes, including drugs, foods, insect bites, and latex
– Mainstay of treatment is IM epinephrine; corticosteroids and antihistamines are also helpful

TABLE 46.1   Function and Components of the Immune System

IMMUNE COMPONENT	FUNCTION
B cells	• Differentiate into plasma cells • Immunoglobulin M (IgM) (acute infection) and IgG (chronic infection, immunity) • Antibodies created against encapsulated organisms
T cells	• Involved in treating fungal and viral infections
Neutrophils	• Serve phagocytic function to ingest bacterial organisms • Organisms are destroyed within the phagosome-lysosome
Complement	• Activated on the surface of infectious organism, particularly encapsulated resulting in cellular destruction

The Five Immunoglobulin (Ig) Classes					
	IgM pentamer	IgG monomer	Secretory IgA dimer	IgE monomer	IgD monomer
			Secretory component		
Percentage of total antibody in serum	6%	80%	13%	0.002%	1%
Crosses placenta	no	yes	no	no	no
Fixes complement	yes	yes	no	no	no
Fc binds to		phagocytes		mast cells and basophils	
Function	Main antibody of primary responses, best at fixing complement; the monomer form of IgM serves as the B cell receptor	Main blood antibody of secondary responses, neutralizes toxins, opsonization	Secreted into mucus, tears, saliva, colostrum	Antibody of allergy and antiparasitic activity	B cell receptor

Figure 46.2: Differentiating the five classes of immunoglobulins. (Table courtesy of OpenStax College.)

TABLE 46.2   B-Cell Immunodeficiencies

IMMUNODEFICIENCY	PATHOPHYSIOLOGY	CLINICAL MANIFESTATIONS	MANAGEMENT
Bruton agammaglobulinemia	• X-linked inherited mutation in Bruton tyrosine kinase gene resulting in arrested development of mature B cells	• Low immunoglobulins of all classes • Absent lymph nodes and tonsils • Recurrent infections with encapsulated organisms **(Streptococcus pneumoniae, Neisseria, Haemophilus influenzae)** • Symptoms present after 6 mo (infant no longer protected by maternal immunoglobulin G [IgG])	• IVIG
Common variable immunodeficiency	• Defective B-cell differentiation	• Less severe form of Bruton agammaglobulinemia • Presents in adolescence and early 20s • Increased risk of autoimmune disease lymphomas	
IgA deficiency	• Isolated deficiency of IgA	• Recurrent sinopulmonary infections • Chronic diarrhea (giardiasis) • Anaphylaxis when exposed to IgA-containing blood products • Increased risk of autoimmune (celiac disease) and atopic disease	• Supportive management • Ensure blood products are washed and come from IgA-deficient individuals

IMMUNOLOGY
Basics of Immunology

Each of the different cell types in the immune system has different functionality to combat the various infectious organisms (Table 46.1). There are also several classes of immunoglobulins, which have unique functions and are released by B cells depending on the acuity, organism, and site of infection (Fig. 46.2). Deficiencies in cell types or antibodies result in immunodeficiencies with increased risk of infection and other unique manifestations (Tables 46.2, 46.3, 46.4, 46.5, and 46.6).

Immunodeficiencies

TABLE 46.3   T-Cell Immunodeficiencies

IMMUNODEFICIENCY	PATHOPHYSIOLOGY	CLINICAL MANIFESTATIONS	MANAGEMENT
DiGeorge syndrome	• Failure to develop third and fourth pharyngeal pouch resulting in absent thymus (site of T-cell synthesis) and parathyroid glands • Deletion on chromosome 22	• Recurrent viral and fungal infection • Cardiac defects • Abnormal facies (hypertelorism, short philtrum, "fish mouth," cleft palate) • Hypocalcemia (tetany) • Absence of thymic shadow on chest x-ray	• Calcium supplementation • Supportive management
Hyperimmunoglobulin E (IgE) syndrome (Job syndrome)	• Impaired differentiation of Th17 cells resulting in impaired recruitment of neutrophils	• Recurrent staphylococcal abscess • Retained primary teeth • Increased IgE levels	• Supportive management • Prophylactic TMP-SMX for severe recurrent infections

TABLE 46.4   Phagocytic Immunodeficiencies

IMMUNODEFICIENCY	PATHOPHYSIOLOGY	CLINICAL MANIFESTATIONS	MANAGEMENT
Chédiak-Higashi	• Microtubule defect preventing fusion of phagosome-lysosome • CHS1/LYST gene mutation	• Partial oculocutaneous albinism • Progressive neurologic disability • Peripheral neuropathy • Recurrent mucocutaneous and pulmonary Staphylococcus and Streptococcus infection • Giant granules in neutrophils	• Hematopoietic cell transplantation
Chronic granulomatous disease	• X-linked recessive defective NADPH oxidase • Decreased ability to form reactive oxygen species and respiratory burst	• Recurrent infection with catalase-positive organisms (S. aureus, Pseudomonas, Nocardia, Aspergillus, Serratia, Listeria) • Nitroblue tetrazolium test remains yellow • Abnormal dihydrorhodamine on flow cytometry	• Antibacterial and antifungal prophylaxis • Interferon gamma • Hematopoietic cell transplantation
Leukocyte adhesion deficiency	• Defective integrin protein preventing neutrophils from extravasating and reaching site of infection	• Delayed umbilical cord separation • Gingivitis, periodontitis • Absent formation of pus/abscess • Absence of CD18 integrin on flow cytometry • Neutrophilia	• Hematopoietic cell transplantation

TABLE 46.5 Combined B- and T-Cell Immunodeficiencies

IMMUNODEFICIENCY	PATHOPHYSIOLOGY	CLINICAL MANIFESTATIONS	MANAGEMENT
Severe combined immunodeficiency	• Adenosine deaminase deficiency (ADA) • Interleukin-2 (IL-2) receptor gamma chain receptor mutation	• Low immunoglobulin (Ig) of all classes • Lymphopenia • Infection with opportunistic organisms (Pneumocystis pneumonia [PCP]) within first few months of life • IL-2R-gamma gene mutation • <2% ADA activity • Decreased T-cell receptor excision circles	• Hematopoietic cell transplantation
Wiskott-Aldrich syndrome	• X-linked recessive WAS gene mutation	• Thrombocytopenia with small platelets • Eczema • Recurrent infections • Increased risk of autoimmune and lymphoma	• Supportive management • +/- prophylaxis for PCP and herpes simplex virus
Ataxia-telangiectasia	• ATM gene mutation • Inability to repair DNA strand breaks	• Cerebellar ataxia • Spider angioma • IgA deficiency • Increased risk of malignancy • Avoid radiation exposure	• Supportive management

TABLE 46.6 Complement Immunodeficiencies

IMMUNODEFICIENCY	PATHOPHYSIOLOGY	CLINICAL MANIFESTATIONS	MANAGEMENT
C1 esterase deficiency	• Deficiency (hereditary) or autoantibody (acquired) against C1 esterase	• Cutaneous swelling • Laryngeal edema • Abdominal pain (gastrointestinal angioedema) • Acquired form associated with non-Hodgkin lymphoma	• Avoid triggering agents (angiotensin-converting enzyme inhibitors) • Plasma derived from C1 esterase inhibitor concentrate
C3 complement deficiency	• Major opsonin of the complement system prevents activation of the classical complement pathway	• Recurrent infections with encapsulated organism *(Streptococcus pneumoniae, Neisseria, Haemophilus influenzae)* • Increased risk of glomerulonephritis	• Supportive management
Terminal complement deficiency	• Deficiency of complement C5-C9	• Recurrent Neisseria infections	

Low total hemolytic complement (THC) or CH50 levels seen in complement deficiencies.

CHAPTER 47 Dermatology

INCIDENTAL AND BENIGN SKIN LESIONS
Incidental Skin Lesions

Incidental skin lesions are commonly found in newborns and have no clinical significance and require no treatment or follow-up (Table 47.1).

Benign Skin Lesions
Strawberry Infantile Hemangioma
- Epidemiology: most common benign vascular tumor in children
- Signs and symptoms
  - Bright red, sharply demarcated violaceous lesion (Fig. 47-1)
  - Initially rapidly grow and self-regresses over months to years
  - Lesions blanch with pressure
- Management
  - No treatment necessary, most cases will self-resolve
  - Propranolol for complicated (periorbital, ulcerated) hemangiomas

INFECTIOUS RASHES

Kasabach-Merritt syndrome: vascular tumor (hemangioma) that sequesters platelets resulting in thrombocytopenia.

Impetigo
- Definition: localized epidermal infection commonly involving the face
- Microbiology
  - Group A Streptococcus
  - *Staphylococcus aureus*
- Signs and symptoms
  - Honey-crusted lesions (Fig. 47-2)
  - Painful pustules
  - Flaccid blisters (bullous impetigo)
  - Negative Nikolsky sign
- Diagnostics: clinical
- Management
  - Localized: topical mupirocin
  - Widespread or bullous impetigo: dicloxacillin or first-generation cephalosporin
  - Handwashing
- Complications
  - Acute rheumatic fever: prevented with antibiotics
  - Poststreptococcal glomerulonephritis
  - Staphylococcal scalded skin syndrome (SSSS)
  - Scarlet fever

SSSS
- Epidemiology: <5 years old
- Microbiology: *S. aureus*
- Pathophysiology: toxin-producing *S. aureus* that targets desmoglein-1 (transmembrane glycoprotein involved in keratinocyte adhesion) resulting in exfoliative skin lesion
- Signs and symptoms
  - Fever, irritability
  - Periorbital erythema

TABLE 47.1   Incidental Skin Lesions

SKIN LESION	KEY FEATURES	IMAGE	MANAGEMENT
Erythema toxicum. (Image courtesy of Mohammad2018; CC BY-SA 4.0 [https://creativecommons.org/licenses/by-sa/4.0])	• Whitish yellow papules • Migratory erythematous rash • Presents in first few days of life		• Self-resolving
Mongolian spot. (Image courtesy of Wierzman; CC BY-SA 3.0 [https://creativecommons.org/licenses/by-sa/3.0])	• Bluish black macules, buttocks, and posterior thigh • Common in neonates of Asian and African descent		• Self-resolving
Simple nevus. (Image courtesy of Gzzz; CC BY-SA 4.0 [https://creativecommons.org/licenses/by-sa/4.0])	• Painless, pale macules located at the posterior neck (stork bite) • May get darker when baby cries		• No treatment, often persists into adolescence
Milia. (Image courtesy of Masryyy; CC BY-SA 4.0 [https://creativecommons.org/licenses/by-sa/4.0])	• Firm whitish papules on the face and nose • Secondary to underdeveloped sweat glands • May involve mucous membranes (Epstein pearls)		• Self-resolving
Neonatal acne	• Erythematous papules on the face secondary to elevated maternal androgens • Presents around 1 wk of birth		• Self-resolving • +/− benzoyl peroxide or topical retinoids in severe cases

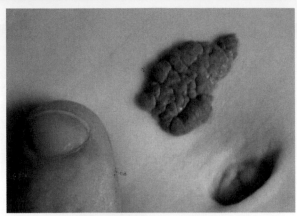

Figure 47-1: Strawberry infantile hemangioma on the abdomen.

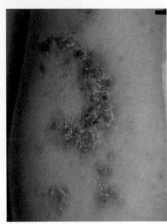

Figure 47-2: Honey-crusted lesions consistent with impetigo on the elbow. (Image courtesy of Evanherk at Dutch Wikipedia; CC BY-SA 3.0 [http://creativecommons.org/licenses/by-sa/3.0/])

- • Superficial flaccid blisters
- • Exfoliation and desquamation of the skin
- • Positive Nikolsky sign (separation of skin upon lateral pressure)
- – Diagnostics: clinical
- – Management
  - • Antistaphylococcal antibiotics
  - • Wound care

Scarlet Fever
- – Pathophysiology: postinfectious (pharyngitis, impetigo) group A Streptococcus toxin mediated rash
- – Microbiology: group A Streptococcus
- – Signs and symptoms
  - • Pharyngeal erythema/exudate
  - • Circumoral pallor
  - • Bright red, strawberry tongue (Fig. 47-3)
  - • Pink, papular, erythematous sandpaper-like rash
  - • Rash starts on the trunk and spreads peripherally within 24 hours
  - • Pastia lines (localized petechiae within skin creases)
  - • Desquamation of the rash after 1 week
- – Diagnostics
  - • Rapid streptococcal test
  - • Throat culture for group A Streptococcus
- – Management: penicillin or amoxicillin

Molluscum Contagiosum
- – Microbiology: poxvirus
- – Signs and symptoms
  - • Waxy, skin -colored papules with central umbilication (Fig. 47-4)
  - • Tend to be grouped due to autoinoculation
  - • Widespread, large, hundreds of lesions indicative of impaired cellular immunity (human immunodeficiency virus)

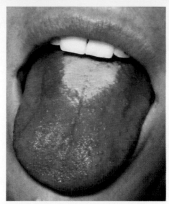

Figure 47-3: Strawberry tongue in a patient with scarlet fever. (Image courtesy of Martin Kronawitter; CC BY-SA 2.5 [https://creativecommons.org/licenses/by-sa/2.5])

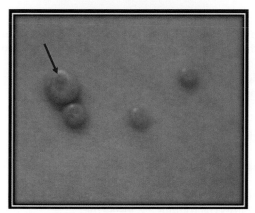

Figure 47-4: Skin lesion of molluscum contagiosum with characteristic central umbilication.

– Diagnostics: clinical
– Management: cryotherapy, curettage, cantharidin

Seborrheic Dermatitis
– Signs and symptoms
  • Erythematous, pruritic, greasy, yellowish scaly plaques involving the areas with multiple sebaceous glands (face, scalp, chest, trunk)
  • Dandruff occurring on the face, eyebrows, and nasolabial folds
  • Chronic cases seen in Langerhans cell histiocytosis
  • Cradle cap in infants
– Diagnostics: clinical
– Management
  • Antifungal shampoo (ketoconazole, ciclopirox, zinc pyrithione, selenium sulfide)
  • Topical corticosteroids for severe cases

Scabies
– Microbiology: Sarcoptes scabiei mite
– Transmission: direct person-to-person contact
– Signs and symptoms
  • Erythematous, pruritic (type IV hypersensitivity reaction to the scabies), burrows involving the web spaces between the fingers, toes, elbows, genitalia, and breasts
  • Excoriations, small pruritic vesicles
  • Highly contagious; likely other household contacts with similar symptoms
– Diagnostics: burrows scrapings (visualization of mites, ova, and feces under light microscopy)
– Management
  • Topical permethrin or oral ivermectin: first line
  • Lindane (however, typically avoided due to neurotoxicity)
  • Wash all clothing and linen used in the last 48–72 hours (mites can only live 2–3 days without a human host)
  • Treat the whole family

Norwegian (crusted) scabies: severe case scabies involving the entire body, associated with immunocompromise; treat with ivermectin.

ITCHY RASHES

Atopic Dermatitis
- Risk factors
  - Family history
  - Change in weather immunity
  - Irritant clothing
  - Environmental exposure
  - Immunodeficiency
- Pathophysiology: mutation of filaggrin gene, which is responsible for strengthening of epidermal cell layers and acts as a natural moisturizing factor
- Signs and symptoms
  - Erythema, pruritus
  - Lichenification (thickening of the epidermis secondary to chronic scratching)
  - Involving the flexor surfaces in adults and extensor surfaces in children
- Associations
  - AAA: atopy, asthma, allergies
  - Wiskott-Aldrich syndrome
- Diagnostics
  - Clinical
  - Elevated immunoglobulin E (IgE) levels
- Management
  - Emollients, moisturizing agents
  - Avoidance of triggers
  - Topical steroids; antihistamines
  - Topical calcineurin inhibitors (tacrolimus, cyclosporine)
  - Severe cases: systemic immunosuppressants, phototherapy
- Complications: secondary to chronic scratching and skin breakdown
  - Superimposed cellulitis: treat with topical mupirocin; oral antistaphylococcal/streptococcal for extensive disease
  - Eczema herpeticum: treat with oral herpes simplex virus antivirals (acyclovir, valacyclovir)

Contact Dermatitis
- Pathophysiology
  - Irritant-type contact dermatitis requires no previous exposure
  - Allergic-type contact dermatitis often requires previous exposure and sensitization; type IV hypersensitivity reaction
- Causes: prolonged and repetitive contact with irritant
  - Latex
  - Detergents, soaps
  - Poison ivy
  - Nickel, copper
  - Medications (neomycin, benzoyl peroxide)
- Signs and symptoms
  - Scaly, erythematous, pruritic
  - Well-demarcated rash involving area of contact (Fig. 47-5)
  - Vesicles, bullae
  - Chronically develop excoriations, hyperkeratosis, fissures, and lichenification
- Diagnostics
  - Clinical
  - Patch testing if etiology is unclear
- Management
  - Avoid offending agent
  - Emollients and other skin-hydrating agents
  - Topical steroids; antihistamines

Urticaria
- Pathophysiology: type I hypersensitivity IgE-mediated reaction resulting in mast cell degranulation of histamine and localized anaphylaxis

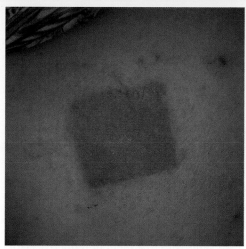

Figure 47-5: Well-demarcated rash in a patient who developed contact dermatitis from a buprenorphine drug patch.

- Causes
  - Drugs
    - Penicillins
    - Sulfa drugs
    - Nonsteroidal antiinflammatory drugs
    - Anticonvulsants
    - Narcotics, radiocontrast dye: both result in direct mast cell degranulation
  - Foods
    - Peanuts
    - Shellfish
  - Infections
    - Acute hepatitis B
    - Strongyloides
  - Insect bites/sting
  - Chronic urticaria triggered by pressure (dermatographism), cold, vibration
  - Systemic disorders (vasculitis, autoimmune, malignancy)
  - Systemic mastocytosis
  - Idiopathic
- Signs and symptoms
  - Prodromal/localized anaphylaxis
  - Sudden-onset wheal and flare reaction: well-circumscribed, erythematous plaques with central pallor
  - Severe pruritus
- Diagnostics: clinical
- Management
  - Epinephrine if there are signs of systemic anaphylaxis (respiratory compromise, hypotension)
  - Antihistamines
  - Oral glucocorticoids for severe unresponsive cases
  - Desensitization for unavoidable triggers

Pityriasis Rosea
- Signs and symptoms: in children, lesion distribution may appear atypical
  - Diffuse, symmetric erythematous pruritic, scaly eruption
  - Preceded by herald patch: oval, rose-colored plaque located on the trunk that resolves followed by multiple smaller lesions; resembles ringworm with central area of clearing
  - Christmas tree distribution on the back: follows cleavage lines on the trunk
  - Diagnostics: clinical
- Management: none, self-resolving

Ensure patient is not pregnant and on appropriate contraception before starting oral isotretinoin due to deleterious fetal side effects.

PIGMENTATION DISORDERS

Albinism
- Pathophysiology: deficiency/decreased function of tyrosinase enzyme preventing conversion of DOPA to melanin
- Signs and symptoms
  - Hypopigmented, chalky, white skin and hair
  - Rough, thickened skin in sun-exposed areas
  - Increased actinic keratoses and freckles
  - Blue/green irises, ocular sensitivity
  - Nystagmus, delayed/decreased visual acuity for age
- Associations
  - Chédiak-Higashi
  - Waardenburg syndrome
- Diagnostics: clinical
- Management
  - Sun protection
  - Periodic comprehensive eye exams with treatment of refractive errors
- Complications: increased risk of skin cancer (most commonly squamous cell carcinoma, increased risk of amelanotic melanoma)

Vitiligo
- Pathophysiology: autoimmune destruction of melanocytes
- Signs and symptoms
  - Patchy, well-demarcated, gradually progressive areas of hypopigmentation (milky, chalky white) (Fig. 47-6)
  - Nonpruritic, nonerythematous
  - Most commonly involves the face
- Associations: other autoimmune disorders (hypothyroidism, pernicious anemia, Addison disease)
- Diagnostics: clinical
- Management
  - Localized disease: topical steroids or calcineurin inhibitors depending on location
  - Extensive disease: oral corticosteroids +/− ultraviolet B phototherapy

---

Many genetic syndromes such as neurofibromatosis, McCune-Albright syndrome, tuberous sclerosis, Sturge-Weber, and others are associated with key dermatologic findings. These specific syndromes are discussed in other sections of the book.

Acne
- Causes
  - Propionibacterium acnes
  - Glucocorticoids
  - Hyperandrogenism
- Pathophysiology (Fig. 47-7)
  - Follicular hyperkeratinization
  - Excessive sebum production
  - Inflammation
  - *P. acnes* proliferation

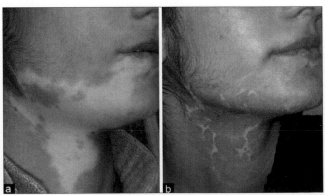

Figure 47-6: Patient with vitiligo of the neck. (Image courtesy of La Verdad; CC BY-SA 4.0 [https://creativecommons.org/licenses/by-sa/4.0])

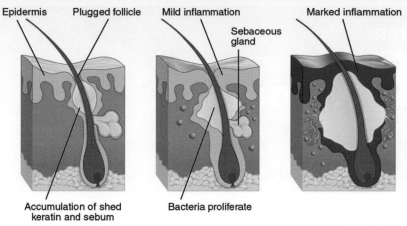

Figure 47-7: Diagrammatic representation of the pathophysiology of acne.

- Signs and symptoms: dependent on the type of acne
  - Inflammatory
    - Erythematous papules, pustules, and cysts
    - Involves the face, upper chest/arms, and back
  - Comedonal
    - Follicular occlusion secondary to hyperkeratosis
    - Blackheads and whiteheads
  - Nodulocystic
    - Large nodules
    - Cystic appearing with sinus tract formation and scarring
- Diagnostics: clinical
- Management: dependent on the type of acne and severity
  - Mild: benzoyl peroxide
    - +/− topical retinoids
    - +/− topical antibiotic (erythromycin, clindamycin)
    - +/− topical salicylates
  - Moderate: benzoyl peroxide + topical retinoids + oral antibiotics (tetracyclines)
  - Severe, unresponsive: oral isotretinoin
  - Alternatives: oral contraceptive pills, spironolactone

Each of the acne medications targets a particular aspect of the acne pathophysiology:
1) Follicular hyperkeratinization: oral/topical retinoids
2) Excessive sebum production: oral contraceptive pills, spironolactone
3) Inflammation: topical salicylates, topical/oral antibiotic
4) *Propionibacterium acnes* proliferation: topical/oral antibiotics

CHAPTER 48 Genetics

INBORN ERRORS OF METABOLISM
Amino Acid Metabolism Disorders

Phenylketonuria
- Pathophysiology: autosomal recessive deficiency of phenylalanine hydroxylase resulting in inability to convert phenylalanine to tyrosine and buildup of phenyl pyruvic acid
- Signs and symptoms: presents within days after birth
  • Intellectual disability
  • Seizures
  • Skin/hair/eyes hypopigmentation
  • Musty/mousy body odor
- Diagnostics
  • Elevated phenylalanine
  • Low tyrosine
  • Newborn screening tandem mass spectrometry
- Management
  • Phenylalanine dietary restriction
  • Avoid artificial sweetener (aspartame)
  • Tetrahydrobiopterin

Maple Syrup Urine Disease
- Pathophysiology: autosomal recessive disorder of impaired branched-chain amino acid metabolism
- Signs and symptoms
  • Feeding aversion, lethargy
  • Vomiting
  • Encephalopathy
  • Hypotonia
  • Sweet maple syrup odor in urine
  • Metabolic acidosis
- Diagnostics: elevated serum and urine branched-chain amino acids
- Management: avoid foods containing branched-chain amino acids

Homocystinuria
- Pathophysiology: cystathione synthase deficiency
- Signs and symptoms
  • Marfanoid habitus
  • Venous thromboembolism
  • Stroke, myocardial infarction
  • Intellectual disability
  • Osteoporosis
  • Downward lens subluxation
- Diagnostics
  • Elevated serum homocysteine
  • Elevated serum methionine
  • Genetic testing
- Management
  • Increased dietary cysteine
  • Methionine-restricted diet
  • Betaine therapy +/− B12 and folate

Alkaptonuria
- Pathophysiology: homogentisate oxidase deficiency resulting in accumulation of pigmented inducing homogentisic acid in tissues
- Signs and symptoms
  - Ochronosis (darkening of joints and connective tissue)
  - Pigmented sclera
  - Early arthritis
  - Early valvular disease
  - Nephrolithiasis
- Diagnostics: blackening of urine when exposed to air
- Management: supportive, no cure

Secondary causes of hyperhomocystinemia include vitamin B12 and folate deficiency.

Carbohydrate Metabolism Disorders
Galactosemia
- Pathophysiology: autosomal recessive deficiency of galactose-1-phosphate uridyltransferase
- Signs and symptoms: presents after initiation of breastfeeding
  - Feeding aversion
  - Vomiting
  - Failure to thrive
  - Liver failure, hypoglycemia
  - Jaundice, hepatomegaly
  - Cataracts
  - Renal failure
  - Increased risk of *Escherichia coli* sepsis
- Diagnostics
  - Absent red blood cell (RBC) galactose-1-phosphate uridyltransferase activity
  - Increased RBC galactose-1-phosphate
- Management
  - Avoid breastfeeding
  - Dietary restriction of lactose and galactose

Fructosuria: deficiency of fructokinase, with elevated urinary fructose; benign disease, no treatment.

Hereditary Fructose Intolerance
- Pathophysiology: aldolase B deficiency resulting in accumulation of fructose-1-phosphate
- Signs and symptoms: onset when attempting to wean from breastfeeding and initiation of formula feeding
  - Diarrhea, bloating
  - Abdominal pain, hepatomegaly
  - Irritability, lethargy
  - Feeding aversion
  - Vomiting
  - Seizures, encephalopathy
  - Frequent hypoglycemia
- Diagnostics
  - Magnetic resonance spectroscopy
  - Genetic testing
- Management
  - Avoid fructose-containing food
  - High-carbohydrate diet and frequent feeding

Glycogen storage disorders are a group of enzymatic deficiencies that result in impaired glycogenolysis. There are many subtypes; however, the four most commonly tested subtypes are included (Table 48.1).

Purine Metabolism Disorders
Lesch Nyhan Syndrome
- Pathophysiology: X-linked recessive mutation of hypoxanthine guanine phosphoribosyl transferase (HGPRT) enzyme → inability to metabolize purine → hyperuricemia

TABLE 48.1   Glycogen Storage Disease (Occurs Secondary to Impaired Glycogenolysis)

GLYCOGEN STORAGE DISEASE	PATHOPHYSIOLOGY	KEY FEATURES	MANAGEMENT
Von Gierke disease (type I)	• Glucose-6-phosphatase deficiency	• Fasting hypoglycemia • Hypertriglyceridemia • Hyperuricemia • Lactic acidosis • Short stature	• Frequent oral glucose
Pompe disease (type II)	• Acid maltase deficiency	• Cardiomyopathy within the first 2 mo of life • Macroglossia • Hypotonia • Glycogen accumulation in lysosomes	• Supportive management, no cure
Cory disease (type III)	• Alpha-1,6 glucosidase deficiency (debranching enzyme)	• Ketotic hypoglycemia with intact gluconeogenesis • Hepatomegaly • Hypotonia • Weakness • Glycogen with short outer chains	• Frequent oral glucose
McArdle disease	• Myophosphorylase deficiency	• Weakness • Myalgias • Myoglobinuria with exercise	• Supportive management

- Signs and symptoms
  - Intellectual disability
  - Self-mutilation
  - Dystonia, choreoathetosis
  - Gouty arthritis
  - Uric acid nephropathy
- Diagnostics
  - Hyperuricemia
  - HGPRT enzyme mutation
- Management: increased fluid intake plus allopurinol

Lysosomal Storage Diseases
Key principles
- Most have autosomal recessive inheritance except Fabry disease and Hunter syndrome, which are both X-linked recessive (Tables 48.2 and 48.3)
- Present within the first few months of life
- Diagnosed via genetic testing
- Treated with enzyme replacement

Gaucher Disease
- Epidemiology
  - Most common lysosomal storage disorder
  - Increased incidence in Ashkenazi Jews
- Pathophysiology: autosomal recessive glucocerebrosidase deficiency → accumulation of glucocerebroside → organ dysfunction
- Signs and symptoms
  - Hepatosplenomegaly
  - Osteoporosis, avascular necrosis of the hip
  - Erlenmeyer flask appearance of distal femur
  - Pancytopenia
  - No neurologic involvement (only lysosomal storage disorder that spares the brain)
- Diagnostics
  - Gaucher cells (lipid-laden macrophages with wrinkled tissue paper appearance)
  - Decreased glucocerebrosidase activity
  - Genetic testing
- Management: enzyme replacement

Fabry Disease
- Pathophysiology: X-linked recessive galactosidase deficiency → accumulation of ceramide trihexoside
- Signs and symptoms
  - Angiokeratoma (tiny maculopapular, nonblanching truncal lesions)
  - Acroparesthesias (burning sensation peripheral neuropathy)
  - Corneal dystrophy, cataracts

TABLE 48.2   Hurler Versus Hunter Syndrome

	HUNTER SYNDROME	HURLER SYNDROME
Inheritance	• X-linked recessive	• Autosomal recessive
Pathophysiology	• Iduronidase deficiency	• Idurontate deficiency
Clinical manifestations	• Corneal clouding • Coarse facial features • Macroglossia • Hepatosplenomegaly • MSK abnormalities (dystosis multiplex, contractures, joint stiffness) • Cardiomyopathy	• No corneal clouding
Diagnostics	• Elevated urine glycosaminoglycan	• Positive urine mucopolysaccharides
Management	• Enzyme replacement	

TABLE 48.3   Tay-Sachs Versus Niemann-Pick Disease

	TAY-SACHS	NIEMANN-PICK DISEASE
Pathophysiology	• Hexosaminidase A deficiency	• Sphingomyelinase deficiency
Risk factors	• Ashkenazi Jews	
Clinical manifestations	• No hepatosplenomegaly • Absent deep tendon reflexes (DTRs) • Cherry red macula (Fig. 48-1) • Blindness • Normal development during first few months followed by developmental delay and regression • Abnormal startle reflex • Seizures	• Hepatosplenomegaly • Increased DTRs
Diagnostics	• Elevated GM2 ganglioside • Lysosomes with onion skinning	• Elevated sphingomyelin • Lipid-laden macrophages (foam cells)
Management	• Supportive, no cure	

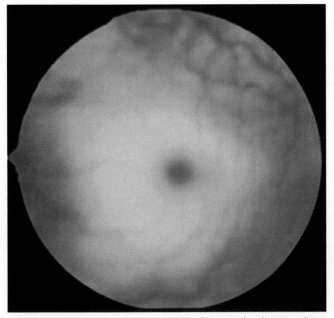

Figure 48-1: Cherry red macula seen in both Niemann-Pick and Tay-Sachs diseases. (Image courtesy of Jonathan Trobe, MD; CC BY 3.0 [https://creativecommons.org/licenses/by/3.0])

– Diagnostics: genetic testing
– Management: enzyme replacement
– Complications
  • Cardiomyopathy
  • Renal failure: most common cause of death

Krabbe Disease
- Pathophysiology: galactocerebrosidase deficiency → accumulation of galactocerebroside and psychosine
- Signs and symptoms
  - Developmental delay
  - Peripheral neuropathy
  - Hyperreflexia
  - Optic atrophy
- Diagnostics: decreased enzyme activity
- Management: supportive, no cure

GENETIC SYNDROMES
Trisomies
Trisomy 21
- Risk factors
  - Family history
  - Robertsonian translocation
  - Increased maternal age (>35 years old)
- Key manifestations
  - Neurologic
    - Intellectual disability
    - Early-onset Alzheimer disease
  - HEENT
    - Flat facies with hypertelorism
    - Slanted palpebral fissures
    - Brushfield spots (speckling of the iris)
    - Hearing loss
  - Cardiopulmonary
    - Endocardial cushion defects
    - Patent ductus arteriosus (PDA)
    - Mitral valve prolapse (MVP)
    - Obstructive sleep apnea
  - Gastrointestinal
    - Tracheoesophageal fistula
    - Omphalocele
    - Pyloric stenosis
    - Duodenal atresia
    - Hirschsprung disease
    - Celiac disease
  - Musculoskeletal
    - Atlantoaxial instability
    - Transverse palmar crease
    - Wide space between first and second toes
  - Hematology: acute lymphoblastic leukemia
  - Endocrinology: hypothyroidism
- Diagnostics
  - Clinical
  - Karyotyping (Fig. 48-2)
- Management
  - Supportive management
  - Genetic counseling
  - Prenatal screening
Trisomy 18
- Signs and symptoms
  - Neurologic
    - Intellectual disability
    - Neurogenic tumor
  - HEENT
    - Microcephaly
    - Low-set, malformed ears
    - Micrognathia
    - Prominent occiput

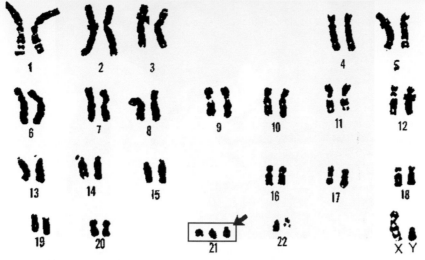

Figure 48-2: Karyotype in a patient with Down syndrome demonstrating three copies of chromosome 21 *(red arrow)*. (Image courtesy of U.S. Department of Energy Human Genome Program)

- Cardiopulmonary
  - Septal defect
  - PDA
- Gastrointestinal: omphalocele
- Musculoskeletal
  - Clubfoot (talipes equinovarus)
  - Rocker bottom feet
  - Clenched fists with overlapping fingers (Fig. 48-3)
  - Hammer toe
- Renal
  - Ectopic/double ureter
  - Polycystic kidneys
  - Wilms tumor
- Diagnostics
  - Clinical
  - Karyotyping (Fig. 48-4)
- Management: supportive, no cure; most patients die within the first year of life

Trisomy 13
- Signs and symptoms
  - Neurologic
    - Intellectual disability
    - Holoprosencephaly
    - Agenesis of the corpus callosum
  - HEENT
    - Microcephaly
    - Microphthalmia
    - Cutis aplasia
    - Cleft lip/palate
    - Cyclopia
    - Coloboma
  - Cardiopulmonary: septal defect
  - Gastrointestinal:
    - Omphalocele
    - Umbilical hernia
  - Musculoskeletal
    - Polydactyly
    - Rocker bottom feet
  - Hematology/oncology
    - Leukemia
    - Teratoma

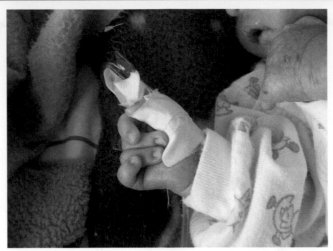

Figure 48-3: Characteristic clenched fist and overlapping third and fourth fingers in a patient with trisomy 18. (Image courtesy of Bobjgalindo; CC BY-SA 4.0 [https://creativecommons.org/licenses/by-sa/4.0])

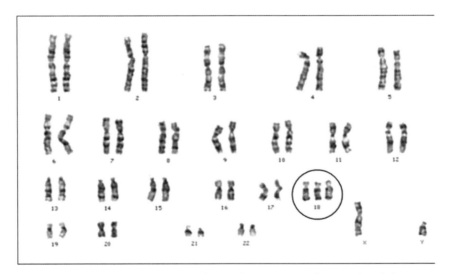

Figure 48-4: Karyotype in a patient with Edwards syndrome demonstrating three copies of chromosome 18 *(circled)*. (Image courtesy of Serra Amoros; CC BY-SA 4.0 [https://creativecommons.org/licenses/by-sa/4.0])

- Diagnostics
  - Clinical
  - Karyotype (Fig. 48-5)
- Management: supportive, no cure; most patients die within the first year of life

Trinucleotide Repeats
Principles
- Group of genetic disorders where patients have repeating trinucleotide sequences that result in coding of abnormal protein and thus abnormal genetic phenotype
- Diagnosed via genetic testing
- No cure, treatment is supportive care for associated complications
Fragile X
- Pathophysiology
  - CGG repeats
  - FMR1 gene mutation on X chromosome
- Signs and symptoms
  - Neurologic

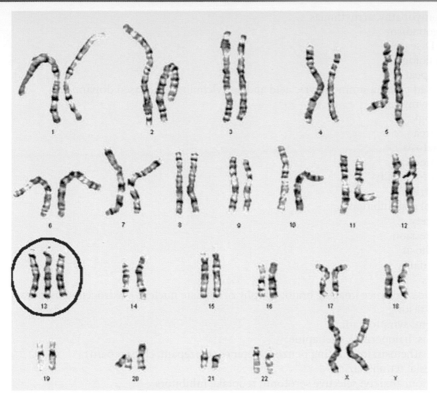

Figure 48-5: Karyotype in a patient with Patau syndrome demonstrating three copies of chromosome 13 *(circled)*. (Image courtesy of CarloDiDio; CC BY-SA 3.0 [https://creativecommons.org/licenses/by-sa/3.0])

- ▪ Intellectual disability: most common cause of disability in boys
- ▪ Attention-deficit/hyperactivity disorder
- ▪ Autism spectrum disorder
- • HEENT
  - ▪ Large ears
  - ▪ Macrocephaly
  - ▪ Prominent jaw
  - ▪ Protruding chin
  - ▪ Recurrent otitis media
- • Genitourinary
  - ▪ Macroorchidism
  - ▪ Premature ovarian failure

Frederick Ataxia
- – Pathophysiology
  - • GAA repeat
  - • Frataxin gene mutation
- – Signs and symptoms
  - • Neurologic
    - ▪ Spinocerebellar ataxia
    - ▪ Dysarthria
    - ▪ Frequent falls
  - • Cardiac: hypertrophic cardiomyopathy
  - • Endocrine: diabetes
  - • Musculoskeletal
    - ▪ Hammer toes
    - ▪ Scoliosis

Myotonic Dystrophy
- – Pathophysiology
  - • CTG repeats
  - • DMPK gene mutation
- – Signs and symptoms
  - • Progressive muscle weakness/atrophy
  - • Cataract

- Cardiomyopathy, arrhythmias
- Hypogonadism

Huntington Disease
- Pathophysiology
  - CAG repeat
  - Decreased gamma-aminobutyric acid and acetylcholine; increased dopamine
- Signs and symptoms
  - Neurologic
    - Chorea
    - Athetosis
    - Dementia
    - Gait instability
  - Psychiatric
    - Social disinhibition
    - Anxiety
    - Depression
    - Psychosis
    - Suicidality
- Diagnostics
  - Magnetic resonance imaging brain: atrophy of caudate nucleus (hydrocephalus ex vacuo)
  - Genetic testing
- Management: symptomatic
  - Psychosis: haloperidol, quetiapine
  - Chorea, athetosis: long-acting benzodiazepines (diazepam, clonazepam)
  - Dyskinesia: tetrabenazine
  - Depression, anxiety: selective serotonin reuptake inhibitors

Anticipation in Huntington disease results in earlier disease presentation in each generation as trinucleotide repeats grow in length.

ANEUPLOIDIES

Klinefelter Syndrome
- Key manifestations
  - Neuropsychiatric
    - Learning disabilities
    - Behavioral disorders
    - Depression
  - Musculoskeletal
    - Slipped capital femoral epiphysis
    - Slim physique with long limbs
  - Gynecologic
    - Breast cancer
    - Gynecomastia
    - Gynecoid appearance
    - Infertility
    - Hypogonadism
  - Cardiac: mitral valve prolapse
- Diagnostics
  - Clinical
  - Karyotyping: XXY (male phenotype)

Turner Syndrome
- Key manifestations
  - Cardiac
    - Bicuspid aortic valve
    - Coarctation of the aorta
  - Reproductive
    - Streak ovaries
    - Lack of secondary female sex characteristics
  - Musculoskeletal
    - Short stature
    - Webbed neck

- • Broad chest with widely spaced nipples
- • Cubitus valgus
- • Endocrine: hypothyroidism
- • Renal
  - • Horseshoe kidney
  - • Double renal pelvis
- – Diagnostics
  - • Clinical
  - • Karyotyping: XO (female phenotype)

Collagen Vascular Disease

Ehlers-Danlos and Marfan syndromes are two collagen-vascular disorders that result in defective collagen synthesis and fibrillin, respectively. As a result there is laxity in various organs and vascular structures (Table 48.4).

Imprinting

Key principles
- • Genomic imprinting occurs when gene on paternal or maternal chromosome is inappropriately silenced (Table 48.5)
- • Uniparental disomy occurs when both normally silenced genes are inherited from the same parent
- • Diagnosed with karyotyping, fluorescence in situ hybridization (FISH) studies, microarrays, or methylation studies

TABLE 48.4 Ehlers-Danlos Syndrome Versus Marfan Syndrome

	EHLERS-DANLOS SYNDROME	MARFAN SYNDROME
Pathophysiology	• Collagen synthesis gene mutation (specific collagen type characterizes clinical manifestations and Ehlers-Danlos syndrome subtype)	• Fibrillin-1 gene mutation
Signs and symptoms	• Rheumatologic: hypermobile joints, kyphoscoliosis • Cardiac: mitral valve prolapse (MVP), valvular regurgitation, aortic aneurysm/dissection • Neurologic: cerebral aneurysm, subarachnoid hemorrhage	• Musculoskeletal: decreased upper limbs to lower limb length ratio, arachnodactyly, pectus deformity • Cardiac: MVP, aortic aneurysm/dissection (cystic medial necrosis) • Ocular: ectopia lentis (downward displaced lens) • Pulmonary: emphysematous bullae, spontaneous pneumothorax • Neurologic: dural ectasia
Diagnostics	• Clinical +/− genetic testing	
Treatment	• No treatment • Screening and management of complications as they occur	

TABLE 48.5 Imprinting Syndrome

GENETIC SYNDROME	PATHOPHYSIOLOGY	CLINICAL MANIFESTATIONS
Angelman syndrome	Maternal imprinting on chromosome 15 Paternal uniparental disomy	Intellectual disability, Random, inappropriate laughter, Hand flapping, Developmental delay, Gait abnormalities ("puppet like"), Seizures
Prader-Willi syndrome	Paternal imprinting on chromosome 15 Maternal uniparental disomy	Poor suckling, feeding difficulties in infants, Hypotonia, Later develop hyperphagia, obesity, Hypogonadism, Almond-shaped eyes, downward sloping mouth
Beckwith-Wiedemann syndrome	Gene imprinting on chromosome 11	Rapid growth, macrosomia, Hemihypertrophy, Macroglossia, Omphalocele, Umbilical hernia, Increased risk of Wilms tumor (periodic screening with abdominal ultrasound)

Chromosomal Deletion

Chromosomal deletions result in unique syndromes with characteristic clinical manifestations, some of which are described in Table 48.6.

Other Inherited Disorders

There is a group of inherited disorders that does not fit in any particular category but has unique clinical characteristics or inheritance patterns (Table 48.7).

TABLE 48.6   Chromosome Deletions

GENETIC SYNDROME	PATHOPHYSIOLOGY	CLINICAL MANIFESTATIONS
DiGeorge syndrome	• Microdeletion on chromosome 22 • Abnormal development of the third and fourth pharyngeal pouch	• Cardiac: tetralogy of Fallot, truncus arteriosus, transposition of the great vessels • Abnormal facies: hypertelorism, micrognathia • Thymic hypoplasia: recurrent fungal and viral infection • Cleft lip/palate • Hypocalcemia (parathyroid hypoplasia)
Williams syndrome	• Microdeletion on chromosome 7 • Elastin gene mutation	• "Elfin faces" • Extremely friendly, social • Supravalvular aortic stenosis • Hyperacusis
Cri du chat syndrome	• Microdeletion on chromosome 5	• High-pitched, cat-like cry • Epicanthal folds, hypertelorism • Intellectual disability • Hyperacusis

Chromosomal microdeletions cannot be diagnosed on karyotype studies, and instead require fluorescence in situ hybridization studies for diagnosis.

TABLE 48.7   Other Inherited Disorders

GENETIC SYNDROME	PATHOPHYSIOLOGY	KEY FEATURES
Noonan syndrome	• RAS/MAPK gene mutation	• Similar to Turner syndrome: webbed neck, peripheral edema, hypoplastic nails • Pulmonic valve stenosis • Craniofacial abnormalities: hypertelorism, downward splinting palpebral fissures
CHARGE syndrome	• Spontaneous mutation	• Coloboma (iris defect) • Heart defects • Choanal atresia • Growth/development retardation • Genitourinary abnormalities • Ear abnormalities
Cornelia de Lange syndrome	• NIPBL, SMC1A, SMC3 gene mutations • Most commonly sporadic mutation	• Single, arched eyebrow • Long eyelashes • Upturned nose • Hypotrichosis • Other gastrointestinal (GI), genitourinary, and neurologic manifestations
Rett syndrome	• MECP2 gene mutation	• X-linked dominant primarily affects females; males die in utero • Normal development followed by regression at 6–12 mo • Flapping tremor
McCune-Albright syndrome	• G-protein cAMP kinase mutation	• Polyostotic fibrous dysplasia • Café au lait spot, "coast of Maine" spots • Endocrinopathies • Precocious puberty
Achondroplasia	• Fibroblast growth factor receptor mutation	• Dwarfism: most common cause • Associated with increased paternal age • Short limbs with relatively longer trunk • Large head, frontal bossing
Mitochondrial myopathies	• Group of maternally inherited mitochondrial disorders affecting all children of affected mother	• Progressive muscle weakness • Lactic acidosis • Myoclonic epilepsy • Strokelike episodes • Optic neuropathy • Encephalopathy
Hereditary hemorrhagic telangiectasia (Osler-Weber-Rendu)	• Abnormally formed blood vessels in skin and mucous membranes	• Bleeding • Arteriovenous malformation: pulmonary, GI • Telangiectasia

CHAPTER 49 Behavioral Disorders

Enuresis
- Definition
  - Continued urinary continence beyond expected age of development
  - >4 years old for daytime incontinence
  - >5 years old for nocturnal incontinence
- Risk factors
  - Males
  - Family history
  - Psychosocial stressors (abuse, birth of a new sibling, starting school, family death)
  - Constipation (large stool burden compresses and irritates the bladder)
  - Diabetes insipidus/mellitus
  - Seizures
  - Obstructive sleep apnea
- Diagnostics: workup organic and psychosocial etiology
  - Thorough health and physical: stressors, family history, neurologic exam
  - Urinalysis
- Management
  - Treat underlying secondary causes
  - Nonpharmacologic
    - Reassurance if patient is still younger than age expected for continence
    - Nighttime enuresis alarm: first line
    - Motivational and reward system
    - Limits nighttime fluid intake
    - Voiding before bedtime
    - Bladder training (timed avoiding)
  - Pharmacologic: only short-term use
    - DDAVP (decreases urine volume)
    - Tricyclic antidepressants

Encopresis
- Definition: fecal incontinence after >4 years old
- Risk factors
  - Chronic constipation (overflow incontinence, retentive encopresis)
  - Psychosocial stressors
  - Intellectual disability
  - Hirschsprung disease
  - Spinal cord abnormalities
- Diagnostics
  - Digital rectal exam
  - Abdominal x-ray
- Management
  - Nonretentive: positive reinforcement, behavioral intervention
  - Retentive
    - Positive reinforcement, behavioral intervention
    - Stool softeners
    - Disimpaction

Nightmares and night terrors have similar presentations; however, they are differentiated based on patient recollection of the events the next morning as they occur in different stages of sleep (Table 49.1).

TABLE 49.1   Nightmares Versus Night Terrors

	NIGHTMARES	NIGHT TERRORS
Signs and symptoms	• Frightening dream • Nighttime arousal • Vivid recall of events	• Nighttime arousal with sudden screaming and shaking • No recall of events
Stage of sleep	• Rapid eye movement	• Slow wave sleep (stage IV)
Diagnostics	• Clinical	
Treatment	• No treatment, self-resolves	• No treatment, self-resolves • Safety precautions

Breath-Holding Spells
- Epidemiology: 6 months to 2 years
- Signs and symptoms
  • Cyanotic subtype
    ▪ Child purposely stops breathing when frustrated or angry
    ▪ Cyanosis
    ▪ Loss of consciousness followed by rapid regain of consciousness and return to baseline
  • Pallid subtype
    ▪ Breath holding associated with minor trauma or frightening event
    ▪ Diaphoresis, pallor
    ▪ Loss of consciousness followed by rapid regain consciousness and return to baseline
- Diagnostics
  • Clinical
  • Rule out cardiac (arrhythmias) or neurologic (seizures)
- Management: no treatment necessary, self resolves by age 8
Pica
- Abnormal urge to ingest nonnutritive substances (sand, dirt, ice)
- Associated with iron deficiency anemia and intellectual disability
- Increased risk of lead poisoning and parasitic infection
Rumination
- Continuous regurgitation and reswallowing food
- Associated with intellectual disability, institutionalization, and psychosocial stressors
- Manage through behavior modification and reinforcing proper eating habits

Attention-deficit/hyperactivity disorder differential diagnosis:
• Absence seizures
• Lead poisoning
• Oppositional defiant disorder
• Depression

Attention-Deficit/Hyperactivity Disorder (ADHD)
- Risk factors
  • Males
  • Family history
  • Preterm birth
- Signs and symptoms
  • Difficulty focusing
  • Impulsivity
  • Hyperactivity
  • Easily distracting
  • Inattentiveness
- Diagnostic criteria
  • Symptoms not explained by other causes
  • Symptomatology onset <12 years old
  • Symptomatology in more than one setting
  • Symptomatology resulting in impaired functioning
- Management
  • Preschool: behavioral modification

- School age: pharmacologic
  - Stimulant medications: first line
    - Methylphenidate
    - Dexamphetamine
  - Nonstimulant medications
  - Atomoxetine
  - Alpha-adrenergic (clonidine, guanfacine)

Side effects of stimulant medications: decreased appetite, weight loss, insomnia, hypertension, tachycardia, decreased growth velocity, and transient tics

Tourette Syndrome
- Definition: anxiety disorder characterized by involuntary motor and vocal tics
- Signs and symptoms
  - Involuntary motor tics
    - Head shaking
    - Eye blinking
    - Jumping, kicking
  - Involuntary vocal tics
    - Throat clearing
    - Coughing
    - Echolalia (repetition of words or phrases)
    - Coprolalia (repetitive use of foul language)
- Diagnostic criteria
  - Symptomatology not explained by another disorder
  - Two or more motor tics
  - One or more vocal tics
  - Tics lasting >1-year duration
  - Tics occurring <18 years old
- Associations
  - ADHD
  - Obsessive-compulsive disorder
- Management
  - Mild: no treatment
  - Moderate to severe
    - Habitat reversal training
    - Tetrabenazine
    - Botulinum toxin
    - Alpha-adrenergic agents (clonidine, guanfacine)

Child Abuse
- Risk factors
  - Maternal/child intellectual disability
  - Young maternal age
  - Caregiver history of abuse
  - Lower socioeconomic status
  - Spousal abuse
  - Substance abuse
  - Single parent
  - Preterm, low birthweight infants
- Signs and symptoms
  - Psychological
    - Failure to thrive
    - Parental neglect
  - Neurologic
    - Retinal hemorrhages
    - Subdural hematoma
  - Bruises
    - Bruises in patterns of objects (cigarettes, iron)
    - Bruises in unusual locations (abdomen, back)
  - Burns
    - Immersion burns
    - Gloves stocking pattern
    - Bathtubs dipping (sparing of flexor increases as child with the legs to avoid burns)
    - Lack of splash burns
  - Fractures
    - Long bone fractures in nonambulating child
    - Spiral fracture (Fig. 50-1)
    - Posterior rib fractures (Fig. 50-2)
  - Other features
    - Delayed presentation after injury
    - Vague history
    - Sexually transmitted disease
- Diagnostics
  - Thorough history and physical exam
  - Skeletal survey
  - Head computed tomography/magnetic resonance imaging
  - Ophthalmologic exam
  - Other laboratory and imaging based on history and physical exam
- Management
  - Admit child to hospital and treat injuries
  - Report to Child Protective Services

Sudden Infant Death Syndrome

If patient survives a sudden infant death syndrome–like event, then it is classified as apparent life-threatening event or brief resolved unexplained event.

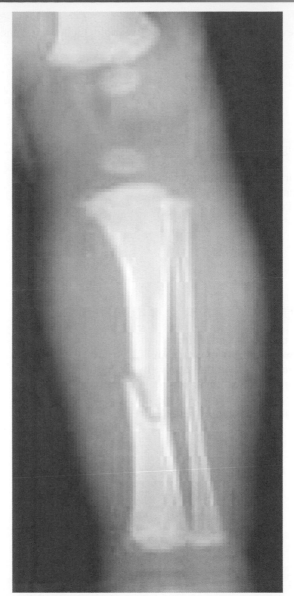

Figure 50-1: Spiral fracture consistent with child abuse. (Image courtesy of National Institute of Health.)

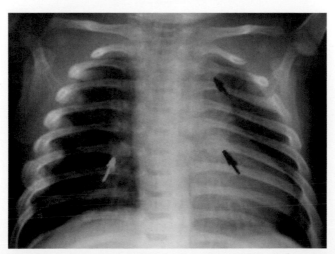

Figure 50-2: Multiple, healing right (green arrow) and left (red arrows) posterior rib fractures in a victim of child abuse. (Image courtesy of National Institute of Health.)

- Definition: sudden unexplained death in a child <1 year old; highest incidence at 2–6 months of age
- Risk factors
  - Prone sleeping
  - Maternal smoking
  - Soft bedding
  - Heating
  - Prematurity
  - Family history
  - Lack of breastfeeding
- Diagnostics
  - Unremarkable history and physical examination
  - Normal labs and imaging
  - Diagnosis of exclusion
- Prevention
  - Supine sleeping
  - Use of pacifier
  - Breastfeeding
  - Avoid overheating
  - Avoid smoking
  - Avoid sleeping with parent

Growing Pains
- Benign condition seen in school-aged children
- Deep, achy bilateral lower extremity muscle pain
- Symptoms most common in the evening, resolve by the morning
- Normal physical examination and activity level
- Not related to growth
- Supportive management, provide family reassurance

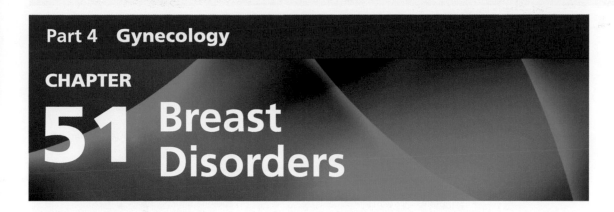

CHAPTER 51 Breast Disorders

BENIGN BREAST MASSES

Breast mass principles
- Common among women especially reproductive age; increased risk of malignancy after 40 years old
- Most have little to no malignant potential and can therefore be observed after one to two menstrual cycles
- If further evaluation is needed, a fine-needle aspiration, core needle biopsy, ultrasound, or mammogram can be performed (Table 51-1)
- Ultrasound is preferred for younger women with suspected cystic masses
- Fine-needle aspiration or core needle biopsy for solid palpable masses
- Mammography for older women (>40 years old), bloody nipple discharge, recurrent cyst after aspiration, concurrent lymphadenopathy, or overlying skin changes

Gynecomastia
- Definition: enlargement of breast glandular tissue
- Pathophysiology: hyperestrinism or hypotestosteronism
- Causes
  - Hyperestrinism
    - Spironolactone, cimetidine
    - Cirrhosis
    - Hyperthyroidism
    - Testicular/adrenal tumors
  - Hypotestosteronism
    - Hypogonadism (Klinefelter syndrome, testicular atrophy, orchiectomy)
    - Hyperprolactinemia
- Signs and symptoms
  - Enlarged breast tissue, single or bilateral
  - +/− tenderness to touch
  - No nipple discharge
- Diagnostics: workup for causes of hyperestrinism and hypotestosteronism
- Management
  - Treat underlying etiology
  - Reassurance for physiologic causes of gynecomastia (i.e., hyperestrinism in neonatal males or pubertal boys)

Self and clinical breast exams are no longer recommended.
Breast cancer commonly metastasizes to the bone, brain, and liver.
Axillary lymph node dissection complications include chronic lymphedema, upper extremity pain, recurrent fungal and bacterial cellulitis.

BREAST CANCER

Breast Cancer
- Epidemiology
  - Most common cancer in women, second most common cause of cancer mortality
  - One of eight women will be affected by breast cancer
- Risk factors
  - Family history with first-degree relative
  - *BRCA1* mutation
  - Age >50 years
  - Ionizing radiation

TABLE 51-1   Differential Diagnosis of Breast Masses

BREAST MASS	KEY FEATURES	MANAGEMENT
Fibroadenoma	• Rubbery, mobile, well demarcated • Premenstrual tenderness • Nonadherent to chest wall	• No treatment • Optional excision
Intraductal papilloma	• Unilateral, serosanguineous bloody nipple discharge	• Core needle biopsy +/− surgical excision
Phyllodes tumor	• Type of low-grade sarcoma • Rapidly growing • Leaflike projections on histology	• Core needle biopsy followed by surgical excision
Fibrocystic change	• Cyclic bilateral breast tenderness • Diffusely nodular breast • Symptoms vary with menstrual cycle	• Symptomatic management: oral contraceptive pills, nonsteroidal antiinflammatory drugs, danazol, tamoxifen

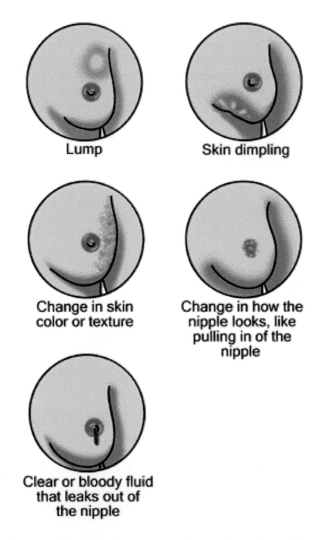

Lump

Skin dimpling

Change in skin color or texture

Change in how the nipple looks, like pulling in of the nipple

Clear or bloody fluid that leaks out of the nipple

Figure 51-1: Illustrations demonstrating the various presentations and early signs of breast cancer. (Image courtesy of National Institutes of Health.)

- • Alcoholism
  • Nulliparity
  • Obesity
  • Hormone replacement therapy
- – Signs and symptoms (Fig. 51-1)
  • Irregular, palpable breast mass
  • Bloody nipple discharge

- Overlying erythema
- Skin, nipple retraction
- "Orange peel" skin
- Axillary lymphadenopathy
  - Diagnostics
    - Mammography
      - Irregular spiculated mass with microcalcifications
      - Asymmetric densities
      - Architectural distortion
    - Breast magnetic resonance imaging or tomosynthesis: indicated for high-risk patients; denser breasts unable to be evaluated by mammography
    - Sentinel lymph node biopsy: positive lymph nodes indicate axillary lymph node involvement requiring axillary lymph node dissection
    - Staging computed tomography abdomen and pelvis
    - Receptor testing: estrogen, progesterone, HER2
  - Management
    - Localized disease
      - Without lymph node involvement: lumpectomy plus axillary radiation
      - With lymph node involvement: lumpectomy plus axillary lymph node dissection
    - Metastatic disease
      - Chemoradiation
      - Hormonal therapy depending on receptor positivity (Table 51-2)
  - Screening: mammography at starting at age 50, every 2 years until 74 years old (US Preventive Services Task Force recommendations)

Breast cancer may present with unique characteristics that should increase the clinical suspicion for a particular subtype (Table 51-3).

INFECTIONS
Mastitis
- Microbiology: Staphylococcus aureus
- Signs and symptoms
  - Unilateral breast erythema/tenderness
  - Fevers, chills
  - +/− fluctuance (indicative of breast abscess)

TABLE 51-2   Hormonal Therapy: Used to Treat Breast Cancer That Is Estrogen, Progesterone, or HER2/Neu Positive

THERAPY	INDICATIONS	MECHANISM OF ACTION	ADVERSE EFFECTS
Tamoxifen	• Estrogen receptor–positive cancer in premenopausal women	• Estrogen receptor antagonist in the breast • Estrogen receptor agonist in the uterus	• Venous thromboembolism • Endometrial hyperplasia/cancer • Hot flashes
Anastrozole	• Estrogen receptor–positive cancer in postmenopausal women	• Aromatase inhibitor	• Osteoporosis • Muscle aches and pains
Trastuzumab	• HER2 receptor–positive cancer	• Monoclonal antibody against HER2	• Reversible cardiomyopathy

TABLE 51-3   Key Features of Breast Cancer Subtypes

BREAST CANCER SUBTYPES	KEY FEATURES
Ductal carcinoma	• Most common breast cancer subtype
Lobular carcinoma	• Associated with contralateral breast cancer
Paget disease of the breast	• Eczematous, scaling dermatitis involving the nipple • Variant of ductal carcinoma
Inflammatory breast cancer	• Overlying erythema/edema with associated lymphadenopathy • Poor prognosis, commonly metastatic upon presentation • Cancer invading dermal lymphatics

- Diagnostics: clinical
- Management
  - Antistaphylococcal antibiotics (dicloxacillin, nafcillin)
  - Continued breastfeeding from affected breast to aid in drainage
- Complications: breast abscess (treat with I&D plus antibiotics)

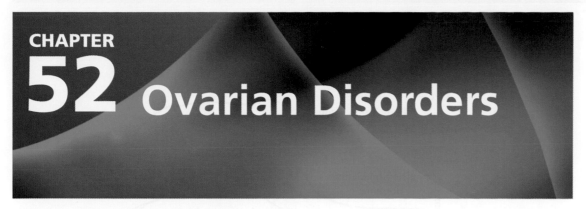

CHAPTER 52 Ovarian Disorders

ANOVULATION AND AMENORRHEA

Basics of amenorrhea
- Divided into primary and secondary amenorrhea
- Primary amenorrhea defined as lack of menses by age 15 years with normal growth and development of secondary sexual characteristics
- Secondary amenorrhea defined as absence of menstruation for 3 months in women who previously had normal cycles or >6 months in women with previously irregular cycles (Fig. 52-1)
- Causes related to abnormal anatomy, hormonal, or hypothalamic-pituitary dysfunction

Anatomic Related

Imperforate Hymen
- Cyclic abdominal pain, uterus, hematocolpos, hematometra
- Clinical diagnosis via visual inspection (bluish bulge on vaginal exam)
- Treatment is surgical excision and evacuation of obstructed blood products

Transverse Vaginal Septum
- Primary amenorrhea with cyclic abdominal pain
- Normal external female genitalia
- Shortened vagina that ends in a blind pouch
- Differentiated from imperforate hymen by presence of hymenal ring below vaginal septum
- Treatment is surgical correction

Vaginal Agenesis (Mullerian Agensis)
- Absence of the mullerian ductal system (vagina, cervix, uterus, fallopian tubes)
- Normal ovaries
- 46XX karyotype
- Associated with other genitourinary abnormalities (renal agenesis, bladder exstrophy, inguinal hernias)
- Surgical correction to restore vaginal patency for the purpose of sexual activity

Asherman Syndrome
- Intrauterine adhesions or synechia secondary to recurrent dilatation and curettages or infections
- Denudement of endometrial surface, increased risk of placenta accreta
- Secondary amenorrhea, dysmenorrhea, cyclic abdominal pain
- Diagnosis and treatment via hysteroscopy with lysis of adhesions

Cervical Stenosis
- May occur secondary to recurrent cervicitis or procedure (conization, loop electrosurgical excision procedure)
- Most commonly asymptomatic
- Secondary amenorrhea, dysmenorrhea
- Crampy abdominal pain relieved by increased menstrual flow
- Treatment is gradual dilation or excision over the external os

Hormonal Related

Androgen Insensitivity Syndrome
- End-organ resistance to testosterone secondary to mutated androgen receptor
- 46XY karyotype: secretion of antimullerian hormone and testosterone results in regression of mullerian structures (vagina, cervix, uterus, fallopian tubes)
- Lack of masculine features due to androgen insensitivity
- Breast development due to peripheral aromatization of testosterone

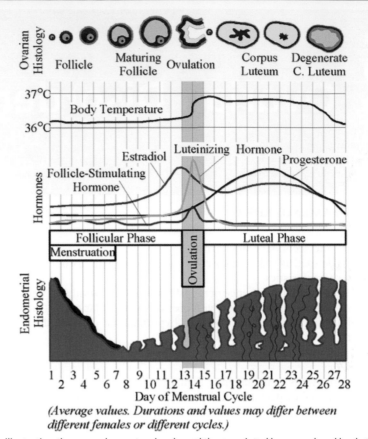

Figure 52-1: Diagram illustrating the normal menstrual cycle and the associated hormonal and body temperature changes. (Image courtesy of Chris 73/Wikimedia Commons; CC BY-SA 3.0 [https://creativecommons.org/licenses/by-sa/3.0])

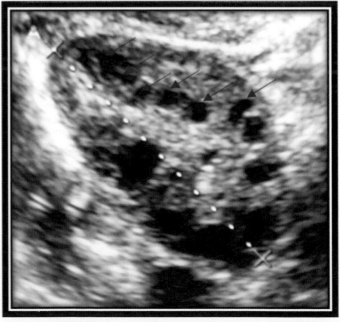

Figure 52-2: Gray scale ultrasound demonstrating polycystic ovaries in a patient with polycystic ovarian syndrome. Red arrows point to multiple ovarian follices. Calipers (dotted white line) demonstrating measurement of enlarged ovary.

Polycystic Ovarian Syndrome
 – Signs and symptoms
   • Hyperandrogenism (hirsutism, acne, male pattern baldness)
   • Ovulatory dysfunction (anovulation, irregular menses)
   • Polycystic ovaries on ultrasound (Fig. 52-2)

- Diagnostics
  - Clinical: two of three previously mentioned signs and symptoms
  - Supporting features
    - Elevated luteinizing hormone (LH) to follicle-stimulating hormone (FSH) ratio
    - Elevated testosterone
    - Acanthosis nigricans
    - Endometrial hyperplasia/cancer
- Management
  - Weight loss: first line
  - Insulin resistance, diabetes: metformin
  - Infertility: clomiphene citrate (ovulation-induction agent)
  - Menstrual irregularities: oral contraceptive pills

Amenorrhea, anovulation, and other menstrual irregularities caused by hypothyroidism or prolactinoma are managed by treating the underlying condition.

HYPOTHALAMIC-PITUITARY-OVARIAN AXIS RELATED

Abnormalities of the hypothalamic-pituitary-ovarian axis results in loss of feedback inhibition or lack of stimulation, which results in elevation or decreased hormonal levels depending on the level of abnormality (Fig. 52-3).

Premature Ovarian Failure
- Definition: menopause prior to 40 years old
- Causes
  - Autoimmune disorder
  - Fragile X
  - Turner syndrome
  - Chemotherapy

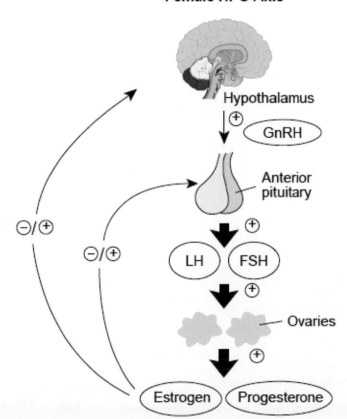

Figure 52-3: Normal hypothalamic-pituitary-gonadal *(HPG)* axis in females. *FSH,* Follicle-stimulating hormone; *GnRH,* gonadotropin-releasing hormone; *LH,* luteinizing hormone. (Image courtesy of Lu Kong, Ting Zhang, Meng Tang and Dayong Wang; CC BY 4.0 [https://creativecommons.org/licenses/by/4.0])

- Signs and symptoms: related to estrogen deficiency
  - Lack of breast development and secondary female sex characteristics
  - Increased risk of osteoporosis
  - Infertility
- Management: estrogen/progesterone placement

Turner Syndrome
- Pathophysiology: streak ovaries → hypoestrogenism → lack of secondary female sexual characteristics
- Key features
  - Cardiac
    - Bicuspid aortic valve
    - Coarctation of the aorta
  - Musculoskeletal
    - Short stature
    - Webbed neck
    - Broad chest with widely spaced nipples
    - Cubitus valgus
  - Renal
    - Horseshoe kidney
    - Double renal pelvis
- Diagnostics
  - Clinical
  - Karyotyping: XO (female phenotype)

Kallmann Syndrome
- Pathophysiology: hypothalamic hypogonadism → gonadotropin-releasing hormone (GnRH) deficiency → decreased FSH and LH
- Signs and symptoms
  - Delayed secondary sexual characteristics
  - Decreased testicular volume
  - Absent breast development
  - Lack of pubic and axillary hair
  - Anovulation
  - Decreased libido
- Other related features
  - Anosmia (involvement of olfactory bulb)
  - Renal agenesis, adrenocortical insufficiency
  - Congenital heart defects
- Management: GnRH replacement

First step when evaluating patients with primary or secondary amenorrhea is a urine pregnancy test.

Hypopituitarism
- Destruction of the pituitary gland secondary to infection, infiltration, infarction, mass effect
- Presents with hypogonadotropism (amenorrhea, decreased libido, infertility)
- Other symptoms related to anterior pituitary hormone deficiencies
  - Hypocortisolism
    - Orthostatic hypotension, tachycardia
    - Hypoglycemia
    - Eosinophilia
  - Hypothyroidism
    - Bradycardia
    - Hypothermia
  - Hyposomatotropism
    - Decreased muscle mass
    - Increased low-density lipoprotein
  - Hypoprolactinemia
    - Failure to lactate
- Diagnosed by hormonal testing
- Treat with hormone replacement

Anorexia Nervosa
- Psychiatric condition characterized by body image disturbance, food aversion, and severe malnutrition

- Signs and symptoms
  - Hypothalamic hypogonadism (inability to produce GnRH)
  - Lanugo
  - Emaciation
- Management includes hospitalization, psychotherapy, and replenishment of nutritional stores
- Important to slowly replenish nutritional stores due to risk of refeeding syndrome

> Refeeding syndrome: replenishment of carbohydrates switches body from catabolic to anabolic state → hyperinsulinemia → increased glucose uptake by cells → increased adenosine triphosphate (ATP) production → rapid uptake of extracellular potassium to keep up with ATP production → hypophosphatemia → cardiopulmonary failure

BENIGN OVARIAN MASSES

Physiologic Cysts
- Associated with normal menstrual cycle, thought to represent exaggeration of normal physiologic response
- Subtypes
  - Theca lutein cysts
    - Stimulated by beta-human chorionic gonadotropin (beta-hCG) and FSH
    - Associated with twin and molar pregnancy
    - Occur in multiples and bilateral
  - Follicular cysts: failure of follicle to rupture during the follicular maturation phase of the menstrual cycle
  - Corpus luteum cyst: failure of corpus luteum to involute at the end of luteal phase
- Signs and symptoms
  - Asymptomatic: most common
  - Tender, unilateral adnexal mass
- Diagnostics: transvaginal ultrasound
- Management
  - Asymptomatic, <7 cm: no further management; most cases will resolve spontaneously
  - Asymptomatic, >7 cm: laparoscopic removal due to increased risk of ovarian torsion
- Complications
  - Hemoperitoneum
    - Secondary to ruptured ovarian cyst
    - Sudden onset, unilateral lower abdominal pain
    - Shoulder pain (phrenic nerve irritation) cyst
    - Pleuritic chest pain
  - Ovarian torsion
    - Pathophysiology: twisting of the ovaries around its supporting structures (suspensory ligament of the ovary) obstructing blood supply to the ovary
    - Signs and symptoms
      - Intermittent, sudden onset, unilateral lower abdominal pain
      - Palpable adnexal mass
      - Nausea, vomiting
      - +/− guarding, rebound tenderness
    - Diagnostics: decreased/absent flow on Doppler
    - Management
      - If ovary remains viable: laparoscopic detorsioning and cystectomy
      - If ovary necrotic: laparoscopic oophorectomy

Teratoma (Dermoid Cyst)
- Definition: benign tumors containing tissue from cells of all three germ layers
- Signs and symptoms
  - Abdominal fullness
  - Palpable adnexal mass
- Diagnostics
  - Transvaginal ultrasound: cystic, complex, calcified mass
  - Histology: multiple germ cell layers
- Management: laparoscopic cystectomy

- Complications
  - Chemical peritonitis: spillage of cyst contents during removal
  - Struma ovarii: hyperthyroidism secondary to ectopic thyroid tissue within the teratoma
  - Malignant transformation: increased risk with immature teratoma

OVARIAN CANCER

Ovarian cancer principles
- Most common cause of gynecologic associated death
- Subdivided into epithelial, germ cell, and stromal tumors
- Epithelial ovarian tumors account for the vast majority of ovarian cancer
- Often diagnosed at advanced stage due to lack of specific signs or symptoms

EPITHELIAL TUMORS

Epithelial Ovarian Cancer
- Epidemiology
  - Accounts for majority of ovarian cancer
  - Seen in postmenopausal women
  - Most common subtype is serous
- Risk factors
  - Increased number of ovulations
    - Nulliparity
    - Early menarche
    - Late menopause
    - Lack of breastfeeding
  - Genetics
    - Family history
    - *BRCA* mutation
    - Lynch syndrome (hereditary nonpolyposis colorectal cancer)
- Signs and symptoms
  - Abdominal pain/fullness
  - Bowel obstruction
  - Adnexal mass
  - Pleural effusion
  - Ascites
- Diagnostics
  - Transvaginal ultrasound: large, multiloculated, solid or mixed consistency mass
  - CA-125
    - Most useful in postmenopausal women as may be elevated by other causes in premenopausal women
    - Useful for assessing response to treatment and/or recurrence
- Management
  - Staging
  - Debulking surgery (total abdominal hysterectomy–bilateral salpingo-oophorectomy, omentectomy)
  - +/− chemoradiation

Protective factors against ovarian cancer include anything that decreases the number of ovulations: breastfeeding, anovulation, multiparity, and oral contraceptive pills.

Other causes of elevated CA-125 occur in premenopausal women: leiomyoma, endometriosis, diverticulitis, and peritonitis.

Germ Cell Tumors
Germ cell tumors:
- Tumor of cells that eventually differentiate into mature gametes
- Most commonly seen in young, premenopausal women
- Most common subtype is dysgerminoma
- Tumor markers include alpha-fetoprotein, beta-hCG, lactate dehydrogenase

SEX CORD STROMAL CELL TUMORS

Sertoli Leydig
- Definition: testosterone-secreting ovarian tumor
- Signs and symptoms: hyperandrogenism
  - Virilization (deepening voice, clitoromegaly)
  - Male pattern baldness
  - Acne
- Diagnostics
  - Transvaginal ultrasound
  - Testosterone levels
- Management: surgical resection

Granulosa theca cell tumor
- Definition: estrogen-secreting ovarian tumor
- Signs and symptoms: hyperestrinism → endometrial bleeding
- Diagnostics
  - Transvaginal ultrasound
  - Elevated estrogen levels
  - Histology
    - Coffee bean–shaped nuclei, Call-Exner bodies
    - Endometrial hyperplasia
- Management: surgical resection

Meigs syndrome: sex cord stromal tumor characterized by triad of ovarian fibroma, ascites, pleural effusion

Latzko triad: profuse watery vaginal discharge, lower abdominal pain, and pelvic mass; associated with fallopian tube cancer

CHAPTER 53 Uterine Disorders

ANATOMIC DEFORMITIES

Uterine anatomic abnormalities occur due to embryonic failure of cleavage, dissolution, and/or fusion (Table 53-1; Figs. 53-1, 53-2, and 53-3).

Secondary dysmenorrhea occurs due to endometriosis, leiomyoma, or adenomyosis.

TABLE 53-1 Uterine Anatomic Deformities

SUBTYPES	EMBRYONIC PATHOPHYSIOLOGY	DIAGNOSTICS	MANAGEMENT	COMPLICATIONS
Septate uterus	• Failure of septum dissolution	• Transvaginal ultrasound • Pelvic MRI • Hysteroscopy	• Surgical correction	• Recurrent pregnancy loss • Breech presentation • Ectopic pregnancy • Preterm labor
Bicornuate uterus	• Failure of fusion of paramesonephric ducts cranially			
Uterine didelphys	• Complete failure of fusion of paramesonephric ducts			

MRI, Magnetic resonance imaging

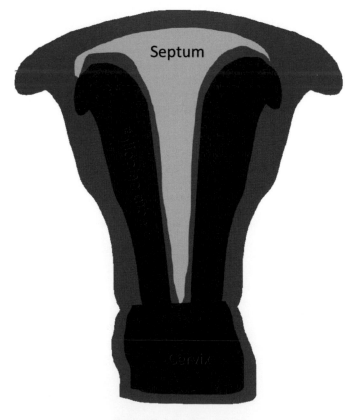

Figure 53-1: Septate uterus

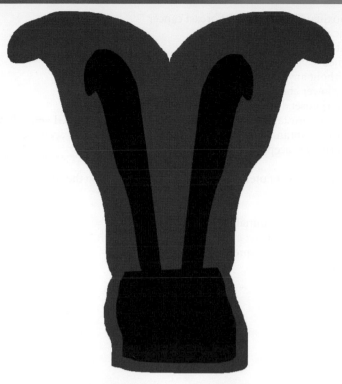

Figure 53-2: Bicornuate uterus

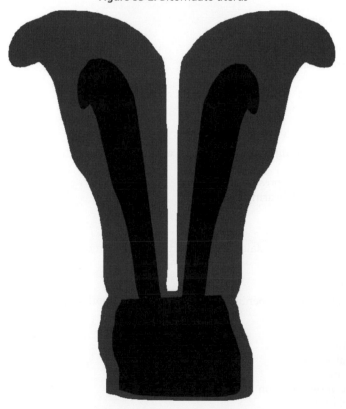

Figure 53-3: Uterine didelphys

UTERINE PAIN AND NONMALIGNANT BLEEDING

Endometrial Polyp
– Definition: benign growth of endometrial tissue with concurrent vasculature
– Signs and symptoms
   • Intermenstrual bleeding in premenopausal women
   • Normal physical exam

- – Associations: tamoxifen for treatment of breast cancer
- – Diagnostics: pelvic ultrasound
- – Management: hysteroscopic resection

Primary Dysmenorrhea
- – Dysmenorrhea without any discernible etiology
- – Recurrent, crampy lower abdominal pain
- – Gastrointestinal (GI) upset during menstruation
- – Secondary to excessive prostaglandin release resulting in uterine and GI smooth muscle contraction
- – Treat with nonsteroidal antiinflammatory drugs (NSAIDs), oral contraceptive pills (OCPs), or alternative hormonal contraception

Endometriosis
- – Pathophysiology: deposition of uterine glands and stroma outside the uterus
- – Signs and symptoms
  - Asymptomatic
  - Chronic, cyclical lower abdominal and pelvic pain
  - Uterosacral ligament nodularity: cul-de-sac
  - Adnexal mass/tenderness, endometrioma
  - Fixed, retroverted uterus
  - Dyspareunia
  - Dyschezia

Bleeding associated with leiomyomas typically subsides after menopause due to lack of estrogen stimulation resulting in shrinking and involution of leiomyomas.

- – Diagnostics
  - Clinical
  - Laparoscopy: definitive diagnosis
    - Adhesions
    - "Chocolate cyst"
    - Powder burn lesions
- – Management
  - Symptomatic: NSAIDs
  - Hormonal
    - OCPs
    - Danazol
    - Gonadotropin-releasing hormone (GnRH) agonist
  - Surgical
    - Laparoscopic ablation: preserve fertility
    - Hysterectomy: if childbearing is complete
- – Complications: infertility

Endometriosis of the ovary results in formation of "chocolate cyst"; this is the most common site for endometriosis.

Leiomyoma (Fibroid)
- – Definition: estrogen-responsive benign growths of uterine smooth muscle
- – Risk factors
  - Black
  - Hyperestrinism
  - Premenopausal
- – Signs and symptoms
  - Asymptomatic: most common
  - Uterine irregularity
  - Menometrorrhagia
  - Dysmenorrhea
  - Abdominal pain/pressure
  - Urinary urgency
- – Diagnostics (Fig. 53-4)
  - Clinical
  - Pelvic ultrasound

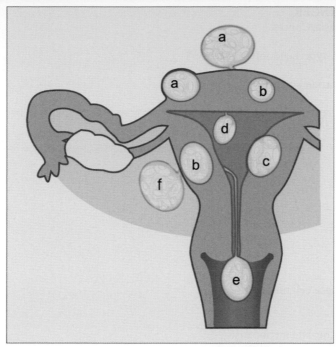

Figure 53-4: Various locations and subtypes of leiomyoma. These result in different clinical presentations due to impingement on adjacent structures and friability. (a) = subserosal fibroids. (b) = intramural fibroids. (c) = submucosal fibroid. (d) = pedunculated submucosal fibroid. (e) = protruding fibroid. (f) = intraligamental fibroid. (Image courtesy of Hic et nunc; CC BY-SA 3.0 [https://creativecommons.org/licenses/by-sa/3.0])

- Management
  - Mild, asymptomatic: observation
  - Moderate
    - Hormonal
      - OCPs
      - GnRH agonists
      - Progestins
      - Danazol
    - Nonhormonal
      - NSAIDs
      - Tranexamic acid
      - Mifepristone
  - Severe
    - Myomectomy: preserves fertility
    - Embolization
    - Hysterectomy: definitive treatment
- Complications: development of any of the following are indications for surgical intervention
  - Iron deficiency anemia secondary to severe bleeding
  - Recurrent miscarriage
  - Infertility

Adenomyosis
- Pathophysiology: deposition of endometrial glands and stroma within the myometrium
- Signs and symptoms
  - Diffuse, bulky, globular tender uterine enlargement
  - Dyspareunia
  - Tenderness before and during menses
  - Dysmenorrhea, menorrhagia
- Diagnostics
  - Pelvic ultrasound
  - Pelvic magnetic resonance imaging
- Management
  - OCPs, progestins: decrease menstrual bleeding
  - Hysterectomy: definitive treatment

ENDOMETRIAL CANCER
Endometrial Hyperplasia/Cancer
- Risk factors
  - Hyperestrinism (type I endometrial cancer)
    - Obesity
    - Polycystic ovarian syndrome

Causes of abnormal uterine bleeding: PALM-COEIN
- Polyp
- Adenomyosis
- Leiomyoma
- Malignancy
- Coagulopathy
- Ovulatory dysfunction
- Endometrial dysfunction
- Iatrogenic
- Not yet classified

    - Granulosa theca cell tumor
    - Tamoxifen
    - Nulliparity
    - Early menarche, late menopause
  - Genetics (type II endometrial cancer)
    - Family history
    - Lynch syndrome
    - Peutz-Jeghers syndrome
- Signs and symptoms: postmenopausal bleeding
- Diagnostic
  - Transvaginal ultrasound: thickening of the endometrial lining
  - Endometrial biopsy: definitive diagnosis
- Management
  - Hyperplasia without atypia: progestins
  - Early-stage adenocarcinoma: hysterectomy
  - Advanced-stage adenocarcinoma: total abdominal hysterectomy–bilateral salpingo-oophorectomy +/−chemoradiation
- Protective factors: reduce hyperestrinism states
  - Multiparity
  - OCPs, progestins
  - Weight loss
- Leiomyosarcoma
- Malignancy of uterine smooth muscle
- Presents with rapidly progressive uterine enlargement and abnormal uterine bleeding
- Increased mitotic activity on histology
- No association with leiomyomas

CHAPTER 54 Disorders of the Cervix

BENIGN CERVICAL LESIONS
Cervical Polyp
- Benign overgrowth of endocervical tissue
- Most commonly asymptomatic
- Presents with intermenstrual bleeding
- Diagnosed on speculum exam by the presence of reddish, purple fingerlike projection from the cervical canal
- Treatment is resection

Cervical Fibroids
- Histologically identical to uterine fibroids, often an extension of intramural uterine fibroids
- Same signs and symptoms as other fibroid subtypes
- May result in pregnancy complications (premature labor) if not removed

CERVICAL CANCER
Cervical cancer principles
- Screening starts at age 21 years regardless of sexually transmitted disease history or first age of sexual activity
- From age 21–30 years, screening every 3 years with Pap smear
- From age 30–65 years, screening every 5 years with Pap smear plus human papillomavirus (HPV) DNA testing
- Screening frequency and age at which to stop screening increases in the presence of abnormal results

Cervical Cancer
- Pathophysiology: HPV infection → chronic inflammation → dysplasia → cancer at the transformation zone or squamocolumnar junction
- Risk factors
  - HPV 16, 18, 31, 33
  - Human immunodeficiency virus
  - Smoking
- Signs and symptoms
  - Friable cervical mass
  - Postcoital bleeding
  - Obstructive uropathy
- Diagnostics
  - Pap smear
  - Colposcopy with biopsy: may be later complicated by cervical stenosis/insufficiency
- Management: see flow chart (Fig. 54-1) of interpretation of Pap smear results
- Prevention: HPV vaccine
  - Girls age 11–26 years
  - Boys age 9–21 years

Indications to stop screening:
- Age >65 years or hysterectomy (not related to cervical cancer) plus no history of cervical intraepithelial neoplasia II or greater plus one of the following:
  1. Two consecutive negative Pap smears with DNA testing
  2. Three consecutive negative Pap smears

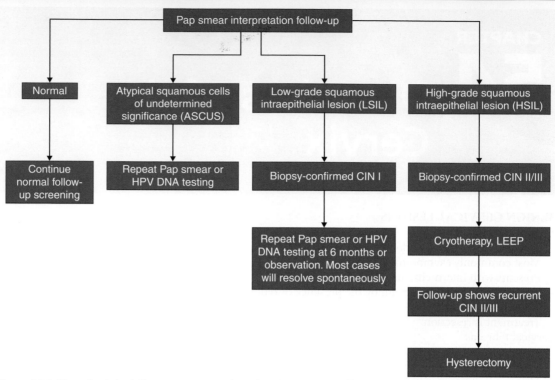

Figure 54-1: Flow chart depicting management based on Pap smear and biopsy results. *CIN,* Cervical intraepithelial neoplasia; *HPV,* human papillomavirus; *LEEP,* loop electrosurgical procedure.

Step-by-step workup for abnormal Pap smear (see Fig. 54-1)
1. Abnormal Pap smear
2. Colposcopy application of acetic acid
3. Visualization of abnormal cervix (punctate lesions, mosaicism, acetic acid staining, abnormal vessels)
4. Biopsy
5. Diagnosis
6. Treatment initiation

Deciding on biopsy technique to evaluate low-grade squamous intraepithelial lesion/high-grade squamous intraepithelial lesion:
- Endocervical curettage: metaplastic epithelium entering endocervical canal
- Cone biopsy: abnormal epithelium entering endocervical canal, biopsy results are worse than Pap smear
- Exocervical biopsy: abnormal epithelium on exocervix

Additional notes regarding cervical cancer screening:
1. Continue screening if patient has history of cervical intraepithelial neoplasia (CIN) II or greater for 20 years after detection.
2. Atypical squamous cells of undetermined significance, low-grade squamous intraepithelial lesion, and high-grade squamous intraepithelial lesion are histologic diagnoses found on Pap smear.
3. CIN I/II/III and cervical cancer are pathologic diagnoses made from biopsy after an abnormal Pap smear.
4. Human papillomavirus infection is associated with multiple malignancies: oropharyngeal cancer, anal cancer, genital warts, vaginal cancer, penile cancer, and cervical cancer.

Vaginal Cancer
Squamous Cell Carcinoma
- Risk factors
  - Age >60 years
  - Human papillomavirus 16, 18
  - Smoking
- Signs and symptoms
  - Postmenopausal bleeding
  - Postcoital bleeding
  - Pruritus
  - Malodorous vaginal discharge
  - Vaginal ulcer, irregularity
- Diagnostics: biopsy
- Management: staging +/− surgical resection +/− chemoradiation

Clear Cell Adenocarcinoma of the Vagina
- Presents in young, menstruating females
- Associated with in utero exposure to diethylstilbestrol
- Similar signs and symptoms, diagnostic workup, and management as squamous cell carcinoma of vagina

Sarcoma Botryoides: type of vaginal/cervical cancer characterized by protrusion of grapelike masses through the vaginal opening; seen more commonly in children

Other Vaginal Disorders
Vaginal Atrophy
- Definition: thinning and atrophy of vaginal tissue secondary to hypoestrinism
- Risk factors
  - Postmenopausal
  - Chemoradiation
  - Smoking
- Signs and symptoms
  - Vaginal pruritus
  - Dyspareunia
  - Urinary urgency/frequency/incontinence
  - Recurrent urinary tract infections
  - Thinned or vaginal tissue
  - Labial regression
  - Decreased vaginal rugae
  - Decreased introitus diameter
- Diagnostics: clinical
- Management
  - Mild: lubricants, moisturizers
  - Moderate/severe: topical estrogen replacement

Lichen Sclerosus
- Definition: chronic inflammation of the vulva and anogenital region
- Risk factors
  - Postmenopausal
  - History of autoimmune disease

- Signs and symptoms
  - Perianal and vulvar pruritus ("figure 8" appearance)
  - Cigarette/parchment-like texture of vulvar skin
  - Introital scarring/stenosis (distortion of external anatomy)
  - Polygonal patches with atrophy
  - Bladder/bowel dysfunction
  - Hypopigmented +/− ecchymosis vulva
- Diagnostics
  - Clinical
  - +/− punch biopsy to rule out squamous cell carcinoma: may represent premalignant lesion
- Management: high-potency topical steroids (clobetasol)

Lichen Planus
- Definition: atrophic inflammatory disorder of the vagina
- Signs and symptoms
  - Erythematous erosions with white borders (Wickham striae)
  - Narrowed introitus
  - Vaginal adhesions
  - Dyspareunia
- Diagnostics: clinical
- Management: high-potency topical steroids (clobetasol)

CHAPTER 56 Gynecologic Infections

Vaginitis is an infection of the vagina, which can be due to bacterial, fungal, or parasitic organism (Table 56-1).

TABLE 56-1 Differentiating Vaginitis

	MICROBIOLOGY	SIGNS AND SYMPTOMS	DIAGNOSTICS	MANAGEMENT
Bacterial vaginosis	• Gardnerella vaginalis	• Gray-white discharge • Fishy odor	• Wet mount: clue cells • pH >4.5 • Positive whiff test	• Metronidazole
Trichomoniasis	• Trichomonas vaginalis	• Yellow-green cervical discharge • Erythematous cervix	• Wet mount: mobile trichomonads • pH >4.5	• Metronidazole for patient and partner(s)
Candidiasis	• Candida albicans	• Thick, curdy white discharge with cottage cheese–like appearance • Vaginal pruritus	• KOH prep: hyphae • Clinical • pH <4.5	• Oral fluconazole or topical antifungals

Cervicitis/Pelvic Inflammatory Disease
- Definition: infection of the cervix, uterus, and the fallopian tubes
- Microbiology
  - Neisseria gonorrhea
  - Chlamydia trachomatis
- Risk factors
  - Unprotected sex
  - Multiple sexual partners
  - Young adults, adolescents
- Signs and symptoms
  - Chronic lower abdominal pain
  - Mucopurulent vaginal discharge
  - Chandelier sign: severe cervical pain on speculum examination
- Diagnostics
  - Clinical
  - Neisseria/chlamydia polymerase chain reaction
- Management
  - Empiric or Neisseria: ceftriaxone + azithromycin
  - Chlamydia: azithromycin
- Complications
  - Ectopic pregnancy
  - Infertility

Endometritis
- Definition: infection of the uterine decidua
- Microbiology: polymicrobial
- Risk factors
  - Postpartum
  - Dilatation and curettage
  - Cesarean section
  - Prolonged rupture of membranes

- Frequent vaginal exams
- Pelvic inflammatory disease
  - Signs and symptoms
    - Uterine fundal tenderness
    - Foul-smelling, mucopurulent lochia
    - Fevers, chills
  - Diagnostics: clinical
  - Management: antibiotics
    - Gentamicin + clindamycin

OR

- Ampicillin/sulbactam

Tuboovarian Abscess
  - Pathophysiology: extension of pelvic inflammatory disease into the ovaries resulting in oophoritis and abscess formation
  - Microbiology: polymicrobial
  - Signs and symptoms: similar to pelvic inflammatory disease plus the following
    - Adnexal mass
    - Fevers, chills
  - Diagnostics: transvaginal ultrasound
  - Management
    - Hemodynamically stable, <7 cm abscess: antibiotics only
      - Second-generation cephalosporin + doxycycline

OR

- Clindamycin + gentamicin
- Hemodynamically unstable, >7 cm abscess: image-guided drainage plus antibiotics

---

Chronic endometritis is treated with doxycycline for 2 weeks.

CHAPTER 57 Menstruation

Premenstrual Syndrome
- Definition: a spectrum of premenstrual disorders characterized by development of gastrointestinal, musculoskeletal, and neuropsychiatric symptoms during the luteal phase of a female's menstrual cycle
- Subtypes
  - Premenstrual tension
  - Premenstrual dysphoric disorder: more severe form characterized by disruption in daily functioning and requiring medication
- Signs and symptoms
  - Emotional lability, irritability
  - Muscle aches, arthralgias
  - Abdominal pain, diarrhea
  - Fluid retention
- Diagnostics
  - Menstrual diary (to confirm symptoms occur at the same time during the menstrual cycle)
  - Recurrence of symptoms in three consecutive cycles
  - Symptoms are not present during preovulatory phase of menstrual cycle
- Management
  - Lifestyle modifications
    - Adequate sleep
    - Avoid caffeine/nicotine
    - Stress reduction
    - Exercise
  - Pharmacologic
    - Selective serotonin reuptake inhibitors (SSRIs)
    - Progestins
    - Drospirenone (progestin analog to spironolactone)

Menopause
- Definition: >12 months of amenorrhea unrelated to any secondary cause
- Causes
  - Natural: hypoestrogenism secondary to ovarian atrophy occurring in late 40 s to early 50 s
  - Early menopause, defined as menopause <40 years old
    - Patient factors
      - Smoking
      - Autoimmune disease
    - Genetics
      - Family history
      - Turner syndrome
      - Fragile X
    - Iatrogenic
      - Oophorectomy
      - Estrogen antagonists
      - Gonadotropin-releasing hormone agonists
      - Chemoradiation
- Signs and symptoms
  - Hot flashes
  - Diaphoresis
  - Insomnia, irritability

- Vaginal atrophy
- Stress incontinence, urinary tract infections
  - Diagnostics: clinical
  - Management: symptomatic
    - Hot flashes
      - SSRI/serotonin and norepinephrine reuptake inhibitor
      - Low-dose hormone replacement therapy
    - Vaginal atrophy: moisturizers, lubricants, topical estrogen
  - Complications
    - Osteoporosis
    - Cardiovascular disease

CHAPTER 58 Sexual Functioning Disorders

Hypoactive Sexual Disorder
- Causes
  - Selective serotonin reuptake inhibitors
  - Oral contraceptive pills
  - Low testosterone levels
- Diagnostics
  - Review patient's medication list
  - Work up for organic pathology (dyspareunia, endometriosis, vaginitis, pelvic inflammatory disease, hypotestosteronism)
- Management
  - Treat organic pathology
  - Flibanserin (serotonin receptor modulator)

Evaluate patient's medication list as several medications are associated with sexual dysfunction:
- Selective serotonin reuptake inhibitors: anorgasmia
- Beta blockers: erectile dysfunction in males
- Alpha blockers: anorgasmia
- Trazodone: priapism
- Dopamine antagonists: decreased libido

Vaginismus (Genitopelvic Pain/Penetration Disorder)
- Risk factors
  - Previous sexual abuse
  - Sexual trauma
  - Lack of sexual knowledge
- Signs and symptoms
  - Pain on attempted vaginal penetration
  - Involuntary adduction upon penetration
- Diagnostics
  - Clinical
  - Work up to rule out organic pathology
- Management
  - Vaginal dilators
  - Desensitization therapy
  - Kegel exercises
  - Psychotherapy

CHAPTER 59 Family Planning

Infertility
- Definition: inability to conceive after >12 months of intercourse in women <35 years old and >6 months in women >35 years old
- Causes
  - Male related
    - Decreased sperm volume
    - Abnormal sperm morphology
    - Cystic fibrosis (absent vas deferens)
    - Varicocele
    - Cryptorchidism
    - Klinefelter syndrome
    - Myotonic dystrophy
  - Female related
    - Endometriosis
    - Polycystic ovarian syndrome
    - Pelvic inflammatory disease (cervical stenosis, tubal scarring)
    - Turner syndrome
    - Anorexia nervosa
    - Mullerian agenesis
  - Both
    - Chemoradiation
    - Hypothyroidism
    - Hyperprolactinemia
- Diagnostics
  - Semen analysis: initial test
  - Work up organic pathology (thyroid-stimulating hormone, prolactin)
- Management: treat underlying etiology; if none is found, augmentation therapies can be utilized
  - Anovulation: clomiphene citrate
  - Abnormal semen analysis or female anatomic disorder (cervical stenosis, tubal scarring): in vitro fertilization

There are multiple types of contraception with different routes of administration, efficacy, and adverse effects. The choice of contraception should be based on patient preference, likelihood of compliance, and underlying diseases that may be worsened by adverse effects (Table 59-1).

TABLE 59-1 Contraception

TYPE OF CONTRACEPTION	PROS	CONS
Oral contraceptives: combination estrogen/ progesterone	• Very effective • Multiple forms of administration (pills, injections, subcutaneous implants) • Regular menses, decreased abnormal uterine bleeding • Decreased risk of ovarian cancer	• Thromboembolic/vascular disease, especially in smokers >35 years old • Worsening hormone-dependent cancer (breast, endometrial) • Worsening hypertension • Worsening migraines (avoid in patients who have migraines with aura) • Headaches, nausea, bloating, mood changes, breast tenderness • High risk of noncompliance for patients taking daily pills
Barrier contraception (condoms, vaginal diaphragm)	• Protection against sexually transmitted diseases	• Not as effective as oral contraceptive • High noncompliance rate
Intrauterine device (IUD)	• Prolonged contraception (5–10 yr) with low maintenance	• Avoid in active pelvic infection (salpingitis, cervicitis) or malignancy • Avoid in abnormally shaped uterus • Increased risk of ectopic pregnancy • Copper IUD contraindicated in Wilson disease • Risk of IUD migration into the peritoneal cavity

CHAPTER 60 Miscellaneous

Pelvic Organ Prolapse
- Definition: protrusion of pelvic organs through the vaginal opening
- Risk factors
  - Multiparity: stretching of pelvic ligaments
  - Increased age: atrophy and decreased elasticity of pelvic ligaments
  - Pelvic surgery: damage to pelvic ligaments
- Subtypes
  - Cystocele: prolapse anterior to the vagina
  - Rectocele: prolapse posterior to the vagina
  - Uterine prolapse: prolapse directly through the vagina
  - Vaginal prolapse: occurs post hysterectomy
- Signs and symptoms
  - Lower abdominal/pelvic pressure
  - Vaginal bulge
  - Urinary urgency
  - Bladder/bowel dysfunction
  - Visualization of protruding organ
- Diagnostics: visualization on speculum exam
- Management
  - Staging of pelvic organ prolapse from first degree (minimal prolapse) to fourth degree (direct visualization of prolapsed organ without straining or speculum exam)
    - Asymptomatic: expectant management
    - Symptomatic
      - Nonoperative
        - Kegel exercises
        - Vaginal pessaries
        - Low-dose vaginal estrogen
      - Operative: surgical correction after failing nonoperative techniques
        - Colporrhaphy
        - Hysterectomy
        - Ligament fixation

Bartholin Duct Cyst
- Pathophysiology: obstruction of the Bartholin glands secondary to infection or thick glandular secretions
- Signs and symptoms
  - Asymptomatic: most common
  - Fluctuant collection seen at 4-o'clock and 8-o'clock positions at the labia majora
  - Tenderness
  - Discomfort with walking, exercise, and intercourse
- Diagnostics: clinical
- Management
  - Asymptomatic: observation
  - Symptomatic: I&D plus word catheter (word catheter allows continuous drainage until tract is healed)

CHAPTER 61 Somatoform Disorders

Diagnosis of any somatoform disorders is only made after exclusion of organic pathology.

Conversion Disorder
- Signs and symptoms: neurologic symptoms that do not follow normal anatomic or physiologic distributions
  - Mutism
  - Blindness
  - Paresthesias
  - Nonepileptic seizures
  - Lack of concern for symptoms: la belle indifference
- Management
  - Patient education
  - Psychotherapy

Illness Anxiety Disorder
- Definition
  - Excessive preoccupation for >6 months with set of symptoms despite reassurance resulting in day-to-day functional impairment
  - Perceive mild symptoms as life-threatening pathology
- Management
  - Frequent scheduled visits with same primary care provider
  - Cognitive behavioral therapy

Somatic Symptom Disorder
- Definition
  - Manifestation of psychological stress as physical symptoms for >6 months resulting in day-to-day functional impairment
  - Excessive thoughts surrounding the physical symptoms
- Management
  - Frequent scheduled visits with same primary care provider
  - Minimize unnecessary testing and procedures
  - Cognitive behavioral therapy
  - Stress management

Factitious and malingering are two disorders with similar presentations that are differentiated based on the type of gain the patient is attempting to achieve (Table 61-1).

Most somatoform disorders have similar risk factors:
1) Female
2) Childhood abuse
3) Recent traumatic experience
4) Underlying stress, anxiety, or personality disorder
5) Low socioeconomic status

TABLE 61-1   Factitious Versus Malingering

	FACTITIOUS	MALINGERING
Definition	• Falsification of physical or psychiatric symptoms to assume the sick role	• Falsification of physical or psychiatric symptoms for personal gain
Type of gain	• Unconscious, internal gain and motivation	• Conscious, external gain and motivation
Goal	• Crave the attention and sympathy received from the medical staff	• Resolution of symptoms after personal gain has been achieved (doctor note, workers compensation)

Factitious disorder by proxy: purposely causing physical symptoms in another individual to receive attention and sympathy from others (e.g., mother inducing symptoms in her child to receive sympathy from the medical staff)

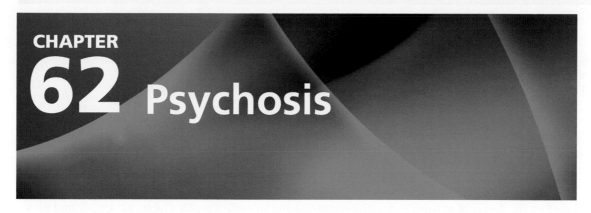

CHAPTER 62 Psychosis

There are many schizo- disorders (Table 62-1) that sound like each other; however, they have specific definitions and unique symptomatology to meet their respective diagnostic criteria (Table 62-2).

Delusional Disorders
- Definition
  - Presence of nonbizarre delusions for >1 month without impairment in daily functioning
  - No impairment in daily functioning
  - Continue to have logical and coherent thought processes
- Several subtypes of delusions
  - Grandiose: delusion of special talents
  - Erotic: delusion that another individual is in love with them
  - Shared: common delusion between two people, often involves one dominant individual imposing delusions on another
  - Jealous: delusion of infidelity
  - Persecutory: delusion others are out to harm them
- Be sure not to confuse with different cultural perceptions
- Management with antipsychotics and psychotherapy

TABLE 62-1 Differentiating Schizo- Disorders

	SCHIZOPHRENIA	SCHIZOPHRENIFORM	SCHIZOAFFECTIVE
Definition	• Presence of two or more for >1 month with total duration from prodromal phase lasting >6 months	• Similar to schizophrenia, except symptoms lasting 1–6 months	• Presence of mania over major depressive disorder with concurrent schizophrenia • Two-week psychosis in the absence of mood symptoms • Mood symptoms tend to predominate over psychotic symptoms
Risk factors	• Substance abuse (cannabis) • Young adults • Family history		
Management	• Antipsychotics • Psychotherapy		• Antipsychotic: initial treatment • Mood stabilizers • Antidepressants • Psychotherapy

TABLE 62-2 Schizophrenia Symptoms

POSITIVE SYMPTOMS	NEGATIVE SYMPTOMS
• Auditory hallucinations: most common • Visual hallucinations • Themed delusions • Thought insertion • Thought broadcasting: others can hear their thoughts • Paranoia: others are out to get them • Guilt: belief they are responsible for several problems • Ideas of reference: cues from external environment applied directly to them • Disorganized speech • Catatonia • Negative symptoms	• Flat affect • Poverty of speech • Apathy • Poor attention • Anhedonia

One of the symptoms must include hallucinations, delusions, or disorganized speech to diagnose schizophrenia.
Brief psychotic disorder: symptoms of schizophrenia lasting <1 month followed by full return of function

Illusion vs hallucination: hallucination is perception without an existing stimulus; illusion is misinterpretation of an existing stimulus

Other nonpsychotic schizo- disorders:
1. Schizotypal: personality disorder characterized by magical beliefs and eccentric thoughts
2. Schizoid: personality disorder characterized by extreme introverted behavior and loss of enjoyment of social activities

Before considering a psychotic disorder as a cause for a patient's psychosis, medical diseases must be excluded as these can have similar presentations (Table 62-3).

Pharmacology

The treatment for psychosis is with antipsychotics, which can be typical or atypical. The choice should be based on the degree of positive vs negative symptoms and side effect profile (Tables 62-4, 62-5, and 62-6). Neuroleptic Malignant Syndrome

– Epidemiology: onset can occur at any time while on antipsychotics
– Signs and symptoms
  • Hyperthermia
  • Lead pipe muscle rigidity
  • Altered mental status
  • Diaphoresis
– Diagnostics: clinical with high index of suspicion
  • Supporting labs
    ▪ Elevated creatine kinase
    ▪ Metabolic acidosis
    ▪ Leukocytosis
– Management
  • Stop antipsychotic
  • Cooling blankets
  • IV dantrolene (ryanodine receptor antagonist)

Tardive Dyskinesia

– Epidemiology: occurs after long-term use of antipsychotics (>6 months)
– Signs and symptoms: uncontrollable, choreiform movements of the face and tongue
– Diagnostics: clinical
– Management
  • Stop antipsychotic, switch to atypical antipsychotic
  • No cure for tardive dyskinesia, most cases are permanent

Neuroleptic malignant syndrome, extrapyramidal symptoms, and tardive dyskinesia can occur with atypical antipsychotics; however, they are more commonly associated with typical antipsychotics.

TABLE 62-3   Medical Diseases Simulating Psychosis

POSTPARTUM PSYCHOSIS	EXAMPLES
Hormones/electrolytes	• Hyperthyroidism • Hypercortisolism • Hyper/hypocalcemia
Drugs/medications	• Cocaine • Amphetamines • Steroids
Central nervous system disorders	• Delirium • Dementia (Lewy body, Alzheimer) • Encephalitis • Meningitis • Seizures/epilepsy
Nutritional deficiencies	• Vitamin B12 • Vitamin B6 • Vitamin B3 (niacin)
Vasculitis	• Systemic lupus erythematosus • Giant cell arteritis

TABLE 62-4   Antipsychotics Pharmacology

	TYPICAL ANTIPSYCHOTICS	ATYPICAL ANTIPSYCHOTICS
Mechanism of action	• Dopamine receptor antagonists	• Combination of dopamine, serotonin, and histamine modulators
Examples	• Haloperidol • Chlorpromazine • Thioridazine • Fluphenazine	• Clozapine • Olanzapine • Quetiapine • Ziprasidone • Lurasidone
Side effects	Extrapyramidal symptoms • Dystonia: muscle spasm • Parkinsonianism: bradykinesia, shuffling gait, tremor • Akathisia Hyperprolactinemia • Decreased libido • Gynecomastia • Amenorrhea Anticholinergic • Dry eyes/mouth • Tachycardia, prolonged QT • Constipation Antiadrenergic • Orthostatic hypotension Antihistamine • Weight gain • Sedation	• Similar to typical antipsychotics except with increased anticholinergic, antiadrenergic, and antihistamine side effects with less risk of extrapyramidal, hyperprolactinemia, tardive dyskinesia, neuroleptic malignant syndrome

Typical antipsychotics are more effective in treating positive symptoms, whereas atypical antipsychotics are better suited for negative symptoms.

TABLE 62-5   Specific Side Effects of Antipsychotics

ANTIPSYCHOTIC	SIDE EFFECT
Thioridazine	• Retinal pigmentation
Chlorpromazine	• Corneal clouding
Clozapine	• Agranulocytosis • Myocarditis • Seizures
Quetiapine	• Cataracts
Ziprasidone	• Prolonged QT
Olanzapine	• Metabolic syndrome
Typical antipsychotics	• Neuroleptic malignant syndrome • Tardive dyskinesia

TABLE 62-6   Extrapyramidal Symptoms

	SIGNS AND SYMPTOMS	MANAGEMENT
Dystonia	• Painful muscle contraction of the neck (torticollis) or eyes	• Anticholinergic (diphenhydramine)
Parkinsonianism	• Shuffling gait • Bradykinesia • Resting pill rolling tremor • Cogwheel rigidity	• Decrease dose or switch to atypical antipsychotic • Anticholinergic
Akathisia	• Inability to sit still with constant need to move around • Fidgety • Restlessness	• Decreased dose or switch to atypical antipsychotic • Benzodiazepine or beta blocker

DEPRESSION AND BIPOLAR

Major Depressive Disorder (MDD)
- Definition: five or more of the following signs and symptoms for two weeks with at least one being depressed mood or anhedonia
  - Change in sleep
  - Loss of interest in previously pleasurable activities (anhedonia)
  - Feelings of guilt or worthlessness
  - Decreased energy
  - Decreased concentration
  - Change in appetite or weight
  - Psychomotor retardation or agitation
  - Suicidal ideation
- Management
  - Determine whether patient requires hospitalization (if patient has suicidal ideations with a plan, then first step would be involuntary hospitalization)
  - Pharmacologic
    - Selective serotonin reuptake inhibitors (SSRIs): first line
    - Alternatives
      - Monoamine oxidase inhibitors
      - Norepinephrine-dopamine reuptake inhibitors (buprenorphine)
      - Tricyclic antidepressants (TCAs)
      - Alpha-2 antagonist (mirtazapine)
  - Psychotherapy: used in conjunction with pharmacologic therapy
  - Electroconvulsive therapy (ECT)

Alternative classes of antidepressants may be beneficial if the side effects can be used to manage the patient comorbidities.

Approach to Suicidal Patients
- Determine whether patient requires hospitalization vs close follow-up
  - If patient has suicidal ideations, but no active plan → ensure close follow-up
  - If patient has active suicidal ideation, with means and a plan → involuntary hospitalization
- Increased risk of suicide if the following are present
  - History of suicide attempt
  - Substance abuse
  - Male
  - Elderly
  - Psychiatric disorder
  - Family history of suicide
  - Social isolation
- Management: ECT for acutely suicidal patients, followed by SSRIs

ECT
- Definition: induces a generalized tonic-clonic seizure lasting between 30 and 60 seconds
- Indications
  - Acutely suicidal
  - Pregnancy
  - Failure of pharmacotherapy
  - Refusal to eat or drink resulting in malnutrition

- Psychosis
- Catatonia
- Adverse effects
  - Transient amnesia: most common
  - Prolonged seizure: increased risk if there is presence of space-occupying lesion or cerebrovascular accident
  - Headache
  - Muscle aches
  - Cardiovascular deterioration if there is severe underlying cardiovascular abnormality (recent myocardial infarction, cardiomyopathy)

Bipolar I and II have overlapping clinical features; however, they are primarily differentiated based on the presence of mania and hypomania, respectively. Other differentiating features are discussed in the chapter (Table 63-1; Fig. 63-1).

Other Mood Disorders

Dysthymia
- Definition
  - Persistent depressive symptoms for at least >2 years in adults or >1 year in children or adolescents; may occasionally meet criteria for MDD
  - No timeframe where patient is without symptoms for >2 months
- Signs and symptoms: two of the following
  - Appetite change
  - Decreased energy
  - Decreased self-esteem
  - Difficulty with concentration
  - Hopelessness
- Management: similar pharmacotherapy as MDD

Cyclothymia
- Definition
  - Swings between hypomanic symptoms and depressed symptoms for at least >2 years without meeting criteria for hypomania or MDD
  - No timeframe where patient is without symptoms for >2 months
- Management: psychotherapy +/− mood stabilizers for hypomanic episodes causing functional impairment

Seasonal Affective Disorder
- Definition
  - Depressive symptoms during winter season with shorter daylight hours
  - Resolution of symptoms during the summer season and longer daytime hours
- Management: bright light phototherapy (exposes the patient to ultraviolet light)

Grief and depression have overlapping clinical features; however, they have key difference that are important to note as they result in significantly different management approaches (Table 63-2).

TABLE 63-1 Bipolar I Versus Bipolar II Disorder

	BIPOLAR I DISORDER	BIPOLAR II DISORDER
Definition	• Mania +/− major depressive disorder (MDD) • Patient will eventually develop an episode of MDD, however is not required for initial diagnosis of bipolar I disorder	• Hypomania + major depressive disorder
Signs and symptoms	• Mania: symptoms must last for seven days or <7 days if hospitalization is required with three of the following: • Increase distractibility • Indiscretion and excessive involvement in pleasurable activities (gambling, shopping, promiscuous sexual behavior) • Grandiosity • Flight of ideas • Increased activity • Lack of sleep • Excessive talking (pressured speech) • MDD (described above)	• Hypomania: same symptoms as mania, however symptoms must last for at least four days with no impairment in daily activity and does not require hospitalization • MDD (described above)
Diagnostics	• Clinical	
Management	• Hospitalization for mania or severe MDD (suicidal ideation with a plan) • Mood stabilizers • Antidepressants for MDD only after initiation of mood stabilizers as antidepressants may precipitate a manic episode	• Same as bipolar I, except hospitalization is not required for hypomania

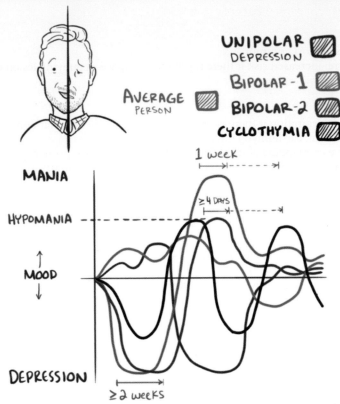

Figure 63-1: Illustration of mood shifts and duration of symptoms associated with bipolar, depression, and cyclothymia. (Image courtesy of Osmosis; CC BY-SA 4.0 [https://creativecommons.org/licenses/by-sa/4.0])

TABLE 63-2   Grief Versus Depression

	GRIEF	DEPRESSION
Similarities	• Decreased sleep • Decreased enjoyment in previously enjoyable activities • Decreased appetite • Crying, tearful	
Differences	• Waxing and waning • Suicidal ideation related to wanting to be with their lost loved one • No significant functional impairment • Enjoy being around family and friends	• Continuous symptomatology • Suicidal ideation unrelated to anything in specific • Functional impairment • No enjoyment regardless who is around
Management	• Support and reassurance	• Selective serotonin reuptake inhibitors

There are three main postpartum mood disorders ranging from benign postpartum blues to severe postpartum psychosis requiring hospitalization of the mother and separation from her newborn (Table 63-3).

Premenstrual Syndrome
– Definition: spectrum of premenstrual disorders characterized by development of gastrointestinal, musculoskeletal, and neuropsychiatric symptoms during the luteal phase of a female's menstrual cycle
– Subtypes
  • Premenstrual tension
  • Premenstrual dysphoric disorder (more severe form characterized by disruption in daily functioning and requiring medication)
– Signs and symptoms
  • Emotional lability, irritability
  • Muscle aches, arthralgias
  • Abdominal pain, diarrhea
  • Fluid retention

TABLE 63-3   Postpartum Mood Disorders

	KEY FEATURES	MANAGEMENT
Postpartum blues	• Emotional lability following childbirth • 2–3 days postpartum	• Emotional support, resolves within two weeks
Postpartum depression	• Sleep disturbances • Depressed mood, anhedonia • Sensation of guilt/worthlessness • Lack of energy • Difficulty concentrating • Appetite changes • Psychomotor agitation/retardation • Suicidal ideation	• Antidepressants (selective serotonin reuptake inhibitorss) • Ensure mother has no thoughts of infanticide
Postpartum psychosis	• Thoughts of infanticide • Hallucinations, delusions • Within two weeks postpartum • Commonly seen in patients with history of bipolar	• Hospitalize mother • Avoid leaving mother and baby alone; may allow for supervised visits • Second-generation antipsychotics (quetiapine, risperidone, olanzapine) +/− mood stabilizer (lithium, valproate)

- Diagnostics
  - Menstrual diary (to confirm symptoms occur at the same time during the menstrual cycle)
  - Recurrence of symptoms in three consecutive cycles
  - Symptoms do not present during preovulatory phase of menstrual cycle
- Management
  - Lifestyle modifications
    - Adequate sleep
    - Avoid caffeine/nicotine
    - Stress reduction
    - Exercise
  - Pharmacologic
    - SSRIs
    - Progestins
    - Drospirenone (progestin analog to spironolactone)

Medical diseases and medications simulating mood disorders
- Depression
  - Endocrinopathies: thyroid, glucose, cortisol
  - Central nervous system (CNS) disorders: stroke, dementia, infection
  - Collagen vascular disease
  - Malignancy: paraneoplastic syndrome, lymphoma, pancreatic adenocarcinoma
  - Alcohol
  - Barbiturate/benzodiazepines
  - Stimulant withdrawal
  - Corticosteroids
- Mania
  - Endocrinopathies: thyroid, cortisol, pheochromocytoma
  - CNS disorders
  - Collagen vascular disease
  - Malignancy
  - Initiation of antidepressants
  - Corticosteroids
  - Stimulants

Pharmacology

There are several classes of antidepressants and mood stabilizers, the choice of which should be determined based on patient preference and using the side effect profile to help manage the patient's comorbidities (e.g., using an antidepressant that has the side effect of weight loss in an obese, depressed patient) (Tables 63-4 and 63-5).

Serotonin Syndrome
- Definition: excessive serotonin levels often due to patient taking multiple drugs that increase serotonin (SSRIs, monoamine oxidase [MAO] inhibitors, serotonin and norepinephrine reuptake inhibitors, TCAs, St. John wort, dextromethorphan)

TABLE 63-4 Antidepressants

CLASS/MECHANISM	EXAMPLES	ADVERSE EFFECTS
Selective serotonin reuptake inhibitors (SSRIs)	• Fluoxetine • Paroxetine • Citalopram • Escitalopram • Sertraline	• Initial increased risk of suicide after initiation • Weight gain • Sexual dysfunction • Serotonin syndrome • Serotonin discontinuation syndrome (flulike symptoms after abrupt cessation of SSRI; treat by slowly tapering medication)
Serotonin and norepinephrine reuptake inhibitors	• Venlafaxine • Duloxetine	• Hypertension • Insomnia
Monoamine oxidase inhibitors	• Selegiline • Phenelzine	• Hypertensive crisis when ingested with tyramine-containing foods (wine, cheese, chocolate cake)
Tricyclic antidepressants	• Amitriptyline • Nortriptyline	• Prolonged QT • Convulsions • Anticholinergic (dry eyes, dry mouth, urinary retention, delirium)
Alpha-2 antagonist	• Mirtazapine	• Sedation • Increased appetite
Norepinephrine and dopamine reuptake inhibitors	• Buprenorphine	• Lower seizure threshold in anorexic/bulimic and patients with electrolyte derangements • Insomnia
Serotonin and adrenergic receptor modulator	• Trazodone	• Priapism • Orthostatic hypotension

TABLE 63-5 Mood Stabilizers

CLASS	EXAMPLES	ADVERSE EFFECTS
First-generation antipsychotics (neuroleptics)	Haloperidol Thioridazine Chlorpromazine	• Weight gain • Sedation • QT prolongation • Parkinsonianism • Akathisia • Neuroleptic malignant syndrome • Tardive dyskinesia
Second-generation antipsychotics	Clozapine Quetiapine Risperidone Olanzapine Ziprasidone	
Unknown	Lithium	• Ataxia • Tremor • Nephrogenic diabetes insipidus • Fetal defects (Ebstein anomaly in newborns) • Thyroid dysfunction • Narrow therapeutic window
Gamma-aminobutyric acid modulator	Valproate	• Thrombocytopenia • Pancreatitis • Hepatotoxicity • Fetal defects (neural tube defect)
Sodium channel inactivator	Carbamazepine	• Syndrome of inappropriate antidiuretic hormone • Fetal defects (neural tube defects) • Stevens-Johnson syndrome • Agranulocytosis
Voltage-gated sodium channel blocker, glutamate modulator	Lamotrigine	• Stevens-Johnson syndrome

See Psychosis chapter for specific side effects and more details regarding antipsychotic side effects.

- Signs and symptoms
  - Hyperthermia
  - Flushing
  - Altered mental status
  - Myoclonus
  - Hemodynamic instability

- Diagnostics: clinical
- Management
  - Cessation of all serotonergic agents
  - Supportive care: cooling blankets, IV fluids
  - Benzodiazepines for sedation
  - Cyproheptadine: serotonin antagonist reversal agent

Other uses for antidepressants
- MAO inhibitors: atypical depression (mood reactivity, leaden paralysis, rejection hypersensitivity)
- Duloxetine: neuropathy
- SSRIs
  - Anxiety
  - Posttraumatic stress disorder
  - Obsessive compulsive disorder
  - Panic attacks
  - Premature ejaculation
  - SSRIs require 4–6 weeks before taking effect
- TCAs: neuropathy
- Buprenorphine: smoking cessation
- Mirtazapine: cachexia
- Trazodone: insomnia
- Carbamazepine
  - Trigeminal neuralgia
  - Seizures
- Valproate: seizures

CHAPTER 64 Anxiety

Panic Disorder
- Definition: anxiety disorder characterized by panic attacks
  - Recurrent, unexpected panic attacks
  - Concern about additional panic attacks for >1 month after a panic attack
  - Change in behavior related to panic attacks for >1 month after a panic attack
- Associations
  - Major depressive disorder (MDD)
  - Agoraphobia
  - Substance abuse
  - Bipolar disorder
- Management
  - Acute: benzodiazepines
  - Maintenance: selective serotonin reuptake inhibitors (SSRIs) +/− cognitive-behavioral therapy (CBT)

Panic attacks are defined as having four of the following signs or symptoms associated with intense fear or discomfort

1. Palpitations
2. Diaphoresis
3. Tremors, shakes
4. Sensation of choking
5. Sensation of shortness of breath
6. Chest pain/discomfort
7. Dizziness, lightheadedness
8. Nausea
9. Paresthesias
10. Depersonalization or derealization
11. Fear of dying
12. Fear of losing control
13. Chills or heat sensations

Mutism may also be a manifestation of severe schizophrenia.

Social Anxiety Disorder (Social Phobia)
- Definition/symptomatology: disproportionate fear of a specific object or situation resulting in the following
  - Avoidance of object or situation
  - Lasts >6 months
  - Results in significant day-to-day impairment
  - Exposure to the object or situation results in intense anxiety due to fear of scrutiny or humiliation in front of others
- Management
  - CBT: first line
  - Benzodiazepines: acute
  - SSRI or serotonin and norepinephrine reuptake inhibitor (SNRI): maintenance
  - Beta blocker (atenolol, propranolol): best for performance anxiety

Phobic disorders are similar to social anxiety disorder except the anxieties are related to a specific object or situation due to irrational fear.

Agoraphobia
- Definition/symptomatology
  - Intense fear of public situations due to fear of difficulty escaping or obtaining help
  - Fear of leaving home alone, close spaces, crowds, lines, public transportation
  - Situation results in fear and anxiety out of proportion to the presumed danger
  - Lasts >6 months
  - Significant social and occupational impairment
  - Highly associated with panic disorder
- Management: CBT +/− SSRI

Selective Mutism
- Definition/symptomatology
  - Failure to speak in certain social situations despite adequate social and language skills
  - Normal communication in other social situations
  - Lasts >1 month
  - Impairment in day-to-day functioning
- Management: CBT

Posttraumatic Stress Disorder
- Risk factors: exposure to life-threatening or severe psychosocial trauma
- Definition/symptomatology
  - Nightmare/flashbacks of traumatic event
  - Avoidance of trigger or site of event
  - Symptomatology >1 month
  - Negative mood/cognition (guilt, anger, anhedonia, detachment, dissociation)
  - Increased arousal (exaggerated startle response, irritability, insomnia, hypervigilance)
  - Significant social and occupational dysfunction
- Management
  - CBT and supportive therapy
  - SSRI or SNRI
  - Prazosin: effective for nightmares

Acute stress disorder is the same as posttraumatic stress disorder, except for presence of symptomatology lasting <1 month and trauma having occurred <1 month ago.

Adjustment Disorder
- Risk factors: change in behavior and increased anxiety following a stressful life event
- Definition/symptomatology
  - Onset of symptoms within three months of stressful life event (loss of a loved one, separation/divorce, moving, birth of a child, marriage)
  - Disproportionate symptomatology in relation to stressor
  - Symptoms resolve within six months after removal of stressor
- Management: supportive psychotherapy

Obsessive-Compulsive Disorder (OCD)

Obsessive-compulsive Disorder (OCD)
- Definition/symptomatology: recurrent obsessions and compulsions
  - Obsessions are intrusive thoughts that provoke anxiety related to safety, germs, guilt, or aggression
  - Compulsions are behaviors that reduce the anxiety-provoking obsessions such as constantly checking locks, washing hands, organizing, and praying
  - Aware that behavior is abnormal, however unable to make the necessary changes
- Associations
  - Tourette syndrome
  - Substance abuse
  - MDD
- Management: CBT plus SSRI

Trichotillomania
- Definition/symptomatology
  - Subtype of obsessive-compulsive–related disorders
  - Frequent hair pulling resulting in hair loss and significant distress
  - Unsuccessful attempts to stop hair pulling
  - Hair pulling thought to be related to anxiety-relieving behavior
- Management: CBT plus SSRI

Body Dysmorphic Disorder
- Definition/symptomatology: exaggeration and preoccupation with perceived flaws or body defects
  - Perceived flaws or defects are often not visible or appear minute to others
  - Spend excessive amount of time trying to resolve perceived flaws with plastic surgery, makeup, and other cosmetic procedures
  - Repetitive behaviors performed in response to perceived flaws (grooming, constant comparison to others): compulsion performed due to obsession
  - Significant impairment in day-to-day activity
- Associations
  - OCD
  - MDD
  - Social anxiety disorder
- Management: CBT plus SSRI

Hoarding Disorder
- Definition/symptomatology
  - Difficulty with discarding possessions regardless of value
  - Accumulation of possessions results in an uninhabitable living space due to congestion and safety risks
  - Significant anxiety and/or excuses when confronted about discarding possessions
  - Social and occupational impairment
- Management: CBT +/− SSRI

Eating disorders can be due to lack of adequate intake or excessive intake and are further defined based on their postintake behavior and duration of this behavior (Table 64-1).

Refeeding syndrome: rapid depletion of extracellular phosphorus and other electrolytes secondary to increased intracellular uptake in the use for adenosine triphosphate synthesis resulting in cardiomyopathy and severe arrhythmias; managed by replacing electrolytes and slowing rate of feeds

TABLE 64-1   Eating Disorders

	DEFINITION/SYMPTOMATOLOGY	DIAGNOSTICS	MANAGEMENT
Anorexia nervosa	• Excessively concerned with gaining weight and body image • Strict dieting and/or excessive exercise • May have binge eating and purging behaviors (e.g., bulimia) • Significant fear of gaining weight • Lack of insight into dangerously low weight	• Hypothalamic hypogonadism → amenorrhea • Body mass index (BMI) <17.5 • Dehydration → orthostatic hypotension • Hypoproteinemia → peripheral edema • Hypochloremia hypokalemic metabolic alkalosis if vomiting • Osteoporosis • Lanugo • Cardiomyopathy, QT prolongation	• Involuntary hospitalization if weight is dangerously low for supervised refeeding • Cognitive-behavioral therapy (CBT) plus supervised weight gain programs • Observe for refeeding syndrome: electrolyte derangements and fluid shifts after feeding severely malnourished patient
Bulimia nervosa	• Binge eating followed by inappropriate compensatory behaviors to prevent weight gain (vomiting, laxatives, diuretics, prolonged fasting, excessive exercise) • At least once a week for >3 months	• Normal to above average BMI • Bilateral enlarged parotid glands • Dental caries/erosions • Russell sign: erosions on the dorsum of the hand due to self-induced vomiting Hypochloremic hypokalemic metabolic alkalosis • Elevated blood urea nitrogen, amylase	• Fluoxetine plus CBT • Caution with bupropion due to lower seizure threshold
Binge eating disorder	• Binge eating associated with lack of control lasting >2 hours: rapid eating, excessive eating when not hungry, eating due to embarrassment, eating until one is excessively full • At least once a week for >3 months • No compensatory behavior • Significant anxiety and distress after binge eating	• Significantly elevated BMI with associated complications (hypertension, diabetes, obstructive sleep apnea)	• CBT • Diet and exercise • Targeted weight loss pharmacotherapy: topiramate, orlistat, phentermine

Do not confuse obesity due to poor diet and sedentary lifestyle with binge eating, as most obese people do not have binge eating disorder.

IMPULSE CONTROL DISORDERS

Pyromania
- Definition/symptomatology
  - More than one episode of purposeful fire setting preceded by anxiety and followed by gratification after setting fire
  - No secondary gain from fire setting (such as monetary gain, anger, recognition, or vengeance)
  - Will often have a criminal record
  - Behavior cannot be explained by another underlying disorder (mania, conduct disorder, antisocial personality disorder)
- Management: no clear treatment, combination of CBT, SSRIs, and mood stabilizers

Intermittent Explosive Disorder
- Definition/symptomatology
  - Recurrent episodes of anger toward people, property, or animals disproportionate to the inciting etiology
  - Episodes occur more than twice per week for three months without physical damage or more than three episodes per year resulting in physical damage
  - Behavioral outbursts are not premeditated with no goal for secondary gain
  - Aggressive behavior not explained by another psychiatric disorder (mania, psychosis, medications)
- Management: CBT plus SSRI

Kleptomania
- Definition/symptomatology
  - Inability to resist stealing objects
  - Objects stolen are not for monetary or personal reasons
  - High anxiety and tension prior to theft, followed by relief after committing theft
  - Theft is not used to express ideology, anger, gain recognition, or vengeance
  - Stolen objects are often returned or thrown away
  - Behavior not explained by another disorder or motive (shoplifting, mania, psychosis, antisocial personality disorder)
- Management: CBT plus SSRI

For most anxiety or anxiety-related disorders, a selective serotonin reuptake inhibitor or serotonin and norepinephrine reuptake inhibitor is the first-line pharmacologic treatment, and cognitive-behavioral therapy is the first-line nonpharmacologic treatment. More often, nonpharmacologic treatment is preferred over pharmacologic.

CHAPTER 65 Dissociation

Principles of dissociative disorders:
- Typically occurs after a significant traumatic event, especially in childhood or after chronic trauma
- Thought to be a coping mechanism for traumatic event
- Mainstay of treatment is psychotherapy +/– pharmacotherapy to treat underlying anxiety disorder

Depersonalization/Derealization Disorder
- Definition/symptomatology
  - Sensation that one is removed/detached from own surrounding and thought processes
  - Sensation of feeling like one is "watching oneself," similar to an out-of-body experience
  - Sensation that one's reality is not actually happening
  - Déjà vu feeling that you have already seen a place that you have never been before
  - Jamais vu: feeling like you have never seen a place even though it is a place where you have been or seen before
- Management: cognitive-behavioral therapy (CBT)

Dissociative Amnesia
- Definition/symptomatology
  - Memory loss of autobiographic information following traumatic event
  - Far away, unexpected travel from home
- Management
  - Ensure patient safety
  - CBT
  - Remove patient from traumatic environment

Dissociative Identity Disorder
- Definition/symptomatology
  - Two or more personalities in different environments
  - Overlap with other dissociative disorders
  - Inability to recall traumatic event or autobiographic information
- Management: CBT +/– selective serotonin reuptake inhibitor (treat underlying anxiety disorder)

CHAPTER 66 Pediatric Psychiatry

ADHD differential diagnosis:
   Absence seizures
   Lead poisoning
   Oppositional defiant disorder
   Depression

Attention-Deficit/Hyperactivity Disorder (ADHD)
- Risk factors
  - Males
  - Family history
  - Preterm birth
- Signs and symptoms
  - Difficulty focusing
  - Impulsivity
  - Hyperactivity
  - Easily distracting
  - Inattentiveness
- Diagnostic criteria
  - Symptoms not explained by other causes
  - Symptomatology onset <12 years old
  - Symptomatology in more than one setting
  - Symptomatology resulting in impaired functioning
- Management
  - Preschool: behavioral modification
  - School age: pharmacologic
    - Stimulant medications: first line
      - Methylphenidate
      - Dexamphetamine
    - Nonstimulant medications
      - Atomoxetine
      - Alpha-adrenergic (clonidine, guanfacine)

Tourette Syndrome

Side effects of stimulant medications: decreased appetite, weight loss, insomnia, hypertension, tachycardia, decreased growth velocity, and transient tics

- Definition: anxiety disorder characterized by involuntary motor and vocal tics
- Signs and symptoms
  - Involuntary motor tics
    - Head shaking
    - Eye blinking
    - Jumping, kicking
  - Involuntary vocal tics
    - Throat clearing
    - Coughing
    - Echolalia (repetition of words or phrases)
    - Coprolalia (repetitive use of foul language)

- Diagnostic criteria
  - Symptomatology not explained by another disorder
  - Two or more motor tics
  - One or more vocal tics
  - Tics lasting >1 year duration
  - Tics occurring <18 years old
- Associations
  - ADHD
  - Obsessive-compulsive disorder
- Management
  - Mild: no treatment
  - Moderate to severe
    - Habitat reversal training
    - Tetrabenazine
    - Botulinum toxin
    - Alpha-adrenergic agents (clonidine, guanfacine)

Autism Spectrum Disorder
- Definition/symptomatology
  - Repetitive and restricted behaviors
  - Excessive interest in inanimate objects
  - Strict adherence to rituals
  - Repetitive motor movements
  - Impaired social and emotional reciprocity
  - Deficits in communication
  - Lack of interest in relationships
  - Neuropsychiatric abnormalities present in early development
- Management: early intervention with multidisciplinary team (speech therapists, behavioral therapists, special educational programs)

Separation Anxiety Disorder
- Epidemiology: 1–3 years old
- Definition/symptomatology
  - Excessive anxiety during separation from loved one
  - Persistent worry about losing major attachment figure
  - Fear of leaving home, going to school, work or being alone
  - Separation results in physical symptoms such as panic attacks, nausea, vomiting and abdominal pain
  - Last >4 weeks in children, >6 months in adults
- Management: family therapy, cognitive-behavioral therapy

Combative Disorders

Oppositional Defiant Disorder
- Definition/symptomatology: four of the following for >6 months toward more than one individual who is not a sibling
  - Easily angered, irritable mood, hostile
  - Constantly breaking rules
  - Arguing and disobedient toward authority figures (parents, teachers)
  - Spiteful
  - Blames and annoys others
- Management: behavioral modification

Conduct Disorder
- Definition/symptomatology: more than three of the following behaviors over the last 12 months with at least one occurring in the past 6 months
  - Disruptive and combative behavior that violates the rights of other humans and animals through physical and sexual means
  - Bullying and intimidation of others
  - Physical and emotional harm inflicted
  - Destruction of property
  - Stay out late at night, absent from school
  - Theft and deceitfulness
  - No remorse for their actions
- Management: behavioral modification

Digestion and Elimination

Enuresis
- Definition
  - Continued urinary continence beyond expected age of development
  - >4 years old for daytime incontinence
  - >5 years old for nocturnal incontinence
- Risk factors
  - Males
  - Family history
  - Psychosocial stressors (abuse, birth of a new sibling, starting school, family death)
  - Constipation (large stool burden compresses and irritates bladder)
  - Diabetes insipidus/mellitus
  - Seizures
  - Obstructive sleep apnea
- Diagnostics: workup organic and psychosocial etiology
  - Thorough history and physical exam: stressors, family history, neurologic exam
  - Urinalysis
- Management
  - Treat underlying secondary causes
  - Nonpharmacologic
    - Reassurance if patient is still younger than expected age for continence
    - Nighttime enuresis alarm: first line
    - Motivational and reward system
    - Limit nighttime fluid intake
    - Voiding before bedtime
    - Bladder training (timed avoiding)
  - Pharmacologic: only short-term use
    - DDAVP (decreases urine volume)
    - Tricyclic antidepressants (TCAs)

Encopresis
- Definition: fecal incontinence >4 years old
- Risk factors
  - Chronic constipation (overflow incontinence, retentive encopresis)
  - Psychosocial stressors
  - Intellectual disability
  - Hirschsprung disease
  - Spinal cord abnormalities
- Diagnostics
  - Digital rectal exam
  - Abdominal x-ray
- Management
  - Nonretentive: positive reinforcement, behavioral intervention
  - Retentive
    - Positive reinforcement, behavioral intervention
    - Stool softeners
    - Disimpaction

Rumination
- Continuous regurgitation and reswallowing food
- Associated with intellectual disability, institutionalized, and psychosocial stressors
- Manage through behavior modification and reinforcing proper eating habits

Parasomnias

Nightmares and night terrors have similar presentations; however, they are differentiated based on patient recollection of the events the next morning as they occur in different stages of sleep (Table 66-1).

Narcolepsy
- Definition: rapid eye movement (REM)–related sleep disorder resulting in decreased REM latency and extension of REM sleep physiology into the awake state
- Epidemiology
  - Onset occurs during adolescence and early adulthood
  - Increased incidence in families
- Pathophysiology: decreased hypocretin (orexin) production from the lateral hypothalamus

TABLE 66-1   Nightmares Versus Night Terrors

	NIGHTMARES	NIGHT TERRORS
Signs and symptoms	• Frightening dream • Nighttime arousal • Vivid recall of events	• Nighttime arousal with sudden screaming and shaking • No recall of events
Stage of sleep	• Rapid eye movement	• Slow-wave sleep (stage IV)
Diagnostics	• Clinical	
Treatment	• No treatment, self-resolves	• No treatment, self-resolves • Safety precautions

- Signs and symptoms
  - Excessive daytime sleepiness
  - Cataplexy: sudden loss of muscle tone following stimulus (laughter, stress, loud sounds, flashing lights)
  - Hypnogogic hallucinations: visual or auditory hallucinations before sleep
  - Hypnopompic hallucinations: visual or auditory hallucinations before awakening
  - Sleep paralysis: inability to move upon awakening due to extended REM sleep (brain is awake, but body is asleep)
  - Vivid dreams
- Diagnosis
  - Daytime multiple sleep latency test
    - Test that measures the amount of time to onset of sleep during five 20-minute daytime napping episodes
    - Shortened sleep latency (<8 minutes to fall asleep) and at least two REM episodes during the five naps
    - Symptoms must be present for >3 months
  - Overnight polysomnography: normal, but may reveal sleep fragmentation
- Management: behavioral modification plus pharmacologic
  - Behavior modification
    - Maintain good sleep hygiene
    - Scheduled naps: prevents sleep attacks
    - Sufficient sleep duration
  - Pharmacologic
    - Modafinil (dopamine agonist), armodafinil
    - Other stimulants: amphetamines, methylphenidate, pemoline
    - Cataplexy prophylaxis: TCAs, sodium oxybate

CHAPTER
67 Personality Disorders

Personality disorders are a group of psychiatric disorders that results in abnormal patterns of thinking and behavior. These are often present since childhood and, thus, are difficult to treat. These behaviors are pervasive throughout all aspects of the patient's life (Table 67-1).

TABLE 67-1   Types of Personality Disorders and Key Manifestations

CLASS OF PERSONALITY DISORDER	TYPE OF PERSONALITY DISORDER	KEY FEATURES
Class A	Paranoid	• Suspicious and mistrust of others • Emotionless • Believe others are conspiring against them
	Schizoid	• Emotionally and socially detached • Avoid intimacy • Interested only in own thoughts and feelings
	Schizotypal	• Magical beliefs and thought processes • Eccentric behaviors • Perceived as being "weird"
Class B	Borderline	• Drastic mood swings going from extremely positive to extremely negative; associated with splitting defense mechanism • Sensitive to abandonment • May threaten suicidal behaviors (wrist cutting)
	Histrionic	• Exaggerated behavior to be the center of attention (bright, revealing clothes) • Seductive and flirtatious behavior • Perceive shallow relationships to be more involved than they actually are
	Antisocial	• Criminal activities that violate human and animal rights • Lack remorse for their behavior regardless of the consequence • Lie and deceit for personal gain
	Narcissistic	• Perceive themselves to be much more important than they actually are • Grandiose characterization of their success • Expects special treatment, admiration, and attention
Class C	Obsessive-compulsive	• Concerned with rules, orderliness, and perfectionism • Highly inflexible and bureaucratic • Detail oriented to the point that it results in difficult relationships and missing deadlines due to loss of the bigger picture
	Avoidant	• Avoid social situations due to fear of inadequacy • Hypersensitivity to criticism • Low self-esteem, overly self-conscious, and highly self-critical
	Dependent	• Excessive need to be taken care of ("clingy") and fear of abandonment • Agree with all decisions to avoid confrontation • Lower initiative, ask permission for all decisions

Personality disorders are divided into class A, B, and C, which have roughly similar characteristics as other personality disorders in the same class.

Definitions
- Dependence: requiring the drug to function normally
- Tolerance: requiring increased dose to achieve the desired effect
- Withdrawal: symptoms that occur after stopping or reducing dose of substance after prolonged or heavy usage

Alcohol
- Mechanism: increases central nervous system (CNS) gamma-aminobutyric acid (GABA) levels
- Signs and symptoms
  - Intoxication
    - Depressed mental status
    - Social disinhibition
    - Slurred speech
  - Withdrawal
    - Tremors
    - Seizures
    - Hallucinations
    - Delirium tremens
- Management
  - Withdrawal (Table 68-1)
    - IV benzodiazepine
    - Banana bag (multivitamin bag including vitamins B1, B9, and B12) prior to giving glucose to prevent Wernicke encephalopathy
  - Maintenance
    - Naltrexone (long-acting opiate antagonist)
      - Long-acting opiate antagonist
      - Decreases desire and pleasure associated with drinking alcohol
    - Acamprosate
      - Glutamate modulator
      - Used to prevent relapse
    - Disulfiram
      - Alcohol dehydrogenase inhibitor
      - Buildup of acetaldehyde results in nausea, vomiting, and flushing

Wernicke encephalopathy triad:
- Ocular dysfunction
- Ataxia
- Confusion

Korsacoff psychosis = Wernicke encephalopathy plus confabulation

Opiates
- Mechanism: CNS opioid agonist
- Signs and symptoms

TABLE 68-1   Timeline of Alcohol Withdrawal Symptomatology

TIMING	SYMPTOMS
0–24 hour(s)	Tremors, irritability
24–48 hours	Seizures, headache
48–96 hours	Delirium tremens

- Intoxication
  - Respiratory depression
  - Altered mental status
  - Pinpoint pupils
- Withdrawal
  - Nausea, vomiting
  - Abdominal pain
  - Headache
  - Diaphoresis
  - Lacrimation
- Management
  - Intoxication: naloxone
  - Withdrawal
    - Methadone (partial opioid agonist)
    - Clonidine (reduces adrenergic symptoms)

Amphetamines
- Mechanism: prevents reuptake of norepinephrine and dopamine
- Signs and symptoms
  - Intoxication
    - Hypertension, tachycardia
    - Hyperthermia
    - Prolonged psychosis
    - Agitation
    - Mydriasis
    - Euphoria
  - Withdrawal
    - Increased appetite
    - Depression, suicidal
    - Anxiety
- Management
  - Intoxication
    - Benzodiazepine
    - Avoid beta blockers: will result in unopposed alpha-agonist action
  - Withdrawal
    - Assess seriousness of suicidal ideation: determine if patient will require involuntary hospitalization
    - Selective serotonin reuptake inhibitors

Phencyclidine
- Mechanism: N-methyl-D-aspartate receptor antagonist
- Signs and symptoms: only intoxication, no significant withdrawal symptoms
  - Extreme combativeness
  - Agitation
  - Nystagmus
  - Hyperacusis
  - Synesthesia
- Management
  - Place patient in a dark room: decreases sensory stimulation
  - Benzodiazepines or antipsychotics: controls agitation

Benzodiazepine/Barbiturates
- Mechanism: increases duration and frequency of chloride opening channel, which potentiates GABA effect
- Signs and symptoms
  - Intoxication
    - Lethargy
    - Ataxia
    - Slurred speech
    - Respiratory depression: more common with barbiturates or when combined with other sedative drugs (alcohol, opioids)
  - Withdrawal
    - Tremors
    - Seizures
- Management
  - Respiratory support
  - Taper with long-acting benzodiazepine
  - Flumazenil: reversal agent with potential to cause withdrawal seizures

Nicotine
- Mechanism: stimulates nicotinic receptors in the autonomic ganglia and increases CNS dopamine
- Sources
  - Cigarette smoking
  - Chewing tobacco
- Signs and symptoms
  - Intoxication: ingested through cigarette smoking
    - Anxiety
    - Insomnia
    - Diarrhea
    - Suppressed appetite
  - Withdrawal
    - Difficulty concentration
    - Increased appetite
    - Weight gain
    - Intense craving
- Management: focused on decreasing dependence
  - Varenicline
    - Partial nicotinic cholinergic receptor agonist
    - Reduces "high" and euphoria
    - Decreases withdrawal symptoms
    - Associated with abnormal dreams and increased suicidality
  - Bupropion
    - Norepinephrine and dopamine reuptake inhibitor
    - Reduces cravings
    - Decreases seizure threshold in anorexic and bulimics
  - Nicotine replacement: administered as lozenge, patch, or gum

Caffeine
- Mechanism: methylxanthine, which acts as an adenosine antagonist and increases release of catecholamines
- Sources
  - Coffee
  - Soft drinks
  - Chocolate
- Signs and symptoms
  - Intoxication
    - Increased arousal
    - Mild euphoria
    - Insomnia
    - Jitteriness
  - Withdrawal
    - Headache
    - Difficulty concentrating

- Nausea, vomiting
- Depressed mood
  - Management: slow tapering of caffeine doses

Marijuana
  - Mechanism: cannabinoid receptor agonist
  - Signs and symptoms
    - Intoxication
      - Conjunctival injection
      - Increased appetite (munchies)
      - Perceptual disturbance
      - Impaired time perception
      - Mild euphoria
    - Withdrawal
      - Anxiety
      - Irritability
      - Headache
      - Insomnia
      - Decreased appetite
  - Management: supportive care

Hallucinogens (LSD)
  - Mechanism: serotonergic agonist
  - Signs and symptoms: only intoxication, no significant withdrawal symptoms
    - Hallucinations
    - Dissociation
    - Mydriasis
    - Synesthesia ("hear" colors, "see" tastes)
    - Impaired judgment
    - Diaphoresis, dehydration
  - Management: supportive care +/− benzodiazepine or antipsychotics for agitation

Inhalants
  - Mechanism: varies depending on the type of inhalant; CNS depression
  - Sources: products easily accessible to young and preadolescents
    - Paint
    - Solvent
    - Glucose
    - Cleaning products
  - Signs and symptoms: only intoxication, no significant withdrawal symptoms
    - Slurred speech
    - Ataxia
    - Euphoria, psychosis
    - Impaired coordination
    - Respiratory depression
  - Management: supportive care

Fibromyalgia
- Epidemiology: involved in young to middle-aged women associated with other medicopsychiatric conditions (migraines, irritable bowel syndrome, chronic pain syndrome)
- Signs and symptoms
  - Chronic musculoskeletal pain involving tenderness of the trigger points (11 of 18 involved; trapezius, medial knee, lateral epicondyle) (Fig. 69-1)
  - Numbness, stiffness
  - Generalized fatigue, weakness
  - Nonrestorative sleep
- Diagnostic
  - Clinical
  - Diagnosis of exclusion
- Management
  - Lifestyle modifications
    - Relaxation, yoga
    - Regular exercise
    - Good sleep hygiene
  - Pharmacotherapy
    - Tricyclic antidepressants (amitriptyline)
    - Gamma-aminobutyric acid agonists: pregabalin, gabapentin
    - Serotonin and norepinephrine reuptake inhibitors: milnacipran, duloxetine
  - Cognitive behavioral therapy

Gender Identity Disorder
- Definition: difference in association between biological sex and identified gender
- Symptomatology/diagnosis
  - Distress between biological sex and identified gender
  - Desire and attempt to change primary and secondary sex characteristics
  - Desire to be treated and viewed as the other gender
- Management
  - Validate patients' feelings and desire to be of the other gender
  - Surgical and hormonal sex change

Sex: biological difference between males and females
Gender: how individuals see themselves in terms of societal roles

Paraphilias: abnormal and/or inappropriate means to obtain sexual satisfaction lasting >6 months and causing impairment of functioning
- Pedophilia: fantasies involving prepubescent children; most common paraphilia
- Voyeurism: fantasy involving watching others engage in sexual activity and undressing
- Exhibitionism: urge to expose oneself to others
- Masochism: fantasy that involves being humiliated and abused by sexual partner
- Sadism: fantasy whereby physical or psychological dominance results in sexual pleasure
- Frotteurism: behavior whereby pleasure is achieved by inappropriately touching or rubbing unsuspecting partner

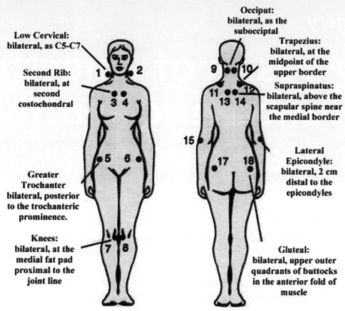

Figure 69-1: Fibromyalgia's 18 tender points

CHAPTER 70 Basics of Anesthesia and Perioperative Medicine

PREOPERATIVE ASSESSMENT

Preoperative assessment is used to determine risk of intraoperative and postoperative complications (Tables 70-1, 70-2, and 70-3). Patient comorbidities and type of surgery both play a role in intraoperative and postoperative outcomes. Higher risk surgeries are highly vascular (substantial risk for blood loss) and require prolonged anesthesia such as abdominal aortic aneurysm repairs and coronary artery bypass graft. Lower risk surgeries are relatively avascular and require minimal anesthesia such as cataract surgery (Table 70-4).

POSTOPERATIVE ASSESSMENT/COMPLICATIONS

Anesthetic Complications

Methemoglobinemia
- Pathophysiology: oxidation of Fe^{2+} to Fe^{3+} resulting in decreased oxygen delivery to peripheral tissues
- Causes
  - Local anesthetics (bupivacaine, benzocaine)
  - Silver nitrate
  - Amyl nitrate
  - Nitroglycerin
  - Dapsone
- Signs and symptoms
  - Cyanosis with normal PaO_2
  - Headaches, dizziness
  - Confusion, seizures
- Diagnostics
  - Elevated methemoglobin levels
  - Chocolate brown blood
- Management: methylene blue

Malignant Hyperthermia
- Causes
  - Halothane
  - Succinylcholine
- Sign and symptoms
  - High fever, >40°C
  - Muscle rigidity
  - Hemodynamic instability
- Diagnostics
  - Clinical
  - Supporting labs
    - Hypercalcemia
    - Hypercalcemia
    - Elevated creatine kinase
- Management
  - Cooling blankets
  - IV dantrolene
  - Correction of acidosis
  - IV fluids

TABLE 70-1   Organ System Approach to Perioperative Medicine

ORGAN SYSTEM	SPECIAL CONSIDERATIONS
Pulmonary	• Increased risk with smoking • Advise to quit smoking and respiratory therapy eight weeks prior to elective procedure • FEV1 is predictive of postoperative pulmonary reserve
Cardiovascular	• General anesthetics decrease inotropy and increase ectopy • Reversible perfusion abnormalities on myocardial perfusion scan predict perioperative risk of cardiac ischemia • Ejection fraction <35% greatly increases risk of mortality • Evaluate for jugular vein distention, recent myocardial infarction (MI), ventricular arrhythmias, valvular disease; optimize medical management with angiotensin-converting enzyme inhibitors, beta blockers, diuretics prior to proceeding • Defer surgery, if possible, for six months after MI
Gastrointestinal/ nutritional	• Sequelae of liver failure (coagulopathy, hypoalbuminemia, hyperbilirubinemia, ascites, and encephalopathy) is associated with significantly increased risk • Severe malnutrition is associated with increased risk; if possible, provide preoperative nutrition (enteral > parenteral) for 1–2 weeks
Endocrine	• Diabetic ketoacidosis: provide adequate IV fluid resuscitation and correction of electrolyte abnormalities • Diabetes and hyperglycemia increase risk of postoperative infections and difficulty with wound healing

TABLE 70-2   Causes of Postoperative Fever

CAUSES	TIMING	KEY MANIFESTATIONS	MANAGEMENT
Malignant hyperthermia	Shortly after initiation of anesthesia	• Hyperthermia >40°C • Muscle rigidity • Metabolic acidosis, hypercalcemia, elevated creatine kinase	• Cessation of anesthesia • 100% oxygen • Cooling blankets • IV dantrolene • Correction of acidosis
Atelectasis	24 hours postoperative	• Asymptomatic	• Pulmonary toilet: incentive spirometry, respiratory therapy • Adequate pain control • Bronchoscopy is last resort
Pneumonia	1–3 days postoperative	• Cough, fever, new infiltrates on chest x-ray	• Antibiotics: treat as hospital-acquired pneumonia (cover pseudomonas and methicillin-resistant *Staphylococcus aureus*)
Urinary tract infection	3–5 days postoperative	• Suprapubic tenderness • Burning with urination • Fever	• Remove indwelling catheter if still present • Antibiotics covering *Escherichia coli*
Deep vein thrombosis	>5 days postoperative	• Unilateral lower extremity tenderness/erythema	• Lower extremity venous Doppler • Anticoagulation • Encourage early ambulation and compression stockings
Surgical site infection	1–2 weeks postoperative	• Surgical site erythema, edema, tenderness, and drainage	• Ultrasound to evaluate for underlying abscess • Antibiotics • I&D or percutaneous drainage if abscess is identified

Increased risk of malignant hyperthermia in patients with ryanodine gene mutation, autosomal dominant mutation.

Propofol-Related Infusion Syndrome
- Cause: prolonged, high doses of propofol infusion
- Key manifestations
  • Hypertriglyceridemia
  • Rhabdomyolysis
  • Metabolic acidosis

- Bradycardia
- Vascular collapse
- Renal failure
  - Management: stop infusion, supportive care

TABLE 70-3 Postoperative Complications by System

ORGAN SYSTEM	CAUSES	KEY MANIFESTATIONS	MANAGEMENT
Neurologic	Delirium tremens	• Altered mental status • Hypertension, tachycardia • Hallucinations	• IV benzodiazepines
Pulmonary	Pulmonary embolism	• Acute onset shortness of breath • Pleuritic chest pain • Hypoxia, tachycardia	• Computed tomography pulmonary angiogram or lower extremity venous Doppler • Anticoagulation, early ambulation • Inferior vena cava filter if contraindication to anticoagulation
	Tension pneumothorax	• Increasingly difficult bag mask ventilation • Decrease in blood pressure; increase in central venous pressure and jugular vein distention	• Needle decompression followed by chest tube
	Aspiration pneumonitis	• Vomiting during intubation	• NPO prior to procedure • Bronchoalveolar lavage
Cardiovascular	Perioperative myocardial infarction	• Chest pain • Elevated troponin • ST elevation	• Percutaneous intervention
Gastrointestinal	Postoperative ileus	• Abdominal distention • No pain • Absent bowel sounds	• Observation • Treat electrolyte abnormalities such as hypokalemia
	Mechanical bowel obstruction	• Abdominal x-ray with dilated loops and air fluid levels • Abdominal pain/distention • Tinkling bowel sounds	• Decompression with nasogastric tube • Bowel rest • +/− surgical intervention for lysis of adhesions
	Fistulas	• Connection of bowel with bowel, bladder, vagina, or skin; fecal material will come out with the connecting organ	• Fistulotomy • Treat/remove aggravating agents such as foreign bodies, epithelialization, tumors, infection, irradiated tissue, inflammatory bowel disease, or obstruction
Genitourinary	Postoperative urinary retention	• Sensation to void, however unable • Suprapubic fullness	• Early ambulation • Bladder scan +/− catheterization • Indwelling catheter after multiple catheterizations
Renal	Electrolyte derangements (sodium, calcium, glucose)	• Altered mental status • Lethargy • Paresthesias (hypocalcemia)	• Treat metabolic derangements
Dermatology	Surgical site infections	• Erythema, edema, tenderness, and fever seven days postoperative	• Antibiotics +/− abscess drainage
	Wound dehiscence	• Leakage of copious serosanguineous fluid from the wound; represents peritoneal fluid mixed with blood	• Tight wound packing • Surgical repair
	Wound evisceration	• Extrusion of abdominal contents from a wound dehiscence secondary to increased intraabdominal pressure (coughing, getting out of bed)	• Cover abdominal contents with sterile dressing and saline followed by emergent repair

TABLE 70-4   Anesthetic Pharmacology

	EXAMPLES	MECHANISM OF ACTION	ADVERSE EFFECTS
Inhaled anesthetics	• Halothane • Sevoflurane • Methoxyflurane • Isoflurane	• Enhancement of inhibitory channels and attenuation of excitatory channels	• Malignant hyperthermia • Hepatotoxicity • Decreased cerebral blood flow • Myocardial depression
IV anesthetics	• Barbiturates: phenobarbital, thiopental	• GABA modulator by increasing duration of chloride channel opening	• CNS depressant • Drug interactions • Contraindicated in porphyria
	• Benzodiazepines: midazolam, lorazepam, diazepam	• GABA modulator by increasing frequency of chloride channel opening	• Risk of dependence • Respiratory depression; however, less compared to barbiturates
	• Propofol	• GABA agonist	• Propofol-related infusion syndrome
	• Fentanyl • Morphine	• Opioid agonist	• Respiratory depression • Allergic reaction
	• Ketamine	• NMDA antagonist	• Increased cerebral blood flow, intracranial hypertension • Disorientation, hallucinations, abnormal dreams
Local anesthetics	• Amides: lidocaine, bupivacaine • Esters: procaine, tetracaine	• Inhibition of activated sodium channels	• Methemoglobinemia (benzocaine, bupivacaine) • Arrhythmias • Allergic reaction (no cross reactivity between amides and esters)
Neuromuscular blockers	• Depolarizing: succinylcholine • Nondepolarizing: rocuronium, vecuronium	• Inhibition of nicotinic receptors	• Malignant hyperthermia • Hyperkalemia • Hypercalcemia

CNS, Central nervous system; *GABA,* gamma-aminobutyric acid; *NMDA,* N-methyl-D-aspartate

Airway Management
- Types of airways
  - Orotracheal: most common
  - Nasotracheal
  - Tracheostomy
- Indications for intubation
  - Altered mental status (Glasgow Coma Scale <8): most common
  - Severe hypoxemia/hypercarbia (i.e., chronic obstructive pulmonary disease exacerbation, congestive heart failure exacerbation, pneumonia) unresponsive to noninvasive ventilation
  - Airway protection: hematemesis, hemoptysis
- Goals
  - Oxygenation: increase FiO_2 and/or positive end-expiratory pressure
  - Ventilation: increase respiratory rate and/or tidal volume
  - Airway protection
- Indications for extubation: underlying reason for intubation has been addressed
  - Improved oxygenation and ventilation
  - Improved mentation

SHOCK
Shock is defined as a state of inadequate oxygenation due to an insult resulting in increased metabolic demands or disruption of normal homeostatic pathways. In response, there are several mechanisms the body employs to restore homeostasis (Table 71-1; Figs. 71-1 and 71-2).

Types of Shock
- Distributive
  - Examples
    - Sepsis
    - Anaphylaxis
  - Pathophysiology: massive vasodilation resulting in third spacing of fluid → high flow state with decreased time for capillaries to extract oxygen from blood → increased heart rate to maintain blood pressure
  - Management
    - Sepsis: IV fluids +/− vasopressors
    - Anaphylaxis: intramuscular norepinephrine
- Cardiogenic
  - Examples
    - Myocardial infarction
    - Valvular disease
  - Pathophysiology: cardiac dysfunction results in decreased cardiac output → low blood pressure and low flow states result in increased time for capillaries to extract oxygen from blood; backup of blood into the pulmonary circuit resulting in pulmonary venous hypertension and pulmonary edema → systemic vasoconstriction and increased heart rate to maintain blood pressure
  - Management
    - Dual antiplatelet
    - Cardiac catheterization
    - Ionotropes (dobutamine, milrinone)
    - Valvular repair
    - Diuresis
    - IV fluids only for right ventricular infarction

TABLE 71-1   Interpreting Shock

TYPES OF SHOCK	CARDIAC INDEX	SYSTEMIC VASCULAR RESISTANCE	PULMONARY CAPILLARY WEDGE PRESSURE (PCWP)	HEART RATE	MIXED VENOUS OXYGEN SATURATION
Distributive	Increased	Decreased	Normal	Increased	Increased
Cardiogenic	Decreased	Increased	Increased	Increased	Decreased
Hypovolemic	Normal/increased	Increased	Low	Increased	Decreased
Obstructive	Decreased	Increased	Increased	Increased	Decreased
Neurogenic	Normal/decreased	Decreased	Normal/increased	Normal/decreased	Normal/decreased

PCWP is a measurement of left atrial pressure.
Cardiac index = cardiac output/body surface area

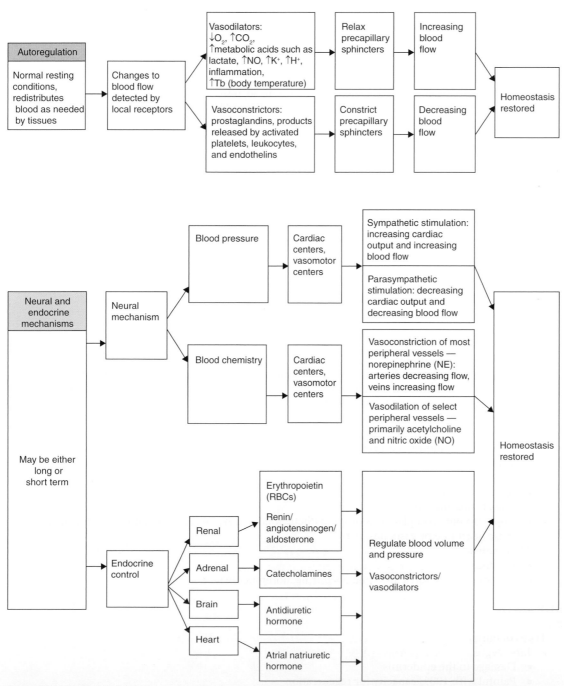

Figure 71-1: Normal regulatory mechanisms for maintaining blood pressure. *RBCs,* Red blood cells. (Image courtesy of OpenStax College.)

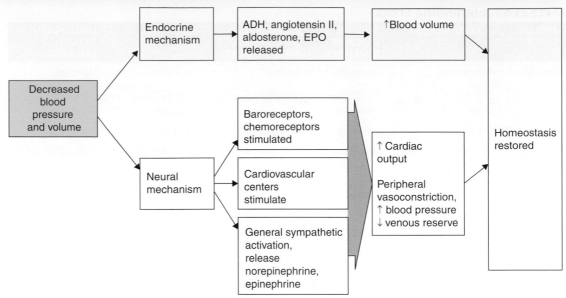

Figure 71-2: Regulatory endocrine and neural mechanisms in response to low blood pressure and volume. *ADH*, Antidiuretic hormone; *EPO*, erythropoietin. (Image courtesy of OpenStax College.)

- Hypovolemic
  - Examples
    - Dehydration (vomiting, diarrhea)
    - Hemorrhage
  - Pathophysiology: low intravascular volume → low flow states and increased time for capillaries to extract oxygen from blood → increased cardiac output, systemic vascular resistance, and heart rate to maintain blood pressure
  - Management
    - IV fluids
    - Blood transfusion if hemoglobin <7
- Obstructive
  - Examples
    - Pericardial tamponade
    - Tension pneumothorax
  - Pathophysiology: physical obstruction to cardiac output → low blood pressure and low flow state results in increased time the capillaries to extract oxygen → increased heart rate and systemic vascular resistance to maintain blood pressure
  - Management
    - Pericardial tamponade: pericardiocentesis
    - Tension pneumothorax: needle decompression followed by chest tube
- Neurogenic
  - Examples
    - Spinal cord injury
    - Spinal cord anesthesia
  - Pathophysiology: complete loss of sympathetic tone → peripheral vasodilation and inability to increase heart rate or vasoconstrict
  - Management
    - IV fluids
    - Systemic vasoconstrictors (phenylephrine, norepinephrine)

BURNS
Burns
- Types of burns
  - First degree
    - Damage to the epidermis
    - Painful with 100% capacity for regeneration
    - Example: sunburn

- Second degree
  - Damage to the epidermis and partial dermis
  - Less painful than first degree due to some nerve damage
  - Examples: blisters
- Third degree
  - Full-thickness damage to epidermis and dermis
  - 0% capacity for generation, will require skin graft
  - Painless due to extensive nerve damage, white/charred appearance
  - Examples: eschar (will require escharotomy to prevent vascular compromise from increasing edema)
- Fourth degree
  - Involvement of muscle or bones
  - Associated with electrical burns
- Determining extent of burns
  - Body surface area (BSA) involved: calculated using rule of 9s and used to estimate how much fluid resuscitation will be required (Fig. 71-3)
  - BSA calculations
    - Head, left arm, right arm account for 9% BSA each
    - Back, chest, right leg, left leg account for 18% BSA each
    - Perineum accounts for 1% BSA
  - Parkland formula for volume resuscitation: (% BSA burned) * (weight in kilograms) * (4 mL/kg)
    - 50% of calculated volume over the first 8 hours
    - 50% of calculated volume over the next 16 hours
    - 50% of calculated volume over the following 24 hours
- Management
  - Admission/transfer to burn unit
  - Aggressive IV fluids: due to extensive fluid loss from third spacing
  - Lower threshold for intubation for burns involving the face: may be indicative of airway injury
  - Topical wound management: side effects in parentheses
    - Silver sulfadiazine (neutropenia)
    - Silver nitrate (electrolyte abnormalities, methemoglobinemia)
    - Mafenide acetate (metabolic acidosis)
  - Nutritional support: due to hypermetabolic state
  - Pain control

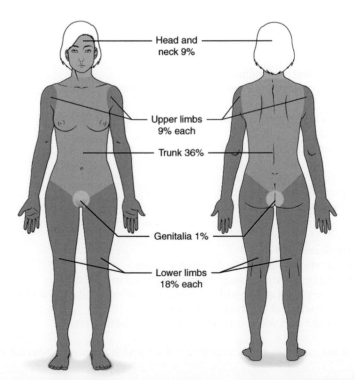

Figure 71-3: Percentage of body surface area involved in burns. (Image courtesy of OpenStax College.)

- Tetanus vaccination
- Skin grafting for third-degree burns
- Complications
  - Sepsis (most commonly from gram-negative rods)
  - Compartment syndrome: secondary to excessive IV fluid resuscitation
  - Hypovolemic shock

Other types of burns
- Chemical burn
  - Secondary to exposure to alkaline products (drainage cleaners, batteries)
  - Treat with extensive irrigation of the affected site
  - Do not neutralize the alkaline agent as it will result in an exothermic reaction and worse burns
- Electrical burn
  - Most significant damage occurs to deeper tissues such as muscle, bone, and fat; associated with fourth-degree burns
  - Extensive severe muscle contraction results in myoglobinemia/myoglobinuria, posterior shoulder dislocation, and fractures
  - Late development of cataracts

> Marjolin ulcer: previously healed extensive burns without adequate treatment resulting in chronic nonhealing ulcer and development of squamous carcinoma

TRAUMA- AND EMERGENCY-RELATED ENTITIES
Heat Stroke
- Risk factors
  - Strenuous activity in extreme heat (military recruit, athletes)
  - Elderly (decreased ability to avoid heat due to mental or physical impairment)
  - Dehydration
  - Medications (anticholinergic, antihistamines, tricyclic antidepressants)
- Pathophysiology: inadequate dissipation of heat
- Signs and symptoms
  - Altered mental status
  - Hemodynamic instability
  - Hyperthermia
  - Dehydration
- Diagnostics
  - Clinical
  - Supporting labs
    - Electrolyte derangements (sodium, potassium)
    - Elevated blood urea nitrogen/creatine, leukocytes, hemoglobin
    - Myoglobinuria
- Management: depends if it is exertional or nonexertional heat stroke
  - Exertional: ice, fluid resuscitation
  - Nonexertional: water spraying, fanning
- Complications
  - Acute respiratory distress syndrome
  - Disseminated intravascular coagulation
  - Multiorgan dysfunction
  - Seizures

Management of traumatic amputation:
1. Amputated limb is wrapped and placed in sterile gauze.
2. Sterile gauze should be moistened with saline and placed in a plastic bag.
3. Plastic bag should be placed on ice without freezing to allow for maximal viability and increased opportunity for reattachment and reimplantation.
4. Order of repair should start with bone, vasculature, and lastly nerves.

Motor vehicle accident associations: specific entities are discussed in surgical subspecialties
- Neurologic
  - Traumatic brain injury
  - Epidural/subdural hematoma

- Diffuse axonal injury
- Coup contrecoup injury
- Concussions
- Pulmonary
  - Pulmonary contusion
  - Pneumothorax
  - Flail chest
- Cardiac
  - Aortic transection/dissection
  - Myocardial contusion
- Gastrointestinal/genitourinary
  - Intraabdominal bleeding
  - Rupture of hollow viscus
  - Bladder rupture

Crush Injury
- Extensive muscle damage (elevated creatine kinase, hyperkalemia)
- Myoglobinemia/myoglobinuria resulting in renal failure
- Treat with aggressive IV fluid
- May be complicated by compartment syndrome of the crushed limb requiring fasciotomy

Drowning
- Hypoxemia from immersion in water; different manifestations occur depending if immersion was in fresh water or saltwater
- Fresh water immersion: hypotonic fluid results in decreased electrolyte levels and red blood cell lysis
- Saltwater immersion: hypertonic fluid draws fluid into the alveoli resulting in pulmonary edema
- Both types result in lung damage and cerebral hypoxia
- Management is supplemental oxygen +/− airway protection

Choking
- Airway aspiration
  - Aspiration of foreign body into an airway; most commonly the right mainstem bronchus due to a less acute branching angle
  - Diagnosed based on history in adults, and sudden onset of wheezing and respiratory distress in young children
  - Chest x-ray is used to identify location, bronchoscopy for retrieval
- Esophageal obstruction
  - Choking can also occur with obstruction of the esophagus
  - If coughing, encourage the patient to continue to cough
  - If patient is not coughing and unable to breathe, perform the Heimlich maneuver
  - May require emergent tracheostomy

Diffuse Axonal Injury
- Pathophysiology: acceleration-deceleration injury resulting in shearing of axons at the grey-white matter junction
- Signs and symptoms
  - Altered mental status
  - Headache, visual disturbances
  - Loss of consciousness, coma
- Diagnostics: computed tomography/magnetic resonance imaging (small hemorrhages with obscuration of the grey-white matter junction)
- Management: lower intracranial pressure to prevent further injury

CHAPTER
72 Neurosurgery

BRAIN BLEED
Intracranial hemorrhage can involve many different spaces of the brain, such as subdural, epidural, subarachnoid, or intraparenchymal (Figs 72-1 and 72-2). Each of these produces a unique set of imaging findings and potential complications (Table 72-1).

Intracranial Hemorrhage
- Risk factors
  - Hypertension
  - Cerebral amyloid angiopathy
  - Atriovenous (AV) malformations
  - Coagulopathy
- Signs and symptoms
  - Headache
  - Nausea, vomiting
  - Altered consciousness
  - Focal neurologic deficits (exact deficits depend on location of hemorrhage)
- Diagnostics: noncontrast computed tomography (CT)
- Management
  - General
    - Lower intracranial pressure: elevate head of bed +/− osmotic diuretics (hypertonic saline, mannitol)
    - Lower blood pressure to 140 mm Hg
    - Anticonvulsants if patient develop seizures
  - Specific
    - AV malformation: coiling/embolization
    - Coagulopathy: reversal with vitamin K and fresh frozen plasma
    - Cerebellar hemorrhage, >3 cm: surgical decompression
    - Intraventricular extension with hydrocephalus: ventriculostomy

Pituitary Apoplexy
- Pathophysiology: untreated pituitary adenoma that undergoes growth, bleeding, and necrosis
- Signs and symptoms
  - Severe headache, altered mental status, confusion
  - Meningeal signs (neck pain/stiffness, photophobia)
  - Acute symptoms of hypocortisolism (hypoglycemia, altered mental status, refractory hypotension)
  - Symptoms of other hormone deficiencies (thyroid, gonadotropins, somatomedin) present days to weeks later
- Diagnostics
  - Neuroimaging (CT head)
  - Lumbar puncture
  - Hormone levels: thyroid-stimulating hormone, adrenocorticotropic hormone, insulin-like growth factor 1 (IGF-1), prolactin
- Management:
  - High-dose steroids to prevent vascular collapse and shock
  - Replacement of other anterior pituitary hormones

536

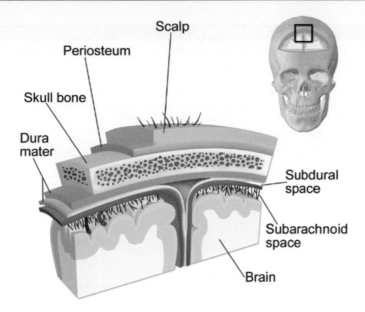

Figure 72-1: Layers covering the brain

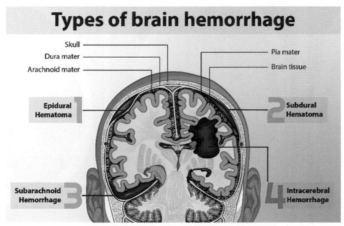

Figure 72-2: Types of brain hemorrhage

BRAIN MASSES
Pituitary Tumors

Acromegaly
- Pathophysiology
  - Insidious, autonomous secretion of growth hormone (GH) → enlargement of soft tissue, cartilage, bones, and visceral organs
  - Growth of long bones will occur if GH excess occurs during childhood prior to fusion of the epiphyseal plates
- Key manifestations
  - Mass effect: headache, visual disturbances
  - Macroglossia, protuberant jaw, widely spaced teeth
  - Coarse facial features
  - Increased hat, ring, and shoe size
  - Carpal tunnel syndrome, early osteoarthritis
  - Obstructive sleep apnea
  - Goiter
  - Cardiomyopathy, hypertension
  - Colonic polyps/cancer, diverticula
  - Diabetes mellitus

TABLE 72-1   Causes of Brain Bleed

	EPIDURAL HEMATOMA	SUBDURAL HEMATOMA	SUBARACHNOID HEMORRHAGE
Pathophysiology	• Temporal bone trauma resulting in rupture of the middle meningeal artery	• Rupture of bridging veins	• Rupture of cerebral aneurysm
Clinical Presentation	• Trauma resulting in loss of consciousness followed by lucid interval, and then rapid clinical deterioration (nausea, vomiting, coma)	• Chronic worsening headache and confusion over days to weeks • May or may not recall minor trauma • Focal neurologic deficits due to mass effect • Elderly, chronic alcoholic	• Sentinel headache that occurs days to weeks prior to subarachnoid hemorrhage • Sudden onset severe headache • Meningismus symptoms • Loss of consciousness
Diagnosis	• Noncontrast computed tomography (CT): lens-shaped hyperdensity that does not cross suture lines	• Noncontrast CT: crescent-shaped density that crosses suture lines	• Noncontrast: hyperdensity filling the subarachnoid space
Management	• Surgical evacuation and decompression	• Surgical evacuation and decompression	• Coiling or embolization • Nimodipine to prevent vasospasm
Complications	• Transtentorial herniation • Ipsilateral pupillary dilation (due to extrinsic compression of cranial nerve [CN] III) • "Down and out pupil" (loss of CN III extraocular muscle function) • Ipsilateral hemiparesis (compression of the contralateral crus)	• Herniation	• Vasospasm • Seizures • Hydrocephalus
Imaging			

- Diagnostics
  - Elevated IGF-1
  - Glucose suppression test: oral glucose load should normally suppress GH; lack of GH suppression indicates autonomous secretion of GH
  - Magnetic resonance imaging (MRI) pituitary
- Management
  - Surgical: transsphenoidal pituitary resection
  - Medical: somatostatin analogues (octreotide, lanreotide), cabergoline, pegvisomant (GH receptor antagonist)

ADULT BRAIN TUMORS
Brain Tumors
Brain tumors arise from specific cell types and therefore have a predilection for certain locations. Each of the brain tumors have imaging characteristics that are suggestive of a particular subtype; however, a biopsy with microscopic evaluation is needed for a definitive diagnosis. Overall, the most common brain tumor is metastasis (Table 72-2).

TABLE 72-2 Types of Brain Tumors

TYPE OF MALIGNANCY	LOCATION	KEY FEATURES
Astrocytoma	Cerebral hemisphere (glioblastoma multiforme)	Glioblastoma multiforme: • Crosses corpus callosum ("butterfly" lesion) • GFAP positive • Graded from 1–4 based on World Health Organization classification: • Grade I: pilocytic astrocytoma • Grade II: low-grade astrocytoma • Grade III: anaplastic astrocytoma • Grade IV: glioblastoma multiforme
Oligodendroglioma	Frontal lobe	• Presents as calcification on imaging • Tumor of cells that myelinate neurons in the central nervous system
Ependymoma	Cauda equina	• Overgrowth of cells lining the ventricles results in signs and symptoms of obstructive hydrocephalus • Common cause of spinal cancer resulting in extramedullary spinal compression
Meningioma	Dural reflection of cerebral hemisphere and parasagittal region	• Tumor that arises from arachnoid cells • Often have dural attachment ("dural tail"), which connects the tumor to the meninges • Benign, slow-growing lesion that tends to recur after excision • Symptoms related to compression of the cortex • Commonly seen in women
Schwannoma	Cerebello-pontine angle	• Peripheral nerve sheath tumor • Associated with neurofibromatosis type II: will have bilateral cranial nerve VIII schwannomas
Pituitary adenoma	Sella turcica	• Bitemporal hemianopia due to compression of the optic chiasm • Endocrine dysfunction: hyperprolactinemia, hypopituitarism

INFECTIONS
Brain Abscess
- Risk factors
  - Human immunodeficiency virus (HIV)
  - Recent neurosurgery
  - Otitis media
  - Sinusitis
  - Endocarditis
- Signs and symptoms
  - Fever
  - Progressive headache
  - Focal neurologic deficits (exact deficits depend on location of abscess)
- Microbiology: polymicrobial with gram negatives and anaerobes
- Diagnostics
  - Noncontrast CT head
  - Stereotactic brain biopsy and aspiration
- Management
  - HIV negative
    - Metronidazole + third-generation cephalosporin
    - Cover for methicillin-resistant *Staphylococcus aureus* if patient had recent neurosurgery
  - HIV positive
    - Empirically treat for *Toxoplasma* with pyrimethamine and sulfadiazine; if abscess improves after reimaging, then retrospective diagnosis of toxoplasmosis is made
    - If abscess does not get smaller after reimaging in 5–7 days, then biopsy must be performed to exclude central nervous system lymphoma

BACK PAIN
Lower back pain is extremely common and increases in incidence with age. Most patients with lower back pain do not require imaging. When presented with the patient with lower back pain, it is important to rule out any acute pathology that may involve the spinal cord, in which case an urgent MRI should be performed (Table 72-3).

TABLE 72-3   Back Pain That May Require Surgical Intervention

	SIGNS AND SYMPTOMS	DIAGNOSTICS	MANAGEMENT
Lumbar spinal stenosis	• Commonly seen in elderly (>60 years) • Associated with degenerative arthritis, thickened ligamentum flavum, spondylolisthesis, and bulging intervertebral discs • Pain worsened lumbar extension (i.e., walking downhill) • Pain relieved with lumbar flexion ("shopping cart sign") • Radiation to the buttocks and thighs • No neurologic deficits	Magnetic resonance imaging (MRI): narrowing of spinal canal with compression of nerve roots	• Nonopioid analgesics • Surgery for persistent/disabling symptoms
Lumbar disk herniation (radiculopathy)	• Herniation of nucleus pulposus through the annulus fibrosis resulting in nerve root compression and radicular symptoms • Acute back pain with unilateral radiation of pain involving a specific dermatome • Positive straight leg test • No vertebral tenderness	Clinical	• Nonopioid analgesics • Surgery for persistent/disabling symptoms
Vertebral fracture	• Associated with osteoporosis, inflammatory arthritis, Paget disease, bony metastasis, hyperparathyroidism • Acute back pain, may be asymptomatic in chronic cases • Point tenderness • Pain worsened with standing, coughing, lying down • Progressive kyphosis • Loss of stature	X-ray	• Nonopioid analgesic • +/− nasal calcitonin • +/− vertebral augmentation (kyphoplasty/vertebroplasty) • Bisphosphonates for osteoporosis
Cord compression (cauda equina syndrome)	• Acute onset lower back pain with neurologic deficits • Lower extremity paralysis • Bladder/bowel incontinence	MRI	• Surgical decompression • +/− high-dose steroids
Infection (epidural abscess, osteomyelitis, discitis)	• Fever, chills • Recent bacteremia • Exquisite point tenderness	MRI	• Antibiotics +/− surgical debridement

Cord Compression
- Pathophysiology: extrinsic compression of the spinal cord resulting in neurologic deficits
- Risk factors
  • History of malignancy (prostate, lung, breast, ependymoma)
  • Epidural abscess/hematoma
  • Vertebral osteomyelitis
  • Trauma
  • Disc herniation
  • Vertebral compression fracture
- Signs and symptoms
  • Neurologic deficits (findings depend on dermatome/sclerotome involved)
  • Upper motor neuron: hyperreflexia, spasticity
  • Lower motor neuron: fasciculations, hyporeflexia
  • Cauda equina syndrome: bladder/bowel incontinence, saddle anesthesia
- Diagnostics: MRI
- Management: surgical decompression +/− glucocorticoids +/− radiotherapy (neoplastic cord compression)

TRAUMA
Cervical Spine Injury
- Should be suspected in any patient who comes in with neck pain after trauma (e.g., motor vehicle accident)
- Immobilize the neck and prepare for possible airway protection

- Evaluate for neurologic compromise
- Obtain CT of the entire cervical spine
  - If fractures are present, evaluate for stability due to associated risk of spinal cord injury in unstable fractures

Skull Fractures

- Occur most commonly secondary to trauma
- Close, linear skull fractures can be managed conservatively
- Depressed or comminuted skull fractures require surgical intervention +/− prophylactic antibiotics
- Basal skull fracture: periorbital (raccoon eyes) and posterior auricular ecchymoses (Battle sign) and cerebrospinal fluid rhinorrhea (fracture of the cribriform plate); managed conservatively

CHAPTER 73 ENT Surgery

EARS

Mastoiditis
- Risk factors
  - Acute or chronic otitis media: extension of infection into mastoid air cells
  - Wegener granulomatosis
- Signs and symptoms
  - Tenderness and erythema of the mastoid bone (Fig. 73-1)
  - Anterior and inferior displacement of the pinna
- Diagnostics
  - Temporal bone computed tomography (CT) scan: loss of trabecular bone
- Management
  - IV antibiotics targeting upper respiratory tract organisms
  - Myringotomy
  - Mastoidectomy if there is presence of bony destruction

Cholesteatoma
- Causes
  - Acquired (chronic otitis media, tympanostomy tubes)
  - Congenital
- Pathophysiology: overgrowth of keratin debris (squamous epithelium) within the middle ear

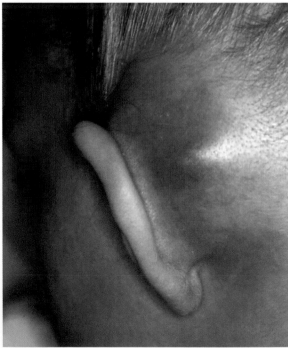

Fig. 73-1: Erythema and tenderness of the mastoid bone consistent with mastoiditis

- Signs and symptoms
  - Conductive hearing loss: erosion of the ossicles
  - Chronic malodorous otorrhea
  - Otalgia
  - Vertigo, tinnitus
- Diagnostics
  - Otoscopy
    - White plaque on the tympanic membrane
    - Retraction pocket behind the tympanic membrane with granulation tissue and skin debris
  - CT/magnetic resonance imaging (MRI): determines extent of extracranial and intracranial involvement
- Management: tympanomastoid surgery with ossicular reconstruction
- Complications
  - Meningitis, brain abscess
  - Cranial nerve palsies
  - Extracranial extension and erosion

NOSE
Nasal Septal Perforation
- Causes
  - Drugs (cocaine, methamphetamine, decongestants, intranasal corticosteroids)
  - Wegener granulomatosis
  - Trauma (piercings, digital trauma)
  - Iatrogenic (postrhinoplasty)
- Signs and symptoms
  - Whistling noise during respiration
  - Crusting, epistaxis
  - Nasal pressure and discomfort
  - Sensation of nasal obstruction: due to turbulent airflow through nasal passages
- Diagnostics
  - Clinical (Fig. 73-2)
  - Biopsy of perforated margin to rule out malignancy
- Management
  - Nasal packing
  - Surgery in severe cases

Nasal septum has poor regenerative capacity due to inadequate blood supply to the nasal cartilage. It primarily receives its blood supply and nutrients via diffusion through the overlying mucosa.

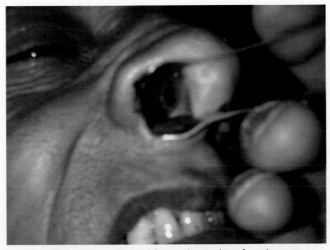

Fig. 73-2: Patient with nasal septal perforation

Nasal Polyps
- Causes
  - Aspirin sensitivity (aspirin-exacerbated respiratory disease)
  - Cystic fibrosis
  - Atopy: asthma, chronic sinusitis, allergic rhinitis
- Signs and symptoms
  - Asymptomatic
  - Dyspnea on nasal breathing
  - Nasal airway obstruction
  - Postnasal drip
  - Rhinorrhea
  - Snoring, anosmia with larger polyps
- Diagnostics
  - Clinical: glistening gray mass in the nasal cavity
  - Biopsy if etiology of nasal polyp is unknown or suspicious for malignancy
- Management
  - Topical nasal steroids (mometasone, fluticasone, budesonide)
  - Surgical resection: polyps tend to recur if not followed up by medical management

Epistaxis
- Definition: bleeding from the nares, most commonly from the anterior septum (Kiesselbach plexus)
- Causes
  - Digital trauma: most common cause
  - Foreign body
  - Bleeding disorders (thrombocytopenia, hemophilia)
  - Sinusitis/upper respiratory infection
  - Nasopharyngeal carcinoma
- Diagnostics: clinical
- Management: increasing level of intervention if previous intervention does not stop bleeding; after bleeding is stopped, address underlying etiology
  1. Most cases resolve spontaneously with nasal pressure
  2. Nasal spray: phenylephrine, oxymetazoline
  3. Anterior nasal packing
  4. Posterior nasal packing for severe cases, may be indicative of bleeding from posterior Kiesselbach plexus
  5. Cauterization

THROAT
Pharyngitis
- Microbiology
  - Viruses
    - Adenovirus
    - Coxsackie
    - Cytomegalovirus
  - Bacteria: group A streptococcus
- Signs and symptoms
  - Rapid onset fever and sore throat
  - Erythematous pharynx
  - Tonsillar enlargement and exudates (Fig. 73-3)
  - Palate petechiae
  - Enlarged and tender cervical lymph nodes
  - Cough, rhinorrhea, and conjunctivitis tend to signify a viral etiology
- Diagnostics
  - Clinical
  - Rapid strep test, if negative confirm with throat culture
- Management: antibiotics to prevent acute rheumatic fever
  - Penicillin or amoxicillin
  - Tonsillectomy: multiple recurrent infections within the past year
- Complications
  - Retropharyngeal abscess
  - Peritonsillar abscess

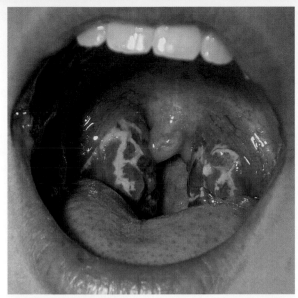

Fig. 73-3: Streptococcal pharyngitis with erythematous pharynx, tonsillar enlargement, and exudates

Retropharyngeal Abscess
- Definition: infection between the posterior pharyngeal wall and prevertebral fascia
- Signs and symptoms
  - Neck pain and stiffness
  - Odynophagia/dysphagia
  - Muffled voice
  - Enlargement of posterior pharyngeal wall
- Diagnostics
  - Neck x-ray: widening of the prevertebral strip (Fig. 73-4)
  - CT scan
    - Ring enhancement with central lucency
    - Anterior displacement airway
- Management
  - Incision and drainage
  - IV antibiotics
    - Third-generation cephalosporin + ampicillin-sulbactam
  - OR
    - Clindamycin
- Complications
  - Airway compromise
  - Posterior mediastinitis, aspiration pneumonia
  - Sepsis, thrombophlebitis
  - Erosion through the carotid sheath, vertebral osteomyelitis

Peritonsillar Abscess
- Signs and symptoms
  - Dysphasia
  - Trismus: painful spastic contractions of the jaw
  - Asymmetric tonsillar enlargement with associated displacement of the uvula away from the affected side (Fig. 73-5)
  - "Hot potato" voice
  - Pooling of saliva
- Diagnostics: clinical
- Management
  - Incision and drainage
  - Antibiotics covering for group A streptococcus and respiratory anaerobes

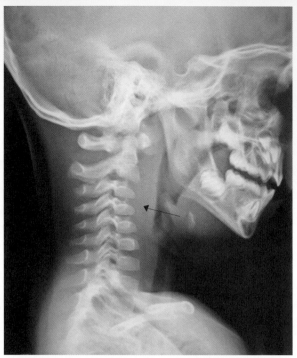

Fig. 73-4: Widening of the prevertebral strip (black arrow) secondary to prevertebral soft tissue swelling in a patient with a retropharyngeal abscess

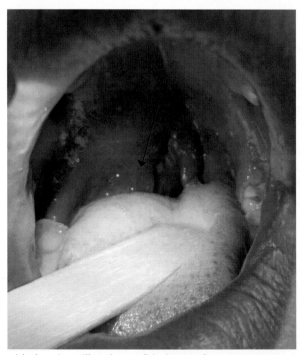

Fig. 73-5: Patient with right-sided peritonsillar abscess (black arrow)

Vocal Cord Polyp/Nodule
- Definition: bilateral, benign masses in the middle one-third of the true vocal cords preventing vocal cords from fully adducting
- Causes
  - Secondary to excessive use of vocal cords (teachers, singers, public speakers): most common
  - Gastroesophageal reflux disease
  - Tobacco abuse

- Signs and symptoms
  - Hoarseness
  - Deepening voice
  - Increased effort to produce similar voice decibel
- Diagnostics: clinical plus laryngoscopy (biopsy of nodule to rule out malignant etiology)
- Management: voice rest +/− surgical excision

Laryngeal Papilloma
- Definition: laryngeal tumor affecting children (multiple masses) and adults (single mass)
- Causes: human papillomavirus (HPV) 6 or 11
- Signs and symptoms
  - Hoarseness
  - Stridor
  - Difficulty speaking
  - Obstruction in severe cases
- Diagnostics: laryngoscopy plus biopsy to rule out malignant etiology
- Management: surgical excision +/− antivirals

NECK
Benign neck masses are characterized based on their location (Table 73-1; Fig. 73-6). Imaging is performed to determine their extent if they are symptomatic and in adult patients to rule out head and neck malignancy.

SALIVARY GLAND
Calculous Sialolithiasis/Sialadenitis
- Definition: formation of stones and obstruction within the salivary ducts
- Signs and symptoms
  - Localized, unilateral painful swelling at the angle of the mandible or in front of the ear
  - Intermittent pain and swelling
  - Palpable calculous
  - Fever if infection occurs secondary to obstruction

TABLE 73-1   Differential Diagnosis of Neck Masses

NECK MASS	CLINICAL MANIFESTATIONS
Thyroglossal duct cyst	• Midline mass, moves with swallowing • May contain ectopic thyroid tissue • May become infected requiring I&D and antibiotics
Branchial cleft cyst	• Lateral neck mass along the sternocleidomastoid • Commonly asymptomatic • May shrink and grow with upper respiratory infections, may become infected
Cystic hygroma	• Posterior to the sternocleidomastoid in the posterior triangle of the neck • Congenital lymphatic malformation • Nonpitting, fluctuant neck mass that transilluminates • Associated with aneuploidies

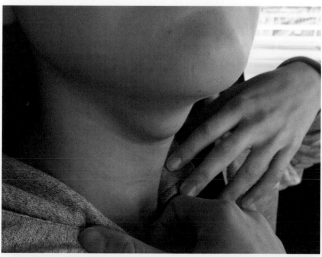

Fig. 73-6: Midline mass, consistent with thyroglossal duct cyst

- Diagnostics
  - Plain films: will visualize most cases of sialolithiasis as most stones are radiopaque
  - Sonogram
  - Sialography: gold standard
- Management
  - Manual compression and manipulation
  - Sialagogues
  - Shockwave lithotripsy
  - Sialoendoscopy

Acute Parotitis
- Causes
  - Infectious (*Staphylococcus aureus*, mumps virus)
  - Chronic vomiting (anorexia, bulimia)
  - Dehydration, poor oral hygiene, xerostomia
  - Debilitated (elderly, postoperative)
- Signs and symptoms
  - Painful, unilateral parotid enlargement
  - Bilateral enlargement may be indication of systemic process (Sjögren, bulimia, mumps)
  - Edema, erythema
  - Fever
  - Purulent discharge from Wharton or Stenson duct
- Diagnostics: clinical
  - Sonogram
  - Radiographs/sialography to rule out calculous sialadenitis
- Management
  - Sialagogues (lemon wedges, hard candy): increase salivation to facilitate expectoration of pus and infectious contents
  - Rehydration
  - Antibiotics covering methicillin-resistant *S. aureus* (vancomycin, linezolid)

Tumors in smaller salivary glands such as sublingual or submandibular are more likely to be malignant; however, overall, most salivary gland tumors are benign.

NEOPLASMS
Head and Neck Cancer
- Risk factors
  - Smoking, alcohol
  - Radiation
  - Betel nut chewing
  - Viral infection: HPV (oropharyngeal), Epstein-Barr virus (EBV) (nasopharyngeal)
  - Immunodeficiency: human immunodeficiency virus, solid organ transplant
- Types: five anatomic locations; most commonly squamous cell carcinoma
  - Oral cavity
  - Pharynx
  - Larynx
  - Nasal cavity
  - Salivary glands
- Signs and symptoms
  - Asymptomatic (results in late detection and poor prognosis)
  - Nontender cervical/submandibular lymphadenopathy
  - Weight loss
  - Dysphasia
  - Neck mass
  - Hoarseness
  - Leukoplakia, erythroplakia
- Diagnostics
  - Panendoscopy (laryngoscopy, bronchoscopy, esophagoscopy) and biopsy: initial test
  - CT/MRI/positron-emission tomography scan for staging

- Management
  - Surgery
  - Radiation
  - Chemotherapy: cetuximab (monoclonal antibody against epidermal growth factor receptor)

Parotid Neoplasia
- Risk factors
  - Smoking
  - Radiation exposure
  - Sjögren syndrome
- Types
  - Pleomorphic adenoma (mixed tumor): most common benign and overall salivary gland tumor; small potential for malignant degeneration
  - Other benign tumors
    - Wharton tumor (more common in men)
    - Oncocytoma
    - Benign lymphoepithelial cysts
  - Mucoepidermoid carcinoma: most common malignant salivary gland tumor
  - Other malignant tumors
    - Adenoid cystic carcinoma
    - Acinic cell carcinoma
  - Lymphoma: develops as a complication of long-standing Sjögren syndrome
- Signs and symptoms
  - Painless unilateral enlargement at the angle of the mandible
  - Facial pain/paralysis: indicative of malignant tumor infiltrating cranial nerve VII
  - Local lymphadenopathy
- Diagnostics
  - Fine-needle aspiration
  - CT/MRI: determine extent of tumor growth and aid with presurgical planning
- Management
  - Benign: superficial parotidectomy with wide margins due to high recurrence rate with incomplete excision
  - Malignant: total parotidectomy with excision of facial nerve

Nasopharyngeal Carcinoma

Frey syndrome: postoperative complication following parotidectomy presenting as gustatory sweating due to aberrant parasympathetic innervation of sweat glands that are divided during surgery

- Risk factors
  - EBV infection
  - Smoking
  - Genetics (Asian descent)
  - Salt cured foods
- Signs and symptoms
  - Epistaxis
  - Rhinorrhea
  - Headaches
  - Cranial nerve palsies
  - Serous otitis media
  - Cervical lymphadenopathy
- Diagnostics: biopsy
- Management: surgical excision +/− chemoradiation

Of note, there is a shift toward a zone-free approach in penetrating neck trauma with improvement in imaging and negative mandatory surgical explorations.

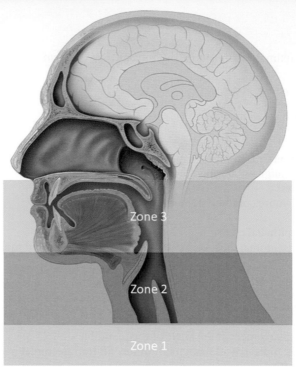

Fig. 73-7: Illustration of the different neck zones

EMERGENCIES
Penetrating Neck Trauma
- Management determined by zone of penetrating trauma
  - Zone I: thoracic inlet to cricoid cartilage
  - Zone II: cricoid cartilage to angle of the mandible
  - Zone III: angle of the mandible upwards
- Management: surgical exploration regardless of zone if there's presence of hemodynamic instability, airway, vascular, or esophageal injury
  - If there are no signs of hemodynamic instability, airway, vascular or esophageal injury, then management is based on zone involved (Fig. 73-7)
    - Zone I: Four-vessel CT angiography plus triple endoscopy (evaluation of pharynx, larynx, trachea, bronchi, and esophagus)
    - Zone II: surgical exploration
    - Zone III: CT angiography
  - Further intervention is determined based on angiographic and endoscopic findings

Ludwig Angina
- Definition: cellulitis and abscess involving the floor of the mouth due to infected dental caries; most commonly involve the mandibular molars
- Signs and symptoms
  - Fevers, chills
  - Dysphagia, odynophagia
  - Drooling
- Diagnostics: clinical
- Management
  - I&D plus antibiotics
  - Close airway monitoring/protection (endotracheal or tracheostomy) due to rapid spread of infection

CHAPTER
74 Breast Surgery

BENIGN BREAST MASSES

Breast mass principles
- Common among women, especially those of reproductive age; increased risk of malignancy after 40 years old (Table 74-1)
- Most have little to no malignant potential and can therefore be observed after one to two menstrual cycles
- If further evaluation is needed, a fine-needle aspiration, core needle biopsy, ultrasound, or mammogram can be performed
- Ultrasound is preferred for younger women with suspected cystic masses
- Fine-needle aspiration or core needle biopsy for solid palpable masses
- Mammography for older women (>40 years), bloody nipple discharge, recurrent cyst after aspiration, concurrent lymphadenopathy, or overlying skin changes (Fig. 74-1)

> Self and clinical breast exams are no longer recommended.
> Breast cancer commonly metastasizes to the bone, brain, and liver.
> Axillary lymph node dissection complications include chronic lymphedema, upper extremity pain, and recurrent fungal and bacterial cellulitis.

BREAST CANCER

Breast Cancer
- Epidemiology
  - Most common cancer in women, second most common cause of cancer mortality
  - One of eight women will be affected by breast cancer
- Risk factors
  - Family history with first-degree relative
  - *BRCA1* mutation
  - Age >50 years
  - Ionizing radiation
  - Alcoholism
  - Nulliparity
  - Obesity
  - Hormone replacement therapy

TABLE 74-1 Differential Diagnosis of Breast Masses

BREAST MASS	KEY FEATURES	MANAGEMENT
Fibroadenoma	• Rubbery, mobile, well demarcated • Premenstrual tenderness • Nonadherent to chest wall	• No treatment • Optional excision
Intraductal papilloma	• Unilateral, serosanguineous bloody nipple discharge	• Core needle biopsy +/− surgical excision
Phyllodes tumor	• Type of low-grade sarcoma • Rapidly growing • Leaflike projections on histology	• Core needle biopsy followed by surgical excision
Fibrocystic change	• Cyclic bilateral breast tenderness • Diffusely nodular breast • Symptoms vary with menstrual cycle	• Symptomatic management: oral contraceptives, nonsteroidal antiinflammatory drugs, danazol, tamoxifen

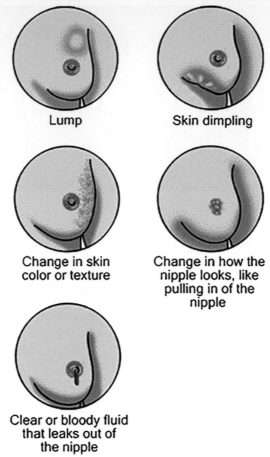

Fig. 74-1: Illustrations demonstrating the various presentations and early signs of breast cancer.

- Signs and symptoms
  - Irregular, palpable breast mass
  - Bloody nipple discharge
  - Overlying erythema
  - Skin, nipple retraction
  - "Orange peel" skin
  - Axillary lymphadenopathy
- Diagnostics
  - Mammography
    - Irregular spiculated mass with microcalcifications
    - Asymmetric densities
    - Architectural distortion
  - Breast magnetic resonance imaging or tomosynthesis: indicated for high-risk patients, denser breasts unable to be evaluated by mammography
  - Sentinel lymph node biopsy: positive lymph nodes indicate axillary lymph node involvement requiring axillary lymph node dissection
  - Staging computed tomography abdomen and pelvis
  - Receptor testing: estrogen, progesterone, HER2
- Management
  - Localized disease
    - Without lymph node involvement: lumpectomy plus axillary radiation
    - With lymph node involvement: lumpectomy plus axillary lymph node dissection
  - Metastatic disease
    - Chemoradiation
    - Hormonal therapy depending on receptor positivity (Table 74-2)
- Screening: mammography starting at age 50 years, every two years until 74 years old (US Preventive Services Task Force recommendations)

Breast cancer may present with unique characteristics that should increase the clinical suspicion for a particular subtype (Table 74-3).

TABLE 74-2   Hormonal Therapy: Used to Treat Breast Cancer That Is Estrogen, Progesterone, or HER2/Neu Positive

THERAPY	INDICATIONS	MECHANISM OF ACTION	ADVERSE EFFECTS
Tamoxifen	• Estrogen receptor–positive cancer in premenopausal women	• Estrogen receptor antagonist in the breast • Estrogen receptor agonist in the uterus	• Venous thromboembolism • Endometrial hyperplasia/cancer • Hot flashes
Anastrozole	• Estrogen receptor–positive cancer in postmenopausal women	• Aromatase inhibitor	• Osteoporosis • Muscle aches and pains
Trastuzumab	• HER2 receptor–positive cancer	• Monoclonal antibody against HER2	• Reversible cardiomyopathy

TABLE 74-3   Key Features of Breast Cancer Subtypes

BREAST CANCER SUBTYPES	KEY FEATURES
Ductal carcinoma	• Most common breast cancer subtype
Lobular carcinoma	• Associated with contralateral breast cancer
Paget disease of the breast	• Eczematous, scaling dermatitis involving the nipple • Variant of ductal carcinoma
Inflammatory breast cancer	• Overlying erythema/edema with associated lymphadenopathy • Poor prognosis, commonly metastatic upon presentation • Cancer invading dermal lymphatics

CHAPTER 75 General Surgery

ESOPHAGUS

Zenker Diverticulum

- Definition: true diverticulum (mucosa, submucosa, and muscularis externa) of the proximal esophagus seen in elderly males
- Pathophysiology: weakness in the cricopharyngeal muscle results in posterior herniation of the proximal esophagus between the muscle fibers
- Signs and symptoms
  - Dysphagia
  - Sensation of food stuck in the throat
  - Regurgitation, halitosis
  - Neck mass
  - Chest discomfort
- Diagnostics
  - Barium esophagram (Fig. 75-1)
  - Avoid esophagogastroduodenoscopy (EGD) if Zenker diverticulum is suspected due to high risk of perforation
- Management: cricopharyngeal myotomy
- Complications: aspiration

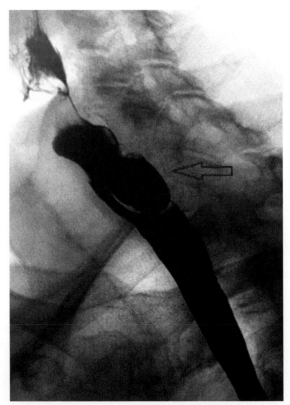

Fig. 75-1: Zenker diverticulum (red arrow)

Other types of esophageal diverticula:
- Traction diverticula
  - Located in the midesophagus
  - Caused by mediastinal adenopathy (pulmonary tuberculosis) and inflammation
  - No treatment necessary
- Epiphrenic diverticula
  - Located in the lower esophagus
  - Caused by achalasia or esophageal spasms
- Managed by treating the underlying cause

Achalasia
- Definition: esophageal motility disorder characterized by incomplete relaxation of the lower esophageal sphincter (LES)
- Causes
  - Idiopathic
  - Adenocarcinoma of the lower esophagus or proximal stomach (pseudo-achalasia)
  - Chagas disease
  - Scleroderma
  - Nissen fundoplication: iatrogenic cause of achalasia
- Pathophysiology: acquired loss of motor neurons in the myenteric plexus of the lower esophageal sphincter
- Signs and symptoms
  - Dysphasia to both solids and liquids
  - Sensation of food stuck in the throat
  - Weight loss
  - Regurgitation
  - Heartburn, chest discomfort
- Diagnostics
  - Barium esophagram: "bird's beak" appearance due to narrowing at the distal esophagus (Fig. 75-2)
  - Manometry: increased resting pressure at the LES
  - EGD with biopsy
    - Loss of motor neurons in the myenteric plexus on pathology
    - Rules out malignant etiologies (pseudo-achalasia)

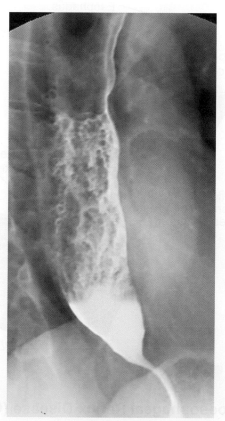

Fig. 75-2: Achalasia

- Management
  - Pharmacologic
    - Calcium channel blockers
    - Nitrates
    - Botulinum toxin injection
  - Surgical: pneumatic dilation, myotomy
  - Alternatives: avoid meals before bed, remain in the upright position while eating
- Complications: aspiration

Gastroesophageal Reflux Disease (GERD)

- Causes
  - Sliding hiatal hernia (herniation of the GE junction above the diaphragm)
  - Gastric outlet obstruction
  - Gastric dysmotility
- Pathophysiology: excessive relaxation of the LES resulting in retrograde flow of stomach acid into the esophagus (Fig. 75-3)
- Signs and symptoms
  - Heartburn, dyspepsia usually after meals
  - Metallic taste in the mouth
  - Nausea, vomiting, early satiety
  - Chest discomfort
  - Belching, regurgitation
  - Nocturnal asthma
  - Chronic cough, hoarseness
- Diagnostics: additional testing only done in unresponsive or atypical cases
  - Clinical: retrospective diagnosis of GERD if patient responds to proton pump inhibitors (PPIs)
  - 24-hour pH monitoring: most sensitive and specific, used in special cases
    - Prior to Nissen fundoplication
    - Patients unresponsive to PPIs
  - Endoscopy with biopsy
    - Assess for changes to esophageal mucosa (Barrett esophagus)
    - Presence of alarming symptoms such as weight loss, gastrointestinal (GI) bleeding, anemia, elderly, signs of obstruction, or persistent vomiting

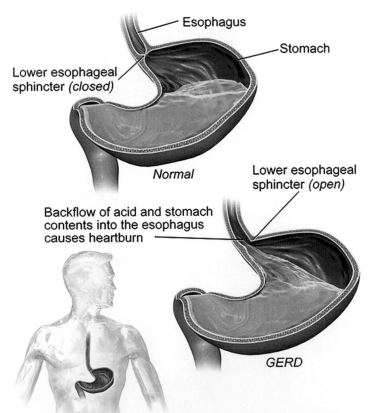

Gastroesophageal Reflux Disease (GERD)

Fig. 75-3: Pathophysiology of gastroesophageal reflux disease

- Management
  - Behavioral modification
    - Avoid spicy/fatty foods, chocolates, peppermints, alcohol, large meals before bedtime
    - Sleep with torso elevated
    - Weight loss
  - Pharmacologic
    - PPIs
    - H2 blockers, antacids
  - Surgical: for cases unresponsive to behavioral and pharmacologic management
    - Nissen fundoplication (laparoscopic or open procedure, which wraps the GE junction around the LES)
- Complications
  - Barrett esophagus: metaplasia of the LES from normal stratified squamous epithelium to columnar epithelium; precursor to adenocarcinoma
  - Esophageal strictures/spasms
  - Aspiration pneumonia
  - Erosive esophagitis
  - Dental erosion
  - Laryngitis

Paraesophageal hernias: herniation of the gastric fundus through the diaphragm resulting in increased risk of strangulation and ulceration; may require surgical repair

Esophageal Rings/Web
- Definition
  - Ring: circumferential protrusion of the esophageal mucosa into the lumen
  - Web: partial protrusion of the esophageal mucosa into the lumen
- Causes: unknown, hypothesized to be from chronic GERD
- Signs and symptoms
  - Intermittent dysphagia to solids
  - Sensation of food stuck in throat
  - Dyspepsia
- Associations
  - Rings
    - Hiatal hernia
    - Eosinophilic esophagitis
  - Webs
    - Plummer-Vinson syndrome: triad of esophageal web, iron deficiency anemia, increased risk of squamous cell carcinoma
- Diagnostics: barium esophagram
- Management
  - Thoroughly chew food
  - Pneumatic dilation
  - Long-term PPIs

STOMACH

Peptic Ulcer Disease
- Causes
  - *Helicobacter pylori* infection
  - Nonsteroidal antiinflammatory drugs, steroids, cholinomimetics
  - Gastrinoma (Zollinger-Ellison syndrome)
  - Burns (Cushing ulcer)
  - Head trauma (curling ulcer)
- Signs and symptoms
  - Gnawing epigastric pain immediately (gastric ulcer) or hours (duodenal ulcer) after meals
  - Nausea, vomiting, belching
  - Hematemesis, black stools
  - Early satiety
- Diagnostics
  - *H. pylori* testing: urea breath test, stool assay
  - EGD: most commonly located on lesser curvature stomach
  - Gastric ulcer should be biopsied to rule out malignancy and followed up with repeat endoscopy to document resolution/improvement in select high-risk cases

Substitute metronidazole for amoxicillin for penicillin-allergic patients.

- Management
  - Avoid causative agents
  - *H. pylori* eradication
    - Triple therapy: amoxicillin, clarithromycin, PPI
    - Quadruple therapy: metronidazole, tetracycline, bismuth, PPI
  - Refractive: selective vagotomy
- Complications
  - Perforation
  - Gastric outlet obstruction
  - Malignancy

Gastric vs duodenal ulcer symptoms:
- Gastric ulcer: symptoms worsen after meals due to stimulation of acid production in the stomach resulting in increased damage to preexisting ulcer.
- Duodenal ulcer: pain of ulcer improves after meals as secretion of bicarbonate increases from Brunner glands located into the duodenum as it prepares for incoming acidic load from the stomach.

  - GI bleed

Gastric Adenocarcinoma
- Risk factors
  - Alcohol
  - Tobacco
  - Preserved foods
  - Chronic atrophic gastritis with intestinal metaplasia (pernicious anemia, *H. pylori*)
  - Adenomatous gastric polyps
  - Ménétrier disease
  - Blood type A
- Signs and symptoms
  - Nausea, vomiting (nonbilious)
  - Succussion splash: sloshing sound heard when stethoscope is placed on patient's abdomen and is rocked back and forth
  - Weight loss, early satiety
  - GI bleed
  - Heartburn
- Diagnostics
  - EGD with biopsy
    - Ulcerating heaped up lesions
    - Linitis plastica (involvement of all layers of stomach, decreased stomach elasticity): poor prognosis
  - Computed tomography (CT) abdomen/pelvis for staging
- Metastatic associations
  - Virchow nodes: left supraclavicular lymph node
  - Sister Mary Joseph nodules: periumbilical lymph nodes
  - Krukenberg tumor: ovaries
  - Blumer shelf tumor: rectum
  - Irish node: left axillary lymph node
- Management: most cases present as advanced disease due to vague nonspecific symptoms
  - Localized disease: surgical resection (gastrectomy)
  - Metastatic disease: chemoradiation, palliative

Dumping Syndrome
- Pathophysiology: rapid emptying of food contents (high osmotic gradient) into the small bowel secondary to gastric bypass, gastrectomy, or pyloric sphincter alteration (Fig. 75-4)
- Signs and symptoms: onset occurs within 30 minutes after ingestion; late dumping syndrome has symptom onset up to three hours after ingestion
  - Cramping, bloating, diarrhea
  - Flushing, diaphoresis
  - Weakness, dizziness
  - Hypotension, tachycardia
  - Hypoglycemia: secondary to insulin oversecretion from large carbohydrate load; seen more commonly with late dumping syndrome

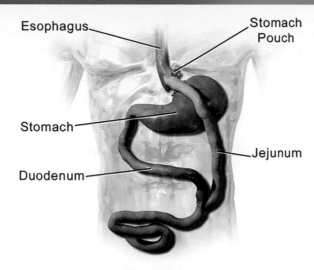

Roux-En-Y

Fig. 75-4: Anatomy of Roux-en-Y gastric bypass where contents from the stomach pouch enter directly into the jejunum. (Image courtesy of Blausen Medical.)

- Diagnostics: clinical
- Management
  - Small, frequent meals
  - Separation of solids and liquids
  - High-protein and high-fiber diet
  - Avoidance of simple sugars; replace with complex carbohydrates
  - Most cases eventually resolve within three months; octreotide or surgical reconstruction (antiperistaltic jejunal loop) for refractory cases

SMALL BOWEL
Appendicitis
- Epidemiology: children and young adults
- Pathophysiology: obstruction of the appendiceal lumen resulting in inflammation, edema, and infection
- Signs and symptoms
  - Abdominal pain
    - Initially periumbilical, followed by right lower quadrant pain
    - Left lower quadrant palpation worsens right lower quadrant pain: Rovsing sign
    - Right leg extension against resistance worsens right lower quadrant pain: psoas sign
    - Internal rotation of right leg worsens right lower quadrant pain: obturator sign
  - Guarding, rebound tenderness
  - Fevers, chills
  - Anorexia
- Diagnostics
  - Clinical
  - CT abdomen and pelvis
  - Ultrasound: preferred in younger children
  - +/− leukocytosis
- Management: appendectomy +/− antibiotics
- Complications: appendiceal perforation
  - Appendicitis symptoms >5 days
  - CT abdomen/pelvis shows walled-off, loculated abscess (phlegmon)
  - Manage with antibiotics, bowel rest, and interval appendectomy

Delayed presentation of appendicitis seen in elderly and pregnancy (due to displacement of the appendix from its natural position in the right lower quadrant).

Mesenteric Ischemia
- Pathophysiology
  - Occlusion of the mesenteric vessels (celiac, superior mesenteric, inferior mesenteric) resulting in intestinal ischemia
  - Deleterious ischemic sequela is reduced due to collateral circulation (marginal artery of Drummond, arc of Riolan)
- Causes
  - Atherosclerotic plaque rupture/thrombosis
  - Cardioembolic
  - Hypercoagulable (inherited, infection, inflammation): commonly associated with venous thrombosis
- Signs and symptoms
  - Abdominal pain out of proportion to physical exam (relatively benign abdominal exam)
  - Peritonitis (seen in late stage after infarction and perforation)
- Diagnostics
  - Abdominal x-ray: may show pneumoperitoneum
  - CT or mesenteric angiogram
- Management: treat underlying etiology
  - General principles
    - Intensive IV fluids: optimizes bowel perfusion
    - Serial abdominal exams, monitor for peritonitis
  - Cardioembolic: anticoagulation +/− embolectomy
  - Atherosclerotic plaque rupture/thrombosis: revascularization or bypass
  - Perforation/infarction: exploratory laparotomy

Chronic Mesenteric Ischemia
- Definition: intestinal angina as abdominal pain occurs 1–2 hours after ingestion of meal due to inadequate blood supply
- Pathophysiology: severe atherosclerosis of the mesenteric vessels prevents optimal blood supply from reaching the bowel to aid in digestion and metabolism when meal is consumed
- Signs and symptoms
  - Food aversion
  - Weight loss
  - Abdominal pain after meals
- Diagnostics: CT or mesenteric angiogram
- Management: revascularization

Small bowel obstruction and ileus have overlapping clinical presentations, and may initially be difficult to differentiate; however, after correction of reversible etiologies and given time, the two should become easier to differentiate as ileus will eventually resolve while small bowel obstruction will persist (Table 75-1).

Carcinoid
- Pathophysiology
  - Serotonin-producing tumor
  - Localized disease is asymptomatic as serotonin is metabolized in the liver to 5-hydroxyindoleacetic acid (5-HIAA)
  - Metastatic disease (especially to the liver) allows serotonin to bypass liver metabolism and enter the systemic circulation
- Signs and symptoms (only seen in metastatic disease)
  - Episodic flushing
  - Wheezing
  - Diarrhea
  - Telangiectasias
  - Tricuspid regurgitation/stenosis (monoamine oxidase enzyme in pulmonary circulation metabolizes serotonin and prevents left-sided valvular involvement)
  - Niacin deficiency causing pellagra (diarrhea, dementia, dermatitis)
- Diagnostics
  - Elevated 24-hour urine 5-HIAA
  - CT or magnetic resonance imaging (MRI) abdomen/pelvis for staging (liver metastases most common)
  - Positron-emission tomography imaging with radiolabeled somatostatin analogues
  - Endoscopy with biopsy

TABLE 75-1   Inflammatory Bowel Disease: Ulcerative Colitis Versus Crohn Disease

	ULCERATIVE COLITIS (UC)	CROHN DISEASE
Epidemiology	Bimodal distribution: age 15–40 years, age 50–80 years	Second and third decades of life
Signs and symptoms	Chronic bloody diarrhea, rectal pain, tenesmus, incontinence Serology: ANCA positive, elevated inflammatory markers, leukocytosis, anemia	Chronic watery diarrhea, abdominal pain, nausea, vomiting Serology: ASCA positive, elevated inflammatory markers, leukocytosis, anemia
Colonoscopy	Continuous mucosal inflammation starting in the rectum and extending proximally Pseudopolyps	Skip lesions: areas of transmural inflammation separated by normal intestine May involve any part of the gastrointestinal tract; most commonly involves terminal ileum
Biopsy	Crypt abscesses	Transmural granulomas
Complications	Toxic megacolon	Fistulas (enteroenteric, enterocystic, intravaginal) Abscesses Obstruction
Extraintestinal manifestations	Erythema nodosum Pyoderma gangrenosum Primary sclerosing cholangitis Arthritis, uveitis, spondyloarthritis	Nephrolithiasis (increased oxalate absorption) Subacute combined degeneration (vitamin B12 deficiency, terminal ileitis) Gallstones (lack of bile acid reabsorption and cholesterol supersaturation) Arthritis, uveitis, spondyloarthritis
Treatment	Acute exacerbation: steroids Maintenance therapy: mesalamine, sulfasalazine Surgery is curative and indicated for disease refractory to medical management	Acute exacerbation: steroids Maintenance therapy: anti-TNF agents (infliximab, etanercept), immunomodulators (azathioprine, mercaptopurine) Surgery for the management of complications such as fistulas, strictures, bowel obstruction
Risk of colon cancer	Increased after 8–10 years of colonic involvement Follow up with colonoscopy every 1–3 years after having UC for 8–10 years Presence of primary sclerosing cholangitis further increases risk	Increased risk only if there is colonic involvement

TNF, Tumor necrosis factor

- Management
  - Localized disease
    - Observation if tumor is <2 cm
    - Surgical resection if tumor is >2 cm; lower threshold if tumor is in the ileum due to high risk of malignancy
    - Most commonly located in the appendix
  - Metastatic disease: somatostatin analogues (octreotide, lanreotide)

PANCREAS
Acute Pancreatitis
- Causes
  - Alcohol, gallstones
  - Hypertriglyceridemia (>1000 mg/dL)
  - Drugs
    - Diuretics (thiazides, furosemide)
    - Valproate
    - Azathioprine
    - Didanosine
    - Pentamidine, metronidazole, tetracycline
    - GLP-1 analogues

- Infectious (cytomegalovirus, mumps, legionella)
- Iatrogenic (endoscopic retrograde cholangiopancreatography [ERCP], cholesterol emboli postcardiac catheterization)
- Trauma
- Signs and symptoms
  - Epigastric pain radiating to the back
  - Nausea, vomiting, anorexia
  - Severe cases
    - Fever, tachycardia, hypotension
    - Hypoxia, tachypnea
    - Cullen sign (periumbilical discoloration: hemoperitoneum)
    - Grey Turner sign (flank discoloration: retroperitoneal bleed)
    - Hypocalcemia (secondary to saponification)
- Diagnosis
  - Two of three required to make the diagnosis
    - Epigastric pain radiating to the back, worsened by food
    - Amylase/lipase more than three times the upper limit of normal
    - CT abdomen/pelvis (pancreatic inflammation, peripancreatic fluid, and fat-stranding) (Fig. 75-5)
    - Abdominal ultrasound or ERCP to diagnose etiology (gallstones)
- Management
  - IV fluid resuscitation
  - Advanced diet as tolerated
  - Pain control often requiring narcotics
  - Laparoscopic cholecystectomy during same hospital admission if gallstones are determined to be the etiology

Imipenem should be avoided in those with seizure disorders as it lowers the seizure threshold.

- Complications: secondary to the release of pancreatic enzymes, cytokines, and other inflammatory markers resulting in inflammation and organ dysfunction
  - Adult respiratory distress syndrome (massive inflammatory response results in widespread vasodilation and leakage of capillaries)
  - Necrotizing pancreatitis (visualized on repeat imaging in patient who continues to worsen and has sepsis physiology)
    - Requires biopsy proven evidence of infection before starting antibiotics

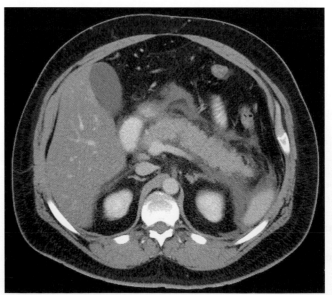

Fig. 75-5: CT abdomen and pelvis in a patient with acute pancreatitis showing pancreatic enlargement, edema, and peripancreatic fluid. (Image courtesy of Hellerhoff.)

- Antibiotics
  - Carbapenem monotherapy (meropenem, imipenem)
    OR
  - Cefepime/fluoroquinolone + metronidazole
- May require necrosectomy
  - Pseudocyst: rule of 6 s
- Develop within 6 weeks
- Observe if <6 cm in size
- Drain if >6 cm in size or if symptomatic
  - Hypotension, acute renal failure (secondary to excessive loss of intravascular volume)
  - GI bleed, ileus

Multiple scoring systems (Ranson criteria, APACHE II, BISAP score) exist as prognostic indicators; however, none have been reported to predict disease severity. There is some utility in triaging patients to determine appropriate level of care.

Chronic Pancreatitis
- Causes
  - Repeated episodes of acute pancreatitis resulting in chronic inflammation → fibrosis → loss of pancreatic exocrine (digestive enzymes) and endocrine (insulin secretion) function
  - Cystic fibrosis
- Signs and symptoms
  - Weight loss, anorexia
  - Chronic epigastric abdominal pain, worsened by meals
  - Malabsorption (fat-soluble vitamin deficiencies), loose greasy stools
  - Hyperglycemia (lack of insulin)
- Diagnostics
  - Imaging: pancreatic calcifications on abdominal CT/X-ray
  - Secretin stimulation test: secretin stimulates the release of bicarbonate-rich fluid; however, in chronic pancreatitis this response will be lacking
  - Normal amylase/lipase
  - Low fecal elastase, increased stool fat
  - Carbohydrate-deficient transferrin: biomarker of chronic alcohol intake
- Management
  - Pancreatic enzyme supplementation (should be taken with PPI or H2 blocker to prevent breakdown of pancreatic enzymes)
  - Alcohol cessation
  - Pain control
- Complications
  - Vitamin deficiencies
    - Vitamin A: blindness, cataracts, dry eyes
    - Vitamin D: osteoporosis, hypocalcemia
    - Vitamin E: spinocerebellar ataxia, hemolytic anemia
    - Vitamin K: bleeding, easy bruising
    - Vitamin B12 deficiency: macrocytic megaloblastic anemia, corticospinal/spinocerebellar tract dysfunction, dementia
      - Pancreatic lipase is required to separate R-binder from B12 and allow B12 to combine with intrinsic factor to be absorbed at the terminal ileum
  - Splenic vein thrombosis: splenic vein runs along the posterior aspect of the pancreas; chronic inflammation can result in thrombosis and development of gastric varices
  - Pancreatic cancer
  - Narcotic addiction

Pancreatic Cancer
- Risk factors
  - Smoking, alcohol
  - Chronic pancreatitis
  - Obesity
  - Genetics (*BRCA*, Peutz-Jeghers, family history)

- Signs and symptoms
  - Weight loss, anorexia, steatorrhea
  - Chronic gnawing abdominal pain, worse at night
  - Courvoisier sign: palpable jaundice (cancer involving head of the pancreas resulting in common bile duct obstruction)
  - Migratory superficial thrombophlebitis
  - New onset diabetes in older patient without risk factors
- Diagnostics
  - CT/MRI abdomen and pelvis (also used for staging)
  - Biopsy
  - Elevated CA-19-9
- Management: dismal prognosis as most cancers have metastasized upon diagnosis
  - Surgery: Whipple procedure (pancreaticoduodenectomy along with removal of common bile duct, gallbladder, and partial gastrectomy)
  - Palliative chemotherapy

PANCREATIC NEUROENDOCRINE TUMOR

Pancreatic neuroendocrine tumors are a group of hormone-producing tumors resulting in symptomatology related to excess hormone production. All are associated with MEN1 syndrome (pituitary, parathyroid, and pancreatic endocrine tumors).

Gastrinoma
- Pathophysiology: autonomously secreting gastrin tumor resulting in hypersecretion of gastric acid and virulent peptic ulcer disease
- Signs and symptoms
  - Abdominal pain, nausea, dyspepsia
  - Anorexia, weight loss
  - Diarrhea, heartburn
- Diagnostics
  - Biochemical studies
    - Elevated serum gastrin (>1000 pg/mL)
    - Secretin stimulation test: normally, secretin should inhibit gastric; however, gastrin levels remain persistently elevated in gastrinoma
  - Localization studies
    - CT abdomen/pelvis to evaluate for metastatic disease
    - Somatostatin receptor scintigraphy
  - Upper endoscopy: multiple, large ulcers extending into jejunum
- Management
  - Localized disease: surgical resection
  - Metastatic disease: PPIs, somatostatin analogues (octreotide)
- Complications
  - Perforated peptic ulcer
  - GI bleed
  - Gastric outlet obstruction

Insulinoma
- Pathophysiology: autonomously secreting insulin tumor resulting in hypoglycemia
- Signs and symptoms: related to hypoglycemia
  - Palpitations, diaphoresis, tremors
  - Headache, visual disturbances
- Diagnostics
  - Biochemical studies
    - Fasting hypoglycemia
    - Low serum glucose, elevated C-peptide
  - Localization studies: CT/MRI abdomen/pelvis to rule out metastatic disease
- Management
  - Acute management: supplemental glucose (IV dextrose, IM glucagon)
  - Localized disease: surgical resection
  - Metastatic disease: diazoxide, octreotide

Glucagonoma
- Pathophysiology: autonomously secreting glucagon tumor resulting in hyperglycemia
- Signs and symptoms
  - Refractory diabetes mellitus
  - Necrolytic migratory erythema
  - Glossitis, stomatitis
  - Abdominal pain, diarrhea, weight loss
  - Venous thrombosis
  - Depression, psychosis, ataxia
- Diagnostics
  - Elevated serum glucagon
  - CT abdomen and pelvis
  - Somatostatin receptor scintigraphy
- Management
  - Localized disease: surgical resection
  - Metastatic disease: octreotide, sunitinib, everolimus

VIPoma
- Pathophysiology: autonomously secreting vasoactive intestinal peptide tumor resulting in activation of intestinal chloride channels
- Signs and symptoms
  - Severe watery diarrhea: commonly referred to as pancreatic cholera
  - Nausea, vomiting
  - Abdominal pain
- Diagnostics
  - Elevated serum VIP
  - Stool osmolality suggestive of secretory etiology (stool osmolar gap <50)
  - Supporting labs
    - Hypokalemia
    - Nonanion gap metabolic acidosis, achlorhydria
    - Hyperglycemia, hypercalcemia
- Management
  - IV fluid resuscitation, electrolyte repletion
  - Localized disease: surgical resection
  - Metastatic disease: octreotide

Somatostatinoma: extremely rare; triad of cholelithiasis, steatorrhea, diabetes

HEPATOBILIARY
Cholelithiasis
- Definition: gallstones within the gallbladder without evidence of obstruction
- Subtypes
  - Cholesterol: most common, occurs due to supersaturation of bile acids
  - Pigmented: secondary to chronic hemolytic process (sickle-cell disease, hereditary spherocytosis)
  - Calcium bilirubinate: chronic infection/inflammation
- Risk factors
  - Obese
  - Female
  - Multiparity
  - Middle age
- Signs and symptoms
  - Asymptomatic: most common
  - Colicky right upper quadrant (RUQ) abdominal pain associated with fatty meals
- Diagnostics: RUQ abdominal ultrasound
- Management
  - Asymptomatic: no treatment
  - Symptomatic: elective cholecystectomy

Cholecystitis
- Pathophysiology: inflammation of the gallbladder wall secondary to obstruction of the cystic duct by a gallstone
- Signs and symptoms
  - Fever
  - RUQ pain (positive Murphy sign)

- Diagnostics
  - RUQ abdominal ultrasound
    - Sonographic Murphy sign
    - Gallbladder wall thickening
    - Pericholecystic fluid
    - Gallstone within the cystic duct
  - HIDA scan
    - Used when ultrasound is equivocal, but suspicion for acute cholecystitis remains high
    - Demonstrates lack of gallbladder visualization due to obstructing gallstone
  - Supporting labs
    - Leukocytosis
    - Mildly elevated liver function tests
- Management
  - Medical
    - IV fluids
    - +/− IV antibiotics depending on severity and risk of complications
  - Surgical
    - Laparoscopic cholecystectomy after stabilization
    - Percutaneous cholecystostomy followed by interval cholecystectomy if patient is a poor surgical candidate
- Complications
  - Emphysematous cholecystitis: severe infection secondary to gas-producing organism (*Clostridium, Escherichia coli*); increased risk of perforation or gangrene
  - Gangrenous cholecystitis: more common in diabetics and elderly who have delayed presentations and treatment
  - Perforation
  - Gallstone ileus: fistula between the gallbladder and duodenum secondary to adjacent inflammation, which allows passage of gallstones into the small bowel; presents with intermittent abdominal pain as a gallstone obstructs various portions of the small bowel before reaching the ileocecal valve; eventually produces signs and symptoms of small bowel obstruction

Other gallbladder entities:
1. Acalculous cholecystitis: seen in severely ill patients with prolonged hospitalizations; requires urgent cholecystectomy or percutaneous decompression.
2. Chronic cholecystitis: associated with chronic irritation of the gallbladder; may result in calcification producing porcelain gallbladder.
3. Porcelain gallbladder: calcification of the gallbladder wall associated with slightly increased risk of malignancy; treatment is elective prophylactic cholecystectomy.
4. Biliary dyskinesia: dysmotility of bile due to hypertonic sphincter of Oddi; diagnosed with HIDA scan showing decreased gallbladder ejection fraction.

Choledocholithiasis
- Definition: obstruction at the common bile duct secondary to gallstone; may be complicated by ascending cholangitis or pancreatitis (refer to Acute Pancreatitis section for more information, will only discuss ascending cholangitis in reference to complicated choledocholithiasis)
- Microbiology: mixed combination of gram negatives and positives (most common organisms are *E. coli*, *Klebsiella*, and *Enterococcus*)
- Signs and symptoms
  - Uncomplicated: intermittent abdominal pain, nausea, and vomiting

Charcot triad: fever, right upper quadrant pain, and jaundice
Raynaud pentad: fever, jaundice, right upper quadrant pain, altered mental status, and hypotension

  - Complicated
    - High fever
    - RUQ pain
    - Jaundice
    - +/− altered mental status
    - +/− hypotension

- Diagnostics
  - RUQ ultrasound
  - Magnetic resonance cholangiopancreatography
  - ERCP: both diagnostic and therapeutic

Supporting labs
- Leukocytosis
- Elevated alkaline phosphatase, aspartate transaminase/alanine aminotransferase

Management
- Uncomplicated: ERCP followed by cholecystectomy
- Complicated
  - Medical: IV fluids and antibiotics
  - Surgical
    - ERCP with sphincterotomy with stone removal +/− stent insertion: decompresses the common bile duct
    - Percutaneous transhepatic drainage: alternative if ERCP is unavailable
    - Cholecystectomy after stabilization

Choledochal Cysts
- Intra/extrahepatic biliary cysts from congenital malformations of the hepatobiliary tree (Fig. 75-6)
- Presents with intermittent jaundice due to obstruction
- Treatment is surgical resection due to biliary obstruction and risk of malignant transformation

Gallbladder Carcinoma
- Risk factors
  - Chronic cholecystitis
  - Choledochal cyst
  - Recurrent infections
  - Porcelain gallbladder

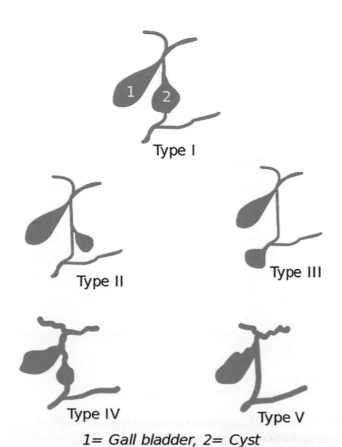

1= Gall bladder, 2= Cyst

Fig. 75-6: Five subtypes of choledochal cyst. Type I: dilation of extrahepatic biliary duct. Type II: cyst from common bile duct (CBD). Type III: choledochocele or dilation of distal CBD. Type IV: dilation of both extrahepatic and intrahepatic duct. Type V: Caroli disease, dilation of intrahepatic duct only. (Image and caption courtesy of I, Drriad; CC BY-SA 3.0 [http://creativecommons.org/licenses/by-sa/3.0/])

- Signs and symptoms
  - Asymptomatic: most common
  - Intermittent RUQ pain
  - Jaundice
  - Weight loss, anorexia
- Diagnostics
  - RUQ ultrasound
  - Cholecystectomy: definitive diagnosis +/− therapeutic depending on cancer stage
- Management: surgical resection; however, most cases are advanced upon diagnosis if symptomatic

Ampullary Adenocarcinoma
- Signs and symptoms
  - Abdominal pain
  - Jaundice
  - Anorexia, weight loss
  - Melena: associated with chronic GI bleed
- Diagnostics
  - RUQ ultrasound: initial test
  - Endoscopy with biopsy: diagnostic
- Supporting labs
  - Microcytic anemia
  - Direct hyperbilirubinemia: obstructive jaundice
  - Positive fecal occult blood test
- Management: surgical resection +/− chemoradiation

Cholangiocarcinoma
- Definition: malignancy involving intra/extrahepatic biliary ducts
- Risk factors
  - Primary sclerosing cholangitis
  - Ulcerative colitis
  - Clonorchis sinensis (liver fluke infection associated with undercooked fish; treated with praziquantel)
  - Choledochal (biliary) cysts
- Signs and symptoms
  - Abdominal pain, palpable abdominal mass
  - Obstructive jaundice: light-colored stools, dark-colored urine, pruritus
  - Weight loss
- Diagnostics
  - Elevated CA-19-9
  - ERCP
  - Percutaneous transhepatic cholangiography
- Management
  - Extremely poor prognosis (<1-year survival after diagnosis) as most tumors are unresectable
  - Palliative stenting for biliary obstruction

Klatzkin tumor: cholangiocarcinoma involving proximal third of common bile duct at the union of the right and left hepatic ducts

Hepatocellular Carcinoma
- Risk factors
  - Any cause of cirrhosis
  - Occasionally hepatitis B can cause hepatocellular carcinoma without evidence of cirrhosis
  - Toxins: aflatoxin, vinyl chloride
  - Hepatic adenoma
  - Infectious: schistosomiasis
  - Metabolic: alpha-1 antitrypsin, Wilson disease, hemochromatosis
- Signs and symptoms
  - Complications of cirrhosis: see Cirrhosis section in gastroenterology
  - Abdominal pain, weight loss
  - Worsening hepatomegaly in a patient with known cirrhosis
  - Paraneoplastic syndromes (hypoglycemia, polycythemia)

- Diagnostics
  - Elevated alpha-fetoprotein
  - Contrast-enhanced CT/MRI: lesion >1 cm, nonrim arterial phase enhancement relative to liver parenchyma
  - Liver biopsy: can be bypassed if classic imaging features are present
- Management
  - Localized disease: surgical resection or embolization
  - Extensive disease: chemotherapy

LARGE BOWEL
Volvulus
- Definition: torsion of the bowel along the axis of its mesentery, most commonly involving the sigmoid colon
- Risk factors
  - Elderly
  - Nursing home patients
  - Younger women: associated with cecal volvulus
- Signs and symptoms
  - Severe, sudden onset abdominal pain
  - Abdominal distention
  - Nausea, vomiting
  - Absence of flatus, constipation
  - High-pitched bowel sounds
- Diagnostic
  - Abdominal x-ray
    - Air fluid levels in the small bowel
    - Severe colonic dilation, lack of haustra
    - Coffee bean sign: seen in sigmoid volvulus (Fig. 75-7)
    - Pneumoperitoneum: seen in advanced cases due to ischemia as twisting bowel cuts off its blood supply
  - Barium enema
    - Parrot's beak sign: distended, air-filled loop of bowel in the RUQ that tapers toward the left lower quadrant
- Management
  - Proctosigmoidoscopy with rectal tube
  - Surgical intervention for recurrent cases or perforation

Large bowel obstruction: unlike small bowel obstruction, often requires surgical intervention; most common causes of large bowel obstruction include cancer and volvulus.

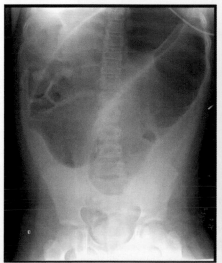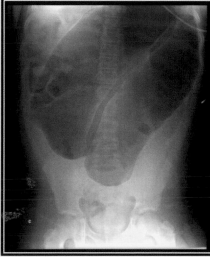

Fig. 75-7: (A) Coffee bean sign in a patient with sigmoid volvulus. (B) Same diagram with overlaid coffee bean.

Ogilvie Syndrome
- Definition: pseudocolonic obstruction secondary to functional bowel dysmotility and adynamic colon; theorized to occur secondary to interruption of parasympathetic fibers
- Risk factors
  - Severe illness
  - Elderly, institutionalized
  - Postoperative
  - Opiates
  - Electrolyte derangements (hypokalemia)
- Signs and symptoms
  - Abdominal distention
  - Mild abdominal pain
  - Bowel sounds present
  - Tympanitic abdomen
- Diagnostics: abdominal X-ray
  - Severe colonic dilation (Fig. 75-8)
  - No air fluid levels
- Management
  - Treat/reverse modifiable risk factors
  - IV neostigmine: avoid if there is suspicion for mechanical obstruction
  - Colonoscopy with decompression
  - Surgical decompression: last resort

Diverticulosis
- Epidemiology: most common cause of lower GI bleed in the elderly (>50 years old)
- Definition: colonic outpouchings that occur secondary to chronic constipation and meat-based Western diet (high protein, low fiber)
- Sign and symptoms
  - Asymptomatic (most common)
  - Chronic constipation
  - Painless hematochezia: outpouchings of the colonic wall cause weakness and results in bleeding in the associated arterial supply
- Diagnostics
  - Colonoscopy (often incidental finding on colonoscopy done for other reasons)
  - CT abdomen/pelvis
  - Barium enema (Fig. 75-9)

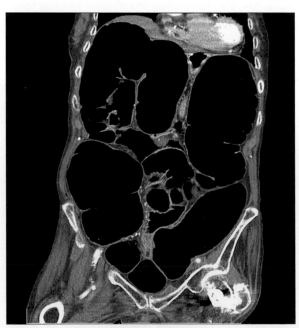

Fig. 75-8: Coronal computed tomography demonstrating diffuse colonic dilation in a patient with Ogilvie syndrome. (Image courtesy of Milliways; CC BY-SA 3.0 [https://creativecommons.org/licenses/by-sa/3.0])

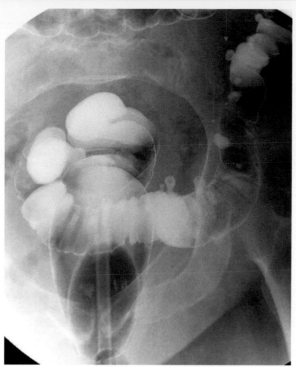

Fig. 75-9: Colonic outpouchings in a patient with diverticulosis on barium enema examination.

- Associations: polycystic kidney disease
- Management
  - Most cases resolve spontaneously
  - Endoscopic or surgical intervention for refractory cases
  - Prevention of complications with a high-fiber diet
- Complications: diverticulitis

Diverticulitis
- Pathophysiology: obstruction and inflammation of a diverticula due to cancer or fecalith
- Signs and symptoms
  - Left lower quadrant abdominal pain
  - Fevers, chills
  - Nausea, vomiting
  - Constipation, diarrhea
  - Increased urgency, dysuria (bladder irritation from inflamed sigmoid colon)
  - Palpable mass in some cases
- Diagnostics
  - CT abdomen pelvis with oral and IV contrast: bowel wall thickening, pericolic fluid collections
  - Upright plain film to rule out perforation
  - Colonoscopy to determine cause of diverticulitis should be done 4–6 weeks after resolution due to increased risk of perforation in the acute setting
- Management: may be treated inpatient or outpatient depending on severity, patient comorbidities, age, and presence of complications
  - Medical
    - IV fluids, bowel rest (NPO)
    - Antibiotics: cover gram negatives and anaerobes
      - Ciprofloxacin + metronidazole
      - TMP-SMX plus metronidazole
      - Amoxicillin-clavulanate
      - Piperacillin-tazobactam
      - Moxifloxacin
  - Surgical
    - If unresponsive to medical therapy
    - Development of complications such as perforation, abscess, obstruction, fistula (colovesical), or toxic megacolon
    - Multiple recurrences

Avoid the use of barium contrast enema if toxic megacolon is suspected due to high risk of perforation and barium-induced peritonitis.

Crohn disease and ulcerative colitis are the two main subtypes of inflammatory bowel disease (IBD). In 10% of cases these may overlap; however, they are differentiated based on the pattern and area of bowel involvement (see Table 75-1, Fig. 75-10).

Both vitamin B12 and bile acids are reabsorbed in the terminal ileum resulting in B12 deficiency in Crohn disease when there is terminal ileum involvement. Loss of bile acids results in increased concentration of bilirubin conjugates and total calcium in the gallbladder. This alters the hepatic bile composition resulting in cholesterol supersaturation and formation of gallstones.

Toxic Megacolon
- Causes
    - *Clostridium difficile*
    - Ulcerative colitis
    - Ischemic colitis
    - Volvulus
    - Diverticulitis
- Signs and symptoms
    - Peritoneal signs (severe ileus, guarding, rigidity, rebound tenderness)
    - Worsening fever (>38°C), abdominal distention
    - Hemodynamic instability
    - Altered mental status
- Diagnostics
    - Abdominal X-ray: initial test (Fig. 75-11)
        - Right colonic dilation >6 cm
        - Haustral folds that do not extend across entire lumen
        - Multiple air fluid levels in the colon
    - CT abdomen and pelvis
- Supporting labs
    - Leukocytosis >10,500
    - Lactate >2.2
- Management: medical emergency due to risk of perforation
    - Medical
        - IV fluids, nasogastric tube (bowel decompression), bowel rest
        - IV corticosteroids for IBD-induced toxic megacolon
        - Antibiotics
            - Third-generation cephalosporin (ceftriaxone) + metronidazole
            - PO vancomycin plus IV metronidazole for *C. difficile* colitis related
    - Surgical: for patients unresponsive to medical management or those who have perforated
        - Subtotal colectomy with end ileostomy

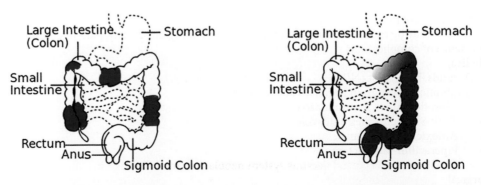

Crohn Disease   **Colitis ulcerosa**

Fig. 75-10: Colonic distribution of Crohn disease *(left)*, and ulcerative colitis *(right)*. Skip lesions seen in Crohn disease versus diffuse colonic involvement starting from the rectum in ulcerative colitis.

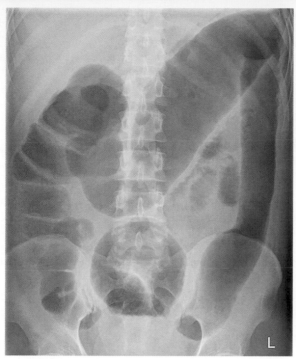

Fig. 75-11: Toxic megacolon in a patient with ulcerative colitis. Abdominal X-ray demonstrating transverse and right colonic dilation, submucosal edema, and loss of haustral folds.

Colon Cancer
- Risk factors
  - Age >50 years
  - Family history
  - IBD (ulcerative colitis)
  - High-fat, low-fiber diet
  - Genetic mutations
    - Hereditary nonpolyposis colorectal cancer
    - Familial adenomatous polyposis (FAP)
    - Peutz-Jeghers syndrome
- Key manifestations
  - Iron deficiency anemia
  - Weight loss
  - Constipation
  - Change in stool diameter (pencil-thin stools)
  - Bowel obstruction
  - Melena, hematochezia
- Associated polyposis syndromes
  - Gardner syndrome
    - FAP variant
    - APC gene mutation
    - Thousands of polyps
    - Colon cancer plus soft tissue tumors (desmoid, lipomas, osteomas, fibromas, sebaceous or epidermoid cysts)
  - Turcot syndrome
    - FAP variant
    - APC gene mutation
    - Thousands of polyps
    - Colon cancer plus central nervous system neoplasms (medulloblastoma, glioblastoma)
  - Peutz-Jeghers syndrome
    - Mucocutaneous pigmentation (lips, perioral, buccal mucosa)
    - Hamartomatous polyps (small intestine): may present as intussusception or small bowel obstruction
    - Increased risk of other cancers (breast, stomach, small intestine, pancreas)

- Hereditary nonpolyposis colorectal cancer (Lynch syndrome)
  - DNA mismatch repair gene mutation
  - Colon cancer without the development of polyps
  - Increased risk for multiple other cancers (endometrial, ovarian, gastric, pancreatic, urothelial, skin)
- Diagnostics
  - Barium enema: apple-core lesion
  - CT abdomen and pelvis
  - Colonoscopy: definitive diagnosis
- Management
  - Surgical resection for localized disease
  - Chemoradiation for advanced disease

ANORECTAL

Hemorrhoids occur due to engorgement of the arteriovenous connections of the anal canal and may be painful or painless depending on their location above or below the dentate line; however, regardless of their location the treatment is similar (Table 75-2).

Anal Cancer
- Epidemiology: most commonly squamous cell carcinoma; rarely adenocarcinoma
- Risk factors
  - Human papillomavirus (HPV) serotypes 16, 18, 31, 33
  - Anal intercourse
  - Smoking
  - Human immunodeficiency virus
- Signs and symptoms
  - Anal pain/mass
  - Rectal fullness
  - Constipation
- Diagnostics: biopsy
- Management: Nigro protocol chemoradiation (5-fluorouracil + mitomycin) preferred over surgery due to preservation of anal sphincter
- Prevention
  - HPV vaccine
  - Barrier contraceptives (chronic)
  - Smoking cessation

TABLE 75-2 Hemorrhoids: Internal Versus External

	INTERNAL HEMORRHOIDS	EXTERNAL HEMORRHOIDS
Definition	Engorgement of arteriovenous connections in the anal canal	
Causes	Low-fiber diet Constipation Increased portal pressures (cirrhosis, obesity, pregnancy)	
Signs and symptoms	Usually painless (visceral innervation) Bright red blood per rectum Classified from grade I (no prolapse) to IV (irreducible) based on degree of prolapse Sensation of perianal fullness	Extremely painful (somatic innervation), especially if thrombosed Bright red blood per rectum or on toilet paper Itchy, mucous discharge
Location	Above the dentate line (lined by columnar epithelium)	Below the dentate line (lined by squamous epithelium)
Diagnosis	Anoscopy Proctoscopy	
Treatment	Medical: High-fiber diet Topical analgesics and steroids: hydrocortisone/lidocaine Antispasmodics: topical nitroglycerin, nifedipine Sitz bath: warm bath used to alleviate anal sphincter spasms; used for acute flares Surgical: Rubber band ligation Sclerotherapy Excision for severe unresponsive cases	

TRAUMA

Key points

- Regardless of blunt or penetrating abdominal trauma, if patient has peritoneal signs, proceed directly to exploratory laparotomy (Figs. 75-12 and 75-13)
- CT abdomen/pelvis should only be done in hemodynamically stable patients
- Injury to abdominal viscera can occur up to T4/T5 as the diaphragm moves superiorly on complete expiration
- Most injured organ causing intraabdominal bleeding is the liver (most common) or spleen; the spleen more often requires surgical intervention due to more significant bleeding
- Other locations of internal bleeding include pericardium, pleural cavity, proximal thighs, and pelvis; bleeding into the proximal thighs and pelvis can result in hemorrhagic shock without obvious physical exam findings
- Intraoperative coagulopathy occurs secondary to multiple transfusions; transfusions must be supplemented with platelets and fresh frozen plasma; a triad of intraoperative coagulopathy, hypothermia, and lactic acidosis necessitate stopping surgery

SPECIFIC TRAUMATIC ABDOMINAL ENTITIES

Abdominal Compartment Syndrome

- Pathophysiology: increased intraabdominal pressure with associated compression of neurovascular structures resulting in neurovascular compromise

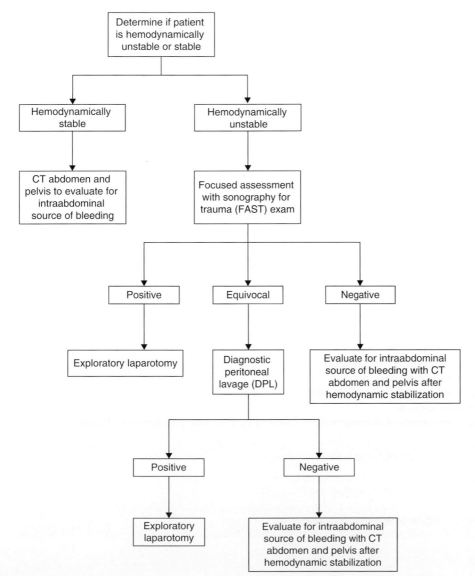

Fig. 75-12: Flow chart for the approach to blunt abdominal trauma; *CT*, Computed tomography

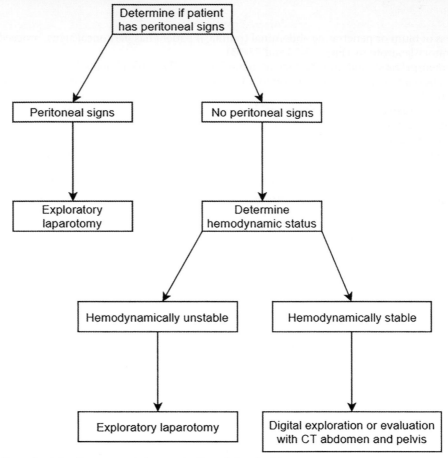

Fig. 75-13: Flow chart for the approach to penetrating abdominal trauma

- Causes
  - Prolonged intraabdominal surgery with excessive fluid and blood resuscitation
  - Trauma
  - Pancreatitis
  - Burns
  - Ruptured aortic aneurysm
  - Large ascites
- Signs and symptoms
  - Tense abdominal distention
  - Tearing of retention sutures
  - Hypotension, tachycardia
  - Elevated jugular venous pressure
  - Decreased urine output
  - Increased intraabdominal pressures
- Diagnostics: clinical
- Management: surgical decompression followed by temporary abdominal closure

Extremity compartment syndrome presents with the 5 Ps:
1. Pain
2. Paresthesias
3. Paralysis
4. Pulselessness
5. Poikilothermia

Diaphragmatic Hernia
- Pathophysiology: herniation of intraabdominal contents into the thoracic cavity secondary to increased intraabdominal pressure; most commonly occurs on the left
- Cause: blunt or penetrating abdominal trauma
- Signs and symptoms
  - Respiratory distress: secondary to compression of lung parenchyma
  - Scaphoid abdomen
  - Nausea, vomiting
  - Enteric tube in the thoracic cavity
- Diagnostics: chest X-ray (bowel loops in the thoracic cavity)
- Management: surgical repair plus exploratory laparotomy

Duodenal Hematoma
- Occurs most commonly in children secondary to blunt abdominal trauma
- Presents with signs and symptoms of small bowel obstruction
- Diagnosed with CT abdomen/pelvis
- Most cases resolve spontaneously with conservative management
- Surgery if unresponsive to conservative measures

ESOPHAGUS

TABLE 76-1   Differentiating Mallory-Weiss Tear Versus Boerhaave Syndrome

	MALLORY-WEISS TEAR	BOERHAAVE SYNDROME
Definition	• Longitudinal submucosal laceration of the distal esophagus or proximal stomach	• Transmural laceration of the esophagus
Causes	• Severe vomiting and retching (due to sudden increase in intraabdominal pressure)	• Severe vomiting and retching • Other causes of esophageal perforation: recent EGD, penetrating trauma
Signs and symptoms	• Self-resolving hematemesis • Epigastric or back pain	• Acute retrosternal chest pain • Subcutaneous emphysema • Crepitus in the suprasternal notch • Odynophagia, dysphagia • Fever, septic shock
Diagnostics	• Clinical: if patient describes appropriate story and is no longer symptomatic at the time of presentation • EGD: longitudinal submucosal laceration	• Gastrografin esophagram: extravasation of contrast through transmural tear • Chest computed tomography/X-ray: pneumomediastinum, left-sided pleural effusion (due to rupture of left posterolateral distal esophagus) • Thoracentesis plus pleural fluid analysis: elevated amylase (due to saliva in the esophageal contents)
Management	• Majority of cases self-resolve requiring no treatment • Persistent bleeding: epinephrine, electrocautery, IV proton pump inhibitors or antiemetics	• Surgical repair • Alternative for surgical repair: drainage, endoscopic stent placement, or esophagectomy (last resort)

EGD, Esophagogastroduodenoscopy.
Barium swallow is generally avoided if transmural tear is suspected, as extravasation into the mediastinum can result in mediastinitis.

Esophageal perforation can be transmural or submucosal often due to severe vomiting. The presence of transmural or submucosal cannot be determined clinically as patients with transmural lacerations will appear acutely ill, while those with submucosal lacerations will have self-resolving symptoms and in many cases may not report to the hospital (Table 76-1).

Esophageal Cancer
– Risk factors
  • Squamous cell carcinoma
    ▪ Smoking
    ▪ Alcohol
    ▪ Elderly
    ▪ Nitrate-containing foods
    ▪ Vitamin/mineral deficiencies (beta-carotene, B1, zinc, selenium)
    ▪ Hereditary: Peutz-Jeghers syndrome, Cowden syndrome (PTEN tumor suppressor gene mutation)
  • Adenocarcinoma
    ▪ Long-standing gastroesophageal disease (Barrett esophagus)
    ▪ Smoking
    ▪ Obesity
    ▪ High calorie and fat intake

- Signs and symptoms
  - Progressive dysphagia to solids, and later liquids
  - Weight loss
  - Gastrointestinal bleed
  - Chest discomfort, dyspepsia
  - Cough, hoarseness
  - Vomiting, regurgitation
- Diagnostics
  - Initial test: barium esophagram (asymmetric narrowing of the esophageal lumen)
  - Biopsy
  - Positron-emission tomography (PET)/computed tomography (CT) for staging
- Management
  - Localized disease: surgical resection
  - Metastatic disease: chemoradiation, palliative stent placement

CARDIAC SURGERY

Coronary Artery Disease
- Risk factors
  - Hypertension
  - Diabetes
  - Dyslipidemia
  - Family history
- Signs and symptoms: substernal chest pain +/− radiation to the neck or jaw
- Diagnostics
  - Electrocardiogram (ECG): initial test
  - Troponin levels: most sensitive
  - Cardiac catheterization: allows for anatomic evaluation of significant stenosis and intervention
- Management
  - General principles: should be optimized prior to and after percutaneous coronary intervention (PCI) or coronary artery bypass graft (CABG)
    - Lifestyle modifications
    - Antihypertensives
    - Antiplatelets
    - Statins
  - PCI
    - Indications
      - Stable coronary artery disease that does not meet criteria for CABG
      - Relief of medically refractive angina
    - Door to balloon time <90 minutes at PCI-capable facility
    - Door to balloon time of <120 minutes at non-PCI-capable facility
  - CABG
    - Indications
      - Left main coronary or left main equivalent disease
      - Three-vessel disease
      - Two-vessel disease with >75% stenosis in left anterior descending artery
    - Complications
      - Bleeding
      - Mediastinitis
      - Acute kidney injury

VALVULAR DISEASE

Left-sided valvular heart disease is far more common than right-sided valvular heart disease (Table 76-2). As valvular heart disease progresses in severity it develops characteristic auscultatory findings, and, combined with patient risk factors, a particular valvular heart disease diagnosis can be made (Fig. 76-1). Echocardiogram is also essential in evaluating the heart morphology, function, and other associated abnormalities that can ultimately guide treatment and determine whether medical or surgical management is needed.

Patients with severe valvular disease undergoing cardiac surgery for other indications should have concomitant valvular surgery.

All nonbioprosthetic valve replacements will require long-term anticoagulation.

TABLE 76-2 **Left-Sided Valvular Disease**

	DIASTOLIC		SYSTOLIC	
	AORTIC REGURGITATION	MITRAL STENOSIS	MITRAL REGURGITATION	AORTIC STENOSIS
Risk factors	• Tertiary syphilis • Ankylosing spondylitis • Aortic dissection • Giant cell arteritis o Endocarditis o Trauma	• Rheumatic heart disease	• Hypertension • Ischemia (papillary muscle rupture) • Mitral valve prolapse	• Ederly • Bicuspid aortic valve (early calcification) • Rheumatic heart disease
Auscultatory location	• Diastolic decrescendo murmur heard at left lower sternal border	• Rumbling diastolic murmur heard in the fifth intercostal space midclavicular line associated with opening snap	• Systolic murmur heard in the fifth intercostal space midclavicular line with radiation to the axilla	• Crescendo-decrescendo systolic murmur heard in the right second intercostal space with radiation to the carotids
Signs and symptoms	• Waterhammer pulse • De Musset sign: head bobbing • Quinke sign: nailbed pulsations • Muller sign: oscillating uvula • Traube sign: systolic/diastolic murmur heard over the femoral arteries • Biphasic pulse	• Atrial fibrillation • High-intensity S1 sound • Left atrial dilation: chest X-ray (straightening left heart border, elevated left main bronchus), esophageal compression (dysphagia), recurrent laryngeal nerve compression (hoarseness)	• Acute: dyspnea, pulmonary edema • Chronic: symptoms related to left atrial dilation	• Syncope, angina, dyspnea • Displaced apical impulse • Pulsus parvus et tardus • Paradoxic splitting with closure of pulmonic valve prior to aortic valve in severe cases • Concomitant angiodysplasia and acquired von Willebrand factor deficiency
Diagnostics	Echocardiogram			
Management	• Medical management: decrease afterload with vasodilators • Surgical indications: symptomatic severe aortic regurgitation (AR), asymptomatic severe AR with ejection fraction <50%	• Medical management only for symptomatic treatment • Surgical indications: severe mitral stenosis (<1.5 cm²), severely symptomatic	• Medical management only for symptomatic treatment • Surgical indications: severe primary mitral regurgitation (MR) with ejection fraction <30%, asymptomatic severe primary MR with ejection fraction 30–60% and/or left ventricular end-systolic diameter >40 mm	• Surgical indications (valve replacement): development of symptoms, decreased valve area (<1 cm²), ejection fraction <50% • Cardiac catheterization prior to surgical repair for possible concurrent coronary artery bypass graft and exclude coronary artery disease as cause of symptoms • Transcatheter aortic valve replacement for poor surgical candidates

Right-Sided Valvular Disease
- Tricuspid regurgitation
  • Associations
    ▪ IV drug users
    ▪ Pulmonary hypertension
    ▪ Systemic carcinoid (may also cause tricuspid/pulmonic stenosis)
    ▪ Complications of pacemaker placement
  • Auscultation: holosystolic murmur at left sternal border, increased with deep inspiration
  • Management: treat underlying disorders, surgical repair

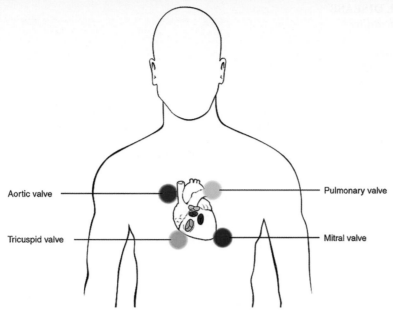

Fig. 76-1: Locations for listening for heart murmurs. Aortic valve: right second intercostal space. Pulmonary valve: left upper sternal border. Tricuspid valve: left sternal border. Mitral valve: left fifth intercostal space midclavicular line.

- Pulmonic stenosis
  - Associations
    - Congenital disorders (congenital rubella infection, tetralogy of Fallot, Noonan syndrome)
    - Systemic carcinoid
  - Auscultation
    - Systolic murmur at the upper left sternal border
    - Increased intensity with deep inspiration
    - Wide splitting S2
    - Pulmonic ejection sound
  - Management: balloon valvuloplasty

Endocarditis
- Definition: infection and seeding of the heart valves or device
- Risk factors
  - Valvular heart disease
  - Prosthetic valve
  - Bacteremia
  - IV drug abuse (*Staphylococcus aureus*)
  - Colon cancer, inflammatory bowel disease (*Streptococcus gallolyticus, Clostridium septicum*)
  - Dental cleaning/infection/cavities (*Viridans streptococci*)
  - Gastrointestinal/genitourinary infection with manipulation (*Enterococci*)
- Signs and symptoms
  - Fever, malaise
  - New murmur or worsening of preexisting murmur
- Diagnostics (Duke criteria)
  - Blood cultures
  - Transthoracic echocardiography, followed by transesophageal echocardiography if necessary
- Management
  - Long-term (4–6 weeks) antibiotics pending culture sensitivity
  - Surgical indications
    - Valve rupture, congestive heart failure CHF
    - Fungal endocarditis
    - Recurrent emboli
    - Abscess formation

PERICARDIAL DISEASE
Constrictive Pericarditis
– Causes
  • Tuberculosis
  • Iatrogenic: cardiac surgery, radiation
– Signs and symptoms
  • Elevated jugular venous pressure
  • Kussmaul sign: increased jugular venous distention (JVD) on inspiration
  • Pulses paradoxus: decrease in systolic blood pressure >10 Hg mm upon inspiration
  • Pericardial knock
  • Signs of right heart failure (hepatomegaly, peripheral edema, ascites)
– Diagnostics
  • ECG: low-voltage QRS
  • CT chest: rimlike calcification around the heart
  • Echocardiogram: equalization of diastolic pressures
– Management
  • Glucocorticoids to decrease the risk of constrictive pericarditis in tuberculosis
  • Pericardiectomy

Other causes of superior vena cava syndrome: fibrosing mediastinitis (tuberculosis or histoplasmosis infection), upper extremity deep vein thrombosis, lymphoma

LUNG SURGERY
Lung nodule principles
• Common incidental finding on lung imaging while working up other pathologies
• It is important to stratify lung nodules to determine further management based on patient risk factors, size, appearance, and previous imaging (Table 76-3)
• This will determine whether patient will require early evaluation, repeat imaging, or no further workup (Table 76-4)
• When lung nodule is detected the most appropriate next step is to examine previous imaging

TABLE 76-3   Comparing High-Risk and Low-Risk Lung Nodules

	HIGH-RISK FEATURES	LOW-RISK FEATURES
Patient risk factors	• Heavy smoker (>30 pack year history) • Previous thoracic radiation (breast cancer, Hodgkin lymphoma, thyroid carcinoma) • >40 years old	• Nonsmoker • No previous radiation • <35 years old
Appearance	• Sparse calcification • Spiculated surface • Subsolid	• Dense calcification • Smooth surface • Solid
Size	>2 cm	<9 mm
Previous imaging	Previously not present or enlarging nodule	Present but unchanged over several years

TABLE 76-4   Management of Lung Nodules Based on Whether Nodule Is Low, Moderate, or High Risk of Being Malignant

TYPE OF NODULE	MANAGEMENT
High risk	• Video-assisted thoracic surgery (VATS) excisional biopsy • Nonsurgical biopsy if patient is a poor surgical candidate
Intermediate risk	• Noncontrast surveillance computed tomography chest • Nonsurgical biopsy: • Bronchoscopy: centrally located lesions • Transthoracic needle biopsy: smaller peripherally located lesions
Low risk	• No further workup

Lung Cancer
- Risk factors
  - Smoking
  - Occupational exposure (asbestos)
  - Previous thoracic radiation
- Key manifestations
  - Cough, fever, weight loss
  - Chest pain, dyspnea
  - Wheezing, tachypnea
  - Pleural effusion, postobstructive pneumonia
  - Phrenic nerve, recurrent laryngeal nerve palsy
  - Pancoast tumor: squamous cell carcinoma of the superior sulcus
    - Horner syndrome: triad of ptosis, miosis, and anhidrosis due to invasion of the superior cervical ganglion
    - Brachial plexus palsies
  - Superior vena cava (SVC) syndrome: carcinoma obstructing the SVC and impeding venous return of blood from head, neck, and arms
    - Facial plethora
    - Ipsilateral neck vein distention
    - JVD
  - Metastases: bone, adrenal, brain
- Types/location
  - Central
    - Small cell lung cancer: all other cancers are considered non–small cell lung cancer
    - Squamous cell carcinoma
  - Peripheral
    - Adenocarcinoma: most common cause of lung cancer in females and nonsmokers
    - Large cell carcinoma
    - Bronchoalveolar carcinoma
- Diagnostics
  - Chest imaging: lung mass with high risk features
    - Squamous cell carcinoma: central cavitation and necrosis
    - Bronchoalveolar carcinoma: mimics pneumonia
  - Sputum cytology
  - Fluorodeoxyglucose-PET scan
  - Biopsy: important to differentiate the different subtypes of lung cancer as this will determine whether patient will require surgery vs chemoradiation (Figs. 76-2 and 76-3)
  - Staging: CT chest/abdomen/pelvis; magnetic resonance imaging brain

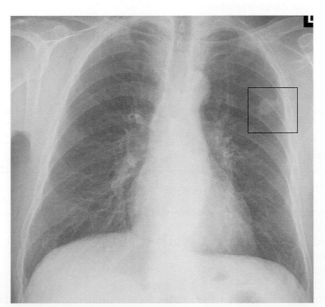

Fig. 76-2: Lung nodule on chest X-ray in the left upper lobe.

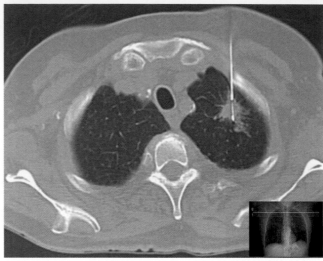

Fig. 76-3: Computed tomography–guided lung biopsy of spiculated left lung mass, highly suspicious for cancer.

TABLE 76-5   Mediastinal Masses Differential Diagnosis

Anterior (four Ts)	Lymphoma ("Terrible lymphoma") Thymoma Thyroid carcinoma Teratoma
Middle	Bronchogenic cysts Pericardial cyst Enteric cyst Esophageal tumor Tracheal tumors Aneurysm of the aortic arch
Posterior	Neurogenic tumors Meningocele Thoracic spine lesion

– Management: overall poor prognosis due to late-stage detection
  • Small cell lung cancer: chemoradiation
  • Non–small cell lung cancer: surgical excision
    ▪ Obtain pulmonary function tests before surgery to determine if patient has the necessary lung reserve to tolerate a pneumonectomy/lobectomy
    ▪ Minimum FEV1 of 800 mL postsurgery is required

OTHER MEDIASTINAL ENTITIES
Determining the location of a mediastinal mass will narrow the differential substantially (Table 76-5).

TRAUMA
Tracheobronchial Injury
– Mechanism: rapid deceleration and chest trauma resulting in rupture at the tracheobronchial junction
– Signs and symptoms
  • Hemoptysis
  • Nonresolving pneumothorax despite placement of thoracostomy tube
  • Persistent air leak
  • Extensive subcutaneous emphysema: crepitus over the upper chest and neck
– Diagnostics: CT thorax or bronchoscopy
– Management: surgical repair
Pulmonary Contusion
– Mechanism: bruising of the lung parenchyma after chest trauma resulting in intraalveolar edema and hemorrhage; may have associated rib fractures

- Diagnostics: chest X-ray (diffuse, patchy, irregular capacities that does not follow anatomic borders)
- Management: supportive with supplemental oxygen, diuresis, and pulmonary toilet
- Complications: acute respiratory distress syndrome (ARDS)

Myocardial Contusion
- Mechanism: severe trauma to the chest at the level of the manubrium, commonly associated with sternal fracture
- Signs and symptoms
  - Sternal chest pain
  - Tachycardia
- Diagnostics
  - ST-T wave abnormality
  - Elevated troponin
  - New onset arrhythmia or bundle branch block
- Management: careful monitoring on telemetry for 24–48 hours
- Complications: cardiogenic pulmonary edema

Cardiac Tamponade
- Complication of pericardial effusion from any etiology (infectious, bleeding, trauma)
- Presents with tachycardia, hypotension, elevated JVP, muffled heart sounds: last three signs make up Beck triad
- Diagnosed by echocardiogram
- Treated by pericardial decompression via pericardiocentesis or surgical pericardiotomy

Rib Fractures
- Common site of fractures after trauma
- Signs and symptoms
  - Localized chest wall tenderness
  - Poor inspiratory breaths
- Diagnosis: chest X-ray
- Management: pain control to prevent hypoventilation → atelectasis → pneumonia
- Complications
  - Atelectasis/pneumonia
  - Pulmonary contusion
  - Pneumothorax (Table 76-6; Fig. 76-4)
  - Organ laceration (liver/spleen if lower ribs are involved)

Hemothorax
- Definition: blood in the pleural cavity from bleeding lung or intercostal artery
- Signs and symptoms: similar to pleural effusion
  - Shortness of breath
  - Ipsilateral decreased breath sounds
  - Dullness to percussion

TABLE 76-6   Tension Versus Spontaneous Pneumothorax

	SPONTANEOUS PNEUMOTHORAX	TENSION PNEUMOTHORAX
Causes	• Preexisting lung disease • Trauma: rib fracture, penetrating wound • Iatrogenic: central line placement, thoracentesis, mechanical ventilation, lung biopsy	
Signs and symptoms	• Sudden, acute onset shortness of breath • Chest pain • Decreased breath sounds on the side of pneumothorax • Tympanitic to percussion	• Same as spontaneous pneumothorax plus hypotension, tachycardia, and elevated jugular venous pressure

Imaging	• Chest X-ray:
	  • Visceral pleural line: most sensitive in the lung apex due to air rising
	  • Absent lung markings peripherally
		• Chest X-ray: same as spontaneous pneumothorax plus the following:
		  • Contralateral tracheal and mediastinal deviation
		  • Ipsilateral flattening of the hemidiaphragm

Management	• Small, simple, and healthy adult: observation, supplemental oxygen • Large to moderate: chest tube • Recurrent: pleurodesis	• Immediate needle decompression followed by chest tube placement

Spontaneous pneumothorax can be divided into primary and secondary types. Primary spontaneous pneumothorax occurs in patients with normal lungs, often seen in tall, thin, athletic males (marfanoid habitus). Secondary spontaneous pneumothorax occurs in patients with preexisting lung disease (chronic obstructive pulmonary disease, asthma).

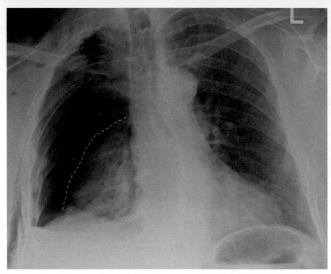

Fig. 76-4: Multiple rib fractures *(red arrows)* resulting in traumatic pneumothorax. (Image courtesy of James Heilman, MD; CC BY-SA 4.0 [https://creativecommons.org/licenses/by-sa/4.0])

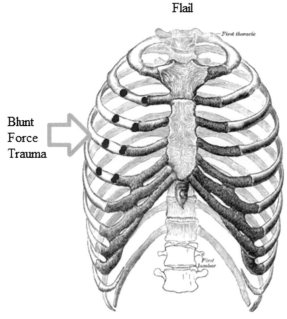

Fig. 76-5: Illustration of a flail chest. Red dots represent sites of fracture. (Image courtesy of Mrnave; CC BY-SA 3.0 [https://creativecommons.org/licenses/by-sa/3.0])

- Diagnostics
  - Chest X-ray
  - Thoracentesis: both diagnostic and therapeutic
- Management
  - Slow bleed: conservative
    - Thoracostomy tube
    - Blood/fluid resuscitation
  - Brisk bleeds: surgical
    - Defined as >200 mL/hour over 4 hours or 1 L drainage upon initial thoracostomy tube placement
    - Requires thoracotomy for surgical expiration
- Complications
  - Empyema
  - Fibrothorax

Flail Chest
- Definition: three or more adjacent rib fractures that fracture in two locations (Fig. 76-5)

– Signs and symptoms
  • Paradoxic chest wall movement (fracture segment retracts inward on inspiration and moves outward on expiration)
  • Shallow breaths
– Diagnostics: chest X-ray
– Management
  • Initial: supplemental oxygen, pain control
  • Respiratory failure: positive pressure ventilation +/− bilateral chest tubes (prevents development of tension pneumothorax)
– Complications
  • Pulmonary contusion
  • ARDS
  • Tension pneumothorax

Abnormalities of the hand occur most commonly due to tendon pathology. Most cases are treated with splinting or surgery for more complicated and refractory cases (Table 77-1).

INFECTIONS
Infectious/Septic Arthritis
- Definition: infection involving the joint space (synovial membrane)
- Pathophysiology: same as osteomyelitis
- Microbiology
  - *Staphylococcus aureus:* most common cause
  - *Neisseria gonorrhea:* young, sexually active
  - *Streptococcus pneumonia:* splenic dysfunction
  - Gram negative: gastrointestinal infection, immunocompromised, IV drug abuse
  - *Eikenella:* human bites
  - *Borrelia burgdorferi* (Lyme disease): bull's-eye rash, hiking, tick bite
- Signs and symptoms
  - Acute, painful, erythematous monoarticular arthritis
  - Palpable effusion
  - Decreased range of motion
  - Fevers, chills
- Diagnostics
  - Arthrocentesis: always initial step in patient with painful, erythematous joint
  - Opaque, purulent fluid
  - >50,000 white blood cells, >75% polymorphonuclear cells, positive Gram stain and culture
  - Polymerase chain reaction if gonococcal arthritis is suspected
  - Imaging (ultrasound or X-ray): joint effusion
- Management
  - Joint washout
  - Empiric treatment with vancomycin (gram-positive coverage) and third/fourth-generation cephalosporin (gram-negative coverage)
  - Antibiotics tailored to Gram stain and culture results

Neisseria gonorrhea septic arthritis is associated with tenosynovitis (wrists, ankles, knees), dermatitis (vesicular pustules, bullae), and terminal complement deficiency. Be sure to check sexually transmitted disease panel (human immunodeficiency virus, syphilis, hepatitis B, chlamydia) in these patients.

Epidural Abscess
- Pathophysiology: hematogenous spread resulting in seeding of the vertebral body or direct invasion from overlying vertebral osteomyelitis
- Risk factors
  - IV drug abuse
  - Recent neurologic procedure (e.g., laminectomy)
  - Epidural anesthesia
  - Spinal steroid injection
- Microbiology: *S. aureus* (most common cause)
- Signs and symptoms
  - Exquisite tenderness over vertebral body
  - Muscle spasms

TABLE 77-1   Hand Abnormalities

HAND DISORDER	PATHOLOGY	SIGNS AND SYMPTOMS	MANAGEMENT
Carpal tunnel syndrome	• Hypertrophy of the flexor retinaculum compressing the median nerve • Associated with rheumatoid arthritis, hypothyroidism, acromegaly, and pregnancy	• Numbness and tingling over the palmar lateral 3.5 fingers • Tinel sign: paresthesias in the median nerve distribution when tapping the flexor retinaculum • Phalen test: symptoms reproduced when wrist is flexed	• Splinting plus NSAIDs • Surgical decompression (release of flexor retinaculum) for refractory cases
Trigger finger	• Stenotic flexor tendon sheath	• Snapping, locking with finger flexion at the MCP joint • Inability to spontaneously extend fingers	• Splinting plus NSAIDs • Glucocorticoid injections • Surgical release of A1 pulley ligament
Mallet finger	• Forceful flexion of extended finger resulting in rupture of extensor tendon at the distal phalanx • Associated with volleyball or baseball injury	• Distal phalanx remains flexed during extension	• Splinting • Surgery for cases associated with fracture, subluxation, or inability to passively extend DIP joint
Jersey finger	• Forceful extension of flexed finger resulting in rupture of flexor digitorum profundus at the distal phalanx • Associated with the jersey-wearing sports	• Inability to flex distal phalanx when making a fist	• Splinting plus surgical repair
Gamekeeper thumb	• Forceful hyperextension of the thumb resulting in injury to ulnar collateral ligament of the thumb • Associated with skiing	• Laxity at the first carpometacarpal joint • Pain and swelling along the ulnar aspect of the thumb	• Splinting • Surgery for cases associated with fractures or complete ligament tear
De Quervain tenosynovitis	• Inflammation and irritation of the extensor pollicis brevis and abductor pollicis longus • Associated with young mothers whose wrists are flexed and thumbs are extended while holding a newborn's head	• Pain along radial aspect of wrist • Finkelstein test: pain reproduced when thumb is held within closed fist and turned in ulnar deviation	• Splinting plus NSAIDs • Glucocorticoid injections
Felon	• Abscess along the palmar side of the distal phalanx secondary to puncture injury	• Fevers, chills • Erythema • Fluctuance	• I&D: delay can result in gangrene and necrosis due to increasing pressures within the small tissue compartment of the distal phalanx
Dupuytren contracture	• Palmar fascia nodularity • Associated with Norwegian men, cirrhotic, and alcoholics	• Inability to place palm flat along a straight surface • Palpation of palmar fascial nodules	• Glucocorticoid or collagenase injections • Fasciotomy for severe cases

DIP, Distal interphalangeal; *I&D*, incision & drainage; *MCP*, metacarpophalangeal; *NSAIDs*, non-steroidal anti-inflammatory drugs.

- • Decreased range of motion
- • Fever, chills
- • +/− neurologic deficits
- – Diagnostics
  - • Magnetic resonance imaging (MRI) spine
  - • Elevated inflammatory markers (erythrocyte sedimentation rate, C-reactive protein)
- – Management
  - • Surgical decompression/drainage
  - • Steroids if acute neurologic deficits are present
  - • Empiric treatment with vancomycin (gram-positive coverage) and third-/fourth-generation cephalosporin (gram-negative coverage). Specific antibiotics pending culture and sensitivities

FRACTURES

Fractures occur most commonly due to trauma such as falls or motor vehicle accidents (Table 77-2). It is important to recognize associated abnormalities, such as neurovascular injury, that may occur with certain

TABLE 77-2 Fractures From Top to Bottom

FRACTURE	KEY FEATURES	MANAGEMENT
Clavicle	• Pain and immobility of the affected arm. Contralateral hand is used to support the affected arm • Majority occur in the middle 1/3 of the bone • Fall on an outstretched arm or direct blow to shoulder • Associated with subclavian artery and brachial plexus injury: may require angiogram if bruit is heard	• Conservative: combination of closed reduction, casting, pain control, and physical therapy • Operative management (open reduction and internal fixation): more appropriate for younger patients, complex fractures, or fractures with increased risk of nonunion
Surgical neck of the humerus	• Bony tenderness, ecchymosis, crepitus at the fracture site • Secondary to direct trauma • Associated with injury to axillary nerve (inability to abduct 15–90 degrees) and posterior circumflex artery	
Radial groove (humerus diaphysis)	• Secondary to direct trauma • Associated radial nerve injury: inability to extend wrist (wrist drop)	
Radial neck	• Most common adult fracture associated with fall on an outstretched hand	
Medial epicondyle	• Avulsion fracture as ligament pulls epicondyle away from the rest of the bone • Secondary to fall on outstretched hand as wrist flexors forcefully contract on the medial epicondyle • Also seen in overhead throwers • Pain, tenderness over the medial epicondyle • Associated with ulnar nerve palsy: decreased risk flexion and sensation to medial hand	
Monteggia	• Direct blow and fracture of the ulna with associated radial dislocation	
Galeazzi	• Direct blow and fracture of the radius with associated ulna dislocation	
Colles	• Fall on outstretched hand with dorsal dislocation of the radial fracture fragment • "Dinner fork" deformity	
Smith	• Fall on flexed hand with palmar dislocation of the distal radial fracture fragment	
Scaphoid	• Tenderness and swelling over the anatomic snuffbox • Initial radiographs may be normal • Associated with high risk of nonunion avascular necrosis if not adequately managed	• Casting even if initial radiographs are normal • Follow-up radiographs in two weeks to confirm fracture or with magnetic resonance imaging on initial presentation
Boxers	• Fracture of the fifth metacarpal • Associated with punching a hard surface	Conservative or operative management depending on severity and complexity of fracture
Femoral shaft	• Secondary to high-velocity trauma • Associated with fat embolism	
Fibular neck	• Associated with peroneal nerve injury: inability to evert or dorsiflex foot (foot drop)	
Stress	• Fracture of normal bone secondary to excessive load • Seen in athletes (especially runners) who suddenly increase their exercise activities • Most commonly occurs in the tibia or calcaneus	• Rest • Gradual increase in exercise activities

Pain under a cast should be promptly removed to evaluate for ill fitting; however, most importantly to allow appropriate physical examination and rule out compartment syndrome.

fractures. Once a fracture has been identified, it is important to identify the type of fracture as this will determine whether a conservative or surgical approach is needed (Fig. 77-1). After treatment, fractures should be monitored for healing changes to ensure proper alignment and stability (Fig. 77-2). Several characteristic fractures are shown in Figs. 77-3 through 77-9, and each displays a specific mechanism or associated injury.

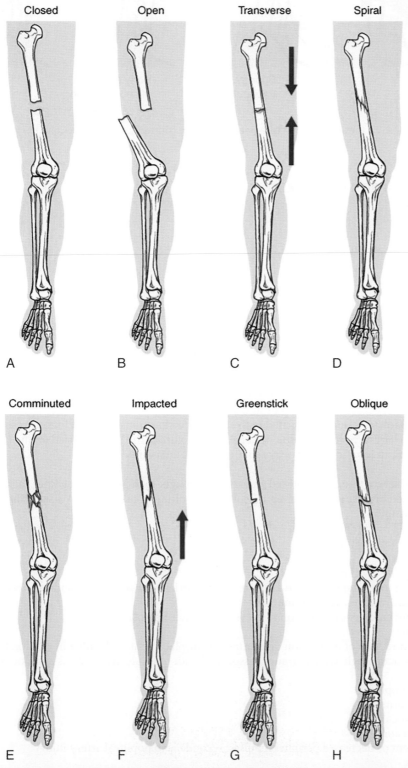

Fig. 77-1: Illustration of the types of fractures. Open fractures must be treated via open reduction internal fixation. Otherwise, depending on the patient, the comorbidities, and complexity of the fracture, treatment options include open reduction internal fixation or conservative management (closed reduction, casting, pain management, physical therapy). (Image courtesy of OpenStax College.)

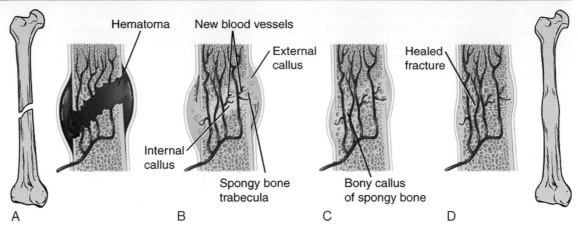

Fig. 77-2: Illustration of the stages of fracture healing. (Image courtesy of OpenStax College.)

X-RAYS OF COMMON FRACTURES

Dislocations

Shoulder Dislocation
- Subtypes
  - Anterior: most common, 95% of cases
  - Posterior
- Mechanism
  - Trauma or direct blow to an outstretched arm: anterior dislocation
  - Severe muscle contraction (seizures, electrocution): posterior dislocation
- Signs and symptoms
  - Abducted arm
  - Externally rotated forearm (may be internally rotated in posterior dislocations)
  - Decreased sensation over the lateral shoulder: secondary to axillary nerve injury
  - Flattened deltoid prominence
- Diagnostics: multiple view shoulder X-ray (Fig. 77-10)
- Management: shoulder reduction plus immobilization

Hillsachs and Bankart lesions: associated with shoulder dislocations. Bankart lesions result in tear of the anterior labrum. Hillsachs lesions result in impaction fracture of the humeral head on the glenoid. Bankart lesions that result in joint instability may require surgical intervention.

Hip Dislocation
- Mechanism: severe trauma to a flexed and abducted thigh, such as impacting knees against the dashboard of a high-speed motor vehicle collision resulting in posterior hip dislocation
- Signs and symptoms
  - Shortening of the affected limb
  - Internal rotation at the hip
- Diagnostics
  - Hip/pelvic X-ray (Fig. 77-11)
  - Computed tomography (CT) to evaluate other injuries after reduction (femoral head and acetabular fractures, vascular injuries)
- Management: emergency reduction to prevent avascular necrosis

Knee Dislocation
- Definition: direction of dislocation determined by displacement of the tibia in relation to the femur
- Mechanism: acute high-velocity trauma associated with multiple ligamentous and potentially vascular injury
- Signs and symptoms
  - Knee deformity
  - Ecchymoses
  - Joint effusion
  - +/− absent or decreased peripheral pulses: secondary to popliteal artery injury
- Diagnostics
  - Knee X-ray (Fig. 77-12)
  - CT angiogram: evaluate patency of popliteal arteries
  - MRI: evaluate ligamentous injury

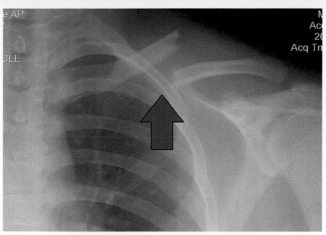

Fig. 77-3: Left mid-clavicular fracture (blue arrow). (Image courtesy of Majorkev at English Wikipedia; CC BY 3.0 [https://creativecommons.org/licenses/by/3.0])

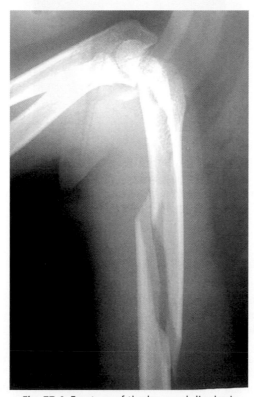

Fig. 77-4: Fracture of the humeral diaphysis

– Management
  • Reduction with follow-up to confirm appropriate reduction technique
  • Management of complications and injuries found on CT/MRI

TENDONS, LIGAMENTS, AND MENISCI
Tendons
Achilles Tendon Rupture
– Definition: rupture of the common tendon for the two heads of the gastrocnemius and soleus at their attachment at the posterior calcaneus
– Risk factors
  • Increasing age
  • Sudden change of direction
  • Fluoroquinolones, glucocorticoids

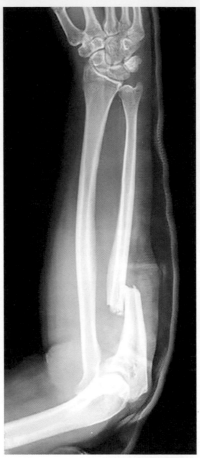

Fig. 77-5: Monteggia fracture. (Image courtesy of Jane Agnes; CC BY-SA 3.0 [https://creativecommons.org/licenses/by-sa/3.0])

- Signs and symptoms
  - Sudden "popping"
  - Limping, swelling
  - Positive Thompson sign: inability to passively plantar flex
  - Hyperdorsiflexion in resting position
  - "Gap" within the Achilles tendon
- Diagnostics: MRI
- Management: surgical repair or casting depending on patient age and comorbidities
- *Rotator Cuff Tendinopathy/Impingement/Tear*
- Definition: tendinopathy or tear of the tendons formed by the supraspinatus (most common), infraspinatus, teres minor, or subscapularis resulting in shoulder pain and instability
- Risk factors
  - Repeated overhead movements: occupational exposure
  - Increasing age: degeneration and repeated ischemia due to impingement
  - Fall
- Signs and symptoms
  - Weakness in abduction
  - Pain with external rotation and overhead activity
  - Positive drop arm test
  - Positive impingement tests (Hawkins, Neer)
  - Positive "empty can" test
  - Subacromial tenderness
  - Painful, normal range of motion
- Diagnostics: MRI or musculoskeletal ultrasound

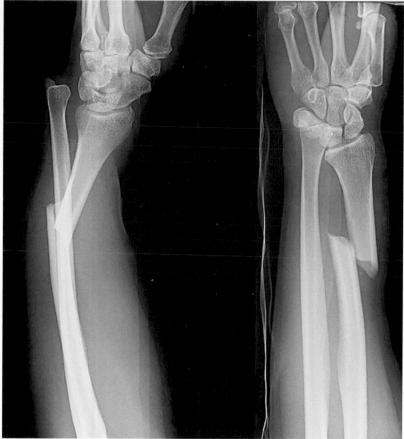

Fig. 77-6: Galeazzi fracture. (Th. Zimmermann; CC BY-SA 4.0 [https://creativecommons.org/licenses/by-sa/4.0])

- Management
  - Rotator cuff tendinopathy: conservative (rest, nonsteroidal antiinflammatory drugs [NSAIDs], physical therapy)
  - Rotator cuff tear: surgical repair (younger, active) or conservative (older, chronic)

In general, tendinopathies and partial tears are managed conservatively, while full tears are managed surgically.

Medial/Lateral Epicondylitis
- Definition: inflammation and irritation of the common flexor (medial epicondylitis) or common extensor tendons (lateral epicondylitis), and they insert into the medial and lateral epicondyle, respectively.
- Risk factors
  - Repeated wrist extension (tennis elbow): lateral epicondylitis
  - Repeated wrist flexion (golfer's elbow): medial epicondylitis
- Signs and symptoms
  - Elbow pain worsened by resistive movements
  - Pain on palpation of the epicondyle
- Diagnostics: clinical
- Management
  - Minimize exacerbating movements
  - Conservative (rest, NSAIDs, physical therapy)

LIGAMENTS
Knee ligament tears: ligaments of the knee function to stabilize the knee in anterior, posterior, lateral, and medial directions. Tears are diagnosed by MRI and often require surgical repair.

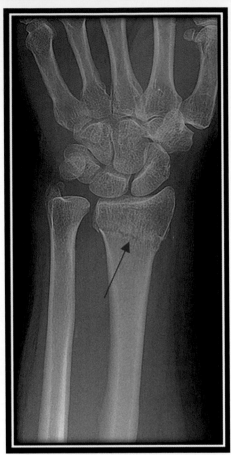

Fig. 77-7: Colles fracture of the distal radius (red arrow). (Image courtesy of Lucien Monfils; CC BY-SA 4.0 [https:// creativecommons.org/licenses/by-sa/4.0])

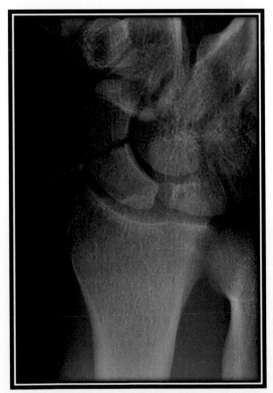

Fig. 77-8: Scaphoid fracture (red arrow). (Image courtesy of Gilo1969; CC BY-SA 4.0 [https://creativecommons.org/ licenses/by-sa/4.0])

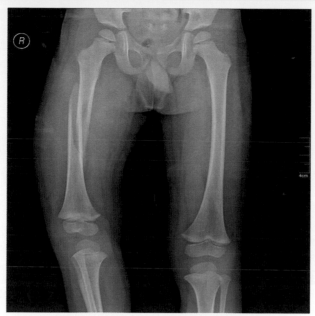

Fig. 77-9: Fracture of the right femoral shaft. (Image courtesy of © Nevit Dilmen; CC BY-SA 3.0 [https://creativecommons.org/licenses/by-sa/3.0])

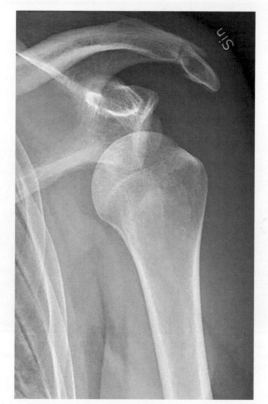

Fig. 77-10: Anterior-posterior view of a left anterior shoulder dislocation. (Image courtesy of Mikael Häggström, MD.)

- Anterior cruciate ligament
  • Deceleration or trauma to the posterior knee
  • Positive anterior drawer sign
  • Positive Lachman test
- Posterior cruciate ligament
  • Trauma to the anterior knee, uncommonly torn, requires severe trauma
  • Positive posterior drawer sign
- Medial collateral ligament

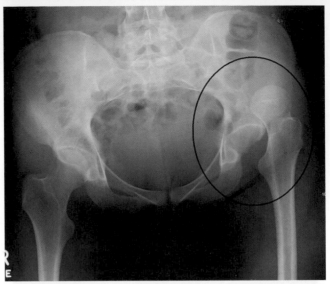

Fig. 77-11: Superior hip dislocation after trauma. (Image courtesy of James Heilman, MD; CC BY-SA 3.0 [https://creativecommons.org/licenses/by-sa/3.0])

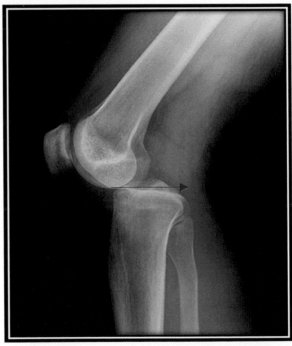

Fig. 77-12: Posterior knee dislocation (red arrow). Be sure to evaluate for vascular injury to the popliteal arteries with computed tomography angiogram. (Image courtesy of Kael Duprey, MD, JD and Michelle Lin, MD; CC BY 4.0 [https://creativecommons.org/licenses/by/4.0])

- • Trauma to the lateral knee
- • Positive valgus stress test
- – Lateral collateral ligament
  - • Trauma to the medial knee
  - • Positive varus stress test

Ulnar collateral ligament tear: commonly seen in baseball players who place excessive valgus stress on the elbow while throwing overhead. Diagnosed by MRI. Chronic or partial tears treated conservatively. Surgical repair for full-thickness tears and high-level athletes.

MENISCI
Meniscal tears

- Menisci are divided into medial and lateral meniscus, with each meniscus further subdivided into an anterior and posterior horn; function as shock absorbers
- Presents with pain and swelling after knee injury; catching and locking of the knee with associated click

Injuries of the knee ligaments and menisci often occur simultaneously.

- Diagnosed by MRI
- Surgical repair is preferred as complete removal of the meniscus results in early osteoarthritis

Trauma
Open Fractures
- Definition: fractures with a bone protruding through the skin
- Management
  • Thorough washout/debridement in the operating room and reduction within six hours of the injury
  • Prophylactic tetanus and antibiotics
  • Analgesia
- Complications
  • Osteomyelitis
  • Deep vein thrombosis/pulmonary embolism: secondary to prolonged immobilization
  • Compartment syndrome
Pelvic Fractures
- Cause: high-velocity trauma
- Signs and symptoms: abducted and internally rotated leg
- Diagnostics: X-ray
- Management
  • External fixation followed by CT angiogram to evaluate for associated pelvic vessels that may be injured

Pelvic fractures are also associated with genitourinary injuries. Findings are further discussed in the Genitourinary section.

Due to prolonged immobility, patients with femoral neck fractures are at increased risk of postoperative deep vein thrombosis/pulmonary embolism.

Pelvis is a space that can hide a significant amount of blood without obvious physical exam findings.

  • Interventional radiology–guided embolization of bleeding vessel if present
  • Conservative management of pelvic hematomas: evaluate for neurologic involvement due to external compression of nerve roots from expanding hematoma

Femoral Neck Fractures
- Causes
  • Trauma
  • Fall
- Signs and symptoms: shortened and externally rotated extremity
- Diagnosis: X-ray
- Management: surgery within 24 hours for medically stable patients; within 72 hours for medically

Femoral neck fractures should be promptly treated to prevent avascular necrosis from disruption of the medial femoral circumflex artery.

unstable patients
  • Femoral neck fractures: screw fixation or arthroplasty
  • Intertrochanteric fractures: open reduction internal fixation
  • Femoral shaft fractures: intramedullary rod fixation

Fat Embolism
- Cause: fracture of long bones (most commonly femur)
- Pathophysiology: fracture results in release of fatty marrow contents into the blood resulting in occlusion of the pulmonary vasculature
- Signs and symptoms
  - Shortness of breath, hypoxia
  - Petechiae
  - Altered mental status
- Diagnostics: clinical
- Management: supportive care until resolution of symptoms

Extremity Compartment Syndrome
- Causes
  - Fracture of forearm or leg
  - Crush injury
  - Burns
  - Excessive IV fluid resuscitation
- Pathophysiology: increased perfusion and edema within a compartment resulting in compression and ischemia of neurovascular structures
- Signs and symptoms: 6 Ps
  - Pain on passive extension
  - Pain out of proportion
  - Poikilothermia
  - Paresthesias
  - Pulselessness
  - Paralysis (late finding)
- Diagnostics
  - Clinical
  - Compartment pressures >30 mm Hg
  - Delta (Δ) pressure (diastolic pressure − compartment pressure) <20–30 mm Hg
Management: fasciotomy

ACUTE AORTIC SYNDROMES
Aortic Dissection
- Risk factors
  - Hypertension
  - Connective tissue disorders (cystic medial necrosis): Marfan, Ehlers-Danlos
  - Congenital anomalies: bicuspid aortic valve, aortic coarctation
  - Trauma
  - Cocaine
  - Large vessel vasculitis (giant cell, Takayasu)
- Signs and symptoms
  - Chest pain with radiation to the back
  - Blood pressure differential in upper extremities: uncommon and cannot be used to rule out aortic dissection
- Diagnostics
  - Chest X-ray: widened mediastinum
  - Confirm with computed tomography (CT) angiography (normal renal function) (Fig. 78-1), magnetic resonance (MR) angiography (nonemergency), or transesophageal echocardiography (abnormal renal function, hemodynamic instability)
- Management (Figs. 78-2 and 78-3)
  - Medical
    - Indicated for descending dissection (Stanford type B)
    - Blood pressure control with beta blockers (labetalol, propranolol, metoprolol) to decrease shearing forces
    - Avoid antiplatelet medication if suspicious due to increased risk of bleeding into the false lumen
  - Surgical
    - Indicated for ascending aortic dissections (Stanford type A)

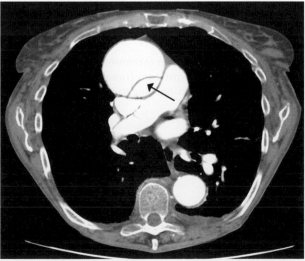

Fig. 78-1: Aortic dissection on axial computed tomography chest. Black arrow points to the true lumen. (Image courtesy of James Heilman, MD.)

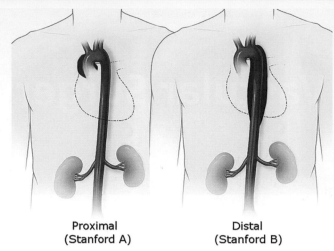

Proximal
(Stanford A)

Distal
(Stanford B)

Fig. 78-2: Classification of aortic dissection using the Stanford classification. (Image courtesy of James Heilman, MD.)

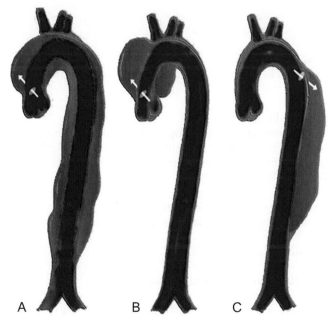

A B C

Fig. 78-3: Classification of aortic dissection using the DeBakey system. (A) type I Debakey dissection involving ascending and descending aorta. (B) type II Debakey dissection involving ascending aorta only. (C) type III Debakey dissection involving descending aorta only distal origin of the left subclavian artery. (Image courtesy of James Heilman, MD.)

- May be indicated for descending dissection (Stanford type B) if the dissection continues to expand or occludes major arteries downstream (renal, iliac)
- Typically avoided in descending dissections due to risk of injuring spinal arteries branching off the descending aorta

Aortic Aneurysm
- Definition: dilation of aorta >3 cm
- Risk factors
  - Smoking
  - Atherosclerosis
  - Hypertension
  - Family history, polycystic kidney disease
  - Connective tissue disorders (Marfan, Ehlers-Danlos)
  - Tertiary syphilis (endarteritis obliterans)
  - Trauma
  - Medium/large vessel vasculitis (giant cell arteritis, Takayasu, Behcet syndrome)
  - Rheumatologic: spondyloarthropathies, rheumatoid arthritis

- Signs and symptoms: depends on location of aneurysm (thoracic vs abdominal)
  - Abdominal aortic aneurysm
    - Asymptomatic (most common)
    - Abdominal/back/flank pain
    - Pulsatile midline abdominal mass
    - Ecchymoses
    - Hypotension, syncope: indicative of impending rupture
  - Thoracic aortic aneurysm
    - Chest pain, shortness of breath
    - Aortic regurgitation murmur
- Diagnostic: typically found on imaging done for other purposes
  - Abdominal ultrasound
  - MRI/CT angiogram
- Management: close monitoring +/− repair depending on size and rate of expansion
  - Medical management
    - Risk factor modification (blood pressure control, smoking cessation, statin + aspirin)
    - Follow-up ultrasound every 6–12 months
  - Surgical management
    - Indications
      ○ Aneurysm >5.5 cm
      ○ Rapidly expanding aneurysm (>1 cm/year)
      ○ Compressive/erosive complications (esophagus, major artery, intestine)
      ○ Rupture (emergent repair)
    - May be repaired via endovascular or open surgery; both have similar outcomes, with choice depending on anatomy and risk of perioperative complications
- Complications
  - Rupture
  - Atheroembolic disease
  - Fistulas (arteriovenous, aortoduodenal)

Penetrating Aortic Ulcer: erosion of the aortic wall secondary to atherosclerotic changes; may result in aortic dissection, hematoma, or perforation.

ATHEROSCLEROTIC-RELATED DISEASE
Carotid Artery Disease
- Definition: narrowing of the carotid arteries secondary to atherosclerosis
- Clinical syndromes/associations
  - Transient ischemic attack (TIA)
  - Amaurosis fugax
  - Stroke
- Diagnostics
  - Carotid artery duplex
  - CT neck angiogram
- Management
  - Medical
    - Aspirin
    - Statin
    - Antiypertensives
    - Antihyperglycemic
    - Smoking cessation
  - Surgical: carotid endarterectomy
    - Men
      ○ Asymptomatic: 60%–99% stenosis
      ○ Symptomatic: 70%–99% stenosis
    - Women: 70%–99% stenosis regardless of symptoms

Peripheral Artery Disease
- Risk factors
  - Same as coronary artery disease as it is a coronary artery disease equivalent
  - Thromboangiitis obliterans (Buerger disease)
- Signs and symptoms
  - Commonly affects lower extremities (buttocks, thighs, calf, foot) with symptoms depending upon peripheral artery involved
  - Intermittent claudication worsened by exertion

- Lower extremity ulcerations involving distal toes
- Decreased peripheral pulses
- Atrophied, smooth, shiny skin, and poor wound healing
- Limb ischemia, rest pain: severe cases
  - Diagnostics
    - Ankle-brachial index (ABI)
      - <0.9 indicative of peripheral artery disease
      - Lower ABI indicates increase disease severity
      - >1.3 indicative of vascular calcification common in diabetics and is nondiagnostic for peripheral arterial disease
    - Toe brachial index: used when ABI is nondiagnostic
    - Arterial angiogram: done prior to surgical intervention to determine severity and location of lesion
  - Management
    - Medical
      - Lifestyle modifications
        - Smoking cessation, strict glycemic control
        - Graded exercise regimen: increases collaterals to improve walking distance and quality of life
      - Pharmacotherapy
        - Antiplatelet (aspirin, clopidogrel), statin: first line
        - Cilostazol: second line
    - Surgical: only if patient has failed medical management
      - Percutaneous revascularization
      - Surgical bypass
      - Thrombectomy if patient develops acute arterial occlusion with limb-threatening ischemia

Leriche syndrome (aortoiliac disease): triad of buttock pain/atrophy, erectile dysfunction, and decreased femoral pulses

Popliteal Aneurysm
- Epidemiology: second most common aneurysm overall
- Risk factors
  - Similar to coronary artery disease
  - Posterior knee dislocation
- Signs and symptoms
  - Asymptomatic: most common
  - Decreased peripheral pulses
  - Enlarging popliteal fossa
  - Exertional claudication
  - Acute limb ischemia
- Diagnostics: duplex ultrasound or angiography
- Management
  - Asymptomatic, small: medical management and risk factor modification
  - Symptomatic, large: endovascular/surgical repair

Atheroembolic Disease
- Pathophysiology: embolization of cholesterol crystals into systemic circulation resulting in occlusion of distant arteries and ischemia
- Risk factors
  - Atrial fibrillation
  - Cardiac catheterization
  - Typical coronary artery disease risk factors
- Clinical syndromes/associations: depends on site of occlusion
  - Central nervous system: TIA, stroke
  - Eyes: amaurosis fugax, Hollenhorst plaques (yellow, refractile plaques in the retinal artery)
  - Kidneys: hematuria, acute kidney injury
  - Gastrointestinal: abdominal pain, bloody diarrhea
  - Skin: livedo reticularis (reticular, lacy rash), cyanotic toes, ulcers
- Diagnostics: clinical
- Management: supportive and treatment of complications

Fibromuscular dysplasia and renal artery stenosis have a similar mechanism in the resulting narrowing of the renal artery; however, they are due to different pathophysiologic mechanisms. Additionally, they differ based on patient epidemiology and associated risk factors (Table 78-1).

Subclavian Steal Syndrome
- Pathophysiology: stenosis at the origin of subclavian artery, which allows for adequate blood supply to the distal arm at rest; however, insufficient supply during activity resulting in decreased blood to the vertebral arteries
- Signs and symptoms
  - Asymptomatic: most common
  - Posterior circulation insufficiency
  - Vertigo
  - Dizziness
  - Syncope
  - Arm claudication
- Diagnostics: duplex ultrasound or angiography
- Management: surgical bypass

As a rule of thumb, in vascular surgery, revascularization is indicated for severe, symptomatic stenosis. Embolectomy is required for acute arterial occlusion. Aneurysms are treated when they become large or symptomatic.

TABLE 78-1   Renal Artery Stenosis Versus Fibromuscular Dysplasia

	RENAL ARTERY STENOSIS	FIBROMUSCULAR DYSPLASIA
Pathophysiology	• Atherosclerotic deposition resulting in circumferential narrowing of renal vasculature	• Abnormal vessel development resulting in formation of aneurysm and functional narrowing of involved vasculature
Signs and symptoms	• Elderly male, severe, resistant hypertension • Diffuse atherosclerotic disease (TIA, angina, peripheral artery disease) • Systolic-diastolic abdominal bruit • Recurrent flash pulmonary edema • +/− renal atrophy • Rise in creatinine (>30%) upon initiation of ACE inhibitor or ARB • Elevated renin and aldosterone levels (secondary hyperaldosteronism)	• Young female, severe, resistant hypertension • Carotid (TIA, amaurosis fugax), vertebral (headache, tinnitus, visual disturbances)
Diagnostics	• Renal duplex Doppler ultrasound • CT/MR angiography	
Treatment	• Risk factor modification: smoking cessation, statins, aspirin, antihypertensives	• Antihypertensives followed by revascularization (percutaneous transluminal angioplasty)

ACE, Angiotensin-converting enzyme; *ARB*, Angiotensin II receptor blocker; *TIA*, transient ischemic attack.

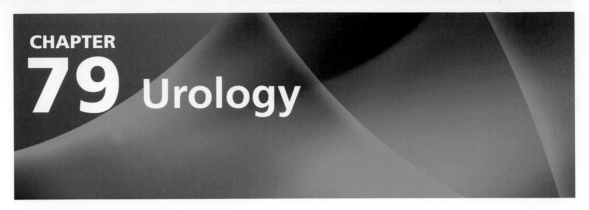

TESTICULAR AND SCROTAL DISORDERS

Testicular Torsion
- Pathophysiology: twisting of the testicular vasculature around its axis resulting in decreased perfusion and ischemia of the testicles
- Signs and symptoms
  - Sudden onset lower abdominal and testicular pain
  - Scrotal swelling
  - Scrotal tenderness
  - Absent cremasteric reflex
  - Horizontal lie of the affected testicle
  - Elevated affected testicle
- Diagnostics: color Doppler ultrasound (absent or decreased testicular flow)
- Management
  - Viable testes: detorsion plus bilateral orchiopexy
  - Necrotic testes: orchiectomy

Higher chance of saving testicle if intervention is performed within the first six hours of symptom onset.

Varicocele
- Pathophysiology: dilation and tortuosity of the pampiniform plexus due to valvular incompetence of the spermatic vein or compression of the left renal vein as it crosses posteriorly to the superior mesenteric artery
- Signs and symptoms
  - "Bag of worms" scrotal mass
  - Scrotal mass increases in size with standing and Valsalva, decreases in size while supine
  - Dull, achy scrotal pain
- Diagnostics: Duplex venous ultrasound
- Management
  - Gonadal vein ligation, percutaneous venous embolization: preserves fertility
  - Conservative management: older men who do not desire fertility
- Complications
  - Testicular atrophy
  - Decrease fertility

Right-sided or bilateral varicoceles should raise suspicion for obstruction secondary to tumor (renal cell carcinoma) or thrombosis.

Testicular vein anatomy: spermatic vein drains into the left renal vein, which subsequently drains into the inferior vena cava (IVC). On the right, the spermatic vein drains directly into the IVC creating a lower pressure system and decreased risk of varicocele.

Hydrocele
- Pathophysiology: peritoneal fluid accumulation in the scrotal sac between the parietal and visceral layers of the tunica vaginalis secondary to incomplete obliteration of the processus vaginalis
- Causes

- Congenital
- Trauma
- Infection (epididymitis, orchitis)
- Signs and symptoms
  - Painless scrotal swelling
  - Positive transillumination: differentiates from solid scrotal mass
- Diagnostics: scrotal ultrasound
- Management
  - Most cases resolve spontaneously
  - Excision of the hydrocele sac for refractory or symptomatic cases

PROSTATE

Benign Prostatic Hyperplasia
- Pathophysiology: prostatic hyperplasia secondary to elevated dihydrotestosterone
- Risk factors
  - Elderly males
  - Black
  - Androgen abuse
- Signs and symptoms
  - Weak urinary stream
  - Nocturia
  - Incomplete bladder emptying
  - Recurrent urinary tract infections
- Diagnostics: clinical
- Management
  - Medical
    - Alpha agonists (relaxes prostatic urethral opening): tamsulosin, doxazosin
    - 5-alpha-reductase inhibitors (decreases prostate size): finasteride
  - Surgical: transurethral resection of the prostate

PENILE DISORDERS

Paraphimosis: retracted foreskin cannot be replaced to its normal anatomic position; results in impaired venous and lymphatic flow; treatment is manual reduction while providing adequate analgesia
Priapism
- Pathophysiology: prolonged erection secondary to occlusion of the corpus cavernosal arteries with resultant ischemia
- Risk factors
  - Medications: trazodone, cocaine
  - Hematologic disorders: sickle cell disease, thalassemia
  - Neurologic injury
- Signs and symptoms
  - Prolonged erection
  - Penile pain and swelling
  - Absence of sexual arousal
- Diagnostics
  - Clinical
  - Cavernosal arterial blood gas or Doppler ultrasonography: differentiates ischemic from nonischemic priapism
- Management
  - First line
    - Corpus cavernosum aspiration: decreases intracorporal pressure
    - Sympathomimetics: dilates corpus cavernosal arteries
  - Alternatives: surgical fistula for refractory/recurrent cases

NEOPLASMS

Renal Cell Carcinoma
- Risk factors
  - Smoking
  - Hypertension, obesity
  - Phenacetin analgesics abuse
  - Autosomal dominant polycystic kidney disease, von Hippel-Lindau syndrome
  - Chronic dialysis
  - Heavy metals (mercury, cadmium)

- Signs and symptoms
  - Abdominal distention, flank pain, hematuria
  - Scrotal varices, testicular pressure (secondary to inferior vena cava or renal vein invasion)
  - Weight loss, night sweat, cachexia
- Paraneoplastic syndromes
  - Syndrome of inappropriate antidiuretic hormone
  - Ectopic erythropoietin, adrenocorticotropic hormone
  - Thrombocytosis
  - Hypercalcemia (parathyroid hormone–like peptide)
- Diagnostics
  - Computed tomography (CT) abdomen/pelvis
  - Chest and brain imaging for staging
- Management
  - Partial/radical nephrectomy depending on the degree of invasion
  - Immunotherapy for advanced disease

Bladder Carcinoma
- Risk factors
  - Smoking
  - *Schistosoma haematobium* infection (chronic cystitis)
  - Pioglitazone, cyclophosphamide (acrolein metabolites)
  - Chemical exposures (painters, metal workers, aniline dyes)
  - Radiation
- Subtypes
  - Transitional cell carcinoma
  - Squamous cell carcinoma (associated with *S. haematobium* infection in North Africa)
- Symptoms
  - Hematuria, dysuria, frequency
  - Abdominal pain, oliguria (secondary to postobstructive uropathy)
  - Suprapubic mass
- Diagnostics
  - Urinalysis for the presence of hematuria and/or cytology
  - CT pelvis
  - Cystoscopy with biopsy
- Management: cystectomy +/− chemoradiation depending on degree of invasion and metastasis

Prostate Cancer
- Epidemiology: most common malignancy in men
- Risk factors
  - Elderly male
  - Black
  - Family history
  - *BRCA1* mutation
- Signs and symptoms
  - Asymptomatic: most common
  - Enlarged, nodular prostate on digital rectal exam
  - Back pain worse at night: indicative of osteoblastic metastasis to the spine (most common site of metastasis)
- Diagnostics
  - Elevated prostate-specific antigen (PSA) levels
  - Ultrasound-guided transrectal biopsy
- Management: based on Gleason scoring
  - Low Gleason (<7/10)
    - Indicative of slow growing, less aggressive malignancy
    - Managed conservatively via observation of PSA level surveillance; patient will likely die from another cause
  - High Gleason (>7/10)
    - Indicative of faster growing, aggressive malignancy
    - Managed via laparoscopic prostatectomy
    - +/− hormonal antiandrogen therapy (flutamide, leuprolide) for metastatic disease

Screening of prostate cancer is controversial due to lack of definitive evidence of improved mortality and associated morbidity with the workup and prostate resection (bleeding, infection, erectile dysfunction).

Testicular Cancer
- Epidemiology: adults to middle-aged men
- Risk factors: cryptorchidism
- Subtypes
  - Germ cell tumor (account for vast majority)
    - Seminomatous
    - Nonseminomatous
  - Non-germ cell tumor
    - Sex cord stromal tumors
    - Lymphomas
- Signs and symptoms
  - Enlarging, firm testicular mass +/− pain
  - Negative transillumination
- Diagnostics
  - Testicular ultrasound
  - Supporting labs
    - Elevated beta-human chorinonic gonadotropin: seminomas, choriocarcinoma
    - Elevated alpha-fetoprotein: yolk sac tumors, embryonal carcinomas
- Management: inguinal orchiectomy plus chemoradiation (seminomas are particularly susceptible to chemoradiation)

TRAUMA
Renal Injury
- Classification: graded from 1–5 with increasing severity of injury
  - Grade I: contusion
  - Grade II–IV: laceration
  - Grade V: shattered kidney
- Signs and symptoms: flank pain, hematuria
- Diagnostics
  - CT abdomen and pelvis
  - Renal angiography: evaluate renovascular injury
- Management: depends on severity
  - Grade I–IV: supportive care +/− embolization
  - Grade V: surgical exploration

Bladder Injury
- Classification
  - Intraperitoneal: rupture of the dome of the bladder with leakage of bladder contents into the peritoneum
  - Extraperitoneal: most common
- Signs and symptoms
  - Diffuse abdominal pain
  - Peritoneal symptoms (seen with intraperitoneal rupture)
- Diagnostics: retrograde cystogram (allows for differentiation between intraperitoneal and extraperitoneal bladder rupture)
- Management
  - Intraperitoneal: surgical repair
  - Extraperitoneal: supportive care (bladder compression)

Urethral Injury
- Classification
  - Anterior bulbomembranous junction
  - Posterior bulbomembranous junction
- Signs and symptoms
  - Blood at the urethral meatus
  - High-riding prostate
  - Penile injury
  - +/− pelvic fracture
- Diagnostics: retrograde urethrogram prior to insertion of a Foley catheter
- Management
  - Anterior bulbomembranous junction: supportive care (suprapubic catheter for bladder decompression)
  - Posterior bulbomembranous junction: surgical repair

Penile Fracture: occurs during vigorous sexual activity; presents with sudden onset penile pain and hematoma. Patient may not provide accurate history due to embarrassment. Management is emergent surgical repair

Ureteral injury is associated with iatrogenic injury due to abdominal or gynecologic surgery.

Ureteral obstruction plus infection: urologic emergency due to rapid decompensation from overwhelming infection; diagnosed on renal ultrasound or CT abdomen and pelvis. Treatment is decompression via percutaneous nephrostomy or ureteral stent.

Fournier Gangrene
- Definition: necrotizing fasciitis of the perineum and genitals
- Signs and symptoms
  - Severe, lower abdominal, scrotal pain
  - Muscle edema
  - Bulla
  - Subcutaneous emphysema, crepitus
- Diagnostics
  - Plain film: initial test
  - CT: evaluate for air within the fascial planes
  - Surgical exploration: both diagnostic and therapeutic
- Management: aggressive IV fluids, broad-spectrum antibiotics, surgical debridement

There are three main cell types that make up the epidermis, each of which has the potential to undergo malignant degeneration (Fig. 80-1).

Actinic Keratosis (also known as solar keratosis)
– Definition: premalignant lesion associated with squamous cell carcinoma
– Signs and symptoms
   • Rough, scaly papules on chronically sun-exposed areas (face, neck, scalp, dorsal hands)
   • Sandpaper-like texture
   • Most common in fair-skinned individuals
– Diagnostic
   • Clinical
   • Biopsy to exclude squamous cell carcinoma for lesions >1 cm, indurated, ulcerated, or rapidly growing
   • Histopathology
      ▪ Parakeratosis (retention of nuclei in the stratum corneum)
      ▪ Acanthosis (epidermal thickening)
      ▪ Thickened stratum corneum, atypical basal keratinocytes
      ▪ Solar elastosis
– Management
   • Medical: topical medications used for multiple lesions
      ▪ 5-fluorouracil
      ▪ Imiquimod
   • Surgical: cryotherapy, curettage

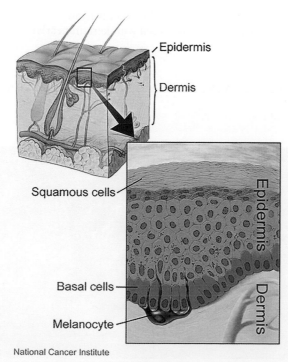

National Cancer Institute

Fig. 80-1: Layers of the skin showing the origin of malignant skin lesions.

Basal Cell Carcinoma
- Epidemiology: most common skin cancer; accounts for up to 75% of all skin cancers
- Risk factors
  - Chronic ultraviolet (UV) exposure
  - Fair-skinned individuals
  - Chronic arsenic exposure
  - Ionizing radiation
- Signs and symptoms
  - Pearly, pink, shiny papule, or plaque (Fig. 80-2)
  - Central depression, telangiectasias
  - Itchy, ulcerating, oozing, crusting, chronically open sores
  - Tends to favor upper lips, nose
  - Locally invasive, metastasis extremely rare
- Diagnostics: biopsy
  - Invasive clusters of spindle cells surrounded by palisaded basal cells
  - Differentiates superficial, nodular, and sclerosing subtypes
- Management
  - Surgical resection (Mohs microsurgery for cosmetically sensitive areas), electrodessication and curettage
  - Topical 5-fluorouracil for superficial basal cell carcinoma

Squamous Cell Carcinoma
- Epidemiology: second most common skin cancer
- Risk factors
  - Chronic UV exposure
  - Fair-skinned individuals
  - Actinic keratosis
  - Smoking/chewing tobacco, alcohol
  - Chronic inflammation/immunosuppression
  - Previous severe burns
  - Chronic arsenic exposure
  - Human papillomavirus infection
  - Cyclosporine
- Signs and symptoms
  - Chronic, ulcerating, irregular lesion (Fig. 80-3)
  - Easily bleeds
  - Scaly, hyperkeratotic, nodular appearance
  - Favors the lower lips
  - Numbness, paresthesia secondary to local perineural invasion
- Diagnostic: biopsy (cords of invasive squamous cell with keratin pearls)
- Management: surgical resection

Marjolin ulcer: squamous cell carcinoma that occurs after a severe burn or chronic wound resulting in chronic inflammation, dysplasia, and invasive cancer
Bowen disease: squamous cell carcinoma in situ

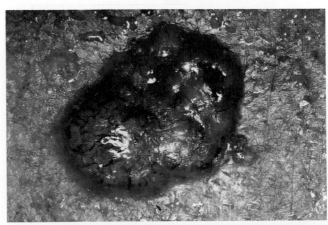

Fig. 80-2: Telangiectatic, pink, shiny lesion consistent with basal cell carcinoma.

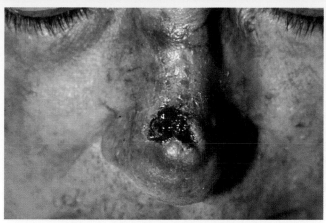

Fig. 80-3: Scaly, ulcerating lesions involving the tip of the nose secondary to squamous cell carcinoma.

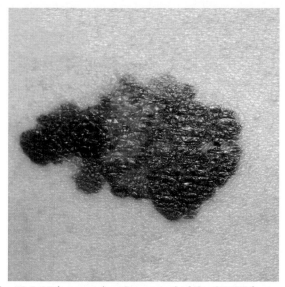

Fig. 80-4: Melanoma showing several of the ABCDE features.

Melanoma
– Risk factors
  • White, fair-skinned
  • Chronic UV exposure, tanning booths
  • Family history
  • Severe, blistering sunburn
  • Dysplastic nevus syndrome
  • Xeroderma pigmentosum (autosomal recessive disease impairing DNA repair caused by UV light)
  • Chronic inflammatory disease (inflammatory bowel disease, autoimmune)
– Signs and symptoms: ABCDE (Fig. 80-4)
  • A: asymmetry
  • B: irregular borders
  • C: color variegation
  • D: diameter >6 mm
  • E: evolving, evolution
    ▪ "Ugly duckling" sign: in a patient with multiple nevi, one or more nevi will look significantly different than the others
– Subtypes
  • Lentigo maligna: more superficial; good prognosis
  • Superficial spreading: most common type; radial spread
  • Acral lentiginous: most common in dark-skinned; involves palms, soles, and subungual regions, and positive Hutchinson sign (darkening of the nail bed and plate extending out to the skin)

- Nodular: vertical growth pattern; worse prognosis
- Amelanotic melanoma
  - Diagnostics
    - Excisional biopsy with 1- to 3-mm margins
    - Breslow staging for depth of invasion: determines prognosis
    - Lymphatic mapping, sentinel lymph node biopsy
  - Management
    - Localized disease: surgical resection
    - Metastatic disease
      - Metastectomy for limited metastatic disease (oligometastatic)
      - Immunotherapy
        - Pembrolizumab
        - Nivolumab
        - Ipilimumab
      - Vemurafenib (BRAF-positive mutation)
      - Alternatives: interferon-alfa, interleukin-2

Chronic ultraviolet exposure, chronic inflammation, fair-skinned, and ionizing radiation are all risk factors for the development of skin cancer.

CHAPTER
81 Ophthalmology

Glaucoma
- Risk factors
  - Blacks, Asians
  - Family history
  - Diabetics
- Causes
  - In most cases of open-angle glaucoma, cause is unknown
  - Drugs (anticholinergic, tricyclic antidepressant, steroids)
- Pathophysiology: excess production or decreased the drainage of aqueous humor → elevated intraocular pressure → compression of the retina and optic nerve head → blindness
- Types
  - Acute angle-closure glaucoma
  - Chronic angle-closure glaucoma
  - Open-angle glaucoma: accounts for 90% of cases
- Signs and symptoms: acuity of symptoms and gonioscopy differentiate the types of glaucoma
  - Red, painful, rock-hard eye
  - Fixed, nonreactive, middilated pupil (Fig. 81-1)
  - Decreased visual acuity
  - Mild visual deficits (loss of peripheral vision)
  - Occasional halos
  - Blindness: seen in cases of acute angle-closure glaucoma or chronic open-angle glaucoma
- Diagnostics
  - Fundoscopic exam: increased cup-to-disc ratio and cupping of the optic disc; normal ratio <0.5
  - Tonometry: increased intraocular pressure; normal pressure 12–20 mm Hg
  - Gonioscopy: measures angle of the anterior chamber
- Management
  - Pharmacologic
    - Acetazolamide (carbonic anhydrase inhibitor): decreases production of aqueous humor
    - Timolol (topical beta blocker): decreases production of aqueous humor

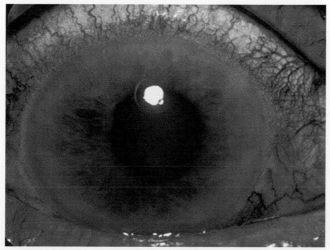

Fig. 81-1: Acute angle-closure glaucoma with fixed, nonreactive middilated pupil.

- ▪ Latanoprost (prostaglandin analog): increases outflow of aqueous humor
- ▪ Pilocarpine (cholinergic analogue): opens canal of Schlemm allowing passage of aqueous from the posterior chamber to anterior chamber of the eye
  - ▪ Mannitol (osmotic diuretic)
- • Surgical
  - ▪ Laser trabeculoplasty
  - ▪ Iridotomy: burns hole in the iris to facilitate flow of aqueous humor

---

Acetazolamide also used in benign intracranial hypertension, altitude sickness. Adverse effects include metabolic acidosis.
 Latanoprost may result in browning of the iris.
 Pilocarpine adverse effects include miosis and cyclospasm.

Aqueous humour: produced from the ciliary body. Flows out from the posterior chamber to the anterior chamber and eventually reabsorbed by a trabecular meshwork and the canal of Schlemm. Its flow becomes obstructed from the posterior to anterior chamber due to a lens that is anatomically more forward.

Cataracts
- – Risk factors
  - • Elderly, diabetic
  - • Smoking
  - • Ultraviolet exposure
- – Associations: commonly a disease of the elderly; however, may be a manifestation of other diseases
  - • Prematurity: disappears within a few weeks
  - • Late manifestation of electrical burns
  - • Congenital: TORCH infection (rubella, varicella), chromosomal abnormalities
  - • Systemic disease
    - ▪ Galactosemia (bilateral)
    - ▪ Myotonic dystrophy
    - ▪ Wilson disease
  - • Drugs: steroids, quetiapine
- – Pathophysiology: oxidative damage of the lens resulting in its opacification
- – Signs and symptoms
  - • Painless blurry vision, often bilateral (one eye may initially be affected before the other)
  - • Glares and halos associated with nighttime driving
  - • Loss of red reflex late in disease
  - • Second site phenomenon: improvement of presbyopia due to myopic shift, which increases the convergence power of the lens (patients note they no longer require their reading glasses)
- – Diagnostics: slit-lamp examination (Figs. 81-2 and 81-3)
- – Management: surgical lens extraction and implantation of artificial lens

---

Acute angle-closure glaucoma: ophthalmologic emergency due to sudden worsening of chronic angle-closure glaucoma. Precipitated by extrinsic factor that causes pupillary dilation (stress, dark room, anticholinergic, sympathomimetic, decongestants). Must be treated emergently with IV acetazolamide and mannitol due to risk of blindness.

Retinal Detachment
- – Risk factors
  - • Trauma, ocular surgery
  - • Exudative age-related macular degeneration
  - • Diabetic retinopathy
  - • Connective tissue disorders (Marfan syndrome, Ehlers-Danlos)
  - • Myopia
  - • Retinopathy of prematurity
  - • Retinitis
- – Pathophysiology
  - • Accumulation of fluid in the subretinal space → separation of the sensory retina from the retinal pigment epithelium
  - • Neurosensory layer of the retina contains photoreceptors with rods and cones, which degenerate upon separation from the retinal pigment epithelium → loss of vision

Eye with Cataract

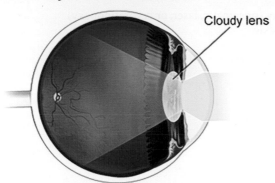

Cloudy lens

Cloudy lens, or cataract, causes blurry vision

Fig. 81-2: Illustration of patient with cataracts.

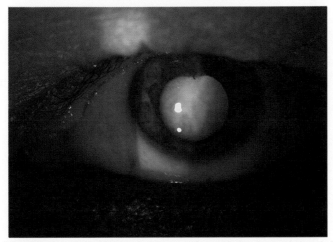

Fig. 81-3: Patient with advanced cataracts showing presence of cloudy lens.

- • Tractional forces on the retina
- • Posterior vitreous detachment
- – Signs and symptoms
  - • Flashing lights
  - • Floaters
  - • Painless unilateral sudden loss of vision (retina lacks pain receptors)
  - • "Red veil" or "curtain coming down"
  - • Leukocoria
- – Diagnostics
  - • Fundoscopy
    - ▪ Vitreous debris
    - ▪ Elevated and detached retina
    - ▪ Weiss ring: white fibrous ring signifying the point of attachment between the posterior vitreous and the round optic nerve
    - ▪ Tobacco dust cells: retinal pigment epithelial cells that have floated into the vitreous humor
  - • Ophthalmic ultrasound
    - ▪ Vitreous hemorrhage
    - ▪ Retinal elevation
- – Management
  - • Conservative management if retinal detachment is due to posterior vitreous detachment as symptoms of floaters will self-resolve

- Surgical
  - Retinopexy (pneumatic, laser, or cryoretinopexy)
  - Scleral buckle

Retinal detachment is an ophthalmologic emergency.

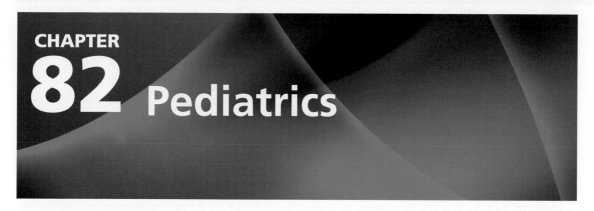

CHAPTER 82 Pediatrics

GASTROENTEROLOGY

Omphalocele is associated with other anomalies and chromosomal disorders. Gastroschisis occurs as an isolated defect (Table 82-1; Figs. 82-1 and 82-2).

STOMACH

Pyloric Stenosis

- Risk factors
  - Firstborn
  - Males
  - Erythromycin
  - Formula feeding
- Signs and symptoms
  - Nonbilious projectile vomiting after feeding (4–8 weeks after birth)
  - Olive-shaped, palpable epigastric mass
  - Peristaltic waves
  - Failure to thrive, dehydration
  - Eager to feed after vomiting

In contrast, nonbilious vomiting in tracheoesophageal fistula occurs after first feed.

- Diagnostics
  - Abdominal ultrasound
  - Hypochloremic, hypokalemic metabolic alkalosis
- Management
  - Initial: IV fluid resuscitation, correction of electrolyte abnormalities
  - Definitive: pyloromyotomy (Fig. 82-3)

"Double bubble" sign is also seen in duodenal atresia.

TABLE 82-1   Omphalocele Versus Gastroschisis

	OMPHALOCELE	GASTROSCHISIS
Pathophysiology	• Failure of herniated bowel contents to return into the abdominal cavity	• Incomplete fusion of the abdominal wall
Signs and symptoms	• Protrusion of abdominal contents outside the abdomen, including the liver, covered by peritoneum • Umbilical cord goes to the defect	• Protrusion of abdominal wall contents outside the abdomen, uncovered by peritoneum • Umbilical cord is normal, the defect is to the right of the cord
Diagnostics	• Postnatal: clinical • In utero: second trimester ultrasound, elevated maternal serum alpha-fetoprotein	
Management	• Immediately cover bowel with saline dressing and plastic wrap to prevent insensible fluid losses • Small defects: primary surgical repair • Large defects: multistep silastic silo surgical repair • IV fluids, nutrition, and antibiotics	

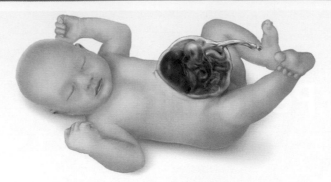

Fig. 82-1: Illustration of omphalocele. (Images courtesy of Centers for Disease Control and Prevention, National Center on Birth Defects and Developmental Disabilities; CC BY-SA 3.0 [https://creativecommons.org/licenses/by-sa/3.0]).

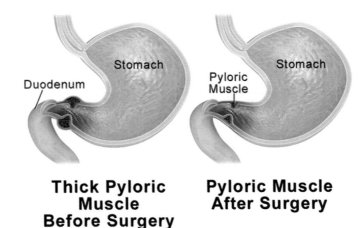

Fig. 82-2: Illustration of gastroschisis. (Images courtesy of Centers for Disease Control and Prevention, National Center on Birth Defects and Developmental Disabilities; CC BY-SA 3.0 [https://creativecommons.org/licenses/by-sa/3.0])

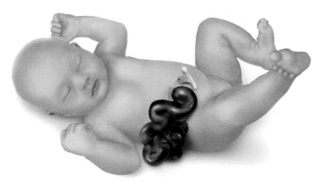

Fig. 82-3: Pyloric stenosis before and after pyloromyotomy. (Image courtesy of Blausen Medical.)

PANCREAS
Nesidioblastosis (Congenital Hyperinsulinism)
– Pathophysiology: hyperinsulinism secondary to beta cell hyperplasia
– Signs and symptoms
  • Jitteriness, lethargy
  • Episodic hypothermia
  • Convulsions
  • Macrosomia in utero
– Diagnostics
  • Persistent hyperglycemia in infants and neonates
  • Glucagon challenge test: inadequate increase in blood glucose after administration of glucagon
  • Molecular/genetic testing

- Management
  - Medical
    - Diazoxide
    - Frequent feedings
  - Surgical: partial pancreatectomy

Annular Pancreas
- Signs and symptoms
  - Bilious vomiting
  - Abdominal distention
  - Hypoactive/absent bowel sounds
- Diagnostics: abdominal X-ray
  - "Double bubble" sign
  - Air fluid levels: secondary to small bowel obstruction
- Management: surgical correction/bypass

HEPATOBILIARY
Biliary Atresia
- Epidemiology: 2–8 weeks old
- Pathophysiology: fibrosis and sclerosis of the biliary system impairing extrahepatic biliary transport
- Signs and symptoms
  - Progressively, worsening jaundice
  - Pale stools (bile unable to reach the gut)
  - Dark urine (conjugated bilirubin excreted through the urine)
  - Hepatomegaly
  - Splenomegaly (portal hypertension)
- Diagnostics
  - Direct hyperbilirubinemia
  - Abdominal ultrasound: absent/abnormal gallbladder
  - Phenobarbital (stimulates bile flow) followed by HIDA scan: lack of bile reaching the duodenum is suggestive of biliary atresia
  - Intraoperative cholangiogram: confirmatory
- Management
  - Surgical repair (Kasai procedure: portoenterostomy) prior to development of biliary cirrhosis to reestablish bile flow
  - Liver transplant: definitive treatment
- Complications: biliary cirrhosis

SMALL BOWEL
Duodenal and jejunal atresia have characteristic imaging findings, associations, and pathophysiology, which allow them to be differentiated (Table 82-2; Fig. 82-4).
Malrotation
- Pathophysiology: abnormal intestinal rotation resulting in compression of the superior mesenteric arteries → intestinal obstruction → bowel infarction
- Signs and symptoms

TABLE 82-2 Duodenal Versus Jejunal Atresia

	DUODENAL ATRESIA	JEJUNAL ATRESIA
Pathophysiology	• Failure of duodenal lumen to recanalize at 8–10 week gestation	• Mesenteric vascular accident in utero (maternal use of vasoconstrictive medications: cocaine, tobacco, nasal decongestants)
Signs and symptoms	• Bilious vomiting following first feeds • Feeding refusal • Polyhydramnios	• Bilious vomiting • Abdominal distention
Diagnostics	• Abdominal X-ray: "double bubble" sign • Upper gastrointestinal (GI) study	• Abdominal X-ray: multiple air fluid levels, "triple bubble" sign • Upper GI study
Associations	• VACTERL syndrome • Down syndrome	• None
Management	• Stabilization: IV fluids, bowel rest • Definitive: surgical correction	

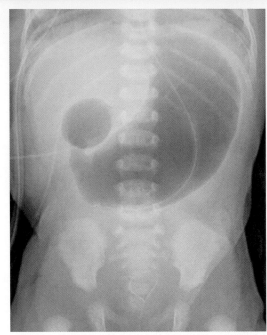

Fig. 82-4: Abdominal X-ray showing dilated stomach and proximal duodenum with atretic distal segment consistent with "double bubble" sign in a patient with duodenal atresia.

- Abdominal pain
- Absent/hypoactive bowel sounds, constipation: mechanical bowel obstruction secondary to development of peritoneal bands (Ladd bands)
- Anorexia
- Bloody, dark stools
– Diagnostics: upper gastrointestinal (GI) study with small bowel follow-through (demonstrates malrotated intestines; ligament of Treitz on right side of the abdomen)
– Management
  - Intestinal obstruction: gastric decompression, bowel rest, IV fluids
  - Intestinal infarction: exploratory laparotomy with resection of infarcted bowel segments

Intussusception
– Epidemiology: 6–24 months old
– Pathophysiology: telescoping of the proximal intestinal segment (lead point) into a more distal segment → intestinal obstruction → ischemia and necrosis (Fig. 82-5)
– Causes: any of the following can act as a lead point and increased risk of intussusception
  - Peyer patches hyperplasia (viral infection, lymphoma)
  - Meckel diverticulum
  - Intestinal polyp/tumor
– Signs and symptoms
  - Episodic, colicky abdominal pain
  - Vomiting, lethargy
  - Sausage-shaped right upper quadrant mass
  - Empty right lower quadrant
  - Currant jelly–like stool: indicative of intestinal ischemia
– Diagnostics
  - Abdominal X-ray: evaluate for perforation and/or obstruction
  - Air contrast enema: coil spring sign
  - Abdominal ultrasound: target sign
– Management
  - Air/contrast enema: both diagnostic and therapeutic
  - Surgery if obstruction unrelieved by enema

Meconium ileus and meconium plugs have unique associations that allow them to be differentiated. Additionally, both are diagnosed and treated with enemas (Table 82-3).

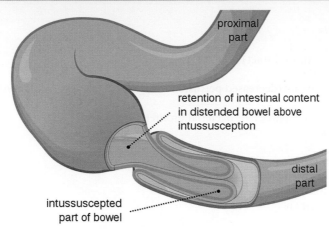

Fig. 82-5: Diagrammatic representation of intussusception demonstrating telescoping of the proximal segment of bowel into a more distal portion and resulting in bowel obstruction. (Image courtesy of Olek Remesz.)

TABLE 82-3   Meconium Ileus Versus Meconium Plugs

	MECONIUM PLUGS	MECONIUM ILEUS
Definition	• Functional obstruction of the lower colon resulting in failure to pass meconium	• Failure to pass first stool (meconium) within the first 24 hours secondary to thickened meconium
Diagnostics	• Abdominal X-ray: intestinal distention	• Abdominal X-ray: same as meconium plug plus "soap bubble" appearance • Contrast enema: microcolon
Associations	• Hirschsprung disease • Infants of diabetic mother • Mothers who received magnesium sulfate • Small left colon syndrome	• Cystic fibrosis (may be first presenting symptom)
Management	• Enema: both diagnostic and therapeutic	

Meckel Diverticulum
– Pathophysiology
  • Ectopic gastric/pancreatic tissue most commonly located in the small intestine resulting in intestinal erosion
  • Remnant of the vitelline duct (incomplete obliteration in utero)
  • True diverticulum with intestinal outpouching
– Signs and symptoms
  • Asymptomatic: most common
  • Painless hematochezia
– Diagnostic: technetium 99 m pertechnetate scan (Meckel scan): localizes heterotopic gastric tissue
– Management: diverticulectomy
– Complications
  • Intussusception
  • Intestinal obstruction
  • Volvulus
  • Iron deficiency anemia

Meckel's diverticulum rule of 2s:
• 2% of the population
• 2 feet from ileocecal valve
• 2 inches long
• 2 types of ectopic tissue (gastric, pancreatic)
• 2 years old
• Males 2:1

LARGE BOWEL

Necrotizing Enterocolitis
- Risk factors
  - Prematurity (immature GI tract)
  - Very low birthweight
  - Congenital heart disease (decreased perfusion to GI tract increases risk for enteric bacterial translocation)
  - Enteral feeding (act as sources for bacterial proliferation)
- Signs and symptoms
  - Fever, lethargy
  - Abdominal distention
  - Abdominal wall erythema
  - Poor feeding, bilious vomiting
  - Bloody bowel movements
- Diagnostics
  - Abdominal X-ray
    - Pneumatosis intestinalis
    - Portal vein gas
    - +/− free air under the diaphragm
  - Supporting features
    - Thrombocytopenia
    - Disseminated intravascular coagulation
    - Metabolic acidosis
- Management
  - Gastric decompression
  - Broad-spectrum IV antibiotics
  - Stop enteric feeds, initiate parenteral nutrition
  - +/− surgery: if there are signs of perforation or bowel necrosis

Hirschsprung Disease
- Pathophysiology: lack of migration of neural crest cells → aganglionic bowel segment → absence of bowel autonomic innervation
- Signs and symptoms
  - Meconium ileus/plug
  - Abdominal distention
  - Bilious vomiting (Table 82-4)
  - Blast sign: expulsion of stool on digital rectal exam
  - Chronic constipation (seen in older infants, adolescents)
- Associations: trisomy 21
- Diagnostics
  - Barium enema: dilated proximal with narrowing of distal segment
  - Rectal suction biopsy: absence of ganglia
- Management: resection of aganglionic segment

MISCELLANEOUS

Umbilical Hernia
- Definition: defect at the linea alba resulting in protrusion of intraabdominal contents through the navel
- Risk factors
  - Hypothyroidism
  - Beckwith-Wiedemann syndrome
  - Prematurity
  - Collagen vascular disease (Ehlers-Danlos syndrome)
  - Black

TABLE 82-4   Differential of Bilious Versus Nonbilious Vomiting and Their Onset

	BILIOUS	NONBILIOUS	ONSET
Tracheoesophageal fistula		+	After first feeds
Pyloric stenosis		+	4–8 weeks after birth
Duodenal/jejunal atresia	+		After first feeds
Hirschsprung disease	+		Weeks–months

- Signs and symptoms
  - Soft, nontender protrusion over the navel
  - Worsens with crying and straining
  - Easily reducible
- Diagnostics: clinical
- Management
  - Vast majority of cases resolve by age 5 years
  - Surgical closure for large, persistent (>5 years), or symptomatic cases

Congenital Diaphragmatic Hernia
- Defects in the diaphragm allowing protrusion of abdominal viscera into the thoracic cavity causing extrinsic compression of the lungs and pulmonary hypoplasia
- Presents with respiratory distress, scaphoid abdomen
- Chest X-ray shows dilated loops of bowel in the chest (Fig. 82-6)
- Secure airway, gastric decompression, followed by surgical repair

CARDIOLOGY
Congenital Heart Disease
Key principles
- Prenatally, right-left heart connections exist to allow blood flow to bypass high pulmonary vascular resistance (Fig. 82-7)
- After birth, pulmonary vascular resistance decreases, right-left heart connections close, resulting in postnatal development of cardiovascular system (Fig. 82-8)
- Persistent septal defects tend to be left-to-right shunts postnatally due to higher left-sided pressures
- Left-to-right shunts may become right-to-left shunts as increased blood flow results in pulmonary hypertension and reversal of pressure gradient (Table 82-5)
- Septal defect predisposes to failure to thrive, congestive heart failure, frequent respiratory infections, endocarditis, and paradoxic embolism
- Cyanotic congenital heart defects are ductus dependent to allow oxygenated blood to reach systemic circulation (Table 82-6)
- Congenital heart diseases are identified on echocardiogram (Fig. 82-9)

Understanding the normal fetal circulatory system and the transitions that occur after birth will aid in understanding cyanotic and acyanotic congenital heart disease.

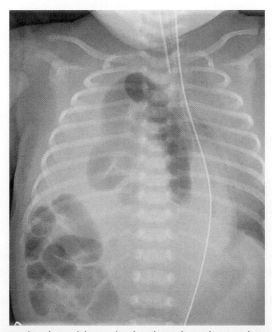

Fig. 82-6: Chest X-ray demonstrating bowel loops in the thoracic cavity consistent with right-sided congenital diaphragmatic hernia. (Image courtesy of Kinderradiologie Olgahospital Klinikum Stuttgart; CC BY-SA 4.0 [https://creativecommons.org/licenses/by-sa/4.0])

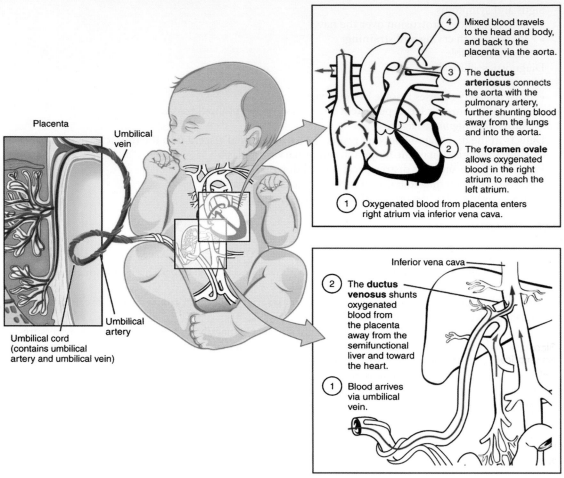

Fig. 82-7: Flow of blood in the fetal circulatory system.

CARDIOTHORACIC
Vascular Rings
- Epidemiology: <1 year old
- Definition: anomalous branch of the aorta surrounds the trachea and esophagus
- Signs and symptoms
  - Biphasic stridor: secondary to narrowing of the extrathoracic airways
  - Stridor improves with neck extension
  - Feeding difficulties
  - Choking
- Associations
  - Congenital heart defects
  - Tracheomalacia
- Diagnostics
  - Barium esophagram: indentation of the esophagus
  - Magnetic resonance (MR) angiography
- Management: surgical division of the vascular ring

UROLOGY
Hypospadias and epispadias are defects along the surface of the penis differentiated based on the location of the opening and associated pathologies (Table 82-7).
Cryptorchidism
- Definition: undescended testicle, most commonly remaining in the abdominal cavity
- Signs and symptoms
  - Unilateral absence of testicle in the scrotal sac
  - Hypoplastic scrotum
  - Poorly rugated scrotum
  - Inguinal fullness

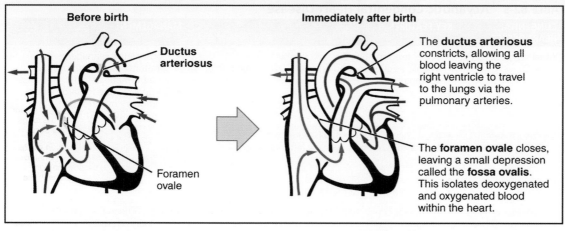

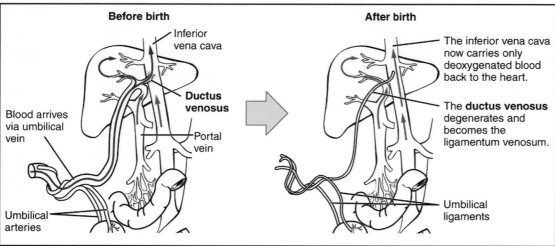

Fig. 82-8: Illustration of the neonatal circulatory system immediately before and after birth.

- Associations
  - Inguinal hernia: secondary to patent processes vaginalis
  - Testicular cancer
  - Hypospadias
  - Epispadias
- Diagnostics: clinical
- Management: orchiopexy before 1 year old if testicles are not descended by 6 months

Exstrophy of the Bladder
- Pathophysiology: abdominal wall defect resulting in protrusion of the urinary bladder over the symphysis pubis
- Signs and symptoms
  - Exposed bladder and urethra
  - Diathesis of the symphysis pubis
  - Low-set umbilicus
  - Inguinal hernia
- Diagnostics
  - Prenatal ultrasound
  - MRI: confirmatory
- Management
  - Cover the exposed bladder after birth
  - Surgical correction and early closure of the bladder

Posterior Urethral Valves
- Abnormal folds of tissue in the distal urethra causing bladder obstruction
- Most common cause of obstructive uropathy in young boys
- Presents with oligohydramnios, suprapubic fullness, weak urinary stream, and recurrent urinary tract infections

TABLE 82-5   Acyanotic Congenital Heart Disease

CONGENITAL HEART DEFECT	KEY FEATURES	MANAGEMENT
Atrial septal defect (ASD)	• Wide, fixed splitting S2 • Systolic ejection murmur at upper left sternal border • Asymptomatic	• Conservative management, spontaneous closure for small asymptomatic defects • Surgical closure for large defect, pulmonary hypertension, arrhythmias, heart failure
Ventricular septal defect (VSD)	• Most common congenital heart defect • Holosystolic murmur over the left lower sternal border	
Atrioventricular canal	• Combination of ASD and VSD • Associated with trisomy 21	
Patent ductus arteriosus (PDA)	• Allows for connection between pulmonary artery and aorta • Continuous machinery-like murmur over the upper left sternal border • Wide pulse pressure • Bounding arterial pulses • Associated with congenital rubella infection	• Isolated defect: indomethacin to stimulate closure • Ductus dependent: prostaglandin to keep open
Coarctation of the aorta	• Narrowing of the aorta after the left subclavian artery • Hypertensive upper extremities (pink), hypotensive lower extremities (cyanotic, decreased pulses) • Rib notching on chest X-ray (collateral circulation from internal memories) • Associated with Turner syndrome	• Prostaglandin to maintain PDA open for severe ductus dependent coarctation • Surgical or balloon angioplasty repair
Ebstein anomaly	• Tricuspid valve displaced into the right ventricle • Triple or quadruple gallop • Tricuspid regurgitation • Right atrial enlargement • Electrocardiography: right axis deviation, tall P waves • Associated with maternal lithium use	• Medical management with loop diuretics, inotropes, prostaglandin • Surgical repair if symptomatic
Aortic stenosis	• Systolic ejection murmur at base • Most commonly due to a bicuspid aortic valve (associated with Turner syndrome) • Severe cases present with congestive heart failure	• Balloon valvuloplasty or surgical replacement if symptomatic
Pulmonic stenosis	• Systolic ejection murmur at the upper left sternal border • Most commonly asymptomatic, congestive heart failure in severe cases • Prominent pulmonary arteries on chest X-ray	• Prostaglandin to maintain PDA in severe cases while pending definitive treatment • Balloon valvuloplasty in severe or symptomatic cases

- Renal ultrasound will show bilateral hydronephrosis
- Diagnosis confirmed with voiding cystourethrogram and cystoscopy
- Treatment is valve ablation

Neuroblastoma

- Epidemiology: primarily affects <2 years old, majority of cases present by 5 years old
- Pathophysiology: N-myc oncogene mutation
- Definition: malignancy of immature neural crest cells along the sympathetic nervous system, most commonly occurring in the adrenal glands
- Signs and symptoms
  - Palpable abdominal mass that crosses the midline
  - Horner syndrome (involvement of superior cervical ganglion)
  - Peripheral neuropathy
  - Proptosis
  - Opsoclonus myoclonus ("dancing eyes and feet")
  - Hypertension
- Diagnostics
  - Elevated homovanillic acid, vanillylmandelic acid levels
  - Computed tomography (CT)/MRI abdomen and pelvis: calcification and hemorrhages of suprarenal mass
  - Bone marrow biopsy

TABLE 82-6   Cyanotic Congenital Heart Disease

CONGENITAL HEART DEFECT	KEY FEATURES	MANAGEMENT
Tetralogy of Fallot	• Pulmonic stenosis • Right ventricular hypertrophy • Overriding aorta (aorta overlying ventricular septal defect [VSD]) • VSD • Chest X-ray: boot-shaped heart • Cyanosis dependent on degree of right-to-left shunting • Increased systemic vascular resistance (valsalva, squatting, knee-chest position, systemic hypertension) decreases right-to-left shunting and improves cyanosis • Decreased systemic vascular resistance (hypotension, exercise, dehydration, crying) increases the right-to-left shunting and worsens cyanosis	• Prostaglandin • Beta blocker • Surgical repair
Transposition of the great vessels	• Separate pulmonary and systemic circulation • VSD • Single S2 • Chest X-ray: "egg on a string" • Associated with uncontrolled maternal diabetes, DiGeorge syndrome	• Prostaglandin to maintain patent ductus arteriosus connection between separate pulmonary and systemic circulation • Balloon atrial septostomy (maintains patent foramen ovale [PFO] prior to definitive surgical repair) • Surgical repair
Truncus arteriosus	• Aorta and pulmonary artery originate from common trunk • Mixing of oxygenated and deoxygenated blood results in mild cyanosis • VSD • Diastolic murmur at apex • Systolic ejection murmur along the left sternal border • Associated with DiGeorge syndrome	• VSD repair • Graft separating aorta and pulmonary artery
Total anomalous pulmonary venous return	• Pulmonary veins drain into systemic circulation → mixing of oxygenated and deoxygenated blood entering right atrium → mild cyanosis • Pulmonic ejection murmur at left sternal border • Chest X-ray: snowman appearance	• Surgical repair
Tricuspid atresia	• Interatrial connection (atrial septal defect, PFO) present to allow for right-to-left shunting • Left atrial dilation + left ventricular hypertrophy • Electrocardiography: deviation, small or absent R waves in precordial leads	• Multistage surgical repair

– Management: staging (commonly metastatic upon initial presentation) +/− surgery +/− chemoradiation

Wilms Tumor
– Epidemiology
  • Most common childhood renal tumor
  • Commonly presents in children <5 years old
– Signs and symptoms
  • Abdominal mass that does not cross midline
  • Hypertension
  • Hematuria
  • Fever, weight loss, night sweats
– Associations
  • Beckwith-Wiedemann syndrome
  • Macroglossia
  • Hemihypertrophy
  • Organomegaly
  • WAGR syndrome
    ▪ Wilms tumor
    ▪ Aniridia
    ▪ Genitourinary abnormalities
    ▪ Mental retardation

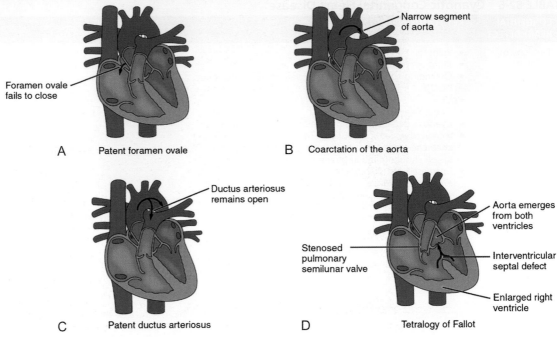

Fig. 82-9: Illustration of various congenital heart defects.

TABLE 82-7 Differentiating Hypospadias Versus Epispadias

HYPOSPADIAS	EPISPADIAS
Urethral opening on the ventral surface of the penis	Urethral opening on the dorsal surface of the penis
Associated with cryptorchidism, inguinal hernias	Associated with bladder exstrophy
Plastic surgery repair using foreskin; do not circumcised	Surgical repair

- Diagnostics
  - Abdominal CT/MRI
  - Tissue biopsy
- Management: staging +/− surgical resection +/− chemoradiation

---

Wilms tumor is a palpable abdominal mass that does not cross midline, in contrast to neuroblastoma that crosses midline.

ORTHOPEDICS
Pediatric Knee
Osgood-Schlatter Disease
- Epidemiology: young, athletic adolescents
- Pathophysiology: osteochondrosis of the tibial tubercle secondary to overuse resulting in chronic traction at the tibial tubercle from the inserting patellar tendon
- Signs and symptoms
  - Tenderness at the tibial tubercle
  - Pain relieved by rest, worsened by activity
  - Recent growth spurt
- Diagnostics
  - Clinical
  - Knee X-ray: avulsion apophysis of the tibial tubercle (Fig. 82-10)
- Management
  - Avoid aggravating activity
  - Symptomatic management: rest, ice, pain control

Patellofemoral Syndrome
- Epidemiology: young, female athlete
- Risk factors

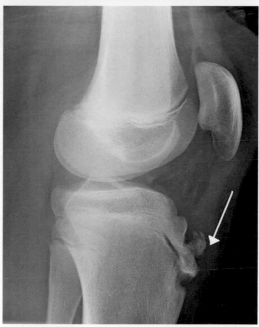

Fig. 82-10: Avulsion of the tibial tubercle (white arrow) in a patient with Osgood-Schlatter disease. (Image courtesy of James Heilman, MD; CC BY-SA 3.0 [https://creativecommons.org/licenses/by-sa/3.0])

- Imbalance of quadriceps muscle
- Trauma
- Meniscal tear
- Signs and symptoms: chronic anterior knee pain worsened by running and squatting
- Diagnostics
  - Patellofemoral compression test: pain worsened with knee extended and patellar compression
  - Knee X-ray: normal
- Management: physical therapy

PEDIATRIC HIP
Pediatric hip abnormalities are commonly tested pathologies and can be differentiated primarily based on the patient's age and imaging characteristics (Table 82-8; Fig. 82-11).

MECHANICAL DEFORMITIES
Genu Varum
- Definition: abnormal bowing of the lower extremity seen in infants and young toddlers
- Signs and symptoms: bowing of the lower extremities
- Diagnostics
  - Clinical
  - Lower extremity X-ray
- Management: conservative, most cases resolve by age 2 years
- Complications: Blount disease (continued genu varum after age 3 years): requires surgical correction due to increased risk of growth disturbances

Clubfoot
- Definition: inward orientation of the feet secondary to genetic syndrome, physical compression in utero (oligohydramnios), or neuromuscular disorder
- Signs and symptoms
  - Plantar flexion
  - Foot inversion
  - Internal tibial rotation
- Diagnostics: clinical (Fig. 82-12)
- Management
  - Early casting and manual manipulation at early age due to increased ligament laxity
  - Surgical correction for refractory cases

Scoliosis
- Epidemiology

TABLE 82-8   Differentiating Pediatric Hip Abnormalities

	DEVELOPMENTAL DYSPLASIA OF THE HIP	LEGG-CALVÉ-PERTHES DISEASE	SLIPPED CAPITAL FEMORAL EPIPHYSIS
Pathophysiology	• Lax articulation of the femoral head within the acetabulum	• Idiopathic avascular necrosis of the capital femoral epiphysis	• Slippage of the femoral metaphysis relative to the epiphysis through the growth plate
Epidemiology	• Newborns	• 4–10 years old	• Overweight adolescentsRecent growth spurt
Signs and symptoms	• Positive Barlow test: easily dislocated hip while in flexion and external rotation with clunking sound • Positive Ortolani test: reducibility of dislocated hip • Galeazzi test: difference in knee height when lying supine with knees flexed	• Insidious onset, painless limp • Antalgic gait • Decreased range of motion • +/− referred knee pain	• Insidious onset hip/knee pain • Limping • Decreased range of motion • Abduction and internal rotation of the hip • External rotation of the thigh while hip is flexed
Diagnostics	• Ultrasound: X-ray is not as useful as bones have not ossified	• Hip X-rayMagnetic resonance imaging: more sensitive	• Hip X-ray
Management	• Abduction splinting with Pavlik harness	• Casting • Bracing • Bed rest	• Surgical pinning of the femoral head • +/− prophylactic pinning of the contralateral femoral head

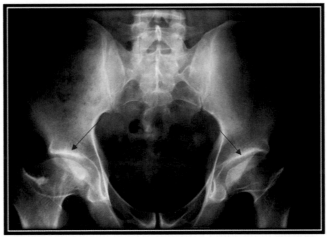

Fig. 82-11: Bilateral flattening of the femoral heads (red arrows) secondary to avascular necrosis in a patient with Legg-Calvé-Perthes. (Image courtesy of Jfrolick; CC BY 3.0 [https://creativecommons.org/licenses/by/3.0]).

- • Adolescence
- • Females
- • Neuromuscular disorders
- • Collagen vascular diseases (Marfan syndrome, Ehlers-Danlos)
- – Definition: abnormal curvature of the spine, most commonly toward the right
- – Signs and symptoms
  - • Asymptomatic: most common
  - • Chronic back pain
  - • Decreased range of motion
  - • Dyspnea: secondary to restrictive lung disease, only seen in severe cases
- – Diagnostics
  - • Abnormal hump while bending forward
  - • Spine X-ray (Figs. 82-13 and 82-14)
- – Management: depends on symptoms and severity of curvature
  - • Asymptomatic: observation

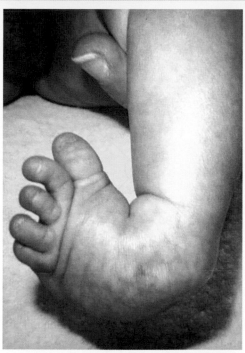

Fig. 82-12: Patient with clubfoot. (Image courtesy of OpenStax College.)

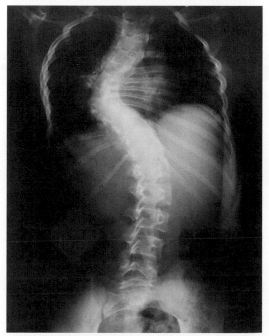

Fig. 82-13: X-ray of a patient with scoliosis. (Image courtesy of Gkiokas A et al; CC BY 2.0 [https://creativecommons.org/licenses/by/2.0])

- Mild curvature: bracing
- Severe curvature: surgical arthrodesis

FRACTURES AND DISLOCATIONS

Fractures involving the growth plate are unique to the pediatric population, as the growth plates are fused in adult patients. These are important to recognize, as injury to the growth plate may result in long-term growth abnormalities and malalignment (Table 82-9; Fig. 82-15).

Supracondylar Fracture

– Epidemiology: most common fracture in children

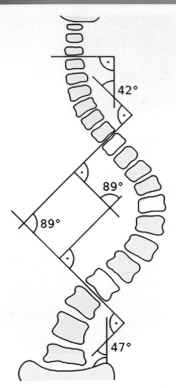

Fig. 82-14: Cobbs angle measurements used to determine the degree of spinal curvature. (Image courtesy of Sko-liose-Info-Forum.de; CC BY-SA 3.0 [http://creativecommons.org/licenses/by-sa/3.0/])

TABLE 82-9   Types of Growth Plate Fractures (Salter-Harris Fractures)

SALTER-HARRIS FRACTURE	KEY FEATURES
Type I	Fracture through the physis
Type II	Fractures through the physis and metaphysis; Most common subtype (75% of cases)
Type III	Fracture through the physis and epiphysis
Type IV	Fracture through the physis, metaphysis, and epiphysis
Type V	Crush fracture where physis is compressed by metaphysis and epiphysis

Operative management is typically required for Salter-Harris fractures types III–V.

- Mechanism: fall on outstretched hand
- Signs and symptoms
  - Elbow pain
  - Decreased peripheral pulses: vascular injury of the brachial artery
  - Numbness and tingling: injury to the median nerve
- Diagnostics: elbow X-ray
- Management: casting
- Complications
  - Compartment syndrome
  - Volkmann contractures
  - Cubitus varus deformity

Radial Head Subluxation (Nursemaid's Elbow)
- Epidemiology: infants and young toddlers
- Definition: slippage of the radial head through the annular ligament and out of its normal position adjacent to the ulna
- Sign and symptoms
  - Sudden onset pain while pulling on child's arm
  - Inability to bend arm at the elbow
- Diagnostics: elbow X-ray

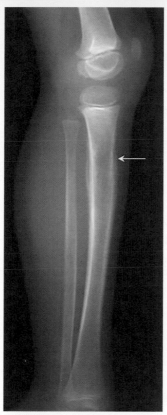

Fig. 82-15: Periosteal reaction and onionskin pattern (white arrow) in a patient with Ewing sarcoma.

– Management: radial head reduction via supination or hyperpronation of a flexed elbow at the forearm (may hear a "pop")

NEOPLASMS

Osteosarcoma
– Epidemiology: most common primary bone tumor in young adults and adolescents most commonly affecting the distal femur (metaphysis of long bones)
– Risk factors
  • Paget disease of the bone
  • Prolonged use of teriparatide
  • Chemoradiation
  • Retinoblastoma gene mutation
– Signs and symptoms
  • Bone pain, muscle aches
  • Tender soft tissue mass
  • Pathologic fractures
– Diagnostics
  • Imaging (MRI/CT):
    ▪ Periosteal elevation (Codman triangle)
    ▪ Spiculated sunburst pattern
  • Staging: CT chest (lung is common site of metastasis)
  • Biopsy
  • Elevated lactate dehydrogenase, alkaline phosphatase
– Management
  • Surgical resection
  • Chemotherapy: methotrexate-based regimen (cisplatin + doxorubicin)

Ewing Sarcoma
– Commonly affects young boys and adolescents
– Malignant anaplastic small blue cell tumor arising from diaphysis of long bones
– Onionskin pattern on X-ray (Fig. 82-16)
– 11:22 translocation

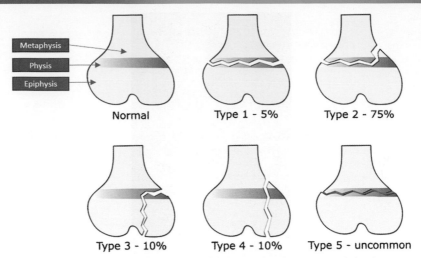

Fig. 82-16: Diagrammatic representation of the types of Salter-Harris fractures and the frequency at which they occur. (Image has been modified and courtesy of Dr Frank Gaillard [MBBS, FRANZCR] [http://www.frankgaillard.com])

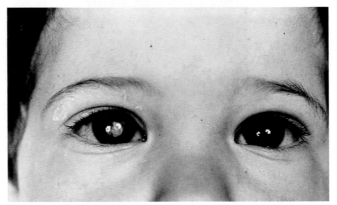

Fig. 82-17: Leukocoria in a patient with retinoblastoma.

OPHTHALMOLOGY

Strabismus
- Definition: misalignment of the eyes
- Pathophysiology: image is suppressed in the deviated eye resulting in permanent cortical blindness
- Signs and symptoms
  - Diplopia
  - Abnormal red reflex
  - Ptosis
  - Decreased visual acuity

Trilateral retinoblastoma = bilateral retinoblastoma + pineal gland tumor

---

- Diagnostics
  - Hirschberg corneal light reflex
  - Cover-uncover test: cover the good eye, which should result in correction of misaligned eye
  - Brighter red reflex in deviated eye
- Management
  - Eye patch over the "good" eye to prevent misalignment of the "bad" eye
  - Surgical correction of misalignment for refractory cases
- Complications: amblyopia

Retinoblastoma
- Epidemiology: most common primary malignant intraocular tumor
- Pathophysiology: retinoblastoma gene mutation resulting in inactivation of retinoblastoma suppressor gene
- Signs and symptoms
  - Leukocoria (Fig. 82-17)
  - Strabismus
  - Ocular pain
  - Glaucoma
- Diagnostics
  - Orbital CT/ultrasound: intraocular calcifications
  - Avoid biopsy due to risk of seeding vitreous fluid
- Management
  - Large tumors: enucleation
  - Small tumors: external beam radiation (may result in secondary tumors)

CHAPTER
83 Transplant Surgery

Transplant basics
- Indication for transplant varies on the type of organ being transplanted and the recipient's comorbidities
- Commonly transplanted organs include kidneys, liver, lungs, bone marrow, pancreas, and heart (Table 83-1)
- Most patients with organ transplants will require immunosuppressive agents and periodic follow-ups to monitor for transplant rejection (Table 83-2)

TABLE 83-1 Indications for Types of Organ Transplant

ORGAN	INDICATION
Kidneys	• End-stage renal disease requiring dialysis • Glomerulonephritis • Polycystic kidney disease
Liver	• Cirrhosis • Chronic hepatitis • Biliary atresia • Primary biliary cirrhosis • Primary sclerosing cholangitis
Lung	• Chronic obstructive pulmonary disease • Cystic fibrosis • Primary pulmonary hypertension
Pancreas	• Type I diabetes
Bone marrow	• Leukemia • Lymphoma • Aplastic anemia
Heart	• Severe cardiomyopathy • May be performed with lung transplant

TABLE 83-2 Types of Transplant Rejection and Management

TYPE OF REJECTION	KEY FEATURES	MANAGEMENT
Hyperacute	• Vascular thrombosis within minutes after establishing blood supply to the organ secondary to ABO incompatibility	• Secondary to clerical error
Acute	• Worsening enzymes (elevated liver function test, creatinine) or symptoms of involved organ • Onset within the first three months	• IV steroid bolus • Increase dose or add additional immunosuppressive agents • Biopsy for confirmation
Chronic	• Similar to acute; however, occurring after several years	• New transplant

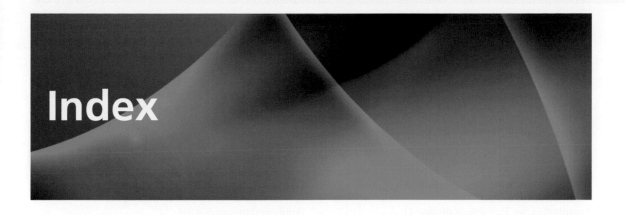

Index

Page numbers followed by "*f*" indicate figures, "*t*" indicates tables, and "*b*" indicates boxes.